Fundamentals of Clinical Practice

A Textbook on the Patient, Doctor, and Society

Fundamentals of Clinical Practice

A Textbook on the Patient, Doctor, and Society

Edited by

Mark B. Mengel, M.D., M.P.H.
Tufts University School of Medicine
Boston, Massachusetts

and

Warren L. Holleman, Ph.D.
Baylor College of Medicine
Houston, Texas

Plenum Medical Book Company • **New York and London**

Library of Congress Cataloging-in-Publication Data

Fundamentals of clinical practice : a textbook on the patient, doctor,
  and society / edited by Mark B. Mengel and Warren L. Holleman.
      p.   cm.
  Includes bibliographical references and index.
  ISBN 0-306-45348-7
  1. Physician and patient. 2. Social medicine.   I. Mengel, Mark
B. II. Holleman, Warren Lee.
  [DNLM: 1. Physician-Patient Relations.   W 62 F981 1996]
  R727.3.F87   1996
  610.69'6--dc21
DNLM/DLC
for Library of Congress   96-46673
                                                         CIP

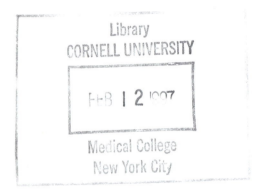
ISBN 0-306-45348-7

© 1997 Plenum Publishing Corporation
233 Spring Street, New York, N. Y. 10013

Plenum Medical Book Company is an imprint of Plenum Publishing Corporation

10 9 8 7 6 5 4 3 2 1

Printed in the United States of America

To those dedicated practitioners of the art who taught us that
the core of clinical practice remains the
doctor – patient relationship

Contributors

Bruce Ambuel, Ph.D., M.S., Assistant Professor of Family and Community Medicine, Waukesha Family Practice Residency, Medical College of Wisconsin, Waukesha, Wisconsin 53188

Elisabeth D. Babcock, Ph.D., M.C.R.P., Executive Director, Lynn Community Health Center, Lynn, Massachusetts 01901

Kristen Lawton Barry, Ph.D., Associate Director of Research for the Serious Mental Illness Treatment Research and Evaluation Center, Veterans Administration Field Unit, Health Services Research and Development, Ann Arbor, Michigan 48113-0170

Alan Blum, M.D., Associate Professor, Department of Family Medicine, Baylor College of Medicine, Houston, Texas 77005

Thomas L. Campbell, M.D., Associate Professor of Family Medicine and Psychiatry, Department of Family Medicine, University of Rochester School of Medicine, Rochester, New York 14620

John L. Coulehan, M.D., M.P.H., Professor of Medicine and Preventative Medicine, State University of New York Health Sciences Center, Stony Brook, New York 11794

Mark R. Cullen, M.D., Professor of Medicine and Public Health, Yale University School of Medicine, New Haven, Connecticut 06510

Larry Culpepper, M.D., M.P.H., Director of Research and Professor of Family Medicine, Department of Family Practice, Memorial Hospital of Rhode Island/Brown University, Pawtucket, Rhode Island 02860

Annette M. David, M.D., M.P.H., Fellow in Occupational Medicine, Yale University School of Medicine, New Haven, Connecticut 06510

Frank Verloin deGruy III, M.D., M.S.F.M., University Distinguished Professor and Chair, Department of Family Practice and Community Medicine, University of South Alabama College of Medicine, Mobile, Alabama 36604

Ronald M. Epstein, M.D., Assistant Professor of Family Medicine and Psychiatry and Director of Predoctoral Education, Department of Family Medicine, University of Rochester and Highland Hospital, Rochester, New York 14620

Laura B. Frankenstein, M.D., Medical Director, Lynn Community Health Center, Lynn, Massachusetts 01901

Joshua Freeman, M.D., Senior Physician, Department of Family Practice, and Director, Faculty Development Center, Cook County Hospital, Chicago, Illinois 60612

Anamari Golf, M.A., Research Associate, Faculty Development Center, Department of Family Practice, Cook County Hospital, Chicago, Illinois 60612

L. Kevin Hamberger, Ph.D., Professor of Clinical Family and Community Medicine, Department of Family and Community Medicine, Medical College of Wisconsin, Milwaukee, Wisconsin 53188

Warren L. Holleman, Ph.D., Assistant Professor, Department of Family Medicine, Baylor College of Medicine, Houston, Texas 77030

James N. Hyde, M.A., M.S., Associate Professor, Department of Family Medicine and Community Health, Tufts University School of Medicine, Boston, Massachusetts 02111

Masie Isabell, M.D., M.S., Senior Attending Physician, Department of Family Practice, and Medical Director, Englewood Family Practice Clinic, Cook County Hospital, Chicago, Illinois 60612

Ann C. Jobe, M.D., M.S.N., Senior Associate Dean, Student Affairs and Academic Programs, and Associate Professor, Department of Family Medicine, East Carolina University School of Medicine, Greenville, North Carolina 27858-4354

Eliana C. Korin, Dipl. Psic., Psychosocial Faculty, Residency in Preventative and Social Medicine/Department of Family Medicine, Montefiore Medical Center, Bronx, New York 10467

Barry S. Levy, M.D., M.P.H., Director, Barry S. Levy Associates, Sherborn, Massachusetts 01770

Julie Lipkin, M.D., Attending Physician, Department of Family Practice, Coordinator of Geriatrics, and Chairperson, Hospital Committee on Bioethics, Cook County Hospital, Chicago, Illinois 60612

Mark Loafman, M.D., M.P.H., Medical Director and Associate Director, Primary Care Community Wellness Center, Loyola–West Suburban, Family Practice Residency Program, Oak Park, Illinois 60302

Christopher J. Mansfield, M.S., Ph.D., Director, Center for Health Services Research and Development, Department of Family Medicine, East Carolina University School of Medicine, Greenville, North Carolina 27858-4354

Susan H. McDaniel, Ph.D., Associate Professor of Psychiatry and Family Medicine, Department of Family Medicine, University of Rochester School of Medicine, Rochester, New York 14620

Monica McGoldrick, M.A., L.C.S.W., Ph.D. (Hon.), Director, Family Institute of New Jersey, Metuchen, New Jersey 08840

Catherine P. McKegney, M.D., M.S., Faculty Member, Department of Family Practice and Community Health, University of Minnesota Medical School, Minneapolis, Minnesota 55408

James W. Mold, M.D., Associate Professor and Director, Research Division, Department of Family Medicine, University of Oklahoma Health Sciences Center, Oklahoma City, Oklahoma 73104

Isaiah Perry, Department of Family Practice, Cook County Hospital, Chicago, Illinois 60612

Roger A. Rosenblatt, M.D., M.P.H., Professor and Vice Chair, Department of Family Medicine, University of Washington School of Medicine, Seattle, Washington 98195

David B. Seaburn, M.S., Assistant Professor of Psychiatry and Family Medicine, Department of Family Medicine, University of Rochester School of Medicine, Rochester, New York 14620

Sara G. Shields, M.D., M.S., Assistant Professor of Family and Community Medicine and Director of Family Medicine Obstetrics Training, Department of Family and Community Medicine, University of Massachusetts, Worcester, Massachusetts 01610

Peggy B. Smith, Ph.D., Professor of Obstetrics/Gynecology and Director, Teen Health Clinic, Ben Taub Hospital, Population Program, Baylor College of Medicine, Houston, Texas 77030

Eric J. Solberg, M.A., Executive Director, Doctors Ought to Care, Department of Family Medicine, Baylor College of Medicine, Houston, Texas 77005

Howard F. Stein, Ph.D., Professor of Department of Family and Preventive Medicine, University of Oklahoma Health Sciences Center, Oklahoma City, Oklahoma 73104

Marlene F. Watson, Ph.D., Assistant Professor and Director, Master of Family Therapy Program, Medical College of Pennsylvania and Hahnemann University, Philadelphia, Pennsylvania 10031

Preface

Fundamentals of Clinical Practice is an introductory textbook focusing on the patient–physician relationship. Formerly closeted behind closed doors, this most intimate of healing relationships is coming under increasing scientific scrutiny. Physicians and other healthcare providers are beginning to understand the critical importance of this relationship to the health of patients, as well as to larger societal relationships, systems, and values.

To facilitate the reader's exploration of the patient–physician relationship, all chapters include numerous illustrative cases and conclude with cases for discussion that allow small groups of learners to tackle these difficult issues. Our hypothesis is that through discussion a deeper understanding of the dynamics of the patient–physician relationship will allow medical students and other future healthcare providers to form more effective therapeutic relationships with their patients.

Part I of this textbook, "The Patient," explores the relationship through the patient's perspective, with chapters on human health and disease and individual and family development. Understanding the patient's perspective is critical to establishing a sound therapeutic relationship. The day when a physician could maintain solely a disease or technological perspective is fading fast under the weight of patient criticism, particularly in primary care fields. Patients judge such a disease or technological perspective as less humane and frequently vote with their feet, finding other physicians who are much better able to balance the caring aspects of medicine with the curing.

Part II, "The Doctor," explores the relationship from the physician's perspective, another perspective often ignored by medical education. The effects of medical training on the personhood of the physician are discussed by McKegney, while Coulehan offers the reader a comprehensive, erudite discussion of what it means to be a physician in today's chaotic healthcare environment. Both offer tips for coping with the challenges and complexities of caring for patients while maintaining a balance with personal values and lifestyle.

The patient–physician relationship is surrounded by a web of other relationships and systems that are explored in the Part III, "Society." Systems theorists have come to understand the importance of context and the dynamics, or behavioral patterns, that are reinforced within that context. Important societal systems such as the family, community, the workplace, public health and the environment, cultural issues, and the healthcare system itself are explored in depth to show the learner how these multiple contexts shape the patient–physician relationship and, thus, the care that is delivered to patients.

The critical role of values within the patient–physician relationship is explored in chapters on "Medical Ethics" and "Health Policy and Economics." It may seem strange to readers that a chapter on health policy and economics is contained within the values section, yet how we spend our money is a firm indication of our values, particularly with regard to healthcare. Despite the fact that health reform recently failed at the federal government level, market forces are changing the healthcare system in dramatic ways, ways that will no doubt affect the patient–physician relationship.

Special societal problems also have a profound effect on the patient–physician relationship. Some of the most difficult issues that physicians face in partnering with their patients around health issues are discussed in the special societal problems section including chapters on "The Tobacco Pandemic," "Alcohol and Drug Abuse," "Violence," "Mental Illness," "Sexually Transmitted Diseases," "Vulnerable and Indigent Populations," and "Maternal and Child Health." These topics have usually been ignored within the medical school curriculum, as they do not fit nicely into the disease-oriented biomedical model. However, recent research indicates that physicians not only have a positive role to play in both the detection of and counseling patients concerning these issues, but that they should also play such a role, as these societal problems profoundly affect health.

Our hope is that these chapters will provide an introduction to the critical role of the patient–physician relationship to the health of patients. We realize that such a textbook cannot be all-inclusive or provide all of the information a physician will need to deal with these issues in the future. Thus, each chapter concludes with a section of recommended readings that allow the student to pursue more in-depth information in areas of particular/ special interest.

Patients are demanding more from their physicians and the healthcare system today, not only in terms of medical services, but also in terms of humane, understanding care. Research has shown that physicians who pay attention to the patient–physician relationship serve their patients better, as evidenced by improved health outcomes. Additionally, paying attention to the patient–physician relationship can serve as a profound source of professional satisfaction for physicians. As physicians pay more attention to the patient–physician relationship, insurers and other third-party payers will begin to understand the vital importance of this relationship and will promote it as a vital part of the therapeutic process. Physicians who understand the importance of the relationship can play a central role in stimulating reform of the U.S. healthcare system.

Mark B. Mengel, M.D., M.P.H.

Boston, Massachusetts

Warren L. Holleman, Ph.D.

Houston, Texas

Acknowledgments

Without the aid of many people this textbook simply would not have been possible. Many of our colleagues have been very supportive of this text, even to the point of being chapter authors. We are especially appreciative of the support of Mac Baird, Howard Stein, Jim Mold, and Ann Jobe. Without the warm support and suggestions of these colleagues, this work would not have been possible.

Special thanks go to our students, who have stimulated us to continually update and improve our ideas on the physician–patient relationship. Particularly first- and second-year medical students have asked the "embarrassing" questions that have prompted us to conceptualize and then reconceptualize our understanding of the physician–patient relationship and how it can be utilized to improve patient health.

The tireless support of our secretaries is gratefully acknowledged. Chapters have to be edited, authors have to be "nagged," and publishers have to be placated. Linda Ready and Terri Woods have performed well and tirelessly in helping us meet deadlines.

We also want to thank the editorial staff at Plenum Publishing headed by Mariclaire Cloutier, who has been very supportive and understanding of our many foibles. They have been particularly helpful in editing our rather long-winded, confusing prose into much briefer, more understandable sentences.

Lastly, we would like to thank our families, without whose support the long hours necessary—usually after work—to put together a book of this size and scope would not have been possible. Our wives, Laura Frankenstein and Marsha Cline Holleman, and our children, Sally, Annie, and Tom, also helped in bringing us back to reality.

Contents

Section B. Values

PART I

The Patient

The premise that the patient is the focus of the physician's efforts is so obvious that it really doesn't warrant stating; however, as physicians focus on disease, the personhood of the patient often gets lost as an irrelevant or insignificant detail. These chapters help to reestablish the focus on the patient—not only their disease, but also their personhood—by explaining the complex nature of human health and disease and also the developmental life cycles that are important for physicians to understand when caring for patients of all ages.

CHAPTER 1

Human Health and Disease

Roger A. Rosenblatt

CASE 1-1

An elderly woman consulted her physician because she was having dizzy spells and couldn't sleep. Her husband had recently died, and her only child lived on the other coast. The results of her physical exam were essentially normal, except for mild hypertension.

The physician, unsure of the diagnosis, ordered a series of tests, which included a 24-hour electrocardiogram searching for arrhythmias, an electroencephalogram, a CT scan of the head, and a variety of blood tests. When these were unrevealing, he referred her to a neurologist, who did some additional tests, again finding nothing abnormal. The neurologist referred her to an otolaryngologist, suspecting middle ear dysfunction, but more tests were not helpful. Medicare paid for about half of the charges incurred, and the patient received sheaves of bills for the balance. Six months later, her symptoms were unchanged.

AMERICAN MEDICINE AS AN ANOMALY

The U.S. medical enterprise is an anomaly on the world stage. Put simply, the United States spends more on medical care than any other nation, yet it has millions of citizens without ready access to even the most basic healthcare services. Despite an enormous investment in healthcare—over 1 trillion dollars in 1995—healthcare status as measured by such conventional measures as infant mortality or longevity is only fair, lagging far behind other countries that invest much smaller shares of their national wealth into medical objectives (Rice, 1994; Schieber *et al.*, 1994).

U.S. medicine has evolved along a path quite different from that taken by other industrialized countries. Although medical care occupies much of our interest and our

3

wealth, the basic strategy for delivering medical care has been left largely to the vagaries of chance and self-interest. Not only is the United States without an organized national health service, it also lacks any financing mechanism that ensures that individuals can obtain needed healthcare without plunging into penury. Healthcare policy is determined primarily by groups that profit from the decisions that they make, namely, insurance and pharmaceutical companies, hospitals, physicians, and other healthcare professionals. Medical care in the United States is a "market-oriented health care system spinning out of control" (Relman, 1994).

Not only is the medical enterprise careening across the social landscape without anyone at the helm, there is also considerable question as to whether the activities on which we spend our time and money contribute to the health of either the individual patient or the society of which she is a part. The woman described in Case 1-1 presents her physician with the problem of dizziness, and he deploys an impressive array of technical gadgets to try to find that part of her anatomy causing her to experience this disquieting symptom. But as is usually the case, her symptom cannot be understood simply as a mechanical failure; it is just as likely to be caused by depression following her husband's death, despair related to social isolation, or a normal consequence of an aging neurological system. The physician's traditional approach generates considerable revenues for those who survey and interpret the tests, but the woman herself does not benefit. In fact, awash in additional bills and made anxious by the cascade of tests, she has actually been harmed by her encounter with the medical care system.

The purpose of this chapter—and this entire book—is to place the medical endeavor in a broader biological, psychological, and social context. Specifically, this chapter will:

1. Introduce readers to the determinants of health, illness, and disease, placing the role and importance of medical care within a broad social, cultural, and economic context
2. Explore the role of the physician in modern industrial society and the potential benefits and harm that derive from the physician's activities
3. Encourage physicians to be parsimonious and skeptical in their approach to medical care
4. Introduce the powerful tools provided by epidemiology and health services research as ways to determine what things physicians do that are most likely to improve the well-being of individuals and society

As practitioners of the healing arts, we have immense capacity to assist people in confronting and addressing the inevitable health problems that are as much a part of life as respiration and locomotion. But we cannot discharge this trust adequately if we become passive parts of a dysfunctional machine.

CASE 1-2

The old black man was found crumpled beside a wall, flaccid and unconscious. When brought to the emergency room, he was awake but unable to talk or move the left side of his body. His blood pressure was elevated and he smelled of alcohol and tobacco. When the ER staff reached his ex-wife, she told them that he had lost his job as a school custodian 6 months earlier when rising Medicaid costs led to a reduction in state funding for schools.

Two days later the patient had a second, more massive stroke and died after a short period on a ventilator. The resident wrote "cerebrovascular accident" in the space on the death certificate reserved for cause of death.

5

HEALTH AND
ILLNESS IN
HUMAN SOCIETY

—— HEALTH AND ILLNESS IN HUMAN SOCIETY ——

THE HEALTH OF THE INDIVIDUAL

Medicine is a reductionist endeavor; we break human beings into organs, cells, organelles, and molecules to gain insight into and power over fundamental biological processes. But as physicians, as patients, and as people, biochemical pathways are less important than psychological states of being. Individuals search for peace, surcease, wholeness, nirvana, and health is the end point of that quest.

Operationalizing health, that is, coming up with a definition that lets us know whether our activities are enhancing the health of individuals, is problematic. The World Health Organization has proffered a lofty but essentially vacuous formula: "Health is a state of complete physical, mental, and social well-being, and not merely the absence of disease or injury." Such a state is both unobtainable and unmeasurable, although it does generate humility in pointing out both how wide of that mark we are as humans and how medicine contributes only a small part to the attainment of such an Elysian state.

A more parsimonious and more useful approach is to define health as the absence of pain and dysfunction. Although there is an element of subjectivity even in this spare yardstick, we can at least measure whether our interventions have made people more comfortable or more functional. From a practical standpoint, it is usually physical or psychological pain that leads patients to consult physicians, and it is only fair that physicians focus their efforts on the identified problems of the individuals seeking help.

The major source of our discomfort in wrestling with all of these definitions is the fact that living is also dying. Aging seems to be woven anarchically into the very process of cell division, so that the embryo as it differentiates sows the seeds of its ultimate dissolution. If we examine human longevity historically, it becomes evident that the total human life span has changed little across the centuries for which we have accurate records, Methuselah and his cousins notwithstanding. The triumph of science—particularly public health interventions—in recent centuries is that a greater proportion of the population survives the random physical and biological agents of destruction to survive into their 70s and 80s, at which point the inexorable limits built into cellular biology override the temporary entropic lacunae that constitute life.

Thus, we as physicians often find ourselves torn in different directions by the desires of our patients and our scientific formulation of the problems with which they present. Patients bring us their symptoms and their sorrows, and we turn them into diseases that we hope can be found in the pages of the texts on which we were weaned. The art of medicine lies in using our scientific knowledge to address the existential needs of our patients, without lapsing into quackery on the one hand or irrelevant technological sophistication on the other. The most powerful tool for doing this is to understand that our patients are part of larger structures that are just as important as the smaller structures of which they are composed.

The resident was "anatomically correct" in assigning the cause of death of our second patient to a cerebrovascular accident. The terminal event occurred when a bit of eroded atherosclerotic plaque from the intimal surface of the carotid artery lost its moorings, drifted downstream, and lodged in the distribution of the middle cerebral artery. Deprived of blood flow and oxygen, part of the brain died, and the patient with it. But was it an "accident"? And was the cause of death cerebral anoxia, or was it the patient's unemployment, alcoholism, or racial heritage? The pathologist who sliced the brain may have ignored these questions, but an accurate autopsy would encompass more than blood vessels and clotting parameters. In the following discussion we will rise above the autopsy table, searching for causation not in end points, but in antecedents.

THE HEALTH OF THE FAMILY

Humans cannot exist as solitary organisms. As Bolman's pioneering work on human development demonstrated, infants raised in hygienic but nonnurturing settings become autistic, physically perfect but functionally flawed (Bowlby, 1983). Even more subtle deprivation can thwart normal development, as the modern epidemics of sexual abuse and the growth of the underclass demonstrate.

With rare exceptions, physicians are constantly reminded of the fact that their patients exist as parts of family units, even though families come in many shapes and sizes. Even as we hone in on the underlying pathophysiology that is the material substrate of disease, we realize that the impact of disease on the individual is mitigated or amplified by the family of which the patient is a part. The aging man whose wife dies is much more likely to join her in death than is his peer with an even worse disease but whose wife is hale and hearty (Gallagher *et al.*, 1982).

It is literally impossible to understand the patient without understanding both his family of origin and the current family structure. This may sound ludicrous when talking about something as cut-and-dried as a fractured ankle, upper respiratory infection, or metastatic breast cancer. But in each of these cases the family structure—in all its variation—is important both in the etiology of the disease and in our ability to help the patient overcome the problem.

The patient with a broken ankle may have suffered the injury on the ski slopes, but his ability to use crutches while the injury heals depends to a certain extent on both the physical and social environments of the family. Who will do the shopping during the 6 weeks in the cast? The child with the URI and repeated ear infections may get them because the mother smokes or because the child spends much of the day in an overcrowded and underventilated day-care center. The patient with breast cancer is likely to have different feelings about aggressive chemotherapy—and different desires about long-term goals—depending on the health of her spouse, the desires of her children, and her own experience watching her mother die from the same disease.

The situation becomes even more graphic when the diseases themselves arise in the cauldron of the family. Certainly emotional disabilities, from garden-variety depression to exotic forms of schizophrenia, have at least some of their roots in the family situation. But the real challenge to the clinician is to remember—and incorporate—the family dimension into even the most mundane of presenting complaints. Although the divorce of the school custodian in Case 1-2 did not "cause" the subsequent stroke, a stable marriage might well have prevented or mitigated the physiological changes that led ultimately to the fatal event. Understanding family dynamics is just as important for the neurosurgeon as for the family physician—all patients come supplied with families, just as all patients come supplied with hearts. And both are needed for human beings to live, function, and thrive.

THE HEALTH OF THE SOCIAL GROUP AND THE EFFECT OF SOCIETY ON HEALTH

Individuals belong to an interlocking series of social groups, from the small circle of the nuclear family to ever-widening circles that include neighborhoods, communities, cultures, and nations. The composition of these social groups—and the person's place within them—has a profound effect on every aspect of life. In the same way that the manner in which a child is raised shapes her intelligence and personality, a person's position within society affects employment, happiness, health, and longevity.

A growing body of evidence demonstrates that a person's health depends on many factors that are frequently ignored by practitioners (Evans *et al.*, 1994). We tend to look for the causes of disease in such things as genetic defects, specific pathogens, deleterious health habits, or harmful accidents. But the health of the individual is also strongly related to much more amorphous social distinctions such as social class, employment, race, and ethnicity. It is the interaction among all of these factors that raises or lowers a person's susceptibility to illness and affects the chances of recovery once illness has begun.

Medical care has a part to play in determining the health status of the individual and the larger society, but the part is relatively small compared with other social forces. Even the most sophisticated diagnostic and therapeutic technologies are of less importance than the basic ingredients of life, such as food, shelter, clothing, and self-respect. The absence of any of these latter factors is just as devastating as most cancers. In addition, most of the medical interventions that have improved the health of populations have little to do with the traditional patient–physician relationship. Safe food and water, the development of vaccines and the implementation of immunization programs, the use of seat belts, and efforts to curb smoking all depend on broad social programs aimed at populations, not individuals (Cluff, 1987).

Thus, it is critical to view medical care as one way in which society attempts to improve the well-being of individuals, as well as the larger population. All too frequently, the immediacy and drama of the individual clinical encounter crowd out the prosaic but effective strategies that concentrate on improving everyone's health rather than the health of one person. This enormous concentration of resources directed at the individual diverts social investment in other interventions—education, social programs, and so forth—that have greater potential to improve the social and physical milieu. The irony is that the enormous resources that we pour into medical care tend to be taken away from services such as education or social services that ultimately have a much greater impact on whether a person lives a healthy life.

We should return for a moment to our hapless patient in the emergency room, terminally ill from a stroke. Although we can and will use sophisticated imaging technologies to locate and describe the lesion in his brain, the real lesion lies in the society from which he sprung. Black men in our society have dismal health prospects, and real improvements in the health of African-Americans will require policies that address racism, employment, social status, and income distribution. Although it may seem artificial to suggest that rising Medicaid costs drain resources from the education budget, this dynamic is being played out in innumerable state legislatures as this book is being written. The physician with an interest in the health of her patients must also become involved in broader social policies that affect the well-being of the entire population, messy and fractious as this arena always is.

THE HEALTH OF THE PLANET

Humanity's ultimate hubris is anointing itself as the pinnacle of creation. In this view, the world exists to further the aims of humankind, and all other species are at best subservient and at worst irrelevant to our pursuit of our own ends. The consequences of this worldview surround us: environmental degradation, wholesale destruction of species and habitat, and rampant pollution.

The root cause of many of these catastrophic effects lies in the tremendous overpopulation of the planet in the last 100 years. Medicine has played a significant part in this most devastating of biological changes (Green, 1992). Just as the industrial revolution created the technological tools to radically alter the biosphere in which we live, the emergence of modern medical interventions vastly increased effective human fertility. The irony of the situation is that the environmental changes have the potential to affect directly the health of individual humans, just as they have already begun to affect the quality of life for us and many of the other species with whom we share this planet (Leaf, 1989).

What role do the medical profession and the individual physician have to play in averting this looming tragedy? The most important step is to acknowledge the problem in all of its depressing enormity and to educate ourselves and our families, colleagues, and patients about its personal and general importance at every opportunity. Denial and repression are perhaps the strongest psychodynamic mechanisms within the human mind. The natural tendency when confronted with a threat to global existence is to consign it to some distant future date, outside our personal realm of interest or control. But the reality is that these changes have occurred relatively quickly and can be reversed just as quickly, given our technological capacity. The difficulty lies in changing two behaviors—reproduction and consumption—that are such powerful goals and motivators that modifying them is considerably more difficult than, say, stopping smoking.

In the clinical arena, the individual physician can certainly have a very real and potentially enormous effect by giving couples the information and the techniques needed to control their own fertility. A very large proportion of pregnancies are unplanned and unwanted, disrupting and impoverishing the families where they occur (Gottlieb, 1995). Simply by eliminating all unintended pregnancies in the United States, we could achieve a dramatic reduction in the overall birth rate, a reduction that if replicated worldwide could have a marked impact on the rate of population rise.

Physicians play an important role in educating children and adolescents about sexual development and fertility control. All primary care physicians—and most specialists— have the opportunity to raise the issue of family planning with their patients as part of routine health maintenance activities. And while most physicians will not perform abortions, the physician has the responsibility to make patients aware that this is a safe and legal procedure, even while trying to provide the patient with the knowledge and the tools to prevent unwanted pregnancies. Even if the individual clinician does not wish to provide these services because of moral or ethical reservations, he should support the right of other members of the profession to include termination of pregnancy in their repertoire.

The physician is sanctioned by society as a healer, and as such has the opportunity to influence the conditions that promote or undermine good health. All of our efforts at helping individual patients deal with their infirmities and diseases will be swept away unless we are part of the process that also restores and protects the health of the earth.

CASE 1-3

The patient, moribund on Friday, had revived by Monday. After conventional chemotherapy had failed to arrest his terminal lymphosarcoma, the attending physician had given him a shot of Krebiozin, heralding the event with a sense of drama and pageantry. Although there was no scientific evidence that Krebiozin was effective, the tumors had melted to half their original size, and the patient returned home for 2 glorious disease-free months. He relapsed and quickly died after the newspaper printed an AMA article stating flatly that Krebiozin was worthless.*

THE PHYSICIAN'S ROLE—WHAT PART DO WE PLAY?

THE PHYSICIAN AS HEALER—SOURCE OF OUR SOCIAL LEGITIMACY

The role of physician has multiple roots, the sturdiest of which is that of healer. In every prehistoric or primitive culture, selected individuals are sanctified by their community as healers, charged with diagnosing and treating the illnesses of individuals or at times groups. Healers are expected to have acute powers of observation, extensive knowledge about the natural realm, and the ability to mediate and intervene between the causes of illness and their impacts on individuals.

In primitive and prehistoric societies, the role of healer was grafted onto and combined with that of religious leader. The mysteries of life and death were intermingled, and it was natural that the role of healer be conferred on that individual who mediated between the natural and the supernatural. Although the shaman or medicine man may have had limited empirical knowledge of disease as we understand it, he was not ineffective. By tapping into a shared communal understanding of life and its travails, he had the trust and belief of the patient and the family (Bloom, 1965). And trust and faith can heal, whether we call this the placebo effect, the inevitable consequence of self-limited illnesses, or the use of "alternative" physical and medicinal agents that promote the restorative functions of normal physiology.

As far as we know, empiricism was first grafted onto the shamanistic role with the emergence of the Greek schools of medicine in the fourth century B.C. (Sigerist, 1960). The schools at Cos and Cnidus developed systematic approaches to the study of human anatomy, physiology, and the coherence of certain types of illness. The Greek physician may still have traveled like a minstrel from town to town, but he was judged more on his diagnostic and prognostic accuracy than on his ability to commune with the gods.

The evolution of the modern role of the physician derives from both of these sources. Medicine emerged as a guild or profession during medieval times, not much more scien-

---

*Adapted from an article by Bruno Klapfer, *Journal of Projective Techniques*, 1957—cited in articles by Anne Harrington, Probing the Secrets of Placebos, *Harvard Medical Alumni Bulletin*, Winter 1995, page 35.

tifically advanced than the early Greeks. The emergence of the scientific method during the fifteenth century enabled a better understanding of basic physical and biological processes. Medicine as a profession benefited enormously. But even though today's physician-technician may interpret genetic patterns and employ lasers, the social role of the physician as healer still undergirds our relationship to patients and our place in society. When we forget these foundations, we unnecessarily limit our ability not only to provide comfort, but also to promote healing (White, 1988).

Physicians in today's society still stand at the interface between the secular and the priestly. Although most patients will not have spontaneous remissions when their cancers are treated with placebos like Krebiozin, we do have the power to heal because of the patient's belief in our skill, expertise, and commitment. In our frenetic world, many problems that patients bring to the physician are expressions of disequilibrium, anxiety, or the cumulative effects of physical, psychological, and social stress. We are most effective in restoring balance and relieving suffering when we use tools such as empathy and concern, when we listen and support rather than probe and test.

CASE 1-4

The child lay on the gurney, seemingly intact, but mute after having fallen off her bicycle. The pediatric emergency room physician did his best to find some remediable cause of the child's coma, but it was clear that the child had a severe closed-head injury, with little chance of recovery. The pediatrician established with the parents that the child had not been wearing a bicycle helmet, trying not to blame them for the injury to their daughter. These cases bothered the pediatrician more than all of the cases of leukemia and meningitis that he saw, because they seemed to be so preventable.

After his shift was over, the pediatrician sat down with some of his colleagues and planned a study to determine the frequency of children's head injuries and what could be done to make helmets more available and more likely to be used. The campaign took several years, but ultimately the proportion of kids wearing helmets increased, and the number of head injuries coming to emergency rooms decreased. After this experience, the pediatrician decided to tackle another problem that brought kids into his ER, namely, gun injuries. He is still working on that one.

THE EVOLUTION OF PUBLIC HEALTH AND ITS RELATIONSHIP TO MEDICAL CARE

One of the great ironies of medicine is that the most effective interventions are directed at populations, while most of the resources go for the care of individuals. We have explored this concept earlier and now must grapple with how this anomaly can be addressed by the individual physician. In the country as a whole, we have done a spectacularly poor job of partitioning resources between curative and public health. Yet the individual physician can help restore the balance not only by paying attention to providing the best care to each patient who walks in the door, but also by keeping in mind the population of patients that could benefit from the skills of the physician.

We acknowledge that most of the work that physicians will do is with individual patients, and much of the job of medical school and residency is to make physicians excel in their care of individual patients. Yet most physicians are motivated by a desire to have an impact on the people whom they treat, and an important way to multiply one's impact is to always be open to interventions at the family, social group, or population level.

The targets of opportunity exist in virtually every segment of medicine, no matter how specialized. One can draw the inspiration to pursue these issues from one's clinical practice and special expertise, as did the pediatrician in Case 1-4. The primary care physician has limitless opportunities, based on the type of practice, from prevention of falls in the elderly to improving vaccination rates among immigrants. But a population-based perspective is by no means limited to primary care. The neurosurgeon certainly can get involved in both the prevention of head injuries by using seat belts for motorists and helmets for motorcyclists and better treatment of patients with head injuries by emergency medical technicians. Oncologists can get involved in reducing the presence of carcinogens in the community or encouraging people to avoid excessive exposure to the sun. Thoracic surgeons may choose to be involved with programs designed to help patents stop smoking or to prevent kids from starting.

Public health is likely to remain weak in the United States, if only because of the relentlessly individualistic focus of our society. One way to redress this imbalance is for all physicians to incorporate the public health perspective in their work and in their lives. Not only will these efforts pay off in better health for the population, and for individual patients, but they are a potent antidote to the burnout and the cynicism that can invade the life of the busy practitioner. You may not be able to get Mrs. Smith to give up cigarettes, even though her emphysema propels her into your office every time the air pollution increases, but you may be able to help her child avoid the same dismal outcome.

For those with a particular interest in population-based medicine, the concept and practice of community-oriented primary care (COPC) may have special appeal (Tollman, 1991). The basic tenet of COPC is that the individual physician can effectively care not only for a collection of individual patients, but also for an entire defined community (Waitzkin & Hubbell, 1992). Even in the disorganized chaos of our disjointed medical care system, most physicians provide care to some group of patients that can be counted and described. For the rural physician, it may be possible to characterize all of the people living in a small town or within the catchment area of a specific rural hospital. For the urban physician, it may be a collection of neighborhoods or a particular suburb.

In all of these cases, the physician—wearing the public health hat—can find out about the prevalence of disease that afflicts this particular group of people. And knowledge confers power, because an understanding of the cause of the disease allows the physician to get involved in organized efforts to intervene. The target can be something as straightforward as making sure that the elderly have flu vaccines or as complex as trying to tackle the problem of teenage pregnancy in a rural high school. But in either case, there are sets of tools and approaches that the physician can use to multiply her effectiveness and combine the mantle of healer with that of physician to the community.

CASE 1-5

The stylish woman flew into the office, trailing an overloaded briefcase, an umbrella, and a few wisps of errant cigarette smoke. "My allergies are killing me," she said, almost before the physician entered the room. "That Seldane you gave me didn't do a thing; haven't you got something better?"

The physician glimpsed the chart: a succession of brief visits for episodic ills, all annoying, none serious. His eyes glanced at the health maintenance form he kept at the front of every chart, unsullied in this case by any entries. He noticed that he'd written "Smoking" on the problem list, but realized that was as far as he'd ever gotten.

"I have just the thing for you," he said. "There's a new steroid nasal inhaler that will knock out those allergy symptoms. But I don't think we'll make a lot of progress until we talk a bit about your smoking. And I also notice that you haven't had a Pap smear or a breast exam in years."

"Oh, doctor, be a dear and write me a prescription for the allergy puffer. I'll be sure to make an appointment to get that Pap smear."

FROM PREVENTION TO CURE TO PALLIATION—WHEN TO INTERVENE?

In the previous section, we confronted the dilemma faced by the physician who is trying to decide what portion of his energy to spend wrestling with the fundamental public health problems that cause disease and what portion to spend with the individual patient who manifests these diseases. In this section, we address a different sort of priority setting: the competition between taking care of the acute episodic problems that patients bring to us and focusing our energies on preventing the appearance of disease.

The patient who breezes into the office wanting a nostrum for her nostrils—but postponing the Pap smear and avoiding any mention of her smoking—exemplifies the dilemma. Many physicians act like outfielders, i.e., the patient hits the ball, the physician fields it briskly, handles it briefly, and tosses it back. And then turns to the next fungo, hoping that it won't go over the fence. The physician lives in the present, and the workday is defined by what gets past the second baseman, or the receptionist in this case.

Although every primary care physician must learn to become a good fielder, the job requires more than the ability to handle whatever ball is hit his way. Although some of the promises of the health promotion/disease prevention approach have been overblown by individual medical disciplines and the popular press, many preventive activities make good sense. In our particular case, the physician can have more impact on the health, longevity, and well-being of this young woman by tackling the smoking issue than by writing a ream of prescriptions.

The unique asset of the primary care physician is that he has the knowledge, the leverage, and the opportunity to interweave curative and preventive medicine together. Our harried young female executive might prefer to avoid discussion of her smoking, but her allergies won't let her. And she has enough faith in her personal physician—faith distilled out of repeated visits in which her physician has solved other problems—that she can be forced to confront the more fundamental issue of smoking. This may not be the visit where she decides to quit, but evidence shows that the concerned physician, probably more than any other person in society, can encourage and sustain smoking cessation.

Our physician is also armed with an extremely powerful tool, namely, the health maintenance protocol. For every patient, there are a handful of health promotion and disease prevention activities that have been shown to be effective in detecting or preventing disease. Customized for each patient—based on her age, sex, racial and ethnic heritage, occupation, family history, and personal behaviors—are a set of health maintenance activities that are inexpensive and efficacious.

13

FROM
PREVENTION TO
CURE TO
PALLIATION—
WHEN TO
INTERVENE?

The key to an effective health maintenance program is a program that is customized for each patient and contains only those elements that are both efficacious and cost-effective, both in the economic and in the social sense. Routine chest X rays and electrocardiograms will occasionally reveal unexpected "pathology" in patients, but to what effect? Many of the tests that are glibly espoused by groups with a particular interest in a disease—from routine prostate-specific antigen (PSA) to mammograms at age 30—may do the individual patient more harm than good, either by exposing them to radiation, finding conditions that either cannot or should not be treated, or simply causing unnecessary cost and anxiety. The key for the primary care physician is to tailor the health maintenance approach to those conditions where early detection will make a difference to the particular patient to whom they are applied.

Fortunately, an enormous amount of superb work has been done in helping to craft such health maintenance protocols. The pioneering work in this field was done by a pair of community family physicians who practice in upper New York State, Frame and Carlson, and their papers have been an inspiration for scores of physicians who have followed in their footsteps (Frame & Carlson, 1975a–d). Their approach, originally presented in 1975 and updated in 1986, subjects each potential test or intervention to six critical criteria (from Frame & Carlson, 1975a):

1. The condition must have a significant effect on the quality or quantity of life.
2. Acceptable methods of treatment must be available.
3. The condition must have an asymptomatic period during which detection and treatment significantly reduce morbidity or mortality.
4. Treatment in the asymptomatic phase must yield a therapeutic result superior to that obtained by delaying treatment until symptoms appear.
5. Tests that are acceptable to patients must be available at reasonable cost to detect the condition in the asymptomatic period.
6. The incidence of the condition must be sufficient to justify the cost of screening.

These six principles are enormously powerful in focusing our attention on areas where prevention works, makes sense, and is economical. This approach is not static: As our understanding of the pathophysiology and natural progression of disease expands, and as new tests are developed, the list expands and contracts. An extremely practical product of this approach has been the recommendations of the Canadian Task Force on the Periodic Health Examination and the U.S. Preventive Services Task Force. Both groups used the Frame and Carlson approach, and both forged practical age-specific guidance to the application of the preventive healthcare in the context of primary care practice (Goldbloom *et al.*, 1989; U.S. Preventive Services Task Force, 1990). See Chapter 15 on Health Promotion and Disease Prevention in *Introduction to Clinical Skills: A Patient-Centered Textbook.*

One of the important ingredients of a successful health maintenance program in primary care is a medical care system that supports such an approach, both financially and organizationally. If the physician works in a community where there are too few health-care providers, care for patients with illness may crowd out attention to situations that may be abstract causes of illness in some distant future. If the physician works for a hospital that has recently acquired a chain of ambulatory clinics that expects each physician to see 25 patients a day to earn a yearly incentive bonus, the tendency will be to write the prescription and ignore the wisps of tobacco smoke. And if the insurance for the patient specifically excludes health maintenance, both the physician and the patient will have to examine the fiscal impact of tests and activities that the insurance company will not cover.

Fortunately, most employers, managed care organizations, and insurance companies have realized that carefully designed health maintenance protocols save money as well as improve the length and quality of life. As a greater portion of medical care—even in that last frontier of competition and individualism, the United States—moves toward some variant of capitated healthcare, health maintenance becomes a more sensible and rewarded activity. The adept and successful physician will blend prevention seamlessly into the more traditional practice of curative medicine.

CASE 1-6

Annie was referred from Port Angeles, a logging town on the Olympic peninsula, after her catastrophic GI bleed sent her into acute renal failure. By the time she arrived at University Hospital, she was in a coma, caused by the combination of profound blood loss, renal failure, and sepsis.

The intern struggled for days to try to restore some semblance of biochemical homeostasis. Dialysis was begun, antibiotics were given, and Annie was monitored in the ICU. One crisis followed another, as one physiological system after another in her aging body was overwhelmed by the illness.

The intern became obsessed with the goal of keeping Annie alive; he slept on a cot in the corridor rather than go home even on the nights he wasn't on call. He was partly goaded on by the troop of relatives who stood around Annie's bed, watching these medical heroics. They were mute, almost sullen, but present for every blood gas, X ray, or dressing change.

On the seventh day of her hospitalization, Annie developed disseminated intravascular coagulation and bled to death. The intern was at her bedside with the family and looked at them apologetically, feeling as if he were a complete failure. The patient's brother looked back at him, bobbed his head wearily, and said, "Thank God it's finally over; we have been hoping she would be spared this torture for days." (This case is a description of one of the author's first patients during his first rotation on the medical service during his internship year.)

PRESERVING CONTEXT WHILE
—— ADDRESSING THE NEEDS OF THE ——
INDIVIDUAL; MARSHALING THE TOOLS

When physicians sit for their board exams in the specialty they have chosen, they will have spent at least a decade mastering material relevant to the exam. From that first premed biochemistry course in college, through anatomy in medical school, to the rigors of residency, physicians are immersed in a series of theoretical and applied scientifically based endeavors to make them reasonably comfortable with taking care of the problems brought to them by patients. Although the medical curriculum has its flaws, U.S. physicians are arguably the best practitioners of the science of medicine since physicians as a recognizable guild or profession emerged during prehistory.

U.S. medicine is far from perfect, however, as we have discussed in this introductory chapter. While the U.S. physician can bring more scientific firepower to bear on the physical problems of any particular patient than most physicians in other countries, it does not follow that the U.S. physician is more effective than his peers. The fault lies both in the organization of the medical care system and in the role of the physician within society.

Although the individual physician cannot remedy these imperfections alone, there is a set of tools that can multiply the effectiveness of physicians. In this section we briefly review a handful of those that can be simply and practically applied in the day-to-day practice of medicine. The three tools are the biopsychosocial perspective, population-based medicine, and clinical epidemiology. They have been touched on in different ways in the discussion thus far in this chapter, but they are so important to effective clinical medicine that it is worth revisiting them briefly in a slightly different way.

15

PRESERVING
CONTEXT WHILE
ADDRESSING THE
NEEDS OF THE
INDIVIDUAL;
MARSHALING
THE TOOLS

TREAT HUMAN BEINGS, NOT PATIENTS

I will never forget Annie, in Case 1-6, because I never knew her when she was alive. She appeared in the ward of our tertiary care hospital, and I did what I had been trained to do: try to restore physiological equilibrium to a body that had been ravaged by disease. I couldn't talk to her—she was comatose. I didn't talk to her family, even though they surrounded me, because it never occurred to me that they would have anything of value to tell me. Had I asked, I would have learned that Annie would have rejected the vain attempt to rescue her from what turned out to be irreversible pathophysiologic processes. I was devastated by her death; her family was relieved.

Annie, unfortunately, was and is a typical hospital patient. The failure in this case was not our inability to forestall death, but the failure to ensure that the medical response was meaningful in terms of the patient's life and illness. She may have been unable to provide any detail, but her family was available and unconsulted. She came from a different culture and a different social class than the physicians who cared for her, and that was a part of the barrier between us. But the major impediment was our narrow focus on vital signs, culture reports, and lab tests. We maintained our distance from the patient to protect ourselves from the overwhelming enormity of her illness. We pursued our own goals and interests by treating her far beyond the point at which the rational response would have been to allow her to die with dignity and in such a way that we would not inflict further suffering on her or her family.

Medicine does not exist in a vacuum, even though the actions of physicians often seem to be unconnected to the larger world. The essential tool for the physician is breadth of vision, the ability to place the patient in a context. It is not a question of injecting humanism into medicine. Rather, medicine needs to be reformulated as a scientific endeavor within the human domain (Schwartz & Wiggins, 1988). The biopsychosocial perspective is just as important to the relevance and effectiveness of the modern physician as the germ theory of disease (Engel, 1977).

POPULATION-BASED MEDICINE: A WAY TO SET GOALS FOR YOURSELF AND YOUR PRACTICE

Unfortunately, we do not always have the luxury of totally separating ourselves from the organizational structures that shape many aspects of the medical encounter. In the rapidly disappearing fee-for-service model of medicine, physicians have subtle (and sometimes not so subtle) incentives to schedule more visits, perform more tests, and do more procedures. Equally pernicious are those managed care systems that install physician gatekeepers, especially when physicians benefit financially from stinting on the care provided to an individual patient. When physicians benefit personally from either giving too much or too little care to their patients, a conflict of interest arises that can undermine the trust that cements the physician–patient relationship.

Retaining a patient-centered focus when dealing with individuals does not, however, release the physician from any concern about the fiscal and social ramifications of his actions. As I discussed in my review of community-oriented patient care, the physician is in a privileged position to focus not only on the problems that patients bring to the medical visit, but also on the underlying public health issues that cause illness and suffering in the population generally. In that respect, the physician also has the responsibility to think about whether medical expenditures would have more impact if spent on other activities, from improvements in the educational system, to bolstering family planning capability, to job creation or environmental protection.

Population-based medicine is in many ways the antithesis of personal medical care. Population-based medicine deals with the denominator, an entire group of people defined by residence, race, social class, or culture; personal medical care deals usually with the individual, although at times the family unit—broadly defined—is the target of the medical intervention. Population-based medicine is a tool used to change social policies, priorities, and programs and sets goals that are met by introducing changes that affect large groups of people. Personal medical care is aimed at individuals, often when they are sick or in an attempt to detect or prevent illness.

Although physicians are not usually trained in the skills of population-based medicine, they need to be active participants in the arenas where these decisions are made. The relatively little attention paid to population-based medicine and public health in the United States does not mean that policies are not articulated. Rather, the healthcare system that has evolved has embedded within it the implicit value that the quality and range of medical services will be determined by patient income, employment, and social status and that many of the fundamental causes of illness, disability, and dysfunction will not be addressed on a societal basis. To the extent that individual physicians do not agree with those decisions, they need to be involved in resetting these broader social goals.

CASE 1-7

The man sat sheepishly in the exam room, a piece of paper in his hand. "My wife sent me in for a PSA test," he explained. "You know, one of those tests that tells me if I have cancer of the prostate. She read about it in **Good Housekeeping.***"*

The physician tried to dissuade the man, who was a vigorously healthy 60-year-old, had normal findings on prostate exam, and had no symptoms, but the wife's instructions prevailed. The test came back elevated, and the physician sent him on to a urologist. The patient underwent a biopsy, which was negative. He began to get annual PSA exams and had several repeat biopsies, each of which was quite painful and left the patient feeling old and weak.

EPIDEMIOLOGICAL PRINCIPLES AS A WAY TO UNDERSTAND THE BALANCE BETWEEN HEALTH AND ILLNESS

Most physicians understand the logic of the biopsychosocial approach to medical care, even if the rigors of daily medical practice may leave them without the time or energy to ask about family and friends. Population-based medicine is even more remote, both because physicians receive little training in its application and because it seems to exist in a realm far removed from the day-to-day hurly-burly of medicine as it is practiced.

Clinical epidemiology provides a tool that ties together many of the themes of this chapter, bridging the world where physicians interpret the tests of individual patients and policymakers try to make decisions about the policies that shape medical practice in this country (Fletcher *et al.*, 1982). Epidemiologists—and their partners in crime, biostatisticians—use their observations of the incidence, prevalence, and natural course of illness and medical treatment to try to extract generalizable rules about both illnesses and treatments. Clinical epidemiology harnesses those observations to the work of the individual physician.

The patient described in Case 1-7 is one you will see a thousand times, with minor variations. Is ordering a PSA logical for this 60-year-old, or would his life have been better if he had gone without? Should one get an exercise tolerance test for the middle-aged man who would like to run a marathon? Should one use expensive pills to reduce the cholesterol level in a 50-year-old woman from 230 to 190? And what does it mean when the alkaline phosphatase reading on the routine blood test is 5% above the normal range?

The individual clinician must become a professional skeptic, armed with enough knowledge of epidemiology to critically evaluate the unending stream of data spewed out by the professional and popular press. Not only are many of the nostrums, tests, and interventions urged on us expensive irritations, many of them are potentially dangerous. The patient in Case 1-7 was lucky. Had the biopsy showed a small focus of cancer, he might have ended up with a radical prostatectomy, which carries a high risk of impotence and incontinence. Those might be acceptable outcomes if the procedure were lifesaving, but we don't know whether prostate cancer in elderly males is even a disease, much less whether lives will be saved by surgery. This hasn't prevented an explosion in the number of radical prostatectomies, largely because physicians and patients alike are much more comfortable with action than inaction, even when evidence is lacking for efficacy.

I would argue that clinical epidemiology is a subject just as essential to the modern physician as a basic understanding of anatomy. We expect physicians to have a fairly precise idea of the locations of the main organs and the way they are interconnected, even though the ability to name all of the metacarpals generally fades as soon as the faintly prurient acronymic ditty is forgotten. By the same token, the physician should have a firm understanding of the concepts of specificity, sensitivity, prevalence, and predictive value, even if the nuances of odds ratios are something that has to be looked up. Health and illness are not pure states of being, but exist as physical, social, and epidemiological constructs. The competent physician will understand health and illness from all of these perspectives.

CONCLUSION: THE HUMAN COMEDY— MAN AS PART OF NATURE

Although Galileo had the intellectual courage to revoke man's place at the center of the universe, he paid a heavy price for his heresy. Although we know with our minds that man is but a mote on a speck of dust lost in the immensity of space, we know with our bellies that we are the masters of creation and that the stars continue to revolve around the earth.

The central challenge of life is accepting the brevity of our individual existence. We are born into pain and shackled to mortality. We spend much of our existence looking for nostrums or diversions to blur this painful reality or deny it by involving magical kingdoms where we will leave our corporeal bodies behind.

Medical care as an organized human activity grows out of our unwillingness to accept passively the anonymous but destructive effects of entropy and accident. Part of the allure of the medical profession is the chance to struggle against the impersonal forces of nature, to deal with our own mortality by mitigating the suffering of others. This book seeks to put this struggle into a broader context, to acknowledge the interrelationships between the individual, the society in which she is embedded, and the entire planetary community of which that society is a part. Most of medical education focuses on the powerful tools of a focused trade. But physicians are more than body mechanics, and we fail in our quest to improve the lives of individuals if we don't also direct attention to the broader social and ecological context in which they lead their lives.

Becoming an effective physician requires more than technical competence or even well-honed interpersonal skills. Although it will be a continual and often frustrating challenge, the physician has a responsibility both to herself and to the species to engage in the broader issues while also responding to the very real existential suffering of the individual.

These two activities will at times exist together and at times proceed in parallel. The goal is not ultimate success—just as with the life cycle of individuals, the art is in the process as opposed to the product. Medicine is a rewarding struggle, but a struggle nonetheless.

———————— CASES FOR DISCUSSION ————————

CASE 1

Mrs. O'Callahan is a 48-year-old clerical worker who lives alone after a painful divorce 3 years ago. Since then she has had a succession of physical problems, including headaches, reflux, insomnia, and foot pain. She comes in to see you now because she has been having twinges of chest pain for about 2 weeks, getting worse particularly in the last 3 days. Her physical exam is unrevealing.

1. *Your initial suspicion is that her chest pain is psychophysiologic, but you know that she has a strong history of heart disease in her family. How would you proceed with the initial workup?*

2. *Although the results of the first tests that you order are normal, the symptoms do not abate. Mrs. O'Callahan becomes more and more concerned about them and asks whether or not she should be referred to a cardiologist. Her managed care plan is structured in such a way that any referrals to outside specialists come out of your capitation (the insurance that you receive monthly for taking care of Mrs. O'Callahan). How does this affect your decision?*

3. *While you are trying to unravel the problem, you learn from another physician that he was sued by the patient because she charged that he was negligent in working up her arthritis. How does this affect your relationship with the patient and the decisions you make regarding her care?*

4. *The patient starts showing up in the emergency room without calling your office and demanding that she be admitted to the coronary care unit. You suggest that she might want to consider psychological counseling, but she rejects that suggestion angrily. What do you do now?*

Phyllis was only 15 when she came into your office, but she wanted to get pregnant. She lived in a housing project not too far from your office with her 35-year-old mother and three younger sisters. She smoked, was doing poorly in school, and fought with her mother and her mother's boyfriends. She also had bad asthma, which got worse in the spring and after she and her mother had been at war. She had been having unprotected intercourse for about 4 months and wondered why nothing had happened.

1. *Your first inclination is to talk to Phyllis's mother, but the teenager doesn't want her mother to know that she's coming in to see you. Are you willing to continue seeing Phyllis without the mother's involvement?*
2. *On further questioning, you find that Phyllis has been suspended from school after getting into a shoving match with another girl during lunch. What responsibility do you have for following up on this?*
3. *Phyllis eventually does get pregnant and asks if you would be willing to deliver the baby. What is your response?*
4. *You are a bit worried about Phyllis's sisters, whom you haven't seen for quite a while. Is there anything you can do about their healthcare?*

CASE 3

Mary, a 42-year-old white woman, has been seeing you for years as her family physician. You've also been taking care of her husband Roy, a 45-year-old black Vietnam veteran with a long-term drinking problem. Mary has terrible headaches that get worse before her periods and also has been having trouble with their teenage son.

1. *Mary comes in one day and asks you what you think of feverfew, a homeopathic headache remedy that one of her friends recommends. What is your opinion?*
2. *Although Mary has been trying to get Roy to stop drinking for years, it has been to no avail. Recently he's told her to shut up or get out. What advice can you offer Mary?*
3. *Roy has worsening hypertension, hypercholesterolemia, and a terrible family history for heart disease. Should you try to get him started on antihypertensive and lipid-lowering agents?*
4. *The teenage son has run away from home, been picked up by the police, and ends up in the youth shelter. Mary calls you in a panic. What is your response?*

CASE 4

You have just gone to work in a small apple-growing town in the eastern part of the state. Although many of the surrounding farm families are well-off, the town itself is decrepit. There is a large population of Hispanic migrant workers, some who still migrate and some who have settled out. There is quite a lot of racial tension between the older white families and the migrants who pick the crops, and everyone drives around with a rifle in their pickup and a handgun in the glove compartment. You are struggling to make your practice a success but also would like to do something to reduce the number of accidents and traumatic injuries from fights that keep you up nights in the emergency room.

1. *You have a sense that the accident rate is much higher in your town than in others like it in the state but aren't sure. What can you do to find out if your appraisal is correct?*

2. *The state comes out with a program to improve emergency medical services in rural towns but requires that the money go to an elected community board. What role do you have in establishing or running such a board?*
3. *The hospital administrator is at his wit's end because the government's healthcare program for migrants doesn't pay for inpatient care. What advice do you offer him?*
4. *Juan, a 32-year-old migrant apple picker, comes in with scabies, which he got from the dirty bedding in one of the shacks provided by a local farmer. What do you prescribe for Juan, and what do you tell your county health department?*

CASE 5

You live in a town in the central United States where there is a large open pit mine, the main industry for that region. You notice that your patients are showing signs and symptoms of lead poisoning, which is confirmed by blood tests. The mine is financially tenuous, with old technology and marginal yields; it seems unlikely that it could afford to install appropriate pollution control equipment.

1. *What do you tell your patients when their children show elevated levels of lead in their blood?*
2. *How do you inform the local industry?*

ACKNOWLEDGMENTS. I would like to acknowledge the helpful suggestions of Theodore Phillips, John Geyman, and Robert Beaglehole.

——————— RECOMMENDED READINGS ———————

Bloom SW: *The Doctor and His Patient: A Sociological Interpretation.* New York, Free Press, 1965.

> The classic—but still relevant—study of the role and function of the physician from the sociologic perspective.

Evans RG, Barer ML, Marmor TR: *Why Are Some People Healthy and Others Not? The Determinants of Health of Populations.* New York, Aldine de Gruyter, 1994.

> A comprehensive and readable analysis of the relationship between social organization and the health of the individual.

Illich I: *Medical Nemesis: The Expropriation of Health.* New York, Pantheon Books, 1976.

> This perceptive social critic details the extent to which the medicalization of ordinary life causes can undermine the health of both the individual and the larger society.

White KW: *The Task of Medicine: Dialogue at Wickenburg.* Menlo Park, CA, Henry J. Kaiser Foundation, 1988.

> A modern reexploration of the biopsychosocial model of human disease.

CHAPTER 2

Individual and Family Life Cycle

Eliana C. Korin, Marlene F. Watson, and Monica McGoldrick

CASE 2-1

A family physician was worried about a patient, a 53-year-old woman whose blood pressure had become progressively elevated despite appropriate treatment; no cause for secondary hypertension or noticeable changes in her life were identified. Mrs. Garcia, the patient, a pleasant and energetic Latina widow, was living with her daughter and two grandchildren. One day, she brought her 18-month-old granddaughter to her physician for a routine medical visit with complaints of sleep problems. The toddler often cried or had temper tantrums at bedtime.

While assessing the child's development, the physician also explored the family situation. The child was the result of an unexpected though welcomed pregnancy of a single mother, a full-time worker, who already had a 12-year-old son. When the grandmother was asked how this unexpected return to childrearing responsibilities had been for her, she confessed that in her enthusiasm to have a granddaughter, she did not anticipate the emotional and physical demands posed by an active toddler at this stage of her life. The patient's stress was exacerbated because of feelings of discomfort in renegotiating childcare arrangements with her daughter, whom she had promised support. Moreover, given the present situation, she could not pursue her plans to spend the winter holidays with siblings in her hometown.

At this point, the physician realized the impact of the family dynamics and life cycle issues on his patients' health. The grandmother's blood pressure and the child's sleep problems were successfully addressed as the physician promoted a dialogue between grandmother and mother focusing on the symptoms as responses to the family's adaptation to a new life-cycle stage.

As Case 2-1 indicates, the individual and family life-cycle perspective provides a useful framework for understanding and addressing everyday clinical problems. Over time, the family moves through various life-cycle stages, and new demands emerge requiring individual adaptation and family reorganization. When individuals and/or families resist or fail to adapt to these changes, symptoms are likely to appear. Therefore, the clinician should always ask: "In which life-cycle stage is this patient and his family? How are they dealing with life-cycle transitions?" As illustrated in Case 2-1, the unexpected birth of a child disrupted the natural cycle of life in the family, resulting in interpersonal conflicts and health problems. The symptoms—the grandmother's blood pressure and the child's sleep problems—were successfully addressed when the physician recognized the symptoms as resulting from the family's difficulty to adapt to a new life stage.

The family life cycle is an important predictor of stress, which is often greatest at transitional points when the family is moving from one developmental stage to another (Carter & McGoldrick, 1989). Medical visits tend to occur at times of transitions, such as the birth of a child, the launching of a child, and the disability or death of a parent. An understanding of family life-cycle stages assists physicians in

- Anticipating medical problems
- Developing preventive and health promotion strategies
- Formulating hypotheses about medical problems
- Designing effective treatment strategies

To assist the student in understanding the impact of the family on the health of its members, this chapter will discuss individual development as it occurs within the family life cycle (FLC), describe the FLC stages in relation to health problems, and illustrate the application of the FLC model in medical practice. To appreciate the FLC, however, we must first understand basic patterns in the life cycle of the individual and the relation between individual and family life cycles.

CASE 2-2

Mary Petlock was already pregnant with her second child when she learned that her first, David, aged 2, who had been developmentally delayed in speech and motor skills, was indeed retarded. As the physician spoke with her about David's diagnosis and prognosis, Mary began to realize that the family would be having to deal with his developmental disabilities throughout their future. She worried about how to deal with the loss of the many dreams and hopes she and her husband had for David's life, and about how the other children might have to sacrifice some of their own interests and activities and assume caretaking roles themselves. Mary also worried about how she and the rest of the family would make these adjustments.

The following year Mary's husband, Joseph Verdun, lost his job as a salesman for a large corporation and was unable to find another job. Because of the financial pressures of the new baby, Sam, their retarded son, David, and Joe's unemployment, the couple moved in with Mary's parents. This new living arrangement put pressure on Mary and Joe's relationship, as Mary felt more like a daughter than a mother in her parental home, subject to her mother's continual comments about how she was handling her children and her "lazy" husband. Joe, who did not feel at home with his in-laws, began staying out more, drinking at the local bar. Joe resented his wife's attention to her parents. He also resented David's disability and refused to help care for him. To help support the family, Mary took a part-time nursing job. The following year, with Joe still unemployed, Mary's mother, Anna, aged 55, was diagnosed with Alzheimer's disease.

—— THE INDIVIDUAL LIFE CYCLE IN CONTEXT ——

Evaluating problems in terms of both individual life cycle and the family life cycle is an important part of the medical assessment. The accomplishment of certain physical, intellectual, social, spiritual, and emotional life-cycle tasks are part of normative development. Each person's individual life cycle intersects with the family life cycle at every point, at times causing conflict of needs. For instance, in Case 2-1, the toddler's developmental needs conflicted with grandmother's life plans. Furthermore, when individual family members do not fit into normative expectations for development, there are repercussions on family development, as indicated in Case 2-2 (see Fig. 2.1). Similarly, a family's adaptation to its tasks will influence how individuals negotiate their individual development.

A suggestive schema for exploring normative individual life-cycle tasks is offered in Table 2.1. There are serious limitations to any attempt to condense the complications of life in an oversimplified framework. Obviously there is an overlap between the physical, intellectual, and social/emotional tasks, so that certain tasks could fit into each realm. Communication, for example, is a physical, intellectual, and social/emotional task of development. Table 2.1 presents a skeletal framework for assessing a person's passage through life. The phases of human development have been defined in many ways in different cultures. This outline is a rough guideline, not a statement of the true and fixed stages of life. People vary greatly in their pathways through life. The schema here is meant to be suggestive rather than definitive. Furthermore, accomplishing the individual tasks of

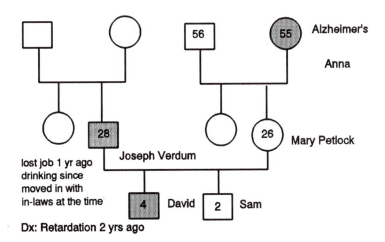

Figure 2.1. Genogram of the Verdum/Petlock family.

Table 2.1
Major Individual Developmental Stages and Tasks

1. **Infancy (approximate ages 0–2)**
   Talk, communicate frustration and happiness
   Learn to make needs known and get them met
   Coordination, sit, stand, walk, run, manipulate objects
   Recognize self as separate person
   Trust others, primarily caretakers
   Overcome fears of new situations
2. **Early childhood (approximate ages 2–4)**
   Speech, language development, ability to relate and communicate
   Coordination, motor skills, eye–hand coordination
   Ability to control one's bodily functions, bowels and urine
   Understand self in relation to the world around oneself, awareness of others in terms of gender, race, and
       disability
   Cooperative play, ability to share
   Ability to obey rules
   Ability to delay gratification
   Development of trusting relationships
   Ability to form peer relationships
   Fantasy play and dramatization to master behavior and control anxieties
3. **Middle childhood (approximate ages 5–12)**
   Increased physical coordination and motor skills
   Ability to play team games
   Skill in reading, writing, math
   Knowledge about nature
   Understanding self in relation to family, peers, community; awareness of "otherness" in terms of gender,
       race, sexual orientation, culture, class, and disability
   Increased ability to conduct relationships with peers and authorities
   Ability to be intimate; to express anger, fear, and pain in nondestructive ways; to develop tolerance
       for difference
4. **Adolescence (approximate ages 13–19)**
   Bodily changes of puberty
   Development of sexual identity
   Increased physical coordination and physical skills
   Increased ability to read, write, think conceptually and mathematically
   Increased understanding of self in relation to peers, family, and community
   Development of a philosophy of life and moral identity
   Ability to handle intimate physical and social relationships as well as increased ability to judge and
       handle complex social situations
   Ability to work collaboratively and individually
5. **Young adulthood (approximate ages 20–40)**
   Ability to care for self and one's own needs
   Discipline for physical and intellectual work, sleep, sex, social relationships
   Ability to caretake one's partner, children, and other family members
   More complex understanding of self in relation to peers, family, community
   Ability to support self and any children one may have
   Focus on life goals, ability to work independently and collaboratively
   Ability to negotiate evolving relationships to one's parents, peers, children, and community, including
       work relationships
   Ability to nurture others
   Ability to tolerate delaying gratification
   Further evolution of one's ability to promote respect for those who are dependent
6. **Middle adulthood (approximate ages 40–60)**
   Handle work, family, community, and social relationships and be accountable for one's responsibilities
   Some waning of physical abilities

Table 2.1

(Continued)

25

THE INDIVIDUAL
LIFE CYCLE IN
CONTEXT

Accept that one cannot do it all and focus on mentoring others
Recognition of one's accomplishments and acceptance of one's limitations
Balance of multiple caretaking responsibilities for those above and below
7. **Late middle age (approximate ages 60s and 70s)**
   Acceptance of declining physical abilities; handle work, family, community, and social relationships and be accountable for one's responsibilities
   Adapting to some loss of intellectual abilities, increasing one's perspective on life
   Attend to one's connections with those who come after
   Recognizing one's triumphs and accepting one's limitations and losses
8. **Aging (approximate ages 80s+)**
   Acceptance of declining of physical abilities and acceptance of diminishing control of over one's life
   Some loss of intellectual abilities, while maintaining wisdom
   Affirming and working out one's legacy to newer generation
   Acceptance of one's life and death

---

a stage depends on resources available to individuals and families to help them develop their abilities.

During the *first stage* (0–2 years) of life, babies need to learn to communicate their needs and have some sense of trust, comfort, and relationship to their caretakers and the world around them. Their needs have to be satisfied consistently so they can develop trust for others and a sense of trustworthiness and security. They learn to coordinate their bodies and begin to explore the world. David, the older son in Case 2-2, was obviously having trouble accomplishing the tasks of this phase. He had been delayed in speech and motor skills, which led to his being evaluated for retardation. His difficulties accomplishing the tasks required extra parental caretaking. All future life stages will be influenced by David's retardation, and extra adaptive skills will be called on from other family members throughout his life to provide him with the special supports he will need. The family will have to do more caretaking and for a longer period than with another child and deal with the lost dreams created by his disabilities for their whole lives. Children not yet born, future siblings and cousins, and even future children of these siblings will need to find the strength to deal with his limitations and offer support to him. The physician will have to help the family to adjust their expectations to David's possibilities while continuing to provide him with the necessary stimulation and support.

The *second stage*, the child's preschool years (2–4), is a time of great development of language and motor skills and abilities to explore and relate to the world around oneself. The child develops cognitive skills with numbers, words, and objects. She becomes more autonomous, learns how to play by herself, and also to share. It is at this time that children begin to form peer relationships and to be aware of themselves as different from others. They start learning to deal with frustration and to accept limits and delay gratification, and also to obey rules. Imagination plays an important role at this stage. Through fantasy play, and later, dramatic play, children learn to master their behavior and to deal with fears and anxieties. Physicians can be helpful to parents by highlighting the value of play and fantasy at this stage, fostering emotional and cognitive development. David in Case 2-2 reached this phase, but his developmental disabilities slowed him down increasingly with age-appropriate skills. He was behind in language and motor skills and in ability to relate to the world around him. He was slower than his peers in developing interpersonal relationships. One might predict that his younger brother, Sam, would outdistance him in developmental skills in the not too distant future. David's ongoing individual developmental difficulties will continue to create extra family life-cycle tasks for other family members in terms of extra caretaking and accommodation to his problems by his brother, who may soon become developmentally more advanced than David. This situation will create a reversal of the expected family hierarchy, where the younger brother and any future siblings will become caretakers to the oldest, while usually it is the oldest who does more caretaking for the younger ones.

The *third developmental phase* might be said to cover the school-age years of childhood, from about age 5 to 12. At this time children typically make many developmental leaps in their cognitive skills, motor skills, and emotional skills. Children expand their social world in terms of their ability to communicate and handle relationships with an increasing range of adults and children beyond their families. They learn how to conduct relationships in terms of fairness, tolerance for others who are different, conflict resolution, competition, collaboration, and intimacy. They begin to understand their identity in terms of gender, race, culture, and sexual orientation and to differentiate themselves from others. They learn to follow directions, to tolerate frustration, and to work independently and with others. Accomplishing these tasks depends both on the child's innate resources and on family and community supports to foster the child's development. If deprived of any of these resources the child may develop either physical, emotional, or social symptoms. Children may develop fears, anxieties, phobias, stomach- or headaches, or aggressive or withdrawn behaviors. In Case 2-2, David's brother Sam and any future siblings will have special tasks at this phase to adapt to a retarded older brother and his special needs.

We might consider the *fourth developmental stage* to be adolescence, a phase that is not universal and was never particularly defined prior to the industrial revolution, which required a lengthier apprenticeship to learn the skills necessary for adult functioning. During this phase, young people go through puberty and develop the ability to function increasingly independently. They renegotiate their identity in relation to their parents as they mature, refine their physical, social, and intellectual skills, develop their spiritual and moral identity, and begin to define who they want to become as adults. Family life-cycle problems may interfere with this individual development. For example, if a mother dies leaving three adolescent daughters, the oldest may sacrifice her own individual development, e.g., forego college plans and her social development to become a caretaker for her father and sisters, out of a sense that they need her as caretaker. At the same time her short-circuiting of her individual development will be influenced by how other family members have handled earlier life-cycle dilemmas and by how they are handling this loss of the mother. Special problems may emerge for the family in Case 2-2 when David becomes an adolescent because of his retardation, since his physical development will outdistance his emotional and intellectual development. Special tasks are common, for example, in helping a retarded adolescent deal with his or her emerging sexuality and wish to connect with peers in ways that are appropriate, given the intellectual limitations.

We might think of the *fifth phase of development* as covering the decades of young adulthood (from about age 20 to 40). Of course there are great differences in the pathways at this phase depending on a person's gender or class, but in general it is the phase of generativity in terms of partnering, work, and raising children. It is the time when adults are expected to function without the physical or financial support of their parents, a time when they begin not only to care for themselves but also to take on responsibilities for the care of others—both children and aging parents who need support. It is at this phase that adults need to have the ability to handle individual work and caretaking responsibilities in spite of frustrations. Joe Verdun, the husband in Case 2-2, obviously got off the track at this stage in his own individual life cycle in terms of his responsibility to contribute to the emotional, physical, and financial support of his wife and children. He had not dealt with his disappointment that David was retarded and was avoiding his parental responsibilities for this son. He resented his wife's attention to her parents and said she was not helping him. His irresponsibility shows that he was off the task in his own life cycle at a time in his life when it was appropriate for him to manage his own frustrations and contribute to the care of others. His individual problems increase the burden on all other family members (his wife, children, in-laws, and his family of origin) in their own life-cycle tasks.

The *sixth stage* of the life cycle might be thought of as midlife (a new stage, since in 1900 the average life span in the United States was 43 years), lasting somewhere between ages 40 and 60. Generally speaking, adults are still in good health, their children are teenagers or being launched at this stage. They are often questioning the meaning of their relationships and work and thinking about the place of whatever success they have in the scheme of things. It is a time when people often do a philosophical reexamination of their lives, or even several reexaminations, and consider major changes in their personal and work lives. It is during this phase that women go through menopause, which often allows them to concentrate their energies on new projects, having been freed up from major caretaking and deciding that it is their "turn." Symptoms might occur when the woman's individual needs do not match family and societal expectations. It is a time when people are coming to terms with the fact that they cannot do it all. They have to let go of certain dreams and recognize their limitations in order to concentrate on what they can do. The family in Case 2-2 experienced individual life-cycle problems as well as family life-cycle problems at this stage, when the wife's mother, Anna, at age 55, who had been increasingly disoriented and forgetful for about a year, was diagnosed with Alzheimer's disease. Her diagnosis obviously interfered with the normative tasks of her middle-age life, in that she would lose her intellectual, physical, and emotional functioning prematurely and require caretaking herself. Her individual developmental problems will increase the burdens on the others in the family as well—her husband, her daughters, her son-in-law, and her grandchildren. Necessarily, when a person has individual developmental problems such as this, there is a double burden on the family, which loses the support of the person and now must devote energy to caretaking her.

The *seventh stage* might be considered the 60s and 70s, late middle age or early aging, a time when adults are beginning to retire, take up new interests, and still, in our times, likely to feel in good health and have the energy for major undertakings. They are by this time freed up from childrearing or financial responsibilities, though they are often now helping the next generation, their grandchildren. At this stage, people have to be concerned about husbanding their financial resources and future healthcare needs. It is a time to work out increasing supports and find ways to manage decreasing physical strength and endurance. It is also a time of facing increasing losses of peers, older friends, and relatives. Grief and feelings of isolation often cause depression and facilitate onset of physical symptoms. Spiritual resources are important to maintain one's health and accept decline of one's abilities.

The *eighth or last stage* of life, aging and death, covers roughly the ages from the late 70s to 100+ as people come to terms with their own mortality and that of their peer group and become prepared for death. It is a time to affirm and work out one's legacy and to complete the organization of relationships with one's legatees. Any pending personal business with one's descendants and with oneself will need to be addressed. At this stage one must face decreasing level of functioning and the increasing dependence on others while continuing to maximize one's abilities.

Recalling Case 2-2, the special individual life-cycle problems of three members of the Verdun/Petlock family, Joseph, David, and Anna, will affect the other family members at both an individual and a family level. These issues, of course, also have extended family implications. Mary's and Joe's siblings and aunts and uncles are also affected by the problems, having to decide how much each of them could or should do to help out. The problems also have community ramifications. David's disabilities will require various community resources throughout his school-age and adult years. The community resources or lack thereof to help Joseph with his alcohol problem and to help Anna and the rest of the family with the disabilities created by Alzheimer's disease will have profound implications for this family's future negotiation of their individual and family life cycle.

FAMILY LIFE-CYCLE STAGES

The stages of the family life cycle are by no means universal markers. In different cultures and historical eras, the demarcation of life-cycle stages will vary from current definitions in our society in terms of timing, importance, and roles expected. In our present classification (Table 2.2) of the life-cycle stages, modified from Carter and McGoldrick (1989), we try to be sensitive to differences in class and ethnicity as well as changes in society influencing family relations. What follows are descriptions of each life-cycle stage and developmental tasks illustrated by clinical vignettes.

CASE 2-3

Lucia, a 24-year-old Italian-American woman, presented to a health center experiencing headaches, stomach and chest pains, nervousness, insomnia, and fainting. Results of her physical exam and lab tests were negative. The treating physician, suspecting social and developmental factors, proceeded with symptomatic treatment and a psychosocial evaluation.

One year previously the patient had begun a management training program of a major company and had relocated to another city, which meant moving away from her family. When the physical symptoms became debilitating she left the training program, moved back home with her family, and took a job with a local company. Lucia's physical symptoms initially lessened but then became worse. She reported experiencing physical distress whenever she anticipated being away from home for a prolonged period with friends, especially her fiancé. Lucia's fiancé was well liked by her family, but Lucia secretly was having second thoughts about the marriage. The physician, realizing that the symptoms were anxiety related, requested a consultation with a family therapist.

YOUNG ADULTHOOD

The "young adulthood" stage is defined as the period between the individual separating from the family and forming a family of her own. This stage varies for families depending on socioeconomic factors, cultural values, and job opportunities as well as on the health status of the individual and family members.

Table 2.2
The Stages of the Family Life Cycle[a]

Family life cycle stage	Emotional process of transition: key principles	Changes in family status required to proceed developmentally	
1. Young adulthood	Accepting emotional and financial responsibility for self	a.	Differentiation of self in relation to family of origin
		b.	Development of intimate peer relationships
		c.	Establishment of self regarding work and financial independence
2. Becoming a couple: partnership and marriage	Commitment to new system	a.	Formation of couple system
		b.	Realignment of relationships with extended families and friends to include partner
		c.	Balancing between individual and couple needs/identity
		d.	Deciding on parenting
3. Families with young children	Accepting new members into the system	a.	Adjusting marital system to make space for child(ren)
		b.	Joining in childrearing, financial, and household tasks
		c.	Realignment of relationships with extended family to include parenting, grandparenting, and other roles
4. Families with adolescents	Increasing flexibility of family boundaries to accept children's independence and grandparents' frailties	a.	Shifting of parent–child relationship to permit adolescent to move in and out of system
		b.	Refocus on midlife personal/conjugal and work issues
		c.	Beginning shift toward joint caring for older generation
5. Midlife stage: launching children and moving on	Accepting a multitude of exits from and entries into the family system	a.	Renegotiation of conjugal system as dyad
		b.	Development of adult-to-adult relationships between grown children and their parents
		c.	Realignment of relationships to include in-laws and grandchildren
		d.	Dealing with disabilities and death of parents (grandparents)
6. Families in later life	Accepting the shifting of generational roles	a.	Maintaining own and/or couple functioning and interests in face of physiological decline; exploration of new familial and social role options
		b.	Support for a more central role of middle generation
		c.	Making room in the system for the wisdom and experience of the elderly; supporting the older generation without overfunctioning for them
		d.	Dealing with loss of spouse, siblings, and other peers and preparation for own death; life review and integration

[a]Adapted from Carter E, McGoldrick M: *The Changing Family Life Cycle: A Framework for Family Therapy.* New York, Allyn & Bacon, 1989.

This phase of the life cycle includes those individuals in their 20s who have established separate dwellings from their families, are postcollege or postmilitary, and, for the most part, are financially independent (Aylmer, 1989). It also includes those individuals who bypassed this stage by marrying young and divorcing within a few years as well as those who are living together without formal commitment. It may also include adult children of any age who have never left home and who, along with their families, engage in the tasks associated with this phase of development. Just as physical separation from the family is not synonymous with emotional differentiation from the family, remaining in the home because of cultural values or limited economic and educational opportunities does not necessarily mean foreclosure of identity formation. In fact, Watson and Protinsky (1988) found that *enmeshment*, a family therapy term meaning overinvolvement and lack of differentiation, was positively correlated with identity achievement for African-American youths. We prefer to name this stage "young adulthood" rather than "leaving home," "unattached adult," or "in-between families" to avoid identifying differentiation and independence with disconnection and emotional distancing from the family. In many working-class families from diverse cultures, unmarried adult children are expected to live at home and contribute a portion of their earnings to the family (Strelnick & Gilpin, 1986). Increasing costs of higher education and limitations in the job market have forced middle-class children to prolong their dependence on the family, especially for housing.

Lucia's experience in Case 2-3 illustrates the conflict created by the overemphasis on male norms and reliance on white Anglo-Saxon Protestant middle-class values as the ideal for individuals and their families. Under this value system, Lucia was expected to leave home in her early 20s and to make career development her single most important goal. The failure to value intimacy and attachment along with individuation and separation seriously complicate the process of defining one's adult identity, especially for women and members of other cultures.

The key tasks (Table 2.1) for the individual at this stage of the life cycle are to become emotionally and financially responsible. To achieve these goals the individual must differentiate the self from the family of origin, develop intimate peer relationships, and establish vocational identity, work, and financial independence (Carter & McGoldrick, 1989). The essential task for the family is to support the young adult in her quest for identity and independence functioning and to accept her adoption of new values and life choices. In this phase, problems may occur because of perceived or actual expectations that the adult child will comply with familial life plans and wishes at the expense of her own. Since the expectations may not come directly from parents but indirectly from grandparents or other extended kin, or be prescribed by the community (Strelnick & Gilpin, l986), it is necessary to think more broadly than the nuclear family when assessing the dynamics of the family.

The developmental conflict faced by the young woman in Case 2-3 also involved her relationships with her brother and grandmother. When her parents divorced and the father abandoned the family, she made an unspoken pact with her brother and mother that they would always take care of each other. Close to her ailing grandmother, Lucia often mediated conflicts between her mother and grandmother. Feelings of guilt and disloyalty to the family of origin competed with her need for autonomy and career advancement. Cultural values, family expectations, and additional stressors such as divorce and illness were important factors in this young woman's transitional conflict.

The impact of parental divorce, illness, and death can be particularly significant at this developmental phase. Although these stressors affect individual and family functioning at all phases of the life cycle, parents who lose their spouse to divorce are likely to expect increased support from their adult children at a time when their children need to invest their energies outside the family. Such a situation places young adults in a difficult bind indeed.

Since ethnicity shapes the family life cycle at every stage (McGoldrick, 1988c), understanding cultural patterns is critical for physicians who wish to provide effective care for young adults. For example, while the dominant culture in United States values the young adult's autonomy and independence, many cultural groups such as Italian-Americans tend to value interdependence among family members. Thus, patients such as Lucia face special challenges differentiating from their families. Individual developmental dilemmas are further amplified as families struggle to assimilate into mainstream American culture while maintaining core values of their cultural heritage. Lucia must negotiate some difficult compromises: "How can I succeed in the outside world and be viewed as an adult while maintaining strong ties with my family?" "How can I continue to be loyal and supportive to my family while allowing myself new life options?" A successful transition at this stage will require that Lucia, or any young adult, learn how to increase emotional distance from the family while remaining connected.

When these issues are presented clinically, the task of the physician is to frame symptoms developmentally and to normalize emotional distancing as a necessary transition while encouraging renegotiation of relationships with family as an alternative to estrangement. Young adults who cut off their parents and families do so reactively and are in fact still emotionally bound to rather than independent of the family "program" (Carter & McGoldrick, 1989). Those who learn to relate in a new way, adult to adult, will be able to maintain an ongoing and mutually respectful relationship in which each appreciates the other as they are.

This is an especially challenging task for homosexual young adults and their families. In a similar case to Lucia in Case 2-3, a young woman's headaches were associated with her fear of family rejection because of her recently self-accepted homosexuality. The experience of treating homosexual AIDS patients makes physicians painfully aware of unfortunate consequences of these cutoffs, having witnessed the distress of patients, and sometimes families. But illness also brings opportunities for rapprochement. Family and individual counseling facilitates healing and, eventually, reconnection between patients and their families.

Except for AIDS patients and others facing chronic illness, medical visits are less frequent at this stage. Healthy young adults tend to come to physicians for work-related reasons, such as health assessment, on-the-job injuries, sickness excuses, accidents, sports injuries, or sexually related problems. These encounters provide the physician an opportunity to address disease prevention and health promotion, including a review of this stage's developmental tasks. Recurrent somatic complaints are often responses to developmental and other social stressors. Young adults with chronic illness, especially men, often present with problems of compliance. Their sense of physical vulnerability is often associated with fear of losing their maleness. A focus on developmental tasks will guide the physician toward an understanding of the patient's situation.

CASE 2-4

Vanessa, a 28-year-old educated African-American woman, married for the first time 6 months ago, went to her physician suspecting she might be pregnant. The physician is surprised to find that Vanessa has missed her menses for 2 months without checking or sharing the possibility of a pregnancy with her husband. Despite their original plan to have children early in their marriage, Vanessa now feels ambivalent because of increasing tensions in the marriage. She reports that their relationship has been changing since they moved closer to his close-knit Jamaican family. Mark, her husband, has become less playful and affectionate, and she has become more withdrawn and intolerant. For the physician, this report reflects a contrasting scenario to earlier visits when the couple seemed happy together.

From Vanessa's earlier visits the physician knew the patient as an attractive, intelligent, and career-oriented woman who was completing an MBA degree when she met her husband. The patient was delighted that Mark was smart, outgoing, and responsible, proud of her achievements, and shared her goals of raising a family. They had lived together 8 months and decided to get married in response to her ailing mother's desire to attend her wedding while in good health.

BECOMING A COUPLE: FORMING PARTNERSHIP AND MARRIAGE

The stage of the new couple is one of the most complex and difficult transitions of the family life cycle (McGoldrick, 1989). The two partners must renegotiate a variety of issues previously defined by each as individuals and by their respective families and cultures. They must decide on the rules that will govern their relationship and the boundary that will define them as a couple.

Recent trends, such as unmarried couples establishing households and the formation of committed homosexual partnerships, require us to explore models of partnership other than traditional marriages. The unifying element to these diverse couples is that they form a partnership with a goal of sharing a future together and deciding whether to have children.

The tasks (Table 2.2) that the new couple must successfully resolve are (1) making a commitment to the marital or partnership dyad, (2) realignment of relationships with the extended family and friends to take the partner into consideration (Carter & McGoldrick, 1989), and (3) balancing the needs of the individual with those of the couple. The ability of the partners to make a commitment to each other will be determined by the extent to which they have achieved emotional differentiation from the family of origin and established an identity of their own. Each partner should view the relationship as a means of enriching one's self, not completing one's self. The couple also needs to achieve a balance between the need for intimacy and the need for individual fulfillment. And finally, each has to grapple with expectations from parents and siblings in view of the partner's expectations. For instance, part of the issue facing the couple in Case 2-4 was that the husband, the only married male sibling, was trying to deal with his brothers' tendency to dismiss his new identity as a married man, expecting him to continue to socialize without his wife.

To support couples in their quest to establish and define a bond, the physician must assess the couple's relationship. The following questions are helpful:

- "What is your idea of what a marriage/partnership should be like?"
- "How has this marriage, or getting together, changed or supported your plans for the future?"
- "In which ways do you feel you are, or are not, complementing each other?"

The physician should explore each partner's desire for intimacy, the couple's decision-making process, contacts with relatives or friends, and the extended family's feelings about the marriage. Differences of education and income should also be explored to determine the balance of power between them.

Cultural differences between the partners regarding styles of socialization, family rituals, and patterns of contact with family of origin need to be identified, revised, and selectively combined in the couple's life. The complexity of marriage may not be fully appreciated by the young couple until they are faced with the challenge of deciding such issues as: how and where to celebrate the holidays; whose family traditions to follow; who does what in the household; and the degree of intimacy in the relationship.

When assessing the dynamics of the relationship, it is important that physicians differentiate the impact of culture from race and class. For example, in another case an African-American wife's physical symptoms were caused by stress resulting from her African husband's differing views on gender roles in the marriage. Because the couple shared the same social and class backgrounds, the physician might have overlooked significant cultural differences contributing to the wife's presenting illness. Case 2-4 describes the increasing marital tension between an African-American woman and her Jamaican-Caribbean husband, which was jeopardizing her pregnancy and perhaps her health. The wife, a woman from a small and middle-class nuclear-oriented family, felt left out because of the husband's inattentiveness since the couple moved closer to his tightly knit Jamaican family. Vanessa's withdrawal and irritability reflected her disappointment that her husband's allegiance and loyalty were to his family of origin and not to her. The ambivalence she felt about the pregnancy was linked to conflict over of her husband's commitment to the couple bond. When interviewed, Mark, the husband, was delighted about the news of the pregnancy, reaffirmed his commitment to the relationship, and criticized her ideas of a social life without family contact. He resented her distant and reserved style with his family and interpreted her request to have meals by themselves as a rejection of his family. The situation called for a compromise across personal styles, family legacies, and cultural background, along with consideration of gender differences.

Societal expectations that the man should be the major wage earner and that the woman's career is secondary in the marriage have significant implications for the health of both men and women in addition to how well the couple can jointly address the predictable crises of this stage. For instance, in Case 2-4, the patient's ambivalence about her pregnancy was related to her conflicts between motherhood obligations and the possible demands of a career. She was reluctant to discuss her conflicts with her husband, being skeptical that, as a man, he would understand her ambivalence. Like many other women, she found herself in a bind—to be a devoted mother or a successful professional—a typical dilemma at this stage, when childbearing decisions must be negotiated. Given our society's expectations for women and the lack of support for parenting, it is not surprising that an increasing number of couples and individuals are deciding to be childless.

The physician in Case 2-4 validated and normalized this patient's ambivalence, acknowledging gender differences and highlighting to the patient and her husband the social implications of childbearing for women. Their mutual expectations and frustrations regarding marriage were also examined and reframed in relation to their different cultural backgrounds. This approach promoted dialogue, understanding, and support. The husband conveyed to his wife her prerogative in making a decision about the future of this pregnancy. She decided to continue with the pregnancy, which unfortunately resulted in an early miscarriage.

Interestingly, these family and cultural differences were not a problem until the couple moved closer to the husband's family. Excessive family participation in a new couple's lives tends to undermine their relationship, whereas physical distance between family members places much more burden on the couple to define relationships by themselves (Carter & McGoldrick, 1989). In the above case, for instance, a change in the couple dynamics would be likely to occur if the wife's family became more present in their lives, bringing a balance between the two family legacies. The genogram (McGoldrick & Gerson, 1985) is a most useful clinical tool for exploring these dynamics (see Chapter 6 on the Family System). In our individual-oriented society, we often forget that marriage involves the joining of two families, not simply two individuals.

Physical closeness to family is an important factor when dealing with cases of spouse abuse, which is quite common at this life stage. Family-of-origin involvement often has a buffering effect against violence, besides providing potential support for the victim.

Violence, sexual dysfunction, somatic complaints, and infertility are some common clinical problems arising at this stage of the family life cycle. Physicians aware of these tendencies will be able to detect these problems and address them in an effective and timely manner.

CASE 2-5

Joseph is a moderately overweight but otherwise healthy 7-year-old boy who was brought to the clinic three times in a period of 7 weeks for episodes of acute abdominal pain. Physical exam and initial ancillary tests revealed no abnormalities. The physician treated the boy for constipation and suggested dietary changes and increased physical activities to address the weight problem. Before considering further exams, he decided to explore more carefully the patient's social and family situation. This shy yet articulate and pleasant boy talked positively about school and friends but became evasive when asked about his baby brother and family subjects. Joseph's mother reported that her son was probably missing the special attention he was accustomed to receiving from his stepfather before the birth of his young brother. Most of his exclusive time with his mother or stepfather was related to homework activities. The family had also moved to a new apartment in an attractive neighborhood. He was sharing his parents' attention not only with the new baby but also with the new demands created by this move. The stepfather was very involved with house repairs and mother seemed overwhelmed.

——— FAMILY WITH YOUNG CHILDREN ———

In Case 2-5, 7-year-old Joseph feels abandoned by the parents when the new baby arrives. The stress he experiences as a result of losing his parents' exclusive focus is manifested in recurrent abdominal pain. The parents face multiple demands as they expand their family and improve their life conditions. Like other couples at this stage, they struggle to meet the emotional needs of each child and their own needs as a couple and as individuals, while fulfilling work, household, and extended family demands. Needless to say, this stage of the life cycle poses a significant threat to individual, couple, and family functioning.

Children's symptoms are often indicators of family stress. Recurrent abdominal pain, along with somatic complaints in general, are problems most commonly seen by physicians working with school-age children. The pediatric literature reports that the majority of children with recurrent pain have real pain that results from the interplay of multiple factors: physiologic, psychological, temperamental, and environmental (Poole *et al.*, 1995). Furthermore, they might be manifestations of stress connected to developmental and life cycle transitions or social stressors experienced by the individual and family.

This stage is a time for family expansion: New members are added requiring more physical and emotional space and more financial resources. New pursuits regarding living conditions, work status, and/or career development are explored. Even when individual and family are both progressing and basic family relations are positive, as in the case of Joseph and his family, symptoms might occur as responses to stressful transitions.

The three main tasks (Table 2.2) of the family with young children are (1) adapting the marital system to include children, (2) sharing in childrearing, financial, and household responsibilities, and (3) realignment of familial relationships to include new roles: parents, grandparents, sibling, aunt, uncle, and so on (Carter & McGoldrick, 1989).

Another key issue at this stage of the family with young children is the formation and strengthening of the sibling system. In this phase, siblings learn how to share, build alliances, and support each other. Questions regarding sibling conflicts are commonly presented in medical visits. Sibling competition is determined not only by the availability of parents but also by how parents relate to the children.

The birth of a child requires a major realignment of family relations. When the first child is born, adults move up a generation and assume caretaking responsibilities for the young generation. The couple's own emotional and sexual intimacy may be placed on the back burner as the couple struggles to meet the demands of parenthood. Parenting styles are defined and differences related to culture and family of origin may become pronounced with the birth of a child. Additionally, the couple or single parent may again have to renegotiate boundary issues with the families of origin to accommodate the child's relationship to grandparents and other extended kin. Grandparents have to move to a less central role, supporting parents' authority. In the case of single parents, grandparents' and other family members' roles are negotiated differently, as they are most often needed for caretaking functions. Depending on cultural and class background, older children are expected to help care for younger siblings.

A crucial issue during this stage of the life cycle is the disposition of childcare responsibilities and household chores. The lack of social provision for adequate childcare in our society (McGoldrick *et al.*, 1993) and the decrease of social support in general often cause children to be left without proper attention or force families, especially women, to make sacrifices to attend to family needs. For instance, Joseph's mother in Case 2-5, a medical technician, decided to quit her job to take care of the children, while her husband continued in his career as a computer manager. Childcare is not affordable for the many two-paycheck or single-parent families with small children. When Joseph was younger, his mother, being a single mother, had to rely on her mother to take care of him to be able to work. As illustrated in Case 2-1, grandmothers are often called on to share childcare responsibilities. Financial pressures also require that the husband/father increase his hours of work, thus decreasing family contact and creating family and marital tension. In Case 2-5, as the physician realized later, the mother's statement about Joseph missing his stepfather's presence also indicated her own need for his attention.

An African proverb says that "it takes a village to raise a child," but these are times in which parents, and mothers in particular, are often left alone to take care of their families. The absence of familial or other support for the parents can lead to role strain and stress for the parents, especially the primary caretaker. Consequently, tension may develop between the couple, between parent(s) and extended family, and between parent(s) and children.

The experience of becoming a parent differs greatly for the couple, depending on each parent's gender. The socially accepted standard that mothers should be the primary caretaker for children can cause tremendous stress and anxiety among employed and career-oriented women. For those women totally involved in home life, depression, somatic complaints, or eating disorders often result. Child abuse or neglect may occur as a consequence of feelings of isolation and lack of a partner's and others' support. Research indicates that the transition to parenthood is accompanied by a general decrease in marital satisfaction and a lowering of self-esteem for women (Cowen & Cowen,1985). Also, this phase has the highest rate of divorce (Carter & McGoldrick, 1989).

Rather than focusing only on the mother–child bond, it is important that physicians make a concerted effort to value, support, and reinforce the inclusion of fathers (McGoldrick *et al.*, l993) and other family or community members. Our clinical experiences and those of other colleagues indicate that among many Latino and African-American families (McAdoo, 1980), men are very involved with childcare in spite of the fact that most often primary caretakers are women primarily responsible to identify and respond to the child's needs. Many children are not raised by their parents for cultural, socioeconomic, psychological, and legal reasons. Grandmothers as primary caretakers are a growing phenomenon (Buchanan & Lappin,1990). In assessing and counseling families, physicians need to be aware that different family configurations tend to be stigmatized by norms dictated by the dominant culture. Moreover, childrearing practices vary enormously among cultures and social classes regarding approaches to discipline, styles of nurturance, and physical contact.

In evaluating family functioning for families with young children, the physician can explore different levels of relations with questions like the following:

COUPLE/INDIVIDUAL: "Do you have time for yourselves as a couple?" "Do each of you find time to respond to your personal needs?" "How satisfied are you with the support and attention received from your partner and others?"

PARENTING: "How did you learn to be parents?" "Are you prepared or skillful as parents?" "What are your sources of support and, if necessary, guidance?" "What are your styles of parenting?" "Do these styles conflict with your extended family, your children's school, or your physician or therapist?"

CHILD/PARENT: "How is the 'fit' between the temperament of parents and children?" "How do parents respond to the children's special needs?" "How is the 'fit' between parent's and child's developmental needs?"

When assessing the child, her emotional, physical, cognitive, social, and neurological development must be considered in terms of family resources and responsiveness (McGoldrick *et al.*, 1993). The child's temperament plays an important role in family life. Joseph's quiet, pleasant, and easygoing way had facilitated the formation of the couple. The acceptance and bonding with the stepfather was facilitated by the fact that the stepfather also missed the presence of a father in his childhood.

Joseph's feelings of abandonment in Case 2-5 were exacerbated by his colicky baby brother's demands on his mother, as well as her adjustment to her new roles. As the physician could observe in their office interactions, he was missing her direct attention.

This is the stage when physicians have the most frequent contact with families. Medical visits—for prenatal and child healthcare, acute illness, family planning, and so on—are very frequent. This is a stage when the physician's role can be most meaningful, as it will affect the course of life for many family members.

37

**FAMILY WITH
ADOLESCENT
CHILDREN**

CASE 2-6

A physician was planning to discharge a 16-year-old Latina adolescent hospitalized for a severe asthmatic attack, when the nurse reported that the patient was planning to run away because of conflicts with her mother, a very religious Pentecostal believer. During the last 6 months, Rose, the patient, a college-bound straight A student, had become less interested in school and more rebellious toward her mother. She complained to the nurse of mother's "unreasonable demands": expecting her to be responsible for household chores; babysitting for three smaller brothers; and forbidding her to visit friends. When talking to the nurse, Rose came across as a reasonable, thoughtful young woman. When interviewed with mother, she became very angry and accused her mother of exploiting her as a servant and always taking sides with her brothers. Her mother responded by saying that she expected more from this daughter because she was the oldest. Rose's mother approached the physician privately requesting a gynecological exam to check her daughter's virginity. The young woman had already shared with the physician that she was seeing a boy from school, sometimes visiting his house, but had denied any sexual involvement.

——— FAMILY WITH ADOLESCENT CHILDREN ———

Adolescence calls for major changes in the family, involving a shift of the adolescent's position within the family and renegotiation of relationships at many levels: parent–child, grandparent–parent, husband–wife, and others.

This is a time of intense emotions and polarizations between family members, especially between the parents and the defiant adolescent. These conflicts typically involve a third person, such as a grandparent, a sibling, an aunt or uncle, a friend, and, frequently, a helping professional. As illustrated in Case 2-5, physicians are often pulled in as the conflict escalates and evolves into a medical event. Common medical events include exacerbation of physical symptoms, poor compliance with treatment of life-threatening illnesses, suicide attempts, drug use, and eating disorders. As in Case 2-6, the physician is often asked by parent or child to intervene. As parents and adolescent attempt to gain control, they often enlist support of others for their position, or in some cases, mediation of the conflict. The physician's timely involvement is often crucial to interrupt escalating conflicts that might ultimately lead to tragic outcomes. Typically, as in Case 2-6, the physician was caught in a power struggle between the adolescent and her mother, precipitated by the adolescent's budding sexuality and her demands for more autonomy and independence. In collaboration with a family therapist, the physician interviewed mother and daughter individually to identify their concerns and needs and to attempt a negotiation between them.

As the adolescent searches for autonomy and independence—a life space beyond the boundaries of the family—parental authority and control are challenged. Old rules and established values are questioned, while new ideals and mores are proposed by the adolescent, causing conflict and challenging the stability of the family. This process is less tumultuous when parents learn to be flexible enough to allow the youngster room for new experiences and autonomy, and yet know when to be firm and clear about limits in order to provide a point of reference for the experimenting adolescent. Developing flexible boundaries that allow the adolescent to move in and out, to be dependent at times of vulnerability, and to be independent to the point of taking serious risks is a stressful task for parents, especially in times of increasing violence in many communities. Parents might also feel hurt or rejected by statements such as, "I don't want to be like my father or mother" or "Get out of my life," which represent the adolescent's attempts to differentiate from the family and define his self-identity.

The youngster's ability to differentiate from others will depend on how well she can handle intense emotions in the context of conflicting social expectations about sexual roles and norms of behavior dictated by family, community, peers, and the media (Garcia-Preto, 1988). The physical and sexual changes that take place at this stage have a dramatic effect on how adolescents see and evaluate themselves and radically alter how they are perceived by others. It is not uncommon for family members to experience confusion and fear when adolescents begin to express their sexual interests. As illustrated in Case 2-6, Mrs. Rodriguez, fearing that her daughter might be sexually active because she had a boyfriend, attempted to control her sexuality by requesting the physician to check her virginity. The family's culture and religion are also significant factors in this case, as they restrict adolescent female sexuality and independence. Sometimes the adolescent's growing sexuality is ignored or rejected by parents, which may affect her self-esteem or lead her into premature rebellious and risky sexual activity. Promiscuous sexual behavior, unwanted pregnancy, and unprotected sex are possible consequences. Rose's acceptance of her mother's religious values along with her own abilities, academic aspirations, and the presence of other supports served as powerful buffers against sexual acting-out and other risky behaviors and facilitated the formation of a positive self-concept.

The process of identity formation at this stage involves the adolescent's gender and sexual identity. Considering society's bias toward heterosexuality, the physician has to be attentive to the particular needs of gay, lesbian, and bisexual adolescents, whose conflicts of identity might be expressed through somatization, repeated visits for unspecific complaints, suicidal ideation, or depressive symptoms. Ethnic minority youths also face conflicts related to their experiences of racism or other prejudice in dating, groups, schools, and work situations.

Parents usually confront the adolescent's demands for autonomy at the same time that they face their own midlife issues (Carter & McGoldrick, 1989), such as reexamining their life experiences and choices and reviewing their life plans as individuals and as a couple. Divorce or career changes are not uncommon at this period. In addition, this is a time when the family is often dealing with frail grandparents or other older relatives, a burden that usually falls on women. Parents are challenged to keep a balance between their availability to the family and to themselves, between the new and old generation's needs. Clinical problems in adult patients at this stage are frequently related to these life cycle stressors (Table 2.2).

Some families become more vulnerable at this stage. Some parents and families are not prepared for changes and feel threatened by the adolescent's developmental needs. They become rigid and controlling and, in response, the child may often escalate rebellious behaviors. As illustrated in Case 2-6, Rose's mother, a single parent, resisted giving her oldest daughter more freedom and time outside the family because of her fear that this would weaken family ties and undermine her authority as a parent with the younger children. As a single parent who had to face many adversities, such as an abusive husband, homelessness, and poverty, she had to maintain strong control over her children and rely on her daughter's help to raise her other children successfully. Her fear of losing Rose's support, companionship, and love did not allow her to recognize and accept her daughter's needs. Like many other parents of adolescent children, she experienced her daughter's requests for autonomy as rejection.

Families that have the most difficulty letting go of their children are those that have come to rely on them for their support (Strelnick & Gilpin, 1986). In single-parent or divorced families, the oldest child often becomes an essential partner to the parent, caught in a parentified position. The adolescent's separation from the family becomes especially difficult if the parent is not able to restructure his life and build new supports. The independence of the youngest adolescent, the last to move on, can also be complicated when the marital bond is fragile and the parents avoid dealing directly with their issues. For instance, the hospitalization of a diabetic young man for ketoacidosis coincided with his discovery of his emotionally distant father's extramarital affair and the son's concerns for his mother. A family life-cycle perspective allowed the physician to understand the importance of getting both parents involved in their son's treatment and life plans.

The adolescent's development does not depend solely on individual abilities and family competence but, to a large extent, on external factors: the economy, the availability of educational and occupational opportunities, community support, and the influence of the media, to name a few. Many families are disempowered by the intrusion of social institutions and, on occasion, well-intended professionals which result in clashes of cultural values that undermine their authority as parents. Their disciplinary approaches are criticized or misunderstood, their cultural legacies are devalued, and determinations about their lives are made without proper family participation.

The adolescent's demands for more autonomy and independence tend to activate unresolved conflicts the parents have within themselves, with each other, and with their own parents. In this regard, questioning parents about their own adolescence will promote understanding and healing across generations and defuse parent–child conflicts. In this case, 2 years after her own mother died, Mrs. Rodriguez, Rose's mother, was thrown out of the house by her alcoholic father when he found out she had a boyfriend. Previous experiences of loss and rejection made her especially sensitive to her daughter's need to separate from the family.

Adolescence marks a period of turmoil and conflicts but also renewal for individuals and the family. In most families, relationships are renegotiated, new life agendas are set, and families continue their developmental trajectory without major disruptions. In some families change cannot occur without a serious crisis. The role of the physician as a family mediator and life consultant is most valuable at this stage.

CASE 2-7

Mr. Johnson is a 55-year-old man who had worked as a regional sales manager for a large company until a massive heart attack, which resulted in a quadruple bypass 2 years ago. Previously well stabilized with diet, exercise, and medication, his recent lab results revealed a high cholesterol value, particularly the LDL component. Interviewing the patient, his physician found out that Mr. Johnson had been careless about his diet. He appeared irritable and less communicative than usual. Further inquiry focusing on possible life changes indicated that the patient was upset at his wife's increased involvement with school work and limited availability to assist in cooking and in planning family meals. Initially supportive of his wife's decision to return to graduate school, the patient was now constantly arguing with his wife about her increased absence while at the same time claiming his support for her educational goals.

FAMILY AT MIDLIFE

At this stage the renegotiation of the marital relationship is a central task. As the parents become less involved with the task of raising children, they can pay more attention to their own needs, assessing their satisfaction with their personal lives, considering new directions, and often revising their marital arrangement. The decision to pursue one's own needs may pose a threat to the conjugal relationship or to the partner who might expect the marriage to be center stage. The couple in Case 2-7 is an example of the partners' different expectations at this phase of their lives. Mr. Johnson's interests are now limited to the home, where he has had to adjust to a life of limited activity after many years of intense driving and traveling. In contrast, after many years of devotion to her family, raising their two daughters and adjusting to her husband's needs, Mrs. Johnson expects now to have her turn at fulfilling her own goals.

There is a tendency for men and women to be going in opposite directions psychologically at this point (McGoldrick *et al.*, 1993). Men tend to become more interested in relationships and intimacy, while women's energies are more directed toward personal needs and experiences in the outside world, often resulting in marital conflicts and estrangement. When one partner is disabled or significantly older, the disparity between each spouse's needs may strain the relationship. When the marital bond has been established on principles of mutual care and respect, and companionship is valued by both partners, the couple has a better chance to renegotiate their needs despite inevitable conflicts. Fortunately, this was the case for the Johnsons once their physician facilitated a dialogue about their mutual expectations and priorities. A family life-cycle perspective helped the physician understand and address Mr. Johnson's health in the context of the couple's developmental issues. While addressing Mr. Johnson's feelings, the physician did not support his formulation for his problem—"my wife does not care"—and was able to diffuse the couple's conflicts by focusing on the developmental issues and encouraging the partners toward understanding this role reversal.

This transition has been seen negatively as a time of physical and psychological distress for women. It is at this time that women typically experience menopause, to which their reaction will depend largely on their social status and opportunities (Neugarten & Kraines, 1965). When women have more control over their lives, they are less likely to become anxious and symptomatic. Certainly, women whose only source of affirmation has been mothering are more vulnerable to depression, though they usually recover after a period of adjustment (Harbin, 1978). A most significant characteristic of this stage is the great number of entries and exits of family members: Children leave, but the family is enlarged by the addition of in-laws; grandparents become ill and die, while grandchildren expand the family.

The renegotiation of the parent–child relationship with consideration of the adult status of the child is another important task at this stage. For many families this is an easy and rewarding period, marked by the possibility of forming positive relationships with grown children and sharing their accomplishments. For others, the changing economics in our society have made launching difficult, when their adult children cannot support themselves. The youngest of the Johnsons' daughters had lived with them off and on and had been unable to find a stable job. Middle-aged parents are also increasingly needed to provide financial or childcare support for younger families, as illustrated in Case 2-1. Problems affecting their adult children, such as marital difficulties, divorce, and unemployment, are often a major source of stress for their parents, eventually resulting in poor health and an increase in medical visits.

This group has been referred to as "the sandwich generation." They are pressed by the needs of the young, who may still be financially and emotionally dependent on them, and are also pressed by the needs of their aging parents, who are becoming increasingly dependent (Asen *et al.*, 1992).

Women are almost always the main caretakers in the family. The physical and emotional demands of caretaking make them more vulnerable to somatic and psychological problems. When a family member has a flare-up of a chronic illness or does not respond to treatment, the physician should be alert to life-cycle issues, including burnout of the caretaker. Stress at this stage may also signal unresolved issues from earlier life-cycle stages. The physician should assess changes in the marriage, marital satisfaction, caretaking of elderly parents, the strength of the family's support system, relationships with adult children and grandchildren, unfulfilled needs and goals, and the impact of losses. These are some relevant questions to address middle-age patients at this stage:

- "How are things with you and your family now that the children are older and more independent?"
- "Thinking about your life, what are the things that make you feel accomplished or happy, and what are the things you wish could be different?" "And what do you think would be your spouse's response to these questions? To your answers?"
- "What do you like about your marriage now?" "What could be different?"
- "How are your parents doing? How much does their life situation affect your own life now?" "How are other family members doing?"

CASE 2-8

Mrs. Casey, a 65-year-old-woman with a past history of well-controlled non-insulin-dependent diabetes mellitus and hypertension who had been quite independent and active, was hospitalized for a stroke, a left-sided cerebrovascular accident. After that, her ability to walk and use her right hand became quite impaired. The patient was responding well to rehabilitation, but her level of activity was very restricted, requiring constant support in all activities of daily living. Mrs. Casey had five children and was living with the youngest, who was feeling overwhelmed by the prospect of being the main caregiver for her mother. Three other children had been involved, visiting their mother regularly. They appeared to be a close and well-functioning family. The physician noticed, however, some tension among the siblings. The daughters resented their brothers' passivity regarding their mother's needs. One day the patient had a fall in the hospital while trying to stand up without help, resulting in a minor injury. The physician was approached by one of the sons, whom he did not know well. The son angrily criticized him for delaying arrangements for discharge and blamed him for the incident. The physician was taken by surprise, considering his positive and close relationship with the patient and other children, who had praised him in the past for his availability to the family.

The family in later life is faced with the painful task of accepting and adjusting to the physical decline of their older members. Adult children are required to make a shift in relational status with their aging parents and to reorganize their lives to provide them with emotional and physical support. Responses of anxiety, anger, and confusion are not uncommon, as the younger generation tries to cope with the new situation. Past unresolved family issues might emerge, amplifying these emotional reactions. Mrs. Casey's son's accusations can be interpreted as a displacement of feelings of anger and helplessness regarding her physical condition. This was exacerbated by unrecognized guilt as a result of his distancing from his family during other critical moments. The physician–patient–family relationship is especially likely to be affected when family members cannot accept the parents' decline or deal with their own conflicts and responsibilities constructively. In this case, the physician scheduled a family meeting with all of the siblings to help them identify and share their feelings and thoughts regarding their mother's condition and to foster mutual support around caregiving responsibilities.

It is distressing to witness a parent who was once active and healthy become frail and dependent. In Case 2-8, this process was especially challenging to the family, given the fact that Mrs. Casey, a vibrant woman, still held a job until the occurrence of this medical event. A proud and independent person, she avoided asking for help and tried to overcome her physical limitations, resulting in an injury. In general, most aging parents are reluctant to ask family members for support in an effort to maintain their dignity and to avoid being seen as a burden in their children's lives. However, some older adults become totally dependent on the next generation, placing excessive demands on their children. Given time constraints, financial pressures, and conflicting multiple demands on families these days, they are especially challenged to fulfill their caregiving obligations to the older generation. When parents have been autonomous and strong figures, adult children may fail to recognize a parent's needs and delay making the required shift of status in their relations with the ailing or aging parent. In these cases, the physician may have a critical role in facilitating support for the patient by taking the initiative to mobilize the children's involvement in the treatment.

Financial and caregiving demands are a major source of stress for the middle generation, at a stage when they still might be involved with childrearing responsibilities as well as facing financial pressures related to older children's education and their own life changes. Geographic distance is often an additional factor limiting availability of support and straining family relations. Women are especially burdened by becoming the sole or main caregiver for their relatives. Physicians need to be alert to the high incidence of depressive and somatic symptoms among caregivers. It is not surprising that Mrs. Casey's youngest daughter was distressed: She was trying to juggle the competing demands of being an attentive daughter, caring mother, and responsible worker. Typically, Mrs. Casey's daughters were more willing to make personal sacrifices to attend their mother's needs than were her sons, and resentment inevitably emerged. This imbalance of responsibilities is likely to be reinforced when the physician minimizes expectations for men as caregivers in their contacts with the family. The physician's role is also crucial when institutionalization needs to be considered. Besides addressing the patient's feelings of rejection and fear, the physician can help the family deal with their guilt and facilitate the decision-making process.

Awareness of ethnic and multigenerational traditions can help physicians distinguish normative patterns of caregiving from dysfunctional responses of detachment or overinvolvement (Rolland, 1994). Latino families, for instance, tend to have strong intergenerational ties and are likely to be closely involved and protective of patients. In the case of terminal illness, they might prefer to "protect" the patient from knowing the diagnosis. African-American families often share responsibility among immediate and extended family members, forming a kin network to support the needs of aging parents.

For the frail or disabled parent, the transition of status is also difficult as the parent has to grieve the loss of the competent self and adjust to the reality of a less independent and active life. In health or in sickness, the aging individual is challenged to find a dignified role in a society where old people tend to be devalued and marginalized. Many people postpone retirement for these reasons.

Grandparenthood can offer a "new lease on life" as it brings opportunities for meaningful interactions and facilitates resolution regarding one's mortality (Walsh, 1989). The acceptance of one's life and death, a major task at this stage, occurs when the individual is able to achieve a sense of integrity versus despair (Erickson, 1968).

Death and terminal illness of the older generation are particularly emotional events for adult children, as they are forced to face their own mortality and aging (Rolland, 1994). For widows and widowers, feelings of loss, disorientation, and loneliness contribute to an increase in death and suicide rates during the first year, especially for men. Advances in medical technology have extended life expectancy and allowed people to be more functional to enjoy life into older age. Physical and psychological well-being will also depend on financial security, access to health services, and social contacts.

A consultation with the family is always advised when treating older patients to assess and enlist family support to the patient and ensure physician–patient–family collaboration. In the event of illness or disability, the physician should assess:

- How is the family understanding and adjusting to the illness?
- Are the adult children prepared to deal with their parents' aging, disability, and increased dependence?
- Are they able to shift roles to respond to the new needs?
- What is the distribution of caregiving responsibilities among family members?

CONCLUSION

This chapter has described how the individual and family life-cycle perspective is a useful framework to address medical problems as it relates typical clinical presentations to predictable stages and specific developmental tasks. However, the life cycle should not be understood as a static concept. It needs to be examined in relation to particular life contexts with special attention to cultural differences, socioeconomic factors, and societal changes. Social stressors such as poverty and migration, and also critical events such as sickness, death, and divorce, have a major impact on the course of the individual and family life cycle.

The application of the individual and family life-cycle models in medicine has been criticized for promoting the idea of "normal" development and the traditional bias against women and different cultural groups (Candib, 1989). When and how families negotiate a life transition vary according to their ethnicity, class, and religion.

It is important that clinicians examine their own cultural values, especially their assumptions about "normality" and the notion of "family" in assessing individual and family development and functioning, to avoid pathologizing patients' experiences. Finally, the physician should be aware of his own family experiences and life-cycle stage to evaluate how these will affect his understanding and identification with each patient and family.

───────────── **CASES FOR DISCUSSION** ─────────────

CASE 1

A 50-year-old middle-class African-American professional woman, a dynamic high-school principal, came for a follow-up visit 6 months after surgery for breast cancer. The physician was struck by the patient's reaction to his good news about the surgery and lab results. This assertive and engaging woman started crying, revealing an unexpected sense of hopelessness and helplessness about her life situation, caused by marital distress after 23 years of a very happy marriage. The physician noticed that her husband, recently retired, did not come with her to the visit as he usually does.

1. *Considering life cycle issues and the impact of her illness, what kind of questions would you ask this patient about herself, her husband, and their relationship to understand her depression?*
2. *What hypothesis would you have regarding her depression and marital distress?*

CASE 2

A 17-year-old man with a history of well-controlled asthma is hospitalized for the second time in a period of 10 months. No major environmental changes seem to justify this exacerbation of his illness. On visiting the patient in the hospital, the physician noticed that the patient seemed distraught after a family visit. This young man, usually cheerful and positive about life, broke down in tears when asked about his distress.

1. *What information would you elicit from this patient to understand his symptoms from an individual and family life-cycle perspective?*
2. *Suppose he comes from a middle-class family whose parents are facing life transitions. What are these possible transitions and how might they be related to the patient's symptoms?*
3. *Now suppose a different situation: he is college bound and from a poor inner-city family. Considering possible issues related to differences of values, formulate some different hypotheses for the exacerbation of his illness and his emotional response. Take into consideration (a) socioeconomic factors, (b) intergenerational conflicts related to cultural clashes, (c) issues of sexual identity.*

CASE 3

A 32-year-old mother brought her two children—a 6-year-old girl and a 4-year-old boy—for a routine visit. While in your office the children started to fight over a toy. The mother lost her temper and slapped the older child, scolding her for reacting to her brother's provocation. She apologized for the incident and asked for your advice.

1. *How do you understand each child's behavior in relation to life-cycle stages and related tasks? Take into consideration gender differences.*

2. *Focusing on this family's life-cycle stage, what would you like to know about this family situation to help this mother to deal with the sibling fights?*

CASE 4

A powerful business executive, a 56-year-old man of German descent, was hospitalized for congestive heart failure. A medical student went to check the patient and found him arguing with his wife, expressing disapproval of his only daughter's decision to marry before finishing law school. The wife, unable to calm her husband, asked the student to talk to him.

1. *Considering life-cycle issues, what questions should the student ask the patient to understand his feelings?*
2. *Using your knowledge of family life cycle, what could be a possible script explaining the patient's reactions and the family crisis?*
3. *What would be each family member's view of the problem?*

CASE 5

A physician was worried about a 35-year-old diabetic patient whose blood glucose levels became increasingly higher during the past 2 months. While focusing on her social situation, the physician learned that the patient, the youngest of three daughters from a Jewish family, was considering postponing her wedding because of her 70-year-old mother's recent disability as a result of a stroke.

1. *How do you understand this woman's dilemma taking into consideration this family life-cycle stage?*
2. *Discuss caretaking issues in relation to gender and sibling order.*

RECOMMENDED READINGS

Asen KE, Tomson T, Canavan B: *Family Solutions in Family Practice.* Lancaster, England, Quay Publishing, 1992.

> This readable book is a practical guide for medical practitioners on how to manage typical problems in primary care practice from a family perspective. It includes many concrete suggestions on how to interview patients, conduct family meetings, and intervene in problem situations.

Carter B, McGoldrick M: *The Changing Family Life Cycle: A Framework for Family Therapy*, ed 2. New York, Gardner Press, 1988.

> A classic text in the field of family systems that presents a well-conceptualized view of the family as it evolves through the life cycle. A must-read for medical providers interested in expanding their knowledge and skills in family work.

Crouch MA, Roberts L (eds): *The Family in Medical Practice: A Family Systems Primer.* Berlin, Springer-Verlag, 1987.

> A short text describing all aspects of a family systems approach to medical care. It also includes a chapter on the history of family in medicine and on the physician's family.

Doherty WJ, Baird MP: *Family Therapy and Family Medicine: Towards the Primary Care of Families.* New York, Guilford Press, 1983.

This pioneer book introduces a family-oriented model to medical practice applying family therapy theory and techniques. It is practical, clearly written, and still remarkably up-to-date even though it was published in the early 1980s.

McDaniel S, Campbell T, Seaburn D: *Family-Oriented Primary Care: A Manual for Medical Providers.* Berlin, Springer-Verlag, 1990.

This excellent book is designed for physicians who want to enhance their skills in family systems medicine. The book provides a useful conceptual framework including relevant research on family systems and a practical guide to clinical practice illustrated with case examples and protocols.

PART II

The Doctor

As with patients, the personhood of the physician often gets lost in the medical training process as physicians in training attempt to assimilate a vast amount of information and then utilize that information for the good of their patients. These chapters will bring the personhood of the physician into focus and also help physicians-in-training understand the effect of the training process on their psyche and values. Without such an understanding, physicians-in-training are at risk for losing their values and becoming less humane.

CHAPTER 3

Becoming a Physician

Catherine P. McKegney

CASE 3-1

Helen, the ward clerk (unit secretary) on Harris 3, was legendary. She had worked at the University Hospital for somewhere between 15 and 50 years, no one knew for sure how long. The house staff figured she had the secretarial equivalent of tenure. She was intelligent and acerbic, and clearly burned-out. Dana was very excited to be beginning her first rotation in the hospital on Harris 3. As her instructor had suggested, she introduced herself to the ward clerk politely and enthusiastically. Helen's response was, "I eat medical students for lunch, you know." Dana responded, "I don't think I'd taste very good," and hurried off to warn the other student on her team.

INTRODUCTION

How do we become physicians? How do we transform ourselves into those mysterious creatures? Although professional transformation can be as idiosyncratic as the initiates who begin it, there are patterns to the process. These patterns are portrayed in popular media, on television shows such as *ER* and *MASH*, and in best-selling books like Samuel Shem's *The House of God* (Shem, 1978). Though popular culture is attending more to the stories of physician development, insights into the intricacies of how professional transformation occurs are rarely found there. Many medical educators and sociologists have written about the transformations that occur in medical trainees, but collapsing their discussions into a coherent story is very difficult.

In this chapter, I will explore the academic constructs offered by these observers within a metaphor of human development in the context of the family. This metaphor is not reality—medical students are not really children—but it illuminates the process and highlights the individuality of the trainee within the commonality of the training experience and the context of the U.S. medical system. If we decide to view the medical system as a family (McKegney, 1989), who is in and who is outside the family? Who takes what roles? What does this family look like? What does it do well? What are some of its pathologies?

Medical students are the newest members of the family. They don't know the rules and therefore depend on their teachers' guidance to avoid mistakes and to learn how learning occurs in this family. In the preclinical years, they are often confused by the political wrangling that involves their faculty and older trainees, hearing the feelings without understanding the issues. In their clinical years, medical students, like kindergartners, want to demonstrate their vast knowledge of (in this instance) basic science only to find that much of it doesn't apply in the new world of the teaching hospital. They recognize that they can learn from everyone in the hospital, from the department chairs to the orderlies, and are hurt, like Dana in Case 3-1, by the trickle-down resentment that lands on them at the bottom of the heap.

Continuing with the family metaphor, interns are school-age children, learning as fast as they ever will, with new responsibilities, new opportunities, and new vulnerability to a system that has little time to accommodate individual talents or shortcomings. Intern mistakes have the potential to be lethal, since their orders no longer must be "cosigned." Some are overwhelmed by the independence, others become cocky, and most muddle through, learning the basic procedures of the system from the nurses, respiratory technicians (nannies and foster mothers), and senior residents (older siblings). The faculty physicians teach, but focus more on large concepts and pathophysiology than the essential basics of night-to-night management of sick patients.

Senior residents, like adolescents, vacillate between deserved confidence in their specialized knowledge and the anxiety of the impending "real world" waiting for them outside the teaching hospital at the completion of their training. On the one hand, they take on the semiparental function of supervising interns and medical students. On the other hand, they worry what they'll do when they need help "on the outside," seeing adulthood as complete independence from interference or assistance.

Fellows are a bit like adult children who still live at home at an age when most of their peers are settled and on their own. They are often the preferred consultant of their younger "siblings," who are less intimidated about asking them questions than asking the attending faculty. Like "big brother" or "big sister" home from college, the fellow is in the most temporary position of all with the shortest time left before true adulthood.

In the medical education "family" there are several generations of adults, and a variety of in-laws. The fledgling attending physicians are like new parents. They are unsure of exactly how to "raise the children," but fairly certain that they can do a better job than their predecessors. Though they require the assistance of their seniors, some of that help feels like interference, and an imposition of old ways. Community-based physicians are less tied to their family of origin. Though they are less available than academic faculty, they exemplify the career goals of most medical students. Senior faculty physicians have been through the challenges of launching a few generations of trainees and have made a few runs at changing the system. They can see that not all of the new tricks are all that new, or necessarily better than the old tricks. Some have grown cynical and have stopped trying to make a difference.

Nonphysician faculty and staff in hospitals and training programs have vital roles in teaching but, like in-laws or stepparents, they are never quite counted as "real members" of the physician family. Teachers of the basic sciences are valued and gain academic status within the university, but they are in the peculiar position of nurturing trainees who are pursuing a different discipline from their own. They usually have a lower status in the hospital. Compared with physicians, they have less hierarchical power and less acknowledgment of their roles as teachers.

Like stepparents, gardeners, nannies, cooks, and maiden aunts in a huge extended household, the nurses, ward clerks, and radiology technicians do most of the work of patient care in the teaching hospital. The power of these unacknowledged teachers to help or hinder the neophyte physician in learning medicine and in performing the required "scut work" is enormous (Lassetter, 1984; Stein, 1967). Operating room nurses make sure that medical students know how to scrub properly and the nursing assistants on the wards take the time to help house staff find essential supplies. Like most groups whose contributions are undervalued, they resent the invisibility of their contributions to patient care and teaching. When they finish training, medical students will be the highest-paid members of the hierarchy, while currently being the most vulnerable because of their dependent state. In these circumstances, they are the obvious target for retaliation, although usually more indirectly than in Case 3-1.

Deans, department chairs, and most senior faculty are like the grandparents. They sometimes usurp the active parenting role of the younger faculty and sometimes step in to balance the system in essential ways that only years of experience can guide. The grandparents know the myths of the family and the history; they have the clearest vision of the family's place in the community at large.

What are the strengths of this family? Its members are all intelligent, dedicated, energetic, and capable. Most come to their chosen work to heal the sick and assuage their patients' pain. The work is exhausting and joyful: It involves participation in the deepest human experiences and offers unparalleled opportunity for personal growth. The training process is both arduous and exhilarating. Though all members of this "family" are doing their best most of the time, the interaction patterns that are the legacy of medical education can be very painful, contributing to physician impairment and burnout. Like parents who raise their children as they themselves were raised, medical educators tend to teach as they were taught, perpetuating patterns of isolation, rigidity, unrealistic expectations, secret keeping, triangulation, blaming, and denial of the pain that they themselves experienced in training (see Table 3.1) (McKegney, 1989).

Growth from infancy to maturity within the medical family involves development in a number of key ways: "managing emotions" (Smith & Kleinman, 1989), "training for uncertainty" (Fox, 1989), facing mistakes, adapting to a new identity, and delineating boundaries. The remainder of this chapter will examine these themes offering clarity for students who are struggling to become physicians in the context of the medical education system.

CASE 3-2

The first semester of the first year of medical school. Gross anatomy. Six medical students to a cadaver, beginning the first day and for the next 4 months, they will skin her, and then take her apart, beginning with her back and arm, ending with her head—deconstructing her completely before they take the formalin-soaked paper towels from her face.

The six of them talk about her as they use her irreproducible body to see, feel, and embed in their memories the intricacies of human construction. They become a team around her, talking little about the repulsion of filleting human flesh, but

Table 3.1
Comparison of Common Dysfunctional Family Patterns
and Similar Dynamics in the Medical Education System

	Family system	Medical education system
Isolation	Insists on minimal interaction with the community	Sets premeds apart from other undergraduates
	Won't let in-laws give suggestions	Discounts criticism from nonphysicians: "How could they understand?"
Rigidity	Continues autocratic parenting long after children are old enough to make their own choices	Maintains overextension of on-call hours despite more intensive inpatient care demands
Unrealistic expectations	Feeds children junk food, neglecting nutritional needs	Requires house staff to work 30-hour shifts
	Leaves a 10-year-old without supervision overnight	Expects students to not make mistakes that are appropriate to their level of expertise
Secret keeping	Avoids revealing family problems to outsiders	Hides physician impairment and student abuse
Triangulation	Mom talks about disappointments in dad with teenage daughter	University professor criticizes community physician to students, not face to face
Blaming	"You're a bad kid"	"A good intern doesn't forget that kind of thing"
Denial	"There's nothing wrong in our family"	"Internship wasn't *that* bad—all of *us* did one"

acknowledging their respect for her donation, as they are initiated into this new mystery of the human reality.

Most teams named "their" cadavers: Across the room, the young man with the cherry red muscles was called "Godzilla" because of his bulk. And everyone visited him when they had trouble finding the smaller muscles of their wizened "80-something" woman. They all speculated whether he had committed suicide with carbon monoxide because of his color. Of course, they never knew. Each team wondered about what had killed their cadaver. The team gathered around the "80-something" woman was grateful she had everything except her gallbladder; it meant they didn't have to lean over another team's shoulders too often to learn. And they named her "Farrah" after a blonde bombshell of the era, in part as a joke about how old and tiny she was, and in part as a grateful accolade.

CASE 3-3

Sandra, a fourth-year medical student on her cardiology rotation, is the acting intern caring for a 45-year-old woman who had a cardiac arrest at home, was resuscitated by the EMTs after ineffective CPR by her husband, and has persistent hypoxic encephalopathy. The etiology of her arrest was idiopathic hypertrophic subaortic stenosis (IHSS). For the 1 year prior to this disaster, she was the breadwinner because of her husband's disabling back pain from a work injury. He visits her constantly, traveling from their home 50 miles away. Over the second week of hospitalization, as the patient's cognitive impairment appears more per-

manent, Sandra notices that the couple verbally deny Mrs. Jones's limitations; all the while, Mr. Jones does so much for his wife that she is not learning the skills she needs to adapt to her disability.

At morning rounds, Sandra recommends a psychiatric consultation regarding the dysfunctional dynamic she sees developing between husband and wife: organizing their relationship yet again around the illness role of one of them. The attending looks in askance, implying that Sandra is overly sensitive, and states that the couple's relationship will have little effect on Mrs. Jones's recovery. Much to her own shock, Sandra begins to cry, and the senior resident guides her into an empty patient room until she can pull herself together, which she does hurriedly in order to join the team as they finish rounds. Neither the resident, the attending, nor any of Sandra's fellow medical students ever mentions this incident. Sandra is left feeling that she became too involved, and worries that her display of emotion will affect her evaluation.

MANAGING EMOTIONS

One of the goals of the medical training process is to exorcise emotional expression by the developing physician. The normal feelings evoked by close contact with another person—shyness, sexual attraction, fear, revulsion, pity—are deemed "unprofessional." When instructors see evidence of these strong feelings, they often fear that the trainee is not in control, and may not be able to do the job. The initiate is expected to panic, in a very minor way, at the beginning of the first year; after that, the student should be able to hide, if not override, intense responses. After all, a physician should keep a cool head, focus on what can be fixed, remaining warm and therapeutic all the while. Medical students, no longer "laypeople" and not yet physicians, are neither fish nor fowl; the transition from obeying normal societal taboos about what is discussed and what is touched and the full breaking of those taboos as physicians is an awkward process (Harper, 1993).

For the physician in training, this acquisition of "affective neutrality" (Smith & Kleinman, 1989) begins at the very beginning: in gross anatomy lab as in Case 3-2. The revulsion felt when facing the formalin-preserved cadaver is commonplace and seldom discussed. To help the new students stay calm, the instructors are strategically matter-of-fact. The students are recognized as being in transition; they have not yet acquired the distance necessary to perform in the medical system, and they are taught by example. In striving to obey the rules of the medical family, they imitate the calm of the professors, even though they have strong reactions which this placid behavior belies. As adults, they feel fear when facing death and revulsion about urine, feces, and other excreta. Many students are left with the sense that they are the only ones who experience conflict and confusion because of the paucity of opportunities to directly address these feelings. Smith and Kleinman (1989) observed that most students would turn an emotionally charged situation into a scientific problem to be solved, ignoring the affective components, both the patient's and their own. Solving problems is vastly more comfortable than facing the reflection of one's own fear of illness in the patient's. Focusing on the details of technique or points to be learned turns the situation into an intellectual puzzle like the ones they have been playing with for their previous 16 years of education. Consciously ignoring that they are crudely cutting up what once was a human being, students also use humor, joking, as in Case 3-2, gently or disrespectfully to dissipate less acceptable feelings of disgust or anxiety (Fox, 1989).

And what about sexual feelings? Physicians have license to touch others in ways usually associated with intimate relationships. Parents with their infants and lovers with each other have this right—and physicians. Even in this day of magnetic resonance imaging and the Human Genome Project, physicians examine their patients. Patients expect it, and information absorbed through the eyes, ears, nose, and hands of the physician is still the fastest, most "cost-effective" to acquire, and most efficiently integrated. Breaking social taboos to gather information during a history and physical examination requires an adjustment (Harper, 1993). Students often express the confusion they feel as if it were only about technique: uncertainty about what the epididymis feels like, or how to move aside a woman's breast to listen to her heart. To admit to the uncontrollable intrusion of sexual feelings during this basic ritual of the profession hints somehow at unfitness for the job rather than an intact hypothalamus.

Discussion of technical details is one way of ignoring the feelings evoked by physical exams; total avoidance is another popular way to manage this problem. House officers supervising medical students will overlook the "rectal deferred" on the physical exam form, ignoring the student's discomfort just as they ignore their own. In some circumstances, the patient's condition is a legitimate reason for delaying aspects of the exam. Most often, the students' discomfort and their supervisors' are the reasons for incomplete histories or examinations. Since the physicians' discomfort is rarely addressed explicitly, the student gets little guidance in deciding when it is truly appropriate to not do a rectal exam on someone, who happens to look like one's mother, and when the student needs to do the exam in order to provide good care, regardless of who the patient looks like.

Calm in the face of crisis is an appropriate goal for a professional who will face pain and death on a regular basis. Recognizing, naming, accepting, and honoring these feelings might better prepare students for their clinical responsibilities. As one study has shown, unrecognized feelings can interfere with the young physicians' performance of the clinical interview (Smith, 1986). Unfortunately, most medical students are taught to ignore their emotions, in a silent curriculum of denial. By the time they finish medical school, most students will exclaim excitedly about the latest "great case," but will be unable to feel the fear of vulnerability, disability, and loneliness that produced Sandra's tears in Case 3-3. The silence that greeted those tears taught her to suppress them the next time.

Though medical students are intentionally trained to suppress emotional expression, they are also expected to learn how to remain warm and compassionate with patients and their families. This empathy with patients is stated as a value by teachers, but students are left to find it within themselves rather than being guided to balance their levelheadedness with compassion. In expressing compassion, students and house staff are expected to draw on precisely those sensitivities that they silently discarded during gross anatomy and their uncomfortable clinical encounters. The chasm between social self and professional self is too deep for some, and they settle into a cool, distant style. This is familiar as the classic style of the university-based consultant who often knows only parts of his patients' lives, those bits that are relevant to his specialty. Since medical students spend most of their time with university-based physicians, this "expert" style is the professional style they often incorporate as their own.

As Renee Fox documented during the 1960s (Fox, 1989), the humanist movement within medicine articulated the value of the warmer, more collaborative physician that the patient advocacy movement also emphasized. When medical students and residents attempt to build a collaborative bridge with their social skills, they can find themselves awash in feelings: patients', families', and their own. They relied on "analytic transformation" and denial to cope during their own initiations, and so have no personal experience on which to draw while caring for their patients. Awkwardly and ineffectively, they resort to reassuring patients and families with intellectual explanations. Or they assume that patients and families will remain so "emotional" and irrational that explanations will be useless. Instructing students in "patient education" may provide skills, but without attention to the emotional scars and habits of denial that remain from training, the skills will be difficult to incorporate into patient encounters. For example, if we follow Sandra in Case 3-3 into her residency, we find that she feels confused about discussing increasing activities after an MI with a patient and his wife. She knows what the equivalences are between activity achieved in cardiac rehab and the effort needed for home activities. She knows that most couples have questions that they rarely ask about sexual activities after a heart attack. In seminar sessions, she practiced eliciting and answering precisely these questions. Still, she hesitates. Her supervisor comments on her hesitation, and she feels ashamed, and gets teary again. After delicate questioning, she remembers the story of her crying on rounds. When her supervisor agrees with her assessment of the Jones's marital style, and congratulates her for her courage in bringing up the subject, she feels enormous relief. After that she is eager to help her patient and his wife with their questions, both spoken and silent.

CASE 3-4

James is enjoying his fourth-year rotation on infectious disease (ID) consult service. The attending, Dr. Janacek, is approachable, smart, and a good teacher. The consults are interesting; James was worried that all he'd see would be patients with AIDS, but there have been some "interesting cases" in people with intact immune systems. The most recent was a consult from the ENT service about a woman with a persistent sinusitis who was HIV negative and had no risk factors. On rounds, the ID team all commented on how the initial outpatient choice of antibiotics made sense, but that when the woman was admitted 2 days before, the ENT service had missed the boat in their choice of parenteral antibiotic coverage. James was honored to be asked to write the consult note in the patient's chart. He worked very hard to display the ID team's thought processes that led to their recommendation of a change in medications.

When Dr. Janacek reviewed the note, she obviously was not pleased. She felt that James had insulted the ENT service in the way he presented the ID team's recommendations. James was confused. He thought that he had accurately described the deliberations of the team. He hadn't realized the importance of editing the condescension that the team had expressed in their discussions.

"TRAINING FOR UNCERTAINTY"

Renee Fox observed what she called "training for uncertainty" in the medical schools of the 1950s. She defined this as "the flow of medical school experiences that successively and cumulatively taught students to perceive medical uncertainty." They were taught to accept uncertainty as the fate of the physician; without the imaging procedures available today, often only pathologists had the ultimate answers, after doing the autopsy. With acknowledgment of the role of uncertainty in clinical decision making, physicians developed "shared, patterned ways of coping with its meaning and consequences as well as its *de facto* existence" (Fox, 1989). She also described training for "detached concern" where some empathy is maintained, but an emotional distance allows effective clinical decision making. Both of these tasks continue to be important for medical trainees to accomplish, but the training in these areas is hampered by a ballooning body of facts to be memorized. The rapid availability of more information than ever contributes to more precise diagnoses (before autopsy), although diagnoses are still based on probabilities, not absolute certainty. The U.S. infatuation with technologically derived "facts" obscures this reality, even while medical educators recognize the importance of inculcating problem-solving processes rather than teaching facts.

Patients used to spend a significant length of time in hospitals. They were diagnosed, treated, and got better or died in hospitals, in full view of medical students and residents. Extended stays had some disadvantages for patients and contributed to the high cost of medical care, but with shortening lengths of stay, medical trainees rarely see the entire process of diagnosis, treatment, and healing in continuity. These disjointed experiences obscure the evolving nature of diagnosis, the use of therapeutic trial as a diagnostic modality, and the iterative hypothesis testing that occurs with patients with complex diagnostic dilemmas. Because they do not follow cases closely for extended periods, each hypothesis seems like a conclusion, a certainty. On the next admission, or outpatient visit, the inaccuracy of that initial guess is lost in the new workup that appears to provide "the answer."

Most people are uncomfortable with uncertainty, but this is particularly the case for the medical student whose premedical training and preclinical training were focused on certainty: Evaluation was often based on multiple-choice exams with "correct answers." Those students who studied arts and humanities were judged in a more subjective fashion, based on essays and research papers, which revealed the student's ability to understand abstract concepts and to express themselves rationally and critically. The criteria for grading were understandings of concepts and demonstration of adept manipulation of the same. Medical students with strong humanities backgrounds have more experience with uncertainty, but even for them the preclinical years are times of memorization of massive amounts of facts and testing on those facts. During this time their skills for coping with uncertainty lie dormant, and they too may feel unprepared to face the challenges of uncertainty on clinical rotations.

What is ironic and tragic about this is that the clinician actually lives in a world of guesses, increasingly educated guesses, but guesses nevertheless. With real people in real-life situations, there are too many independent variables for any clinician, or any extant computer, to know with certainty what is "the cause" of an illness, or which is "the right" treatment for that illness. The intellectual process of integration is also idiosyncratic to the specialty of the physicians involved: Surgeons do see things differently from endocrinologists. For the medical student, the integration is a new process, and its accompanying uncertainty discomfiting. Fox classifies the students' uncertainty into three types. First, the uncertainty inherent in the students' "incomplete mastery" of Western medicine; for example, the complexities of thyroid function testing take more than one glance before the results can be analyzed correctly. Second, the uncertainties inherent in medicine as a discipline; for example, the ongoing clinical trials for the treatment of various cancers demonstrate the lack of a definitive treatment strategy for these cancers. And third, the uncertainty about which uncertainty is applicable in any given situation (Fox, 1989). Regarding the first two types of uncertainty, my biochemistry professor used to describe the dichotomy as "it is known, I do not know" versus "it is not known." For a student, knowing on which side of the dichotomy a given answer lies is nearly impossible. The modeling that occurs on most rotations is more aimed at hiding unknowing than exploring it.

In Case 3-4, James transcribed the certainty that the ID consulting team expressed in their discussion into the consult note in the patient's chart. Some of this certainty stemmed from his inexperience and his lingering assumption that most of the time there is one correct answer to the questions asked in clinical medicine. When the team members, especially the senior resident and fellow, spoke with conviction, James reveled in the clarity of their recommendations; it was a joy finally to be part of "it is known." Unfortunately, that clinical "certainty" was colored by specialty loyalties, lending the recommendations a deeper intensity than the simple facts allowed, and much deeper intensity than was politic.

As a system, the large teaching hospital is not characterized by smooth communication patterns between all specialties. The competition for research funding, clinical and office space, "good students" for residencies, and patient revenues contributes to intense "clan" rivalry between specialty departments. Communication patterns reify the loyalties typical of turf wars. Attending physicians in academic centers rarely discuss openly differences of opinion across specialty barriers in view of their supervisees. More common is the somewhat pejorative or condescending discussion with the "home team" of the way the other specialty team or "LMD" (local medical doctor) handled the case. As a consequence, many graduating residents are ill prepared for fruitful discussions that are possible in the less rarefied atmosphere of the community hospital.

Comfort with uncertainty comes later now than it did when Fox studied medical students. Often, physicians don't develop it until they have been in practice for many years. Many factors contribute to this developmental delay. The expanding knowledge base means that more time in training is spent with facts than with patients. The expanding technology allows for more facts to be collected about each patient. Finally, Americans have unrealistic expectations of their medical system. They have begun to believe the medical system's "PR." After all, hospitals issue press releases about how modern medicine can keep 500-gram babies alive and transplant livers. The implication for the physician in training is that their uncertainty must be of the "it is known, I do not know" variety. Clearly those of us in medical education have systematically obscured from our students and ourselves that there are only two things in medicine that are absolutely certain. The first is that every patient, and every physician, dies. The second is that no pregnancy lasts forever. Everything else is at best a "current truth," not a permanent one.

CASE 3-5

Maria dreaded her first night of call as an intern, but it went smoothly, with her senior resident helping with the things about which she was uncomfortable. The second night seemed less daunting. However, it turned out to be very busy, with everything taking her three times too long. The senior resident on call, Michael, helped her talk to an elderly man with pneumonia about whether he would want to be resuscitated, and guided her through writing the "do not resuscitate" order. A few hours later his blood gases became a bit confusing, but she remembered about how to give oxygen to patients with COPD, and after an agonizing 20 minutes with the lab sheet, made her decision about adjusting his oxygen, and stumbled off to bed.

The next morning the old man's primary care physician, Dr. Walker, ap-

proached her about her care of his patient in the 3 hours before his death. Dr. Walker gently pointed out Maria's mistake, noting that it probably was not what killed him.

CASE 3-6

Medical students in surgery spend most of their time holding retractors, often from a vantage point where they can see nothing but the backs of blue-robed surgeons and terrifying OR nurses. As the procedure ends, sometimes they are flattered by being required to cut sutures after knots are tied. Surgeons are more than a bit idiosyncratic in their preferences regarding the preferred length of suture left beyond the knot, and one individual may seem, particularly to the uninitiated, to be inconsistent in her or his preferences, sometimes growling "too long," and at other times, "too short."

So, the story goes that one day a particularly bold medical student responded to the surgeon's impatient "Cut!" with an obsequious "Do you want this one cut too long or too short?"

Medical students on their surgery rotations find this story very funny.

FACING MISTAKES

Mistakes in medicine are very difficult to talk about. Physicians are human beings, so of course they make errors. On the other hand, physicians' mistakes have lethal potential, and so are viewed as intolerable. This quandary is particularly acute for the physician trainee, who presumably makes more mistakes than the experienced physician and is less certain whether those mistakes are because of the inherent difficulty of the problem or personal ignorance.

After 18 months of observing surgeons in an academic community hospital, Charles Bosk developed a typology of medical errors and delineated the consequences of mistakes for physicians at different levels of the hierarchy (Bosk, 1979). He recognized two general categories of mistakes: what he called "errors in technique" and "moral errors." Errors in technique can be "technical" or "judgmental" and moral errors can be "normative" or "quasinormative."

Technical errors are mistakes in performance of medical care. While they may not be minor, they are forgivable, in part because they are inevitable in trainees. Examples such as incorrectly tied sutures that lead to a wound dehiscence, a slip of the scalpel, or a pneumothorax because of an attempted subclavian catheter placement are all simple technical errors. Technical errors continue to be forgivable if they are reported to supervising physicians and addressed promptly. In addition, they shouldn't be repeated. The practical rationale for these criteria is that rapid revelation of error allows for prompt corrective measures to minimize the complications induced: packing of the wound, repair of the tissue, or placement of the chest tube can be effected swiftly. Ideally, the supervising resident will know about the blunder and will have initiated the corrective action before the attending is told. The pressure to have begun repairing the mistake before the attending finds out about the error is intense, but any delay in reporting the unforeseen event must be invisible.

Single technical mistakes are considered a natural consequence of inexperience as well as the solution for that inexperience. A mistake is made, the correct action is taught, and the mistake is not repeated. Though the one patient has suffered, *if* the student learns from the experience, future patients will be spared the suffering. On the other hand, a pattern of similar mistakes leads to a different conclusion: that the trainee is not learning. Since the assumption is that all students and house staff are bright, well prepared, and immune to the effects of sleep deprivation, repeated errors seem to indicate that the trainee lacks motivation to learn. Some are said to "not care enough about the patient." These failings fall in the realm of what Bosk designates as "moral errors."

Judgmental errors are mistakes made in decision about a course of treatment. Since medical students and house staff rarely have complete independence in their decision making, they rarely make serious judgmental errors. Maria's mistake in Case 3-5 could be seen as an example of an error in judgment that had serious consequences. Like the attendings in Bosk's study, Dr. Walker saw her error as serious but within the realm of intern mistakes. (As we shall later see, she made the additional normative moral error of not calling for help when she was uncertain.) Dr. Walker assumed that she was careful but inaccurate in her decision to turn down the old man's oxygen, and generously acknowledged that the patient may have died even if she had responded more appropriately. He did not react as to a "moral error" in the way Bosk describes.

"Moral errors" happen when the "surgeon has, in the eyes of others, failed to discharge his role obligations conscientiously" (Bosk, 1979). The assumption is that the trainee doesn't care enough about the patient, the other colleagues on the team, or the profession of medicine to do the best job she or he can. Accurately diagnosing a moral error is more complicated than understanding what technical and judgmental mistakes are. Communication about moral errors is less explicit and the criteria for moral errors are often more idiosyncratic. Bosk separates moral errors into the normative and quasinormative. The former term encompasses mistakes with which any of the surgeons would have taken issue. He uses the latter term to describe the "breaches of standards of performance that . . . are eccentric and attending-specific" (Bosk, 1979). Both types of moral errors are dealt with quite differently from technical errors. Where the errors in technique are met with specific correction and monitoring for patterns, a single normative or quasinormative error can bring down a public shaming on the offender. Technical errors are seen as reflecting the inexperience of the trainee; moral errors are seen to reflect character flaws such as dishonesty or not caring about the patient or the team. Supervisors respond to moral errors by scolding the offender ("What this patient needs is a *real* doctor"), by sarcastically instructing in excruciating detail, and by publicly forbidding further independence until remedial work has been performed.

The most explicit normative rule is "no surprises." "No surprises" means that the physician in charge of any individual trainee is kept informed of changes in the patients' status so that he or she is not blindsided by a problem. The rule applies all the way down the hierarchy: The attending expects no surprises from the chief resident's performance, the chief resident expects none from the junior residents, and on down the line. If the intern caring for a laboring woman fails to inform the supervising physician soon enough for her to arrive before the delivery, that is a surprise. If, as in Case 3-5, the intern fails to ask for help when the patient gets sicker, and patient care suffers, that too is often seen as a normative error. If not calling for help was interpreted by Dr. Walker as indicative of overconfidence or sloppiness, Maria would have been more forcefully reprimanded to "get her attention." In this instance, Dr. Walker chose to view her mistake as a judgmental error. He does not impugn her character or motivation, but corrects her, checking that she understands her mistake.

Quasinormative errors are even more difficult to predict. By definition, what is considered standard procedure by one attending or in one institution is considered "wrong" in another. The apocryphal medical student in Case 3-6 is suggesting that his error, whether "too long" or "too short," will be a quasinormative one. The concrete difference between one way of closing a surgical wound and another is more obvious than the distinction between one antibiotic regimen and another, so quasinormative errors are probably easier to distinguish on surgical services than on medical or pediatric services. Strong opinions are not, however, limited to surgeons. Doing something the correct way on the wrong service may be seen as a judgmental error or as a moral error in the sense that the offending house staff has assumed that he has better judgment than the supervising resident or attending. This would reveal the character flaw of excessive pride, and a public reprimand would be deemed necessary to ensure no repetition.

Since the "no surprises" rule is clear, and the consequence is a dreaded public dressing-down, why do normative errors still occur? Because it is an equally clear though less explicit rule that "doing" things independently is both the mechanism of learning and the signal that progress has been made. "See one, do one, teach one" is the traditional methodology of medical education. Supervising a trainee takes considerably longer and is more difficult and more anxiety producing than doing the procedure or patient evaluation oneself, a fact trainees often don't quite believe. If the trainee seems to be taking too long, or asks for too much supervision, she will not get the opportunity to practice and will fall further behind in acquiring skills. The trainee then has two motivations to avoid calling for help: loss of an opportunity to learn and loss of face, which means she has not yet learned all that was expected. The supervisor, on the other hand, wants to allow as much independence as is safe because independent performance is highly valued in physicians.

The dynamic within the trainee when faced with these two conflicting rules is almost never discussed across hierarchical lines. Performance expectations are seldom specified in advance. Medical students and house staff compare their performances to the chief residents' or attending physicians'—both unrealistic standards for comparison. Since the feedback they usually receive is vague and rarely based on direct observation of performance (Ende, 1983; Bucher & Stelling, 1977), they rely on these grandiose external or inadequate internal standards. These inappropriate expectations mean that the students and house staff usually feel inadequate and overwhelmed. Exacerbating this is their chronic fatigue, which saps their psychological reserves (Eberle, 1988; Gordon et al., 1986; J. W. Smith et al., 1986). Some trainees have trouble discussing their confusion even with peers and end up feeling lonely and stupid. Since the punishment for a publicly found mistake is blame, and asking for help too much may curtail their learning opportunities, trainees often retreat within themselves and learn to keep secrets.

Successful keeping of secrets has obvious dangers for patients, and less obvious risks for students and house staff. Secrets kept about developmentally normal mistakes are particularly insidious: They prevent the reality check offered by a peer or supervisor who points out the inappropriateness of using more advanced physicians as standards of comparison. Peers can and should help each other sort out the technical and judgmental errors from the moral errors. They often do not have the experience to differentiate between normative and quasinormative; more experienced house staff must provide this information. Bosk's study was done in the mid-1970s and since then more attention has been paid to how medical students are treated. The harshness of the shaming he describes has been condemned, but still occurs (Sheehan et al., 1990). His typology of errors provides a vocabulary that is useful in discussions aimed at making sense of the system's responses to mistakes. Occasionally, an attending can articulate the difference between the general and the idiosyncratic, but such a degree of self-revelation to subordinates in the hierarchy is delicate and can further confuse the trainees.

It is crucial for students and house staff to continue to speak about their confusions within peer groups and with supervisors, like Dr. Walker in Case 3-5, who have demonstrated their willingness to examine the reality of mistakes in medical education. Though Bosk delineated his typology of technical and moral errors as though the distinctions were clear, his clarity may have resulted from his being an outsider, a sociologist. Many of the errors classified by the surgery teams he observed as normative could also have been simple errors in technique or judgment. Few medical trainees don't care about their patients but many become so stressed that they have trouble caring about much of anything, much less attending to all of their patients' needs. If "not caring" is the result of being overwhelmed and not having personal physiologic needs met, it is a normal response, a coping mechanism, not a moral failing (Eberle, 1988). Shaming is not an effective or ethical teaching technique. Yet, as Bosk demonstrated, it is frequently used in place of one. In its use of blame and scolding as coercive techniques of behavior control, medical education mimics a neglectful and abusive family system (McKegney, 1989).

Healthy survival in such a system necessitates breaking the rules about keeping secrets, making judicious, but not paranoid, choices of confidants. Sharing enough so that no one stays alone with fears and uncertainties helps prevent the ego-destroying doubts that prevent learning. Maria's mistake was treated as an error in judgment by her supervisor, as it should have been. Though she was not shamed for her error, she will feel guilt and sadness, both of which should be shared. Trusted colleagues must form the "compassionate community" that Howard Brody describes as crucial to our ability to attend "to the sufferings of . . . patients" (Brody, 1992, p. 267). Open communication is risky in any large system with a history of discomfort with uncertainty. Though medicine is ultimately a discipline steeped in uncertainty, it still seems to hold omniscience as a realistic goal (Dubovsky & Schrier, 1983). Treating uncertainty as the exception rather than the rule contributes to the difficulties found in distinguishing normative and quasinormative errors. When residents and attending physicians can explain their opinions as either widely applied standard operating procedure or idiosyncratic preferences, the important consistencies will become apparent and students will know what to remember for the long haul.

CASE 3-7

It is midnight and David has been sent to draw blood on Mrs. Marten—she insisted on "Mrs."—for cardiac enzymes. As he moves quietly in the half-light, arranging the tourniquet and the Vacutainer tube, she querulously asks, "Young man, are you practicing on me?"

CASE 3-8

Calvin is finally finishing his internship. He thought it would never end. Next month he will be expected to teach, but how can he? He feels that this has been the longest, most grueling year of his life, but he dreads his first night of call as a G2, the questions that the G1s will have, and responsibility for the patients! He feels he doesn't know enough, that all the other soon-to-be G2s are better pre-

pared than he, that something awful will happen, and his incompetence will be discovered. He considers asking for more rotations as a G1, but is nauseated at the thought of a longer internship, and more nauseated at the shame he would feel at admitting his inadequate knowledge.

ADAPTING TO THE IDENTITY

In all training programs, fledgling professionals go through several transitions of identity between their initial "lay" status and being a professional "with all its privileges and obligations." At each transition, disequilibrium occurs with uncertainty about how many of the privileges are deserved, and how many of the obligations can be met. For students focused on education as a preprofessional process, being accepted to medical school is like approaching the top of a steep slope of a mountain. At first it appears to be very near the summit. As one clambers over what appears to be the final lip, one discovers that a taller and steeper slope is still ahead.

The first 2 years of medical school are generally grounded in the familiar process of classroom study, examination, and grading based on those exams. The small sliver of the "privilege" that accompanies putting on the short white coat excites, while trying to stuff the tools of the trade in its pockets frustrates, the neophyte. For students who have come straight through school, this is probably their first professional role. The recurrent adolescence of the highly educated is in its penultimate stage. For students who have had other professions, their chosen regression to apprenticeship begins to have results. As the excitement fades, confusion encroaches: How do I introduce myself to patients? How do I respect patients' rights to have experienced care and at the same time learn enough to provide good care when I'm done? What is my role on this team, anyway?

As a medical student, to be called "doctor" holds a thrill tinged with dishonesty. One is not yet a doctor, and truthfulness demands that the distinction be acknowledged. Excessive emphasis on student inexperience is unfair to both the student and the patient, since it increases anxiety without increasing safety. A compromise must be reached. The term "medical student" is actually confusing to many patients; after all, nurses and PT students study "medicine" in the minds of some outside the medical professions. Introducing oneself as a "student doctor" seems to be clear to most English speakers in the United States. It has the advantage of being free of jargon, acknowledges the training status of the student, and indicates which training program he or she is in.

So, what should David in Case 3-7 say? On the one hand, fairness and honesty demand that he assent to his relative inexperience but not undermine both himself and the patient by harping on it. There is probably no one right answer. Different schools and hospitals will have cultural norms that need to be respected. Discussing this with fellow medical students and house staff will clarify local norms. Lying about one's inexperience rarely works anyway, as patients are very attuned to the demeanor of those who may cause them pain. In addition, lying reinforces the trainee's sense that not knowing is somehow shameful, rather than being "appropriate for gestational age," perpetuating further the pattern of secret keeping that hampers learning. For both the trainee and the patient, clarifying the degree of supervision and naming the supervisor can provide reassurance based on honesty and trust.

Many trainees, at many levels of training, express fear that their inexperience will be discovered. Medical students fear that their less-than-perfect understanding of the basic sciences will be glaringly obvious on rounds. The meaning attached to these errors depends on many factors: the ego strength of the student, the atmosphere on the ward team, and whether the supervising physician employs "pimping" to exert power (Brancati, 1989). In situations where supervision does not include direct observation of patient care, secret self-awareness of knowledge gaps engulfs the sense of mastery over what is known. Their sense is that they have successfully fooled everyone for a time, but that they are impostors who will eventually be discovered and ejected from the profession.

Printed in black and white, the fear sounds melodramatic. This "impostor" syndrome is more common among women than men, but there is considerable overlap. Because of the decline in bedside ward rounds as technical information is relied on more and more for diagnosis, students and residents are observed even less than previously. Since they know they have not been directly observed, they find their superiors' evaluations arbitrary and actively discount them. Without feedback based on direct observation, trainees use internal criteria, sometimes idiosyncratic, for evaluating their own performances (Bucher & Stelling, 1977).

Calvin in Case 3-8 is scared for at least two reasons. He faces a role transition with an abrupt increase in independence and responsibility. Without adequate feedback regarding the specifics of his performance, he is uncertain whether he is sufficiently well trained to take on his new responsibilities. When he is on call his first night as a G2, he will be surprised at how much he has learned in the last year, and he will discover that he is not alone in the hospital. Once he is over the top of the steep slope of internship, he can see ahead. Not only is there another slope, but there are climbers ahead of him who can be consulted about the right path to take.

Obtaining clearer feedback before the transition can facilitate the awareness that progress has been made. Structuring this feedback is difficult from the trainee's position of relative powerlessness, but the trainee is the one who is motivated to obtain the specific information needed about his performance. Since most teachers in medicine did not have clear, specific feedback during their training, they are unfamiliar with giving it. It can shock teachers to have students ask for specific information, but particularly those immediately higher in the hierarchy will usually answer the questions if they are posed explicitly: What is one thing you think I do well? What is something I need to work on? And, how would you suggest I do it differently? If needed, handing the supervisor a copy of Ende's article (Ende, 1983) will clarify the request.

Some of the anxiety of adopting the identity of "physician" can be alleviated by more specific information. If the feedback is provided properly about behaviors, rather than inferred personality characteristics, performance is separated from identity and self-worth. This is a crucial process for maintaining health as a physician. If one chooses to "be" a physician, rather than choosing to "practice" medicine, one is far more vulnerable to the devastation that results from physician error and patient morbidity and mortality. After all, the mortality rate is eventually 100%. Healthy physicians are not sanguine about illness and death, but they must recognize that they have worth as human beings outside of their roles as physicians.

For trainees, especially in a university rather than a community hospital setting, the distance from their teachers mitigates against learning much about how "grown-up" physicians maintain their "detached concern" (Fox, 1989). Medical students in particular are so awash in their uncertainty about whether something is known, Fox's third category of uncertainty, that they can't get a perspective on how their observations of their teachers relate to their own goals. After all, relatively few students and house staff will be attending physicians in teaching hospitals when they finish their training. Programs that use community physicians as part-time teachers do much to bridge this gap. The community physician provides a model for balancing life and work without the perplexing intrusions of research, tenure, and university politics that affect university-based physicians. Students and residents may not be able to articulate what is distracting their teachers from patient care and teaching, but they recognize the orbital distortion induced by academic gravitational forces. Contact with community physicians clarifies which sources of the distraction are part of university life and which are inherent in medical practice.

CASE 3-9

Philip couldn't help but join the other interns in gossiping about Tina and Dr. Hank Corcoran, the cardiologist. He feels that, as an intern, she is being singularly stupid to "date" an attending physician old enough to be her father, and a married one at that. It is true that he only does morning report occasionally to fill in when one of the regular internists is gone, so he isn't technically her supervisor, but it still doesn't seem right.

Philip has noticed that since she and Dr. Corcoran began making eyes at each other, Tina has stopped going out for pizza and beer with the other interns and the ER nurses. Corcoran seems underfoot all the time on the medicine units, but he isn't very open to questions about patients, unless Tina is the one asking the questions. Philip is furious with Corcoran for giving Tina special attention, and angry with Tina for agreeing to pay the price. She probably thinks she is in love with him. Doesn't she know he's going to drop her as soon as he is bored? Why doesn't Arthur Stein, the department chair, take Corcoran aside and tell him to keep his pants zipped? Philip thinks Dr. Stein would have to be blind to not notice what's occurring.

CASE 3-10

Gail is finishing her fellowship year in geriatrics. Most of her clinical time has been spent caring for the elderly, but she has had two sessions a week in the family practice clinic, where 28-year-old Lindsey became her patient 10 months ago. Lindsey has had over a dozen physicians in the last 5 years: internists, a gynecologist or two, three neurologists, an orthopedist, and a handful of psychotherapists. Gail carefully sent for old records, and Lindsey's first progress notes are in volume three, the first two volumes being full of scratchy copies of handwritten notes from the clinicians who responded to the release of information forms. All of her visits with Lindsey confuse Gail: She can't figure out why the patient came to the clinic. Lindsey always shows up for her appointments with long lists of concerns and authorization forms to be completed and "walks in" at other times without an appointment. On the other hand, she clearly isn't taking her anticonvulsants: The last time she was brought into the ER seizing, her blood level was negligible. The time before that, her level was in the therapeutic range and should have prevented the seizure. Her last neurologist said that her family physician could handle her anticonvulsants, effectively dumping her in Gail's lap. Her current neurologist thinks that Lindsey has psychogenic seizures, and that's why the meds don't work.

Gail feels saddled with tasks beyond her expertise. She feels that Lindsey is dependent on her, expecting Gail to be her social worker as well as her physician. In addition, Lindsey has begun to comment on Gail's increasingly obvious pregnancy, which makes Gail very uneasy for reasons she cannot articulate. In a visit when Gail tried to make a clear contract with Lindsey about how many visits and phone calls per week were feasible, Lindsey dropped the comment that she now lives near Gail and walks by her house every other day. This rattled Gail so much that she didn't finish their discussion of the contract.

Gail talked to Dr. Scott, one of the faculty who is known for her skill in caring for difficult patients. Gail asked Dr. Scott for advice, or permission to terminate as Lindsey's physician, anything to help her feel less trapped. Lindsey's comments about Gail's pregnancy and Gail's house frighten her. She is afraid that Lindsey will "do something." She doesn't feel she has the right to quit as Lindsey's physician unless Lindsey breaks a specific contract. In discussion with Dr. Scott, she realizes that she has taken on social worker as well as physician functions, that Lindsey can't always tell which professional is right to handle which problems, and that Gail can do more delegating. She also realizes that she has not told her husband about her anxiety about this unstable patient walking by their house, and resolves to bring him in on her decision making. The fear dissipates some as her goals of her relationship with Lindsey are clearer to Gail, but none of her discussions with Dr. Scott can completely eliminate the feeling that Lindsey is constantly pulling at the hem of Gail's white coat.

FINDING THE BOUNDARIES

In Case 3-9, Philip is in a quandary: He feels profoundly uncomfortable with Tina's romantic relationship with Hank Corcoran, but isn't sure it's any of his business. In some ways, he sees their relationship as between consenting adults, but on the other hand, their relationship seems wrong. Some of the interns are whispering about it among themselves, but no one is talking to Tina, and there has been no official response from the department head. If we apply the family metaphor introduced at the beginning of this chapter, this cross-generational love affair looks like incest between uncle and niece.

Very few writers have discussed sexual relationships between trainees and teachers in medicine. Recognizing the power inequities and the potential for exploitation, a number of universities have addressed relationships between students and teachers with varying degrees of proscription. How these rules should apply to physicians in training and their supervisors is unclear. The guidelines regarding intraoffice romance developed for businesses are also not quite pertinent. House staff are often students and always employees, but they are employed by the hospital, not the department chair. In university and business settings, mixing a direct supervisory relationship, especially if it involves job or academic performance evaluation, with a romantic relationship is the most taboo of dual relationships because one person's power to consent is assumed to be compromised (Peterson, 1992). In the medical system, the supervisory lines are less rigid; attending physicians have variable supervisory and teaching roles within their own departments and other departments within the hospital or university. House staff are in a unique position; they are neither students who are vulnerable to the whims of their professors, nor are they full-fledged physicians. On the other hand, their professional status is still very dependent on the evaluations of their supervisors.

In Case 3-9, the incest metaphor falls apart in several ways. Tina is not a child, she is a grown woman. Dr. Corcoran is not her blood relative, and not her direct supervisor. On the other hand, she is isolated by the time demands of internship and vulnerable because of the stresses of internship in ways that are not true of an attending physician (Gordon *et al.*, 1986). She is also vulnerable to his authority and privilege, even if he does not have direct supervision over her. The isolation of the couple from her social context, the other interns, the mixture of resentment and pity felt by the uninvolved "siblings," and the silence and blindness on the part of the parental generation are all typical patterns found in families with incest.

Close mentoring in educational settings is a personal as well as a professional process. Good teacher–student relationships involve support aimed at developing the helping professional. Healing professionals need emotional balance and reserves in order to be with their patients in illness and pain. Like Dr. Walker and Dr. Scott, good teachers do not stick to teaching just the facts, they bring their *selves*, with their human forgiveness and compassion to aid their students in expanding their own forgiveness and compassion. In an isolated system like the teaching program, this educational intimacy can be confused with an emotional or sexual one. Exploitation occurs when two crucial precepts are ignored. First, the teacher–student relationship is essentially asymmetrical, and must be. Second, the goal of the relationship is the benefit of the student. When the relationship is operating for the benefit of the "instructor" more than the benefit of the student, the relationship has become exploitative. In a functional teaching relationship, teachers certainly benefit. Helping a student become a fine physician is personally as well as professionally satisfying. Being part of another human being's growth is a real high, and we teach because of that high. Our sources for meeting our own needs for love, self-esteem, and sex must be outside of our teaching and patient care relationships (Bograd, 1992; Peterson, 1992).

In addition to the educational intimacies inherent in medical education, the hierarchy is temporary. The "generations" are so short as to seem almost arbitrary. In Case 3-10, Gail is distressed because Lindsey is a challenging patient and because she is near enough to Dr. Scott's "generation" that she won't get a simple answer. In a few months, Gail and Dr. Scott will both be "parents" and the asymmetry of their relationship will be more a function of their personal relationship than of the hierarchical teacher–student relationship. Dr. Scott will begin to consult Gail at times, and they will gradually become colleagues.

Within the medical education "family," Gail is functioning like a young adult still living at home. She is board certified and capable of practicing on her own, but has chosen to continue her training to obtain more expertise. At some level, she feels she should be able to make it on her own without help. Part of her worry is in anticipation of the upcoming time when she won't have Dr. Scott to ask for advice. In actuality, she will have senior partners in practice who will be available for consultation, and Dr. Scott will welcome telephone consultations from Gail as she has from other residents who graduated before her. As noted in the section on "Adapting to the Identity," Dr. Scott's clarifications that Lindsey is challenging, that Gail is not incompetent because she is having difficulty, and that Dr. Scott will not disappear off the face of the earth on the day Gail graduates are all reassuring.

The reasons that Lindsey is difficult to care for are myriad. As this is not a neurology textbook, this discussion will focus on the challenges in the physician–patient relationship. As trainees move from their identities as laypeople to professionals, they acquire the habits and values of the profession. As noted earlier, they distance themselves emotionally in order to keep a cool head in the presence of death and pain. They become more comfortable with probabilities rather than certainties, and recognize mistakes as (dreaded) learning opportunities. As Fox described, they begin to develop detached concern (Fox, 1989). Medical students often have the role of intermediary between the "real doctors" on their teams and the patients because they are only partly trained and therefore only partially acculturated. In this role, their empathy with and understanding of the patient is often greater than that of their senior colleagues. Medical student explanations of phenomena are frequently more understandable to the patient than professorial explanations. This makes sense: Patients are more likely to ask their real questions of the student, who is less intimidating, and the students have a better memory of the transition between not knowing and knowing.

One of the hazards of this proximity of understanding between students and patients is that with the narrower gap, the emotional boundary between patient and student is less well defined. That boundary need not be huge, but its existence will become increasingly important as the trainee gains more responsibility. The empathy that is crucial to providing humane care is a double-edged sword. If the distinction between professional and patient is obscured, the asymmetric intimacy that is the kernel of the healing relationship will be lost. For medical students, keeping the necessary asymmetry is difficult, but is also an essential part of their learning how to create and maintain a therapeutic relationship.

With some patients, boundary maintenance is fairly easy. They have expectations of what the medical professionals in their lives can and cannot do. They have sufficient emotional and intellectual resources to obtain consultation about medical issues and look to other resources in their social circles or public services to meet their other needs. For families with catastrophic or chronic illnesses, the medical consultation may be quite global in its scope: Do I need to make out my will? Can we have sex? Will my dad need to live with us? But even when the consultation is global with respect to the patient's world, it is restricted with respect to the physician. The relevant part of the physician's world is that which includes the physician–patient relationship. How much of the physician is revealed within that relationship is variable, depending on the community norms, the style of the physician, and the specifics of that physician–patient relationship.

As Gail observed in Case 3-10, some facts about the physician's life are impossible to keep private, like advancing pregnancy. Gail generally felt comfortable with patients' comments on her pregnancy, but with Lindsey something was different. Lindsey's incapacity, whether because of intellectual deficits or personality disorder, to structure the relationship from her end left Gail to deal with an emotional as well as a medical morass. Gail's goal of being open and responsive to her patients' needs backfired. Her tactic of being patient-centered in her care is the appropriate ideal for a physician. Her advancing skills left her open to the chaos of Lindsey's life. Dr. Scott's greater experience with patients with boundary problems provided her with an algorithm for structuring the relationship and bringing the chaos to a level with which Gail could cope. Gail is left with the discomfort inherent in choosing to stay in a clinical relationship with someone who cannot tell where the limits of the asymmetric intimacy should lie. By consulting with someone else, she can make sense out of the chaos and define her own working parameters. She can also learn about her own countertransference, in this case regarding the sense of physical vulnerability associated with pregnancy.

When working to maintain appropriate boundaries with "difficult patients" such as Lindsey, or "difficult attendings" like Dr. Corcoran, it is important to keep five simple guidelines in mind (McKegney, 1993):

1. Don't do it alone.
2. Get a life.
3. Don't do it alone.

4. Take it seriously, but *not* solemnly.
5. Don't do it alone.

Although these guidelines appear obvious, implementing them breaks many of medicine's family rules.

CONCLUSION

As noted throughout this chapter, the essential tactic for healthy development in the medical family is to break the rule about secrets, whether those secrets are about feelings, uncertainty, or errors. Emotions can't be controlled and will not be denied. Strong feelings are inevitable, not evil. They can immobilize the neophyte or can be the source of insight and empathy when acknowledged, discussed, and addressed. Uncertainty is likewise the clinicians' home territory, albeit an uncomfortable dwelling. Despite the challenges of time constraints and technocracy that are so much a part of modern medicine, physicians in training come to know that they often will not know what will happen next, and may never know why. Mistakes are human, learning from them is expected, and the pain of making them can be ameliorated by avoiding blame. The identity transitions are easier if taken stepwise, with support from peers and trusted mentors. Clear boundaries in relationships with patients, colleagues, and supervisors don't always come easily. We each need to know our own identities, accept our feelings, and make choices about our behavior, keeping in mind the goals of the relationship. And when in doubt, get a consult.

Like adults who are recovering from child abuse, the process of becoming a physician has many stages. Though an individual proceeds from one step to the next, the path is more of a spiral than a direct ascent. The first step is to remember the incidents. The second is telling the stories, which may also be an inextricable part of remembering. One colleague had to elaborate on the story of his internship several times before he remembered the "punch line." A simple recitation of the facts is not sufficient, the feelings evoked need to be revealed; apparently irrelevant details can hold the key to emotional content. Next, we must let go of responsibility for having been hurt. Lastly, refusing to deny our perceptions and avoiding blame, we take up the challenge of doing it differently (McKegney, 1989). These tasks seem daunting, but with the companionship of friends and colleagues, becoming a physician is the process of becoming more fully oneself.

CASES FOR DISCUSSION

CASE 1

Sam Hines (medical student) and Ray Leo (intern) are reporting to the senior resident, Petra Cahill, about the night's many admissions. After discussing the two admissions to the intensive care units, they briefly summarize the admittedly incomplete workup of the woman with abdominal pain who was transferred from the ER to the medicine floor at 7:00 AM, an hour ago. Petra hears that Sam has not yet done a pelvic exam on the patient, and promptly tears into him, implying that his evaluation will reflect his "incompetence." Ray tries to defend Sam, pointing out how busy they have been, the unavailability of a nurse to chaperone the pelvic at change of shift, and that Petra is being inappropriately cruel.

1. Who is who in this medical "family"? If Sam is the "kid brother," what role does Ray have? and Petra?
2. What dysfunctional family behavior patterns are evident in this story?
3. How can Sam and Ray soothe their injured self-esteem?
4. What would be the potential problems or solutions if Sam or Ray tried talking to the chief resident about Petra's threats about Sam's evaluation?

CASE 2

Lois Sorenson just joined the Department of Ob/Gyn after finishing her residency in another state. On her first month as ward attending she supervised G1s and G2s from her own department and a G2 from the family practice program, Frank Gagne. She found him very attractive, and he seemed to respond in kind. They chat, briefly because of his schedule, over lunch whenever they run into each other in the cafeteria. About 3 weeks after the end of the rotation, he asks her out for dinner.

1. Is it right for Lois to accept Frank's invitation? Why or why not?
2. If they become romantically involved, would you see this relationship as "incestuous"?
3. Would it make a difference if she were older? if the sex roles were reversed?
4. How would your assessment of the relationship be different if she were one of the family practice faculty?

CASE 3

Esther is working with Dr. Lawler for her fourth-year outpatient pediatrics rotation. The next patient is a 5-year-old, Greg Rollin, brought in by his father for a kindergarten physical. Esther introduces herself to them as "the student doctor working with Dr. Lawler" and asks if she can begin the office visit while Dr. Lawler finishes some phone calls. Mr. Rollin replies, "Of course, anything for a girl as cute as you." Esther feels put down, but isn't sure if she feels worse about being a medical student or about being a woman.

When she presents the case to Dr. Lawler before they go back in the room to see Greg, she mentions his father's remark. Dr. Lawler apologizes to Esther for Mr. Rollin's poor boundaries and at the end of the visit he takes Mr. Rollin aside and tells him that his comment to Esther was inappropriate.

1. Should Esther have made a comment to Mr. Rollin herself? Why or why not?
2. What elements in Dr. Lawler's handling of the situation contributed to Esther's feeling respected? as a medical student? as a woman?
3. If a patient makes a similar comment to Esther when she is a third-year resident, how might her response be different? How does her process of identity formation contribute to the difference?

CASE 4

Larry Martin is on his first clinical rotation as a third-year medical student, the family practice inpatient service. Constance Orvieti is his G2, and Patrice Haas is the attending. The second day on rounds, after Constance finishes presenting the case, Dr. Haas asks Larry about the differential diagnosis of lung nodules based on chest X ray appearance. He is very flattered, and does his best to cover the bases. When she starts pushing him to rank the most likely diagnoses for the patient *admitted last night, he feels confused and trapped. He doesn't remember ever reading anything that specific in the pathology textbook. Dr. Orvieti stares at the wall, and Larry can't tell whether she is ashamed of him because he doesn't know or if she doesn't know the answers to Dr. Haas's questions either.*

1. *Which dysfunctional family behavior patterns do you see in this case?*
2. *What are the sources of Larry's uncertainty?*
3. *How can he get a sense of what realistic expectations are for him at his stage of training?*

CASE 5

After the resuscitation, Dr. Kim Pierce felt like she was going to cry right there in front of everybody. On one level, she knew that the baby's apnea was not something she could have prevented. After all, she wasn't called until 10 minutes or so before the delivery, and she ran from the pediatric call room to L&D as fast as she could. The obstetrician handed her the blue baby, and she intubated and bagged him until he got pinker, and put in the umbilical line. Despite all that, he was still limp and making no respiratory effort when the team from the university Level III nursery arrived 20 minutes later.

Later that morning in the office, she told the story to her partners, George and Sharon, not sure of what she was looking for. She just needed to tell someone. And she cried, and they hugged her, and she went on with her day.

1. *Has Kim failed to develop "detached concern"? What behaviors suggest that she has or has not?*
2. *What factors influenced Kim's decision to let herself cry where she did?*
3. *How do you express strong feelings? How do you adapt to the constraints inherent in the medical system?*
4. *What elements of place and characteristics of companions provide you with the safety you need to get emotional support?*

RECOMMENDED READINGS

Bosk CL: *Forgive and Remember: Managing Medical Failure.* Chicago, University of Chicago Press, 1979.

Bosk is a medical sociologist who spent 18 months studying how surgeons respond to error. This complete write-up of his study is dense, but offers the unique outsider's eye on medical ritual.

Ende J: Feedback in clinical medical education. *JAMA* 250:777–781, 1983.

Ende succinctly delineates criteria for effective feedback and evaluation.

Fox RC: *The Sociology of Medicine: A Participant Observer's View.* Englewood Cliffs, NJ, Prentice–Hall, 1989.

Renee Fox has been studying medicine for four decades; her insights into how physicians are trained and cope with their training and practice are summarized in this book.

McKegney CP: Medical education: A neglectful and abusive family system. *Fam Med* 21:452–457, 1989.

In this theoretical discussion, the metaphor of a family system is applied to medical education.

Sheehan KH, Sheehan DK, White K, *et al.* A pilot study of medical student "abuse." *JAMA* 263:533–537, 1990.

This paper reports on one of the first formal surveys of medical student abuse.

Smith AC, Kleinman S: Managing emotions in medical school: Students' contacts with the living and the dead. *Soc Psychol Q* 52:56–69, 1989.

One of the few recent observational studies of medical student acculturation illuminates coping strategies over the course of training.

CHAPTER 4

Being a Physician

John L. Coulehan

In 400 B.C. on the Greek island of Kos a young man consulted a physician because of shaking fevers and chest pain. He had gotten sick with cough and fever several weeks earlier, seemed to get better, but then the illness recurred. The physician observed his patient in a kindly but businesslike manner. The patient was a thin man, breathing rapidly, and splinting the left side of his chest. There was a deep look of fear in his eyes, hollowed cheeks, and a grimace of pain. The patient sat on a stool, facing away from the light. There was a broad, soft lump over one area of the lower rib cage, appearing warmer and redder than the surrounding skin. When he shook the young man, the physician expected to hear "a wave and a noise," but there was no sound. He took this to be a sign of pus in the chest. An assistant smeared the back of the young man's chest with a thin, watery slip of clay. At the place where the clay dried first, the warmest point, the physician made an incision and quickly inserted a hollow tin tube. Brownish fluid began to drain. An assistant secured the tube. It remained in place draining fluid for several days while the patient's fevers disappeared. Meanwhile, the physician prescribed a liquid diet, herbs, and purgatives for his very weak, but grateful, patient (modified from Majno, 1975, pp. 156–157).

INTRODUCTION

Case 4-1, written nearly 2500 years ago, is easily understandable to us. While the specific methods may differ, the physician's role and behavior are remarkably contemporary. The Hippocratic physician used his hand, his mind, and his heart to help the young man recover. Hand, heart, and mind. Together, these words signify the calling and the full personal commitment that has characterized the profession of medicine throughout history. While the manifestations and proportions of each have changed with changing times, hand, mind, and heart are all essential to medicine. In ancient Greece, the physician used his hands to gather data and to intervene, as in Case 4-1. He understood the physical findings within a mental framework that explained illness as a natural phenomenon, rather than a random or supernatural occurrence. For example, Hippocratic physicians tasted the patient's urine to determine its sweetness in cases now known as diabetes mellitus, and they explained epilepsy as an imbalance of humors, rather than a message from the gods. The physician's heart was also committed to healing. Medicine was a life work dedicated to helping others, not just another craft or business. In the Hippocratic *Precepts* the author was explicit about the connection between caring and medicine: "For where there is love of man, there is also love of the art." And, of course, the *Epidemics* contains the best-known (albeit distorted) of all the Hippocratic sayings: "As to diseases, make a habit of two things—to help, or at least to do no harm."

Mind and hand have not always necessarily been synergistic in the history of medicine (King, 1970). After the Roman era, rational theories were long emphasized at the expense of the "hand" or empirical dimension. For example, the comprehensive theory of physiology and medicine developed by the Roman physician Galen was fossilized during the Middle Ages and used as the basis of medical practice for nearly 1500 years. The Christian era in Europe was associated with the ascendancy of religious values at the expense of skeptical thinking and natural science. Authority replaced observation as a source of truth. While Galen himself was a keen observer, his system became an unquestioned authority that stifled subsequent generations' creativity and investigation. Later theorists tinkered with Galen's theory by developing gizmos and codicils to update it. Other physicians, however, rejected rational systems that didn't seem to jibe with reality. These empiricists, like the seventeenth-century Englishman Thomas Sydenham, confined themselves to recording systematic clinical observations, rather than trying to figure out the big picture (King, 1970). In the eighteenth and nineteenth centuries, hand and mind began again to work together, leading to the development of modern medicine.

Medicine's heart has endured, though, despite the vicissitudes of mind and hand. By "heart," I mean the personal experience of medical practice, as well the physician's motivation and commitment. These, too, have varied according to history and culture. For example, the Common Era brought an infusion of Judeo-Christian values, which transformed and deepened the Greek and Roman virtues of medicine. In the realm of the heart, however, there are striking similarities between today's practitioner and Hippocrates, who wrote:

> The dignity of a physician requires that he should look healthy, and as plump as nature intended him to be. . . . He must be clean in person, well-dressed, and anointed with sweet-smelling unguents that are not in any way suspicious. . . . In appearance, let him be of a serious but not harsh countenance. . . . The physician must have at his command a certain ready wit, as dourness is repulsive both to the healthy and to the sick. (Jones, 1923)

Sounds pretty familiar, doesn't it?

In this chapter, I want to investigate medicine as a practice of the heart. What is it like to be a physician? How does it feel? What are the satisfactions, the stresses, the motivations? Some might argue that these topics are too vague to discuss in a meaningful way. Medicine is so complex and fragmented that generalities about "doctoring" may no longer be anything but platitudes. A pathologist and nuclear medicine specialist. An anesthesiologist and occupational medicine specialist. A staff internist in an HMO and a solo practitioner in Wyoming. What do these women and men have in common? There appear to be more differences than similarities among specialties. Moreover, medical practice is changing so rapidly that doctoring in 5 or 10 years will undoubtedly be experienced much differently than it is today.

Nonetheless, though change is hard upon us, there are commonalties in doctoring that might be called the moral phenomenology of medical practice. These features include elements of motivation, character, psychology, skills, satisfaction, and moral legitimacy. In the next section I present a sketch of this phenomenology. In later sections I focus on the potential for abuse of power and conflicts of interest in medicine. Finally, I describe serious health risks, including burnout and substance abuse, that sometimes arise from the demands of medical practice.

CASE 4-2

In 1972 T. P. was the physician assigned to an Indian Health Service facility that served a large boarding school, as well as several thousand Navajo people scattered over 400 square miles of arid steppe in northern Arizona. He and his wife lived with their two young children in a trailer nestled in a stand of cottonwood trees near the clinic. T. P. would frequently see 70 to 80 patients in a day, many of whom were quite ill, but some of whom had merely come to "town" to socialize a few hours at the trading post and pick up a bottle of "big red pills" for their aches and pains. As the day progressed, he would see an amazing variety of patients: tuberculosis, pneumonia, conjunctivitis, acute rheumatic fever, mitral stenosis, broken bones, alcoholism, an epidemic of hepatitis.

Sometimes T. P. would walk home at the end of the day with his heart singing, "This is the life for me!" He felt like he had accomplished a lot. His work was interesting, important. The patients liked him. Other days he would trudge home feeling dull, angry, incompetent, and overworked. Many patients simply wouldn't take their medicines. Screaming kids got on his nerves. His medical backup was some 60 miles away. He felt he was being manipulated. Because few people in the community had phones and everyone knew where the physician lived, patients would appear at T. P.'s trailer at all hours of the night and weekends—mothers with sick kids, drunks beaten up on the way home from bars in Holbrook. The administrator at the regional hospital said, "Well, you should just turn those people away. Don't treat them. Clinic hours are nine to five." T. P. couldn't turn patients away, but often on weekends he and his family would drive 3 hours to Flagstaff to stay in a cheap motel, cook their meals on a Coleman stove, and sleep gratefully without the threat of a staccato knock at midnight.

EXPERIENCE, VIRTUE, AND SATISFACTION IN MEDICAL PRACTICE

In Case 4-2, T. P. was learning what it means to be a physician—not in the abstract, but in the day-to-day events that make up a life. He was discovering that his life wasn't entirely his own anymore: He had obligations to patients, to the Navajo community, and to the medical profession itself. Sometimes the thought of these duties made him grateful and proud. Yet, at other times they seemed insufficient to alleviate his fatigue or quench his anger. Medical students tend to be both romantic and cynical in their views of professionalism. Early in medical school, they romanticize the power and virtue of medicine; later, when they begin the lived experience of taking care of patients, they sometimes become cynical when the reality doesn't live up to their expectation (Becker *et al.*, 1961). Medicine as a profession is difficult, complex, personally demanding. Often, the answers are unclear and the physician's ability to help is limited. In medicine one encounters suffering that is unfair, intractable, and meaningless. The physician experiences the thrill of healing, but also feels the impotence of failure. She experiences the gratitude of some patients, but also encounters anger, ignorance, and dislike. It is easy to become cynical if you approach medicine with messianic expectations, or without much understanding of your own motivation, needs, and limitations.

ENGAGEMENT, EMPATHY, ENJOYMENT

Most surveys show that physicians derive great satisfaction from taking care of patients. For example, in one study of California physicians, 80% indicated that they were satisfied with their jobs and over 90% reported enjoying their relationships with patients. Interestingly, nearly two-thirds (63%) characterized their work as "fun," a telling observation in this period of considerable change and presumed stress in medicine (Chuck *et al.*, 1993). Satisfaction with medical practice requires that you enjoy its day-to-day activities. An abstract sense of "doing good" by helping others is not enough. When asked about their motivation, applicants to medical school usually say they like science, they want to help people, and they enjoy interacting with others. These three motivations come in different mixtures and sizes. All are necessary, but enjoying "working with people" is the most basic. Both scientific interest and humane motivation are mediated through encounters with patients, families, colleagues, and other health workers.

In Case 4-2, the joys of T. P.'s practice came from his successful interactions with patients. These may have been successful in one or more of a variety of ways—medically (the patient got better), intellectually (the case was interesting), emotionally (the patient's response was personally gratifying), or socially (he simply enjoyed interacting with the patient). At this point in his career, T. P. did not experience some of the other major satisfactions of medicine; for example, he had little financial reward, prestige, or perception of power. Conversely, most of T. P.'s dissatisfactions arose from unsuccessful physician–patient encounters. In his case, cultural difference played a big role. T. P. expected a clear separation between his personal and professional life, but the Navajo community was unused to that type of distinction. Likewise, Navajo patients had trouble understanding the need to keep taking medication once they were feeling better. They believed that the real cause of illness was an underlying personal disharmony that could only be cured by a Navajo *haatali,* or medicine man. Thus, they sought out traditional healing ceremonies as well as Anglo medications. When the appropriate ceremony had been performed, they believed there was no point in continuing to take the Anglo pills.

Yet, despite such cultural differences, much of the time T. P. understood how his patients were feeling and he was able to "connect" with them. They, in turn, felt that he really cared about them, even though he knew little about their culture. In other words, T. P.'s successes were based as much or more on his care and feeling of *empathy* as they were on technical knowledge.

Empathy is a chameleon concept; various observers describe its colors quite differently (Aring, 1958; Basch, 1983; Hoffman, 1984; Spiro, 1992; Zinn, 1993). Some writers emphasize its *intellectual* or *cognitive* aspect, arguing that empathy is primarily a type of knowledge about other people's feelings and experience; in other words, a method of projecting yourself into their place—getting under their skin, so to speak. We learn what others are thinking or feeling by interpreting various verbal and nonverbal cues. Some people are better at this than others. At one end of the spectrum, there are autistic persons who do not seem to be able to form this type of human connection. In fact, autism can almost be defined as a global lack of empathy. People who choose medicine as a career tend to be closer to the other end of the continuum. They enjoy interacting with other people and, therefore, might well be expected to have a high natural degree of empathy.

Some writers stress that empathy is *affective* (Spiro, 1992; Halpern, 1993). They argue that you can't know how a patient is feeling in a given situation without, in some sense, actually experiencing that feeling yourself. Let's say a patient comes to see you for treatment of chronic osteomyelitis in his left foot. He is a contractor whose osteomyelitis developed as a result of stepping on a nail while working at a construction site. His antibiotic treatment has been intermittent and ineffective because of financial and personal problems: His wife left him, his business went bankrupt. You can tell by dozens of signs—the way he sits, the look on his face, the tone of his voice—that he is depressed, frustrated, angry, even overwhelmed. These conclusions are hypotheses (tentative knowledge) about his condition, yet at the same time they are associated with feelings. You don't feel as depressed or overwhelmed about the situation as he does, but you do feel something. You are not a detached observer. This affective aspect of empathy is an essential component of a physician's experience.

A third definition focuses on the *skills* required to be empathic. This operational approach says, "Look, let's not be vague. Let's take the mysticism out of empathy. What we're really talking about here is a set of interactive skills." Thus, empathy results from good eye contact, active listening, facilitative responses, and other communication techniques. The physician learns to be more empathic, simply and precisely, by using and perfecting these skills (Coulehan & Block, 1992).

Finally, some writers elevate empathy to the level of *virtue* (Reich, 1989). This is a complex topic that cannot be covered here, but it is important not to confuse empathy itself with the motivation or personal attributes that lead a person to develop empathy. In medicine the motivation is presumed to be good or virtuous: benevolence, care, compassion, sympathy. I discuss these motivations in the next section. One may, however, have nonvirtuous motivations for developing empathy. Consider the con artist, for example, who wins people's trust because of his charismatic skills, but then uses their trust for his own nefarious ends. Consider also the charismatic cult leader who drives his followers to destruction.

The affective nature of empathy leads to a curious paradox between engagement and detachment in medicine. Medical educators have long taught that physicians should learn to keep their distance from patients (Fox, 1957; Aring, 1958; Becker *et al.*, 1961; Blumgart, 1964). This stance of emotional detachment has been called *clinical distance* or *detached concern*. William Osler explored this issue when he wrote that physicians should adopt a "judicious measure of obtuseness" by which they become relatively "insensible" to the slings and arrows of involvement with patients. He called this ability *aequanimitas,* the virtue by which physicians maintain the inner calmness required in their work (Osler, 1932).

Why is emotional detachment thought to be necessary? For two reasons; first, it protects the physician from being overwhelmed by his patients' pain and suffering. The layperson who faints at the sight of blood becomes an accomplished surgeon at least in part by learning to "disconnect" from the emotional side of the experience. Perhaps in this context "barrier" is a better metaphor. While physicians are physically close to their patients, they must (metaphorically) wear protective clothing, gowns and masks, to shield themselves from emotion. This barrier begins in gross anatomy laboratory and develops over many years of socialization in the culture of medicine. The second reason for detachment is to protect the patient. Medical decisions ought to be objective and not influenced by feelings and biases. An emotional response may lead to biases in clinical judgment that compromise patient care.

Despite the emphasis on detachment, there is virtually universal agreement that physicians ought to be compassionate, develop good rapport with patients, cultivate bedside manner, and demonstrate "the art of medicine." An abstract motivation for doing good is not sufficient; physicians ought in addition to be concerned about their patients as individuals. In order to connect with patients, the emotional barrier must also be porous and the distance amenable to bridging.

Rather than pairing the terms *detachment* and *concern* to describe the physician's professional stance, I prefer to borrow the words *steadiness* and *tenderness* from Thomas Percival. In his *Medical Ethics* (1803), this British Enlightenment physician discussed the tension between objectivity and subjectivity in medicine when he enjoined physicians to "unite tenderness with steadiness" in their care of patients. Under "steadiness" Percival included the intellectual virtue of objectivity or reason, along with the moral virtue of courage or fortitude. By "tenderness" he meant humanity, compassion, fellow-feeling, and sympathy. These are sentiments, moral virtues, and, to use more contemporary terminology, complex emotional attitudes. In another place, Percival contrasted the "coldness of heart" that often develops in practitioners who do not cultivate these virtues with the "tender charity" the moral practice of medicine requires. The ability to combine tenderness and steadiness in physician–patient interactions requires *emotional resilience*, rather than emotional numbness.

Fortunately, in Case 4-2, T. P.'s practice situation did not allow him to become detached. Whatever he learned in medical school about keeping his distance was soon forgotten. He fully experienced his emotions and those of his patients. Thus, he was faced with the necessity of developing an emotional resilience that would allow him to practice objectively, while still being open to the subjective component of each interaction.

CASE 4-3

S. R. is a 40-year-old oncologist who belongs to a small group practice in a medium-sized Midwestern city. S. R. also directs the Cancer Center at the local hospital. He is known in the medical community as a very aggressive physician who takes pride in saying that he never gives up on a patient. When a patient dies he considers it a personal defeat. He frequently speaks up in support of concepts like palliative care and hospice, but in practice he rarely uses them because he is convinced that his patients are "fighters" who want a "full court press." S. R.'s medical colleagues are divided in their assessment of his practice style. Some like to refer patients to him because they know he provides the most aggressive and up-to-date chemotherapy available. Others are concerned because of his reputation as an aggressive, no-nonsense physician who focuses "too much on the tumor, too little on the patient."

BENEVOLENCE, COMPASSION, CARING

The relief of suffering is a fundamental goal of medicine. The ability to implement this goal by prolonging life is a relatively new phenomenon. Throughout most of history, physicians didn't have the tools to cure disease or prolong life, except perhaps in a few surgical situations, e.g., amputation of a gangrenous limb. Medical practice has always been focused on caring, even though curing is a recent benefit. In this context the oft-cited dichotomy between *caring* and *curing* makes little historical sense. Nowadays, some writers contrast the professions of nursing (caring) and medicine (curing) in just this way. This description is perhaps understandable in that medicine has *added* curing to caring. Nonetheless, caring is a prerequisite for medicine or any healing profession.

The term *care* is used in two ways. Its external dimension consists of the sequence of things physicians do for patients, the aggregate of professional services they perform. In this sense care is a list of items or behaviors. "He received the best medical care" often means he received everything the latest technology had to offer. The internal dimension of care, on the other hand, is the personal quality or emotional attribute that motivates the physician to perform the services in the first place. Another word for this internal aspect of care is *compassion*. People who choose to become physicians do so in large part because of a general commitment to help others (benevolence), but they are unlikely to be satisfied with medicine in the long run unless they also have compassion for individual suffering people, many of whom are bothersome, unpleasant, or even downright unlikable.

A third-year medical student on her obstetrics clerkship recently presented to me the case of a 23-year-old pregnant diabetic woman who smoked crack cocaine two to four times daily. The patient had been admitted to the hospital for aggressive insulin management, but was very hostile to the staff and eventually left against medical advice. She had abused and abandoned her first two children, who had subsequently been taken by Child Protective Services. When the student had tried to convince this patient to remain in the hospital, she was rebuffed and insulted. "Why should I be empathetic in a case like this?" the student asked. "This woman doesn't even care about her own children." I explained that she shouldn't confuse empathy and compassion with liking. Empathy is simply the attempt to understand her; compassion, the energy that drives the attempt. It may not be possible to "get through" to this particular patient, but the attempt should be made regardless of like or dislike.

The psychologist Carl Rogers listed three attributes he believed essential in any healing relationship. These therapeutic core qualities include empathy (already discussed), genuineness or honesty (discussed in the next section), and unconditional positive regard (Rogers, 1961). Positive regard is the ability to suspend your moral or personal judgment about the patient's behavior, to set aside your negative feelings (if you have some) and work in the patient's best interests. Positive regard is a function of compassion, based on an understanding of human connectedness: We are all ultimately in the same boat, we all make mistakes, we are all in need of help. Compassion like any virtue can grow or diminish over time. Physicians become more compassionate by practicing empathy and trying to do the best job they can. Alternatively, compassion can be largely "snuffed out" if external stress, the emergence of other priorities, or professional burnout lead the physician to approach patients as objects, rather than subjects.

In Case 4-3, something went wrong with S. R. Instead of caring for his patients, he seems to be marching to a different drummer. His approach to medicine could be characterized by a military metaphor: Disease is the enemy, the physician is a warrior, the goal of medicine is to fight and conquer disease. We use a number of different metaphors or models in describing the physician–patient relationship. Robert Veatch, for example, has written of the *priestly model,* in which the physician controls the access to beneficial power, while the patient has no say and is kept in the dark, and the *engineering model*, in which the physician acts like a technician or engineer, while the patient is simply a broken machine (Veatch, 1972).

William May has described the metaphors of physician as parent, fighter, technician, and teacher (May, 1983). Each metaphor implies a different type of relationship. If the physician is a parent, for example, patients must be children. This implies a benevolent despot who acts in the patient's best interest without consulting the patient, or even against his wishes (*paternalism*), much the same as in Veatch's priestly metaphor.

The military metaphor is a particularly popular one today. Witness the "war against cancer" and our frequent characterization (as in Case 4-3) of good patients as "fighters." When S. R.'s colleagues comment that "he treats all his patients aggressively," many of them, at least, are paying him a compliment. Or at least a mixed compliment. We use the word *aggressive* frequently. Aggressive in tumors means bad, but in physicians it generally means good. We train physicians to fight, to hold on, never to yield. "Don't back down," we tell our students, "treat your patients aggressively. Take risks. Push to the limit. You must often inflict new damage—incisions, tubes, toxic medications—to conquer your patient's disease and alleviate his pain." Unfortunately, if disease is the enemy and the physician is a warrior, the patient, to continue the metaphor, tends to be thought of as a battlefield rather than a person.

Sometimes we admire aggressiveness in physicians even when, as in Case 4-3, it conflicts with other important values, like compassion or honesty. Naked aggression would make more sense, of course, if medicine were literally a war. In some cultures, the warrior role is, in fact, almost literal. Shamans in Central Asia believe that most serious illness is caused by spirit possession. To cure the patient the healer must fight the spirit and vanquish it. Likewise, Navajo Singers (*haatali*) believe that some sickness is caused by soul loss. In these cases the medicine men are obliged to wrestle with dark powers in order to restore their patients' souls. For these traditional healers, medicine is a perilous enterprise that puts them at personal risk. If they prove weaker than their opponent, they might be injured or destroyed. Interestingly, there is also a threat of injury in scientific medicine: The aggressiveness and emotional distance of the war metaphor can lead physician-warriors toward the cycle of professional stress, abuse of power, and burnout.

Each of these metaphors sheds some light on the physician–patient relationship, but also casts a shadow. While capturing one characteristic of illness or healing, each fails to account for other features. Perhaps we need several such images to sketch the whole truth about medicine. However, some metaphors are far more useful than others. In particular, those that capture basic medical values like empathy, care, and compassion, e.g., physician as parent, friend, or teacher, ought to be emphasized more than those that embody less humane values, e.g., physician as warrior or technician. Veatch (1972) characterizes the ideal physician–patient relationship as a *contract model,* while May (1975) uses the term *physician's covenant.** Both of these are grounded in compassion and respect. Both specify duties far more complex than winning a war. S. R. might have chosen a career in oncology because he wanted to "beat" cancer, but he needs to learn that aggression is justified only in the service of compassion.

CASE 4-4

L. C. is taking care of an elderly patient with multiple medical problems, including a stroke that left her with right-sided paralysis and aortic stenosis, i.e., narrowing

---

*May contrasts "covenant" with "contract," stressing the connotation of gift and indebtedness in the former. To him "contract" exemplifies the marketplace. On the other hand, Veatch uses the marriage contract as an example of a contract that is really a covenant. To him the two models are similar. This controversy is important here only in that both writers stress the donative and fiduciary nature of the relationship.

of the aortic valve in her heart. She begins to complain of fatigue and shortness of breath. L. C. examines her two or three times over a period of several weeks and orders some diagnostic tests. The findings on physical examination, as well as the results of an echocardiogram, convince her that the patient's symptoms are the result of severe depression, precipitated by her stroke. She tells the patient and her family that the heart problem is not responsible. Despite antidepressant treatment, the patient continues to get worse and winds up in the Emergency Department where the cardiology consultant concludes that she has "critical" and life-threatening aortic stenosis. This could have been diagnosed and treated several weeks ago, but L. C. simply made a mistake.

PRACTICAL JUDGMENT, HUMILITY, HONESTY

Problem solving is part of the joy of medicine. Physicians are blessed almost every day with the personal and intellectual satisfaction that comes from helping to solve significant human problems. No wonder medical school applicants say that the intellectual stimulation of medicine is one of the profession's most attractive features. Among practicing physicians, the satisfaction of solving medical problems is one of the major motivations for a medical career (Schwenk *et al.*, 1989). It is exhilarating to make an obscure diagnosis or to discover that your patient has the classic findings of a disease you just read about. In fact, some students believe that generalist practice must be less stimulating than subspecialty practice because the latter provides more intellectual challenge by "going deeper" into a specific field. The generalist, this line of reasoning goes, doesn't have any really interesting cardiac or GI patients; only a cardiologist or gastroenterologist is equipped to manage them. This, however, is a misconception on two accounts. First, patients with complex medical problems probably have more need for a primary care physician than patients with minor complaints because they need someone to coordinate their care and help them focus on maintaining function and a healthy perspective. Second, primary care, perhaps counterintuitively, can be more stimulating than a subspecialty because the human problems that patients present in ordinary practice are often more difficult, and certainly every bit as challenging, as diseases dealt with by subspecialists.

The flip side of a profession that revels in problem solving is uncertainty. All diagnostic and therapeutic decisions are, in a sense, experiments. As we evaluate patients we formulate hypotheses, refine the hypotheses, test them, and try to confirm them by seeing what happens when we embark on a certain course of action. While we may take into consideration benefits, risks, probabilities, clinical experience, pathophysiological knowledge, and opinions of experts and peers, medical decisions are still based on hypotheses. These may at times be very well supported, but they are still not certain. Is disease X really causing the patient's symptoms? Will medication Y really help relieve the symptoms? Learning to accept and work within uncertainty is a major part of the physician's professional education. Expert knowledge about a particular disease or specialty is not enough. Sound *clinical judgment* also requires a logical, empathic, and honest approach to decision making within a framework of uncertainty.

Renee Fox distinguished three types of uncertainty in medicine: the physician's incomplete mastery of available knowledge, inadequacy of the state of the art itself, and uncertainty of where the boundary lies between the two (Fox, 1957). L. C., in Case 4-4, relied on an imperfect test, the echocardiogram, in deciding that her patient's symptoms were more related to depression than to aortic stenosis. Is that a state-of-the-art error or a culpable mistake? Should she have pursued another test or consulted a cardiologist? In a case like this it is difficult to know the answers; you can always second-guess when a bad result occurs. The important issue here, however, is to understand that physicians have to learn to deal with their mistakes.

Because misjudgments and mistakes are inevitable in medicine, *humility* (or self-acceptance) and *honesty* are especially important character traits. When we talk about honesty in medical ethics, it is usually with reference to how much to tell our patients. How do we tell patients "the bad news"? When should we withhold information? Should we ever lie to patients? Such discussions are grounded in the tension between our respect for autonomy and the, usually wrong, perception that sometimes truthfulness may not be in the patient's best interest. However, honesty with oneself precedes honesty with patients. Self-delusion is rampant everywhere, but physicians are perhaps particularly vulnerable for a variety of reasons. Our motives are noble; our mistakes, after all, are usually made in the interest of helping others. We carry high responsibilities and work long hours—again in the interest of our patients. Society looks to us as authorities and pays us lots of money and high respect. Thus, it is easy to fall into the comforting delusion that our decisions are always justified and our errors minimal.

In Case 4-4, L. C.'s misjudgment as to the importance of her patient's aortic stenosis was an understandable mistake. After all, the clinical findings were conflicting. The echocardiogram suggested that the aortic valve narrowing was not as severe as it ultimately turned out to be. Yet, the patient was harmed. Could L. C. have done better? Perhaps so, perhaps not. Regardless, it is essential that she accept responsibility for making the misjudgment. In his 1905 valedictory address to the medical students at McGill University, William Osler said, "Learn to play the game fair, no self-deception, no shrinking from the truth; mercy and consideration for the other man, but none for yourself, upon whom you have to keep an incessant watch" (Osler, 1932).

Honesty with oneself leads as night and day to humility or *self-acceptance*. John F. Christensen *et al.* (1992) recently published a study of physician mistakes under the perceptive title, "The Heart of Darkness: The Impact of Perceived Mistakes on Physicians." These investigators interviewed 11 community hospital physicians about errors they had made in caring for patients. These physicians reported two main strategies for coping with mistakes. One was problem-focused: They used the opportunity to obtain new knowledge and learn from the mistake. The second strategy was emotion-focused: They shared their feelings with their spouses, colleagues, or sometimes the patients involved. Being truthful with the patient or family was a particularly helpful way of dealing with the mistake, although the process itself was extremely anxiety-provoking. While this emotion-focused strategy was seen as beneficial, the physicians complained that there was too little support for it in medicine. Peer review structures, like Morbidity and Mortality Conferences, tend to be solely problem-focused. Colleagues often tend to minimize feelings or give facile reassurance, rather than thoughtful emotional support. In addition to these specific ways of coping, the investigators also found that physicians who accepted medicine's limited control over illness and acknowledged the inevitability of making mistakes were better able to understand and profit from their own errors.

CASE 4-5

On "ethics rounds" a subintern in medicine presented the case of an HIV patient with Pneumocystis pneumonia just transferred to the MICU. The patient was agitated, delirious, coughing, and gasping for breath. The students on the unit expressed their concern about their own risk of infection. While they used univer-

sal precautions, they were still uncomfortable with the slim chance that they might contract HIV. "After all," one said, "it seems like we're always drawing blood or putting in another tube."

We began to discuss the physician's ethical obligation to treat HIV patients. Our talk soon gravitated to the medical school's policy that students be required to participate in the care of patients suffering from HIV. "Coercive," one of them called this policy. "It infringes on our basic rights," another said. In fact, most of the students believed the policy to be wrong.

"I don't have any problem with treating AIDS patients," one of them said. "I think it's the right thing to do for me, *but you can't* force *someone else to treat a patient if she doesn't want to."*

"There's too much risk," another claimed. "It's an individual decision. Every doctor has the right to treat or not treat whomever he pleases."

DISCIPLINE, FIDELITY, COURAGE

While the HIV epidemic has led to a reexamination of fidelity and courage in medicine (Daniels, 1991), the drama of HIV may in a sense be a "red herring." The exclusive focus on a physician's duty to provide care despite the risk of infection obscures the need for fidelity and courage in all aspects of medical practice. It is true that HIV brings back into focus the profession's ethical tradition that requires heroism in the line of duty. This tradition is reflected in the AMA's Code of Ethics, which requires physicians to discharge their duties without regard to their own safety. History, however, presents us with a more sober and realistic view of physician behavior. Some physicians have acted selflessly and courageously in times of plague; others have fled from danger. Courage, like other virtues, must be viewed in light of competing values. It seems unreasonable to hold that physicians are morally required to take great risks for their patients, thereby sacrificing their own lives and harming their loved ones. On the other hand, fidelity to our patients, in the case of already established relationships, and fidelity to the profession itself, in the case of sick people who have no physician, demand that we take smaller degrees of risk as part of our professional obligation. The risk of infection with communicable diseases, like tuberculosis and hepatitis B, is an expected and reasonable occupational hazard.

The emergence of HIV made risk to health workers highly visible because of HIV's mysterious (at least, initially) and fatal nature. Nonetheless, the probability of patient-to-physician transmission through fingerstick or mucosal contamination is very low, especially with the use of universal precautions. There is now a wide consensus that the level of risk in caring for HIV patients is well within the reasonable range, even for surgeons. Therefore, physicians have a duty not to refuse to treat patients on the basis of their HIV status. The medical student in Case 4-5 was wrong: Physicians do not necessarily have the right to treat or not treat whomever they choose (see Daniels, 1991, for a further discussion of this complex topic).

The issue of fidelity to patients and the requirement for courage in medical practice is actually much more pervasive than the risk of communicable diseases. Fidelity means sticking with the patient even when the going gets tough: when treatment isn't working, when the cancer is bound to be fatal, when the patient is angry and demoralized. Fidelity also means serving as the patient's advocate in various interactions with employers, insurance companies, state agencies, and so forth. Sticking with patients through the ordinary ups and downs of illness requires a certain amount of courage, a willingness to put your reputation on the line for the patient. The good physician doesn't hide behind job descriptions or bureaucratic limits when the interests of her patient are at stake. She is willing to dive in and do what she can. This day-to-day courage is far more important to medical practice than is the occasional act of heroism.

CASE 4-6

In the lobby of a University Health Center sat an architectural model of the Center as it will look in the twenty-first century. Beside the model, a group of curious people watched a videotape on which a soothing baritone voice announced that he is about to reveal "tomorrow's medicine today." The model showed existing buildings in dull gray, but demonstrated the future in various brighter colors: a basic science building anchored in the clouds, a magnificent new patient care tower, an extraordinary subterranean parking facility. The hypnotic voice described dramatic achievements in organ transplantation and nuclear magnetic resonance, new ways of treating cancer by "enhancing the body's own immune response," comprehensive programs in sports medicine and in geriatric care. The tape showed physicians, nurses, and technicians going about their serious business with very serious expressions. A radiologist stared mournfully at an impressive machine. A nurse frowned at an IV infusion pump.

As medical students and house officers passed through the lobby, they frequently stopped to joke about this heavy-handed promotion film. For weeks the elevators were full of humorous comments about their friends and professors shown on the tape, and about the aura of pomposity and self-importance the tape conveyed.

PLAYFULNESS, HUMOR, CREATIVITY

Physicians have always tried to balance the heavier aspects of their work with humor and lightness. Hippocrates, for example, wrote about the importance of a serious and respectable mien, but also that physicians should be witty, because "dourness is repulsive both to the healthy and to the sick."

Even in these days of dramatic change in the profession, surveys show that the great majority of physicians enjoy their work and characterize it as "fun." The media, of course, portray medicine as an extremely serious business, indeed: a constant treadmill of life-and-death decisions, a volatile mix of fatigue and principle, emotion and science. No wonder physicians might be tempted to take themselves too seriously and become humorless and self-important.

One type of humor often encountered in medicine is *gallows humor*, the pervasive joking we do about the ugliness and pain of clinical situations. Joking about one patient's horrible wound or another patient's bad breath is a type of defense mechanism. Professional distance allows us, at least momentarily, to defuse our own bad feelings by objectifying patients and making light of them. Gallows humor tends to be indiscriminate, however. We sometimes poke fun at our teachers, colleagues, and subordinates as well. The emotional intensity of medical training, combined with long hours and chronic fatigue, promotes this type of defense—sharp, sarcastic wit as a way of coping with one's feelings, thereby avoiding having to "feel" them. The problem with gallows humor is that it can become a pernicious habit, rather than just an occasional emotional outlet. If used extensively, it can lead to permanent detachment and emotional numbness.

A more healthy type of humor is based on empathy and compassion. Medical practice makes us privy to more human foibles and personal stories than are encountered in most other professions. One of its biggest lessons is, or ought to be, that we are all basically in the same boat: "There, but for the grace of God, go I." Humor based on this understanding is gentle, rather than sarcastic; it tends to connect us, rather than separating us. Yet it still serves the helpful function of looking obliquely, rather than directly, at our pain, anger, anxiety, or sadness, thereby helping us to cope with these feelings. Case 4-6 illustrates another form of humor. The young physicians enjoyed making light of the fundraising tape because they well understood how fallible the Health Center's professionals were and had little patience with the air of omnipotence the tape conveyed. They turned the discrepancy between their real life knowledge of medicine and the tape's pomposity into a fertile source of humor. Not taking oneself too seriously is an important habit for physicians to acquire.

CASE 4-7

The Chief of Medicine at a world-renowned Medical Center was held in great awe by the medical community at large, but he was despised and feared by his nurses, medical students, and house officers. He commonly harassed, exploited, and humiliated them on daily rounds. In some cases he would tell students that they shouldn't become physicians because they were too "ignorant" or "unobservant." His temper was legendary, leading him, at times, to throw patient charts to the floor and stomp out of rounds when someone had forgotten an important laboratory value. It was well known that when the Chief himself made mistakes, he generally blamed them—often in public—on his assistants. Interestingly, former students and residents sometimes look back on their time with the Chief and romanticize it; they tend to visualize him as a hero of the days when medicine was stronger and more rigorous than it is today.

THE PHYSICIAN'S POWER

The relationship between physicians and patients has traditionally been viewed as benign and caring, a fiduciary relationship in which a stronger, more knowledgeable party (the physician) agrees to provide medical assistance to a weaker, more vulnerable party (the patient). More contemporary models of the patient–physician relationship stress reduction of the power imbalance by means of joint decision making, patient education, and informed consent. In today's prevalent marketplace metaphor, the physician becomes simply a "provider" who puts a certain type of service on the market; the patient is a "consumer" of this service. A related metaphor considers the physician to be a technician or engineer who provides technical assistance according to the patient's specifications. It is true that enhancing the patient's power, particularly the right to make informed choices about treatment, has been an extremely important development in U.S. medicine over the last 40 years. Yet this development should not obscure the fact that physicians continue to wield tremendous power and that, in fact, there is an intrinsic imbalance of power between physician and patient (Brody, 1992).

In *The Healer's Power* Howard Brody considers three types of medical power (Brody, 1992, pp. 16–17). The first is the *Aesculapian* power that physicians have by virtue of their knowledge and training. This is the impersonal content of medicine, the knowledge and skills peculiar to the profession. A second type is the *charismatic* power that physicians wield based on their personal qualities and interpersonal skills. Characteristics like empathy, compassion, fidelity, honesty, courage, and practical judgment contribute to this type of authority. Comments like "He has a wonderful bedside manner!" or "She has truly mastered the art of medicine!" reflect one's charismatic power. Finally, physicians have enormous *social* or *cultural* power. Part of this arises from the fact that society gives the medical profession authority to determine what counts as illness and medical disability. Illness exempts people from certain social obligations and gives them access to benefits. In turn, the ill person is expected to act in specified ways, e.g., follow the physician's orders, try to get better, and the like. Thus, physicians hold the power to determine whether a patient's experience or behavior constitutes "illness," rather than, for example, laziness, cheating, or moral failure. This social power generally leads to high prestige and socioeconomic status. It also has a spillover effect in that physicians' opinions in nonmedical areas like education, social welfare, and politics tend to be weighted more heavily than they deserve.

Power in the physician–patient relationship can be viewed as a drama in which "the extraordinary power of sickness to make patients susceptible to change at all levels of the human condition is matched by the equal power of this benevolent relationship with its unseen but powerful connection" (Cassell, 1991, p. 73). Thus, the physician's power is necessary to combat (note the war metaphor) the enemy and to strengthen the weakened victim. Power should be used solely for these purposes. However, the physician's power may also be abused. One type of abuse is when physicians use social power to gratify their own emotional needs. In Case 4-7 the Chief of Medicine, a narcissistic, emotionally immature man, was abusing his position in the social system of the profession itself. He typically enhanced his own sense of self-worth by attacking and diminishing those under his professional control. Unfortunately, the socialization process in medicine during the middle part of the twentieth century tended to foster this pattern. Medical education was, and is still, hierarchical in nature; trainees were expected to work long hours with little immediate reward, except for the privilege of working with certain "great" clinicians, and these senior clinicians had often devoted their lives to climbing the ladder in a medical social system that gave them few emotional outlets. As physicians were socialized into the "culture of medicine," they began to excuse the Chief's behavior as an example of necessary rigor. They reinterpreted the past as not-so-bad because it was, after all, *their* past and they turned out to be good clinicians. Future physicians, they reasoned, would benefit by passing through the same type of initiation.

CASE 4-8

A surgical subspecialist saw large numbers of patients for whom he regularly prescribed narcotics, barbiturates, and benzodiazepines in large quantities. One morphine-addicted nurse had gone to him for years as her primary care physician. After completing a detoxification program, she admitted that many years previously she had learned from her classmates in nursing school that this physician would prescribe whatever was requested. In return for yielding to his sexual advances, he had been providing her with morphine and diazepam for more than a dozen years.

This case of a surgeon who sold narcotics prescriptions and sexually exploited his patient illustrates egregious abuse of power in the physician–patient relationship. The surgeon's state-regulated authority to prescribe controlled substances (Aesculapian power) allowed him to engage in the profitable exercise of selling prescriptions for narcotics and other psychotropic drugs. In this he betrayed his professional commitment to prescribe only "that method of treatment which, according to my ability and judgment, I consider for the benefit of the patient" (Hippocratic oath). Moreover, he may well have used his personal charisma and the social power of his position to manipulate this particular patient and others like her.

This case also raises the issue of intimacy and *boundaries* in the physician–patient relationship. How close a personal relationship may we as physicians develop with our patients? In some cases we may feel sexually attracted to patients. Strong transference may lead patients to feel especially attracted to their physicians. Though the American Academy of Psychiatry strongly condemns the practice, surveys have shown that 5% or more of psychiatrists admit to having had sexual relations with patients. While sexual intercourse between patients and physicians has been discussed most openly in psychiatry, it certainly can, and does, occur in all fields of medicine. Physicians who engage in this type of behavior have tried to justify it in one of two ways. Some argue that the sexual relationship is therapeutic for the patient. This implies that the physician is sufficiently in control (i.e., powerful) to use his or her sexual urge as an instrument. Thus, the physician's claim that he or she is trying to help the patient is simply an appeal to medical power. In fact, the physician is preying on the patient's vulnerability and gratitude.

The second type of justification is an appeal to love: The physician is, in fact, in love with the patient; the patient, in love with the physician. This assertion of love, insofar as it can be separated truthfully from the imbalance of power issue, goes counter to the heart of the physician–patient relationship. Physicians must maintain objectivity, despite their closeness and connection to patients. Earlier in the chapter I rejected the term "detached concern" because it suggests *emotional numbness* rather than the *emotional resilience* that is required for good patient care. I suggested rather that we use more heartfelt, less sanitized words to describe the physician's professional stance: the balancing of steadiness with tenderness. Steadiness is essential for objective decision making. Intimate personal relationships with patients undermine steadiness and impair medical care. Thus, physicians typically ought not to provide medical care for their own parents, spouses, and children. Of course, the level of steadiness required, and therefore the appropriateness of treating family members, depends on how much is at stake in the given situation. Thus, a pediatrician treating his child for an ear infection is far different from a husband treating his wife for multiple sclerosis. Because the need for objectivity in clinical judgment precludes intimate relations, the claim that sex with patients is justified because of "love" is either self-delusion or indicates willingness to enter a situation in which objective decision making will be impaired.

CASE 4-9

Dr. F. D. and her colleagues in Sunnydale Internal Medicine Associates are considering whether they should enroll as participating physicians in EconoCare, a for-profit managed care organization in their state. Managed care is rapidly growing in their area. If Sunnydale Internal Medicine Associates does not partici-

pate, the group may well lose a large portion of its patients. In reviewing the contract, Dr. F. D. notes that it includes a requirement that participating physicians agree not to reveal to their patients any disagreements they might have with EconoCare policy, or to recommend therapeutic options that are not covered by EconoCare. Dr. F. D. believes that such "gag rules" are unethical and recommends that the group not join, unless EconoCare is willing to change the contract language.

CONFLICTS OF INTEREST

Professional conflicts of interest arise in medicine, first, because the patient's and physician's interests are not identical, and, second, because medicine is a social system in which many other parties play a role: employers, insurance companies, governmental agencies, and so forth. Many people today have a romantic idea that the physician–patient relationship in the past was free of such conflicts. Not so. However, the "business" of medicine and conflicting professional obligations are more visible now than they were in the past because health professions are more complex and their impact on society greater. I want here to sketch three foci of potential professional conflict: managed care arrangements, where financial incentives may cause physicians to offer less than optimal care; defensive medicine; and ownership of health facilities and defensive medicine, where financial incentives may cause physicians to provide unnecessary care.

MANAGED CARE, HMOs

We tend to think that in the traditional physician–patient relationship, as exemplified by fee-for-service private practice, the physician acted solely in the patient's best interest, while submerging her own needs and desires. The subsequent availability of health insurance brought a third party into this relationship. Until recently this third party was largely a facilitator and passive observer, providing reimbursement for services the physician ordered. Neither the patient nor the physician had to worry much about money; the patient obtained needed care, and the physician was paid for services rendered. In such a setting it was inevitable that "more" would tend to be "better." These dynamics led to unnecessary surgery and overutilization of services (Franks *et al.*, 1992). Such overutilization represents a type of conflict of interest that we don't usually consider: patients systematically exposed to excess risks and costs. These errors of commission are often just as damaging to the patient's interest as errors of omission.

The pressing need for cost control has dramatically changed the role of the third party. In *managed care* arrangements, the health insurer decides which services are justified in a given setting and restricts access to specialty referral and testing. With regard to financing, a specific amount may be paid to the physician during a set time period. Additionally, the generalist physician returned to center stage as the coordinator of care because patients usually have to obtain approval from their primary physician prior to receiving specialty services. Ideally, the primary care physician provides patients with services that range from prevention and health promotion through the management of most acute and chronic problems. This system is more rational, efficient, and cost-effective than an open market in which people choose specialist physicians according to the symptoms they develop. Yet, the strengths of managed care can also be seen as at one another.

The "management" in managed care limits the patient's autonomy in choosing providers. In practice, the primary physician becomes a *gatekeeper*, who at times is forced to take an antagonistic role when patients request medically unwarranted services or referrals. In fact, some HMOs provide monetary incentives for primary care physicians *not* to refer to specialists, thereby introducing a financial conflict of interest with patients. Managed care arrangements also limit physician autonomy. They can only refer to certain specialists, for example. Case 4-9 illustrates one particularly unethical requirement that some managed care organizations have used to restrict physician autonomy. In this case, the physician clearly becomes an agent of the corporate entity, required to conceal from patients relevant information about therapeutic options.

Physicians in HMOs may have patient visit quotas and other restraints. Compared with those in private practice, primary care physicians in HMOs report having less time to spend with individual patients and less freedom to control their own work schedules (Baker & Cantor, 1993). Yet, thus far, perhaps because of voluntary job selection, there is little or no reported difference in career satisfaction between physicians in traditional fee-for-service and managed care settings (Baker & Cantor, 1993).

The essential point is that managed care does not necessarily conflict with good patient care, nor with physician satisfaction. The physician's duty to be an advocate for her patients doesn't disappear in this new environment. The obligation to provide the best care we can sometimes runs afoul of managed standards. A test or treatment that the physician considers essential may be disallowed by the insurance program. Advocacy then demands that the physician explain the situation to the patient, appeal the decision, and even recommend that the patient obtain the service despite nonapproval. This takes time, energy, and negotiating skill. It may not be the cup of tea for a traditionalist who says, "That's not why I went to medical school." However, solidarity with the patient demands that such skills be developed.

DEFENSIVE MEDICINE

The term *defensive medicine* is usually used to describe a pattern of practice that is strongly influenced by the desire to avoid malpractice liability. Instead of making clinical decisions based solely on benefits and risks to the patient, the physician considers perceived liability risks in the decision-making process. Many studies demonstrate that physicians do, in fact, alter their practices in response to the threat of liability. The emergency medicine physician, for example, may routinely order CT scans on all head injury patients, even if clinical circumstances do not warrant the scan. Similarly, the internist or neurologist may order an MRI on all patients who present with headache, knowing, of course, that the vast majority of such scans are not clinically justified. In one study, internal medicine residents reported "defensive medicine" as the main reason for ordering 8% of laboratory tests and 14% of X rays in their practice (Dewar, 1994). Defensive medicine is thought to be a particular problem in the United States because of the excessive number of malpractice suits. Reynolds and colleagues estimated the total annual cost of defensive medicine in the United States to be about $10 billion (1984–1995 data), representing nearly 11% of expenditures of physician services (Reynolds *et al.*, 1987).

Defensive medicine constitutes a professional conflict of interest because it leads physicians to compromise their patients' best interests because of liability risk to themselves. Malpractice liability is discussed more thoroughly in Chapter 17, "Reducing Malpractice Risk," of *Introduction to Clinical Skills: A Patient-Centered Textbook*. Here, however, I want to make three points about defensive medicine as it relates to the psychology and phenomenology of medical practice. First, the specter of liability is not always a negative influence. So-called "defensive" measures may sometimes improve the quality of medical practice. For example, in some studies physicians report spending more time with patients, hiring more office staff, and obtaining more complete informed consent because of the threat of malpractice liability (Dewar, 1994). Whatever the initial motivation for adopting these measures, it seems likely that they may result in better patient care. Medicine is no longer a solitary profession in which practitioners practice independently, assured of noninterference by colleagues or the state. Peer review and other quality-control measures are now the norm. In the United States the pervasive fear of malpractice appears to serve as a mechanism of social control that in some ways enhances and in other ways works to the detriment of patient care.

Second, fear of liability is only one of several factors that contribute to the overuse of laboratory tests and therapeutic interventions. Surveys in Britain and The Netherlands, where malpractice litigation is far less frequent than in the United States, have demonstrated similar patterns of overutilization (Dewar, 1994; Veldhuis, 1994). In these studies, fear of peer disapproval, physician discomfort with medical uncertainty, absence of clear guidelines for appropriate care, and a tendency to adhere to the "technological imperative," i.e., the availability of a new technique tends to make its use appear desirable, were all listed as factors contributing to overutilization.

Physicians have an emotional commitment to action. They are often tempted to act even in situations when they know, or ought to know, that simply watching and waiting would most benefit the patient. Similarly, while the probability of reducing medical uncertainty by performing a certain test might be very small, the *desire* to reduce uncertainty is often great enough to cloud a physician's probabilistic reasoning. For this reason *errors of commission* in medicine have typically been considered less blameworthy than *errors of omission*. The resident knows that if she performs an unnecessary bone marrow on a patient with mild anemia she is less likely to be humiliated at Morning Report than if she fails to perform the bone marrow when the Chief of Medicine actually thinks it was indicated. Physicians often talk of ordering certain tests "for completeness's sake." A right upper quadrant ultrasound may confirm the physician's clinical impression of cholelithiasis, but the physician may also order an abdominal CT scan, just in case. While the first test explains the clinical findings, the second is performed solely for completeness's sake. For these reasons, defensive medicine is, in fact, synergistic with the medical tendency to err on the side of doing too much.

Third, good physician–patient interaction is, in fact, the best defensive medicine. For some years now malpractice insurers have sponsored seminars for physicians on how to reduce their risk of being sued. A major reason for these seminars is to improve physician communication skills. An empathic, compassionate approach with good interactive techniques leads to better diagnosis and therapy. This approach also enhances patient satisfaction. Satisfied patients generally do not bring malpractice suits against their physicians. In fact, if an adverse outcome of care occurs, the strongest predictor of a malpractice action being brought against the physician is a preexisting poor physician–patient relationship (Beckman *et al.*, 1994; Vincent *et al.*, 1994).

Dr. Mark Korsakoff is a neurologist on the medical staff of your hospital. Last year he assumed a large debt when he joined several other physicians in purchasing an MRI machine and establishing a new diagnostic center (Health Scan, Inc.) near Suburban Mall. Health Scan initiated a major advertising campaign including frequent commercials on local television stations. Consumers were urged to contact Health Scan ("where we offer you the most advanced new scanning equipment") if they had headaches, injury, joint pain, or other persistent symptoms. The enterprise has been very successful, so successful in fact that the hospital administrator, Mr. R. Tape, complained that Health Scan was siphoning off patients and reducing the volume of MRI use at the hospital's diagnostic facility. You are aware that some of the medical staff are unhappy with Korsakoff and a little envious because of his glittering financial success.

DIAGNOSTIC FACILITIES

While physicians who work in HMOs and other institutional settings may experience pressures to underutilize medical services, physician entrepreneurs who own diagnostic and other medical facilities tend to overutilize services by too frequent referral of patients for tests or procedures. This type of conflict of interest may seem at first to compromise patient care less than practice arrangements that promote fewer referrals and less testing. After all, here the error, if there is one, lies on the side of being more careful and doing tests "just in case," even if they are not technically indicated.

Many studies, however, have shown that physicians who own facilities overutilize them. The AMA's Council for Health Policy found that approximately 10% of physicians in the United States have ownership interests in diagnostic laboratories, hospitals, nursing homes, or other facilities that might involve self-referral. Moreover, for important classes of services, "patients of physicians who self-refer have higher utilization rates than other patients" (Council on Ethical and Judicial Affairs, 1992). For example, self-referring physicians sent patients to obtain laboratory testing at a 45% higher rate than other physicians. Another study concluded that physicians with a financial interest in imaging facilities referred patients for diagnostic studies 4.0 to 4.5 times more frequently than did other physicians (Hillman *et al.*, 1990).

As a result of such studies, the AMA's Council on Ethical and Judicial Affairs recommended in 1992 that "physicians should not refer patients to a health care facility outside their office practice at which they do not directly provide care or services when they have an investment interest in the facility." The main exception to this recommendation is in cases where "there is a demonstrated need in the community for the facility and alternative financing is not available." The bottom line is that, consciously or unconsciously, financial self-interest conflicts with patient interest in these situations. Thus, self-referral at the very least gives the appearance of impropriety; at worst it is a blatantly unethical practice. The federal government has accepted this professional judgment by creating Medicare regulations against referral to self-owned facilities.

In Case 4-10 Health Scan, Inc. was in the MRI business to make money. There is nothing in the case to suggest that the hospital's scanning facilities were overburdened, inadequate, or inconvenient to patients. As a neurologist, Dr. Korsakoff would naturally refer many patients for MRI studies. The decision about whether or not to get an MRI for a patient with headaches or dizziness is a complex one; different neurologists might decide differently. Nonetheless, data indicate that physicians like Korsakoff who own such facilities order many more MRIs than other physicians.

CASE 4-11

Dr. A. T. has practiced oncology in a small northeastern city for 20 years. He initially belonged to a small group practice, but has been working on his own for the last 5 years. Dr. A. T. is well known for his aggressive approach to treatment, his commitment to patients, and his willingness to teach medical students from State University. He has always prided himself in the ability to work 16 hours a day for the benefit of his patients. Since his divorce 6 years ago, Dr. A. T. has had little contact with his three children because they moved with their mother to another city. Dr. A. T. used to be active in various church groups, but no longer finds the time to get involved. In fact, his friends have been worried about him for the last couple of years. To them, he seems tired, irritable, distant, and somewhat depressed. Newer members of the hospital staff have never seen the optimistic and energetic man A. T. used to be.

SATISFACTION, PROFESSIONAL STRESS, AND BURNOUT

There are two paradoxes in the U.S. folk image of the kindly general practitioner who loved his profession, worked long hours, was permanently on-call, and became the town's font of humane wisdom. The first has to do with the limits of medical power. During the early twentieth century, physicians had far fewer tools and far less ability to alter the natural history of disease than their 1990s' counterparts. The friendliness, accessibility, wisdom, and moral authority that characterizes our image of general practitioners in the "good old days" contain a healthy mixture of fact and fiction. Nonetheless, the cultural belief that those "old days" were "good" is paradoxical, given their lack of medically effective tools and technology.

The second paradox has to do with the character of the physician himself. Kindly, yet firm. Intensely practical, yet committed to virtue. Accessible at all hours of the day and night. Married to his practice, yet also a family man. Always having the time to share part of himself with patients, friends, or students. From where did this prodigious level of energy come? The truth is that few flesh-and-blood physicians ever really met this cultural standard. Physicians have always had to juggle the stresses of their personal and professional lives, hopefully managing to achieve a satisfactory and healthy outcome.

Some recent surveys indicate that most physicians are satisfied with their work and feel professionally fulfilled (Baker & Cantor, 1993; Chuck *et al.*, 1993). Other surveys reveal more evidence of physician disaffection (Cohen *et al.*, 1990). Nonetheless, in recent years a perception has developed that there is widespread dissatisfaction in the medical community (Glick, 1990; Schroeder, 1992). Physicians have been speaking out, perhaps more than in the past, about their personal and professional concerns: heavy workload, long hours, fatigue, bureaucratic interference, alienation from families and social networks, commercialization of medicine, difficult physician–patient relationships, and the expense and stresses of medical education. More recently, managed care and other arrangements that limit physician autonomy are said to cause high levels of dissatisfaction. In some specialties, oncology and emergency medicine, for example, physicians are highly vulnerable to emotional exhaustion and burnout. Recently, 46% of Canadian emergency physicians reported medium to high levels of emotional exhaustion while feeling low levels of personal accomplishment (Lloyd *et al.*, 1994). In a survey of U.S. oncologists, over half expressed some sense of professional burnout (Whippen & Canellos, 1991). In Case 4-11, one particular oncologist, Dr. A. T., appears to be heading toward burnout, if he is not there already. Long hours, time pressure, and on-call commitment are important stressors in medicine, although the need to maintain medical knowledge and repeated exposure to life-and-death situations also create stress (Richardson & Burke, 1991). Among oncologists the most frequent reason cited for emotional exhaustion was insufficient personal or vacation time. Other factors cited were continuous exposure to fatal illness, frustration with limited therapeutic success, and reimbursement problems.

Some observers argue that internal factors are responsible for most physician dissatisfaction. Among these are a movement in physician motivation away from service and toward self-fulfillment as the primary goal. Glick contends that today's physicians have a greater sense of entitlement than past physicians did, corresponding to the rampant growth of entitlement and "rights" in our culture (Glick, 1990). Moreover, Glick claims that there has been a change in the nature of physician satisfaction that has created dissonance between physicians and patients. The patient simply wants to feel better and to be treated in a personal and supportive way. However, the physician, especially the subspecialist, no longer looks for satisfaction in the give-and-take of human relationships, but wants to achieve disease-oriented goals. This often involves technical matters that are only indirectly of interest to the patient.

While the dynamics that Glick outlines are undoubtedly present in today's medicine, giving service and interacting with people remain sources of great satisfaction for most physicians. Burnout occurs not because people find themselves in the wrong profession, but because they fall into a vicious cycle of internal and external factors that leaves them emotionally exhausted. Figure 4.1 summarizes this cycle. First, physicians have high career expectations. These include both internal (caring, curing, intellectual stimulation) and external (status, financial rewards) goals. To accomplish their goals, physicians expend large amounts of physical and emotional energy. In doing this, they are vulnerable to the five "Ds" of emotional stress: depletion, detachment, depersonalization, denial, and depression. A sense of being drained or depleted first manifests itself in social life. The physician simply doesn't feel that he or she has time to spend with family or friends. Social engagements decrease. There is less energy for personal or social causes. This leads to emotional detachment from family and friends, as well as from patients. In Case 4-11 Dr. A. T. illustrates this continuum. In the process of depersonalization, patients become objects—organs, body parts, or "the gallbladder in room 1017." Because of their high expectations of themselves, physicians are often reluctant to admit that things are not going well for them. While most physicians have learned to cope with mistakes in clinical practice, it is more difficult to admit failure to meet personal goals. The need for objectivity in medicine may also lead to emotional numbness, which creates an internal barrier (denial) to experiencing one's own feelings and personal needs.

Finally, the physician may reach the stage of emotional burnout and depression with diminished social attachments; feelings of inadequacy, cynicism, and victimization; and proneness to disruptive behavior, chemical dependency, depression, and suicide. Because burnout adversely affects professional performance as well, the physician is also more

HIGH CAREER EXPECTATIONS

STRONG MOTIVATION

LONG WORK HOURS

EXPENDITURE OF PHYSICAL AND EMOTIONAL ENERGY

PHYSICIAN BECOMES:

Depleted

Detached

Depersonalized

In Denial

BURNOUT

Reduced social involvement

Feelings of victimization

Feelings of lack of accomplishment

Focus on money and power

Disruptive behavior

High malpractice risk

Figure 4.1. The physician stress and burnout cycle.

vulnerable to malpractice suits. In Case 4-11 Dr. A. T. is irritable, withdrawn, and depressed. What effect has this had on his ability to care for his patients?

Table 4.1 presents a list of risk factors or early signs of emotional distress that lead to burnout. Many of these factors can be summarized by the term *indispensable person syndrome*. Many of the personality characteristics that foster good medicine can also become distorted if not counterbalanced by other qualities. For example, a passion for helping others, the desire always to do a good job, and willingness to accept responsibility are all qualities of a good physician. These can be distorted, however, by the grind of practice into messianic and perfectionist patterns of behavior. The indispensable physician values high achievement, but wants to go it alone. While she can't say "no" to new responsibilities, neither can she rely on others to help her accomplish the work. It is

Table 4.1
Risk Factors for Physician Burnout

95

SATISFACTION,
PROFESSIONAL
STRESS, AND
BURNOUT

Is highly motivated to succeed
Likes to be considered indispensable
Likes to work alone
Has difficulty saying "no"
Chronic sense of work overload
Dislikes accepting help from others
Dislikes delegating responsibility
Dislikes discussing problems
Dislikes discussing feelings
Externalizes blame
Personal identity merges with professional identity
Has little time for family and friends

difficult or impossible to ask for help. Yet the indispensable physician is often angry because she is always giving, while others are always taking.

An important factor in maintaining good professional and personal health is to avoid becoming indispensable. Listen carefully to the advice that *you* typically give to fatigued and harried patients: Be sure to take time for yourself. Enjoy your family. Go on vacations. Develop outside interests. Slow down. Change your schedule so that you have time for exercise and meditation or other relaxation techniques.

Does that advice sound familiar?

CASE 4-12

A. K. was a subintern in surgery at University Hospital. She was on call with S. D., a second-year resident. Unexpectedly, S. D. took advantage of an early evening lull to leave the hospital for a quick dinner. When he returned, the senior resident sent him to speak with Mrs. L., a 70-year-old woman who had been admitted through the emergency room and was scheduled for an exploratory laparotomy the next morning. A. K. accompanied S. D. to the patient's room. She noticed that S. D. had alcohol on his breath. His manner was strangely uninhibited and jocular in dealing with Mrs. L., who appeared agitated and a bit confused. His preop interview and examination were hurried and superficial. When Mrs. L. seemed ambivalent and continued to ask questions he had already answered, S. D. became impatient and said, "Look, you need this goddamn operation. Just sign the forms!" Embarrassed, Mrs. L. signed.

The next day at the operation, A. K. noted that S. D. was subdued, but as far as she could tell, assisted the surgeon quite adequately. However, disturbed by his behavior the night before, A. K. took the opportunity to talk with L. R., another surgical resident, who reported that S. D. graduated near the top of his class in a very competitive medical school. During his internship there had been a story of a driving while intoxicated (DWI) incident, but S. D. simply joked about it. More recently, L. R. had heard that S. D.'s long-time relationship with a woman he had known since medical school broke up in a somewhat violent and disturbing way. She knew no details. His clinical work was generally good, but he was often rather avuncular and distracted on morning rounds.

L. R. suggested that A. K. relate the incident with Mrs. L. to the surgery residency director. A. K. wasn't sure what to do.

AM I MY BROTHER'S KEEPER? THE IMPAIRED PHYSICIAN

There is good evidence in Case 4-12 that S. D. was drinking while on duty (alcohol on his breath), that his performance was significantly impaired (rude and angry behavior), and that he had a history of prior alcohol abuse (driving while intoxicated). When presented with the story of S. D., however, medical students have great difficulty trying to figure out what A. K.'s responsibility is. Part of this difficulty arises from A. K.'s status as a medical student. In the hierarchical field of medicine, persons on lower levels may well believe that they should not take it on themselves to judge the behavior of their higher colleagues. After all, reporting S. D.'s behavior may somehow damage their grade or their chance for a good recommendation. However, this also illustrates a more general concern: Whistle-blowers have a rather ambiguous position in our society. We admire them. We tout their integrity and courage. Yet, there is a second, usually subterranean, perception regarding whistle-blowing. The concept of "telling" on our colleagues or friends is a little repugnant to us, evoking memories of childhood breaches of trust and tattletales. In S. D.'s case the feature that generally tips the balance for students is the observation of alcohol on his breath. This is the "smoking gun" that eventually leads students to say that A. K. should report S. D. to the residency director. Many argue that they would first confront S. D. and give him a chance to seek help voluntarily for his presumed drinking problem. Others defer a personal confrontation because of the power imbalance between A. K. and S. D.

The American Medical Association is unambiguous about a physician's responsibility regarding impaired colleagues: "A physician should expose, without fear or favor, incompetent or corrupt, dishonest or unethical behavior on the part of members of the profession." This statement from the AMA's *Current Opinions of the Judicial Council* (1984) specifies a wide range of impairment, as well as other immoral or unprofessional conduct. Our moral obligation in this regard is based on both (1) individual integrity and commitment to patient welfare and (2) allegiance to the community of professionals to which we belong. In return for the trust and privileges it receives from the community, the medical profession must set and monitor its own standards of professional behavior. Yet, Case 4-12 illustrates the dynamics that have led to a poor record in the medical profession of monitoring incompetence, substance abuse, and unprofessional behavior.

Physicians may become unable to perform their duties for a wide variety of reasons, including disease, mental illness, dementia, and substance abuse. The syndrome of burnout contributes directly because it may be a factor in mental illness, and indirectly through demoralization and lowering of personal standards. The term *impaired physician* is usually used, however, to refer to impairment as a result of substance abuse or chemical dependency. To quote Dr. Richard Blondell, "Without help, physicians who become chemically impaired face the possibility of premature death and may cause harm to their patients. Knowledgeable physician colleagues are the most significant factor in any strategy to prevent these tragic events" (Blondell, 1993).

In the past physicians have often been reluctant to confront and openly challenge their impaired colleagues. This situation is well illustrated in William Carlos Williams's wonderful story "Old Doc Rivers" (Williams, 1984). Doc Rivers is a compassionate, dedicated physician who for 30 years has taken care of anyone in town who needed help, "doing something, mostly the right thing, without delay and of his own initiative. . ." Rivers's patients are "a population in despair, out of hand, out of discipline, believing in the miraculous. . ." Everyone knows, however, that Rivers has a tragic flaw: dope addiction. The narrator of the story (another physician) believes that the addiction arose from Rivers's inability to set limits on pouring himself into the medical work. He thinks that the problem reflects more the flawed world of human suffering than the physician's personal shortcomings. He and the other physicians in town clearly admire Rivers, even though they have serious questions about his behavior. Sometimes, for example, Rivers passes out during operations. The narrator's wife asks, "Why do you doctors not get together and have his license taken away?" But the narrator reflects, "I doubted that we could prove anything. No one wanted to try." In the end Rivers kills a patient by compressing her strangulated hernia, but none of his colleagues reports him. The story demonstrates a mistaken understanding of professional ethics, in which admiration for, and solidarity with, the man outweigh one's duty to help a colleague and prevent harm to his patients.

In chemical dependency, individuals habitually use a mood-altering substance despite adverse consequences. Most authorities believe that the prevalence of such dependency among physicians is roughly the same as in the general population (Centrella, 1994). Some studies suggest, however, that patterns of alcohol and drug use are different in that physicians more frequently abuse controlled drugs like opiates and benzodiazepines because of the opportunity for self-prescription, while less frequently using illegal drugs like cocaine and psychedelics. Overall, the AMA estimates a lifetime prevalence of 6–8% for alcohol abuse and 1–2% for other drug abuse or dependence. Each year about 100 deaths of U.S. physicians are directly attributed to chemical dependency. Certain specialties appear to be at higher risk than others for chemical dependency, including anesthesiology, emergency medicine, psychiatry, and family practice (Centrella, 1994).

Table 4.2 lists a number of risk factors for chemical impairment, as well as signs and symptoms of established dependency. As is the case with other professionals, impaired physicians tend to "protect" their work performance as long as possible, even after family and other personal relationships have suffered. However, because chemical dependency is a progressive disorder, clinical judgment and physician–patient relationships eventually suffer. The fact that professional impairment tends to occur in the late stages of dependency complicates early diagnosis and treatment, at least on the basis of professional monitor-

Table 4.2
Signs of Chemical Dependence among Physicians

Risk factors and early signs	Late signs
Alcoholic family members	Family dysfunction
Regular use of alcohol	Depression
Drinking to relax or sleep	Drinking while "on call"
Drinking while studying	Auto accidents
Drinking alone	Memory impairment
Frequent intoxication	Needle marks
Cigarette smoking	Missed work
No religious affiliation	Negativism
High grades in medical school	Poor patient care

ing. Physicians may discuss their concerns with friends and colleagues on a strictly personal basis, but if such help is turned down (e.g., the physician denies that he has a problem), there is often reluctance to take the next step and report the impaired physician to appropriate professional or state authorities. This approach almost ensures that patients will be harmed, perhaps seriously, before intervention occurs. Case 4-12 illustrates a middle ground in which effective action might be taken prior to serious injury. S. D. showed clear evidence of drinking while on duty and subsequent inappropriate behavior. The harm in this case may have been relatively small (rudeness to a patient), but certainly sufficient to warrant reprimand and investigation of alcohol abuse.

The medical profession has generally taken a therapeutic, rather than a punitive, approach to physician impairment. Many state and local medical societies have organized voluntary and confidential programs that promote treatment for impaired physicians and monitor their subsequent performance. In some cases these programs have a nonvoluntary component in that continued medical staff privileges might be linked to successful completion of rehabilitation. While the medical society's goal is to rehabilitate the physician, the state licensure board's main goal is to protect the public. Thus, the licensure board traditionally responds to physician misconduct by limiting or revoking the medical license. However, these goals are not mutually exclusive and in many jurisdictions a good working relationship has developed between professional societies and state licensure boards (Blondell, 1993).

Treatment for chemically dependent physicians is most effective when it involves the support of colleagues, includes well-defined intervention goals, is based on documentation of specific impaired behaviors, and begins soon after the crisis situation that has precipitated intervention (Centrella, 1994). Initial detoxification, which usually lasts about 1 month, may involve either outpatient or inpatient treatment. Extended care of 6 months or more may be required in some cases. An essential part of any long-term therapeutic plan is a mechanism for monitoring future professional performance. Overall, physicians who enter drug rehabilitation programs have better treatment outcomes with less recidivism than the general population of drug abusers, with reported recovery rates without relapse ranging up to 84% (Centrella, 1994).

CONCLUSIONS

The virtues, pleasures, and responsibilities of being a physician are closely intertwined. While medicine is rapidly changing in many respects, certain major features of medical practice endure. The major goals of medicine include caring for the sick and relieving their suffering. These goals can generally be accomplished only in the context of interpersonal relationships. Thus, the patient–physician relationship lies at the core of the physician's responsibility (competent, trustworthy care), skill development (empathic communication), and professional satisfaction (helping, social interaction, problem solving). In particular, clinical empathy, a complex skill that has cognitive, affective, and motivational components, is an essential ingredient for effective medical practice. Personal qualities important in doctoring include benevolence, compassion, caring, practical judgment, honesty, humility, discipline, fidelity, courage, playfulness, humor, and creativity.

Physicians are powerful by virtue of their medical knowledge, social role, and personal qualities and interpersonal skills. Patients are vulnerable by virtue of their illnesses and lack of knowledge. Physicians should use medical power to promote the interests of their patients. In some cases, however, physicians abuse their power or otherwise engage in activities that conflict with their patients' best interest. Engaging in intimate relationships with patients is a clear example of abuse. Conflict of interest may manifest itself in unnecessary or inadequate medical care. Physician ownership of health facilities and defensive medicine are associated with provision of unnecessary services. In some cases managed care arrangements may lead to less than adequate medical care by restricting appropriate services.

Most physicians enjoy their work and find it personally and professionally fulfilling. The dynamics of medical practice, however, may lead to chronic emotional stress and, eventually, to burnout. Physicians sometimes deplete themselves emotionally, detach from family and friends, depersonalize their patients, deny their problems, and become depressed. Physicians who consider themselves indispensable and fail to make "space" for their families and personal development are particularly vulnerable to burnout. Burnout harms not only physicians, but their families and patients as well. Abuse of drugs or alcohol is another possible response to emotional stress. While the prevalence of substance abuse among physicians approximates that in the general population, the pattern of drug use differs with specialty. Physicians have a professional duty to help their impaired colleagues. The first step toward helping impaired physicians is to identify them and facilitate appropriate treatment. Professional organizations, in concert with state agencies, work to foster a therapeutic response that helps physicians while minimizing harm to their patients.

CASES FOR DISCUSSION

CASE 1

Dr. Heigh Tech seems to have it all. After completing an orthopedic surgery residency at a prestigious medical center, he joined a well-known multispecialty group practice. Over the next few years his practice grew by leaps and bounds. His aggressive surgical approach and good outcomes led to referrals of "hard cases" from all over the region. Initially, Tech loved his work. His colleagues had trouble understanding how he could be so consistently pleasant and enthusiastic, given his characteristic 12- to 14-hour workdays. He seemed always ready to help others, but he never accepted any help in his own practice. More recently, however, Tech has begun to complain about overwork: He never gets to take a vacation; patients won't leave him alone; as soon as he leaves the hospital, everything goes to pot; his wife just doesn't seem to understand how much pressure he's under. "I don't know why other people can't pull their share of the work!"

1. *Discuss the satisfactions and dissatisfactions Dr. Tech finds in medical practice.*
2. *Discuss personality characteristics that may make Dr. Tech vulnerable to professional burnout.*
3. *Where do you think Dr. Tech is on the stress–burnout cycle? What would you advise Dr. Tech to do at this point?*

CASE 2

Your patient D. K. has chronic osteoarthritis of his knees. After a spurt of yard work last week, he developed severe pain and swelling of his right knee. You diagnose inflammation and a small effusion secondary to osteoarthritis. You plan to inject a corticosteroid preparation to reduce the inflammation. However, you accidentally use the wrong vial and inject methylprogesterone instead. Later, the nurse brings the mistake to your attention when she notices the empty vial. (This medication has no beneficial effect on arthritis; on the other hand, a single intra-articular injection is probably not harmful.) Three days later D. K. returns for his scheduled follow-up visit. He tells you that his knee is "100% better." In fact, you note that the erythema and swelling are largely gone.

1. *What type of mistake is this? Would you consider it a culpable error? Explain.*
2. *Should you have tried immediately to call D. K. and explain the mistake to him? What would you say?*
3. *Let's say you were unable to reach D. K. Now that he has returned to your office and his arthritis is "100% better," what should you do?*

CASE 3

At 74 years old Dr. T. is still going strong. He practices obstetrics–gynecology full-time, including a full surgical schedule. He is well known among the staff for his high energy and gruff manner. Dr. T. is definitely not "politically correct": He calls a spade a spade, and his positions on social mores are "Victorian," as one of his younger colleagues put it. Dr. Agra, a new general internist on staff, comments to you that she would never refer a patient to Dr. T. because he is "incompetent and abusive to women." In conversation, Dr. Agra reports that Dr. T. doesn't seem to understand newer concepts of endometriosis and premenstrual syndrome. Moreover, he refers to patients as "girlie." In the last couple of years you have heard other physicians make remarks about Dr. T.'s somewhat outdated medical concepts, but his patients, who are mostly older women, seem to love him. You have, however, heard several patients in your practice make negative comments about Dr. T.'s personality and skills. You wonder if the old guy is still competent.

1. *How do you judge the competence of a practicing physician?*
2. *Should physicians be required to pass periodic tests of their knowledge and skills? Should physicians be required to retire at a certain age? Explain.*
3. *What should you or other members of the hospital medical staff do at this point to help Dr. T. or his patients?*

CASE 4

You are a 45-year-old female urologist in a large-staff model HMO. H. S. is a 38-year-old patient with chronic prostatitis. He also suffers from anxiety attacks and depressive episodes since his wife died in a tragic accident 4 years ago. As part of your medical care, you spend time giving him supportive counseling. You have the feeling that he is physically attracted to you, as you are to him. At one point he asks you out for lunch, but you refuse, explaining that your work schedule would not permit it. A couple of months later, the computer software company H. S. works for switches to a different health insurance program, so that your services are no longer covered. He calls you the next month and tells you that he has arranged to see a urologist in the new plan. He also tells you that he really enjoys your company and asks you out to dinner, noting that it would be "okay" since you are no longer his physician.

1. *Is the physician–patient relationship compatible with outside social relationships with patients? with close friendship? with intimacy? Where does one draw the line?*
2. *Describe some of the dynamics that might lead H. S. to be attracted to you, his physician. What might lead you to be attracted to him? Would these dynamics be different if you were a male gynecologist and he were a woman with endometriosis?*
3. *Are there professional or moral reasons not to "get involved" with H. S. when he is still your patient? What about now? When does he stop being your patient? That is, when do the dynamics described in question #2 no longer exist or become morally irrelevant?*

One of your young colleagues in anesthesiology, Dr. Ernest Barr, has had a difficult year, having just gone through a bitter divorce. Because of the divorce he moved from upstate New York to your town and joined the medical staff in your hospital about 8 months ago. Recently, he has appeared more distant and withdrawn than usual. While he has never seemed very social, he is now outright irritable. He has also uncharacteristically called in sick several times in the last few weeks, necessitating last-minute changes in the operating room schedule. You have never heard any complaints before about the quality of Dr. Barr's medical care, but you recently noted him to fall asleep briefly during an operation and, later, to make a mistake in medication dosage. Fortunately, the error was caught and corrected by the assisting nurse anesthetist. You mention this incident to a fellow surgeon who reports a similar occurrence the previous week during a cholecystectomy. In that case, the patient became hypotensive for no apparent reason and the surgeon suspected an anesthesia error. You wonder what is going on with Dr. Barr and whether you should try to do something about it.

1. Dr. Barr's performance seems to be impaired. What are the possible diagnoses? List the features of the case that suggest each one.
2. What should be done? Do you, as a colleague on the medical staff, have any responsibility to do something? If so, why?
3. Barr denies any problems when you raise the issue with him. He tells you to mind your own business. He reminds you that we all sometimes make mistakes. What should you do next?
4. Describe the epidemiology and characteristics of substance abuse among physicians.
5. There are two systems available to sanction unprofessional behavior. Describe the characteristics of each. Which system would you now approach in Dr. Barr's case? Why?

RECOMMENDED READINGS

Brody H: *The Healer's Power.* New Haven, CT, Yale University Press, 1992.

In this book Howard Brody investigates the nature, sources, and implications of the physician's power. Acknowledging that this power has both positive and negative sides, Brody develops a medical ethic based on the interactive process of doctoring. Chapter 16 on "The Physician's Character" is an excellent discussion of virtues in medicine.

Cassell EJ: *The Nature of Suffering and the Goals of Medicine.* London, Oxford University Press, 1991.

In this book Eric Cassell investigates the human meaning of suffering and develops an understanding of medical practice in which relieving that suffering is a major goal.

Williams WC: *The Doctor Stories.* Compiled by Robert Coles. New York, New Directions, 1984.

This book brings together many of William Carlos Williams's short stories about taking care of patients. They illustrate many of the experiences, virtues, and abuses of doctoring discussed in this chapter. In particular, "Old Doc Rivers" is a fine story about an impaired physician.

PART III

Society

The patient–physician relationship is set in a societal context. Understanding that context facilitates the growth of the relationship, while ignoring it can result in many problems, including misunderstandings, miscommunications, conflict, and ultimately the dissolution of the relationship itself. In order to understand the societal context of the patient–physician relationship, this part has been divided into three sections—relationships, values, and special problems.

A. RELATIONSHIPS

Relationships can have a profound effect on the health and clinical care of patients. Although relationship issues and dynamics have been previously ignored by traditional biomedicine as irrelevant, recent research clearly demonstrates the importance of relationships, especially the physician–patient relationship and relationships within the family system, to the health and care of patients. Arising from many perspectives and theoretical models, this research also indicates that physicians, if they can take relational information into account when formulating a therapeutic plan with patients, can to a much better degree improve the patient's health or at least come to a better understanding of the barriers to improving the patient's health.

B. VALUES

As technology has expanded the boundaries of life, what patients hold near and dear and how they view the world have come to assume more importance, especially as society is learning that resources devoted to medical care are not inexhaustible. Although patients clearly want top-quality, easily accessible, low-cost healthcare, the extension of life at all costs is clearly not a top priority for many patients. Learning to recognize where the values of the patient and the physician conflict and then negotiating an effective solution that respects the values of both parties is becoming as important a skill as the medical management of patients. Likewise, understanding the resources available for care and how to use them wisely is essential in this new age of cost containment.

C. SPECIAL PROBLEMS

Physicians are increasingly being confronted with patients who have suffered the effects of seemingly intractable societal problems, problems that often frustrate physicians into lethargy. This section will help physicians in training understand these problems, recognize how their patients are affected by them, and choose appropriate interventions to help patients cope with them. It is also our hope as editors that some future physicians will be stimulated to deal with these problems from a societal perspective to reduce the heavy toll they bear on our patients and the fabric of our society.

CHAPTER 5

A. Relationships

The Patient–Physician Relationship

Ronald M. Epstein

The good physician knows his patients through and through, and his knowledge is bought dearly. Time, sympathy and understanding must be lavishly dispensed, but the reward is to be found in that personal bond which forms the greatest satisfaction in the practice of medicine. One of the essential qualities of the clinician is interest in humanity, for the secret of the care of the patient is caring for the patient. (Peabody, 1984)

Doctors never meet symptoms adjusted to suit their knowledge, [rather] they meet human beings who try through their symptom presentations to communicate signals from within their own bodies. (Rudebeck, 1992)

The whole procedure was just what he expected, just what one always encounters. There was the waiting, the doctor's air of importance . . . the tapping, the listening, the questions requiring answers that were clearly superfluous since they were foregone conclusions, and the significant look that implied: "Just put yourself in our hands and we'll take care of everything; we know exactly what has to be done—we always use one and the same method for every patient, no matter who." . . . The celebrated doctor dealt with him in precisely the manner [Ivan Ilych, the prosecutor] dealt with men on trial. (Tolstoy, 1981)

CASE 5-1

Joyce Samuels had chronic joint pains, shortness of breath, difficulty urinating, abdominal pains, and several other illness episodes over the past 8 years about which she was very anxious. Her husband had regarded these as minor concerns. Diagnostic testing revealed no cause, and she felt either that her physicians were not taking her concerns seriously or that they were withholding information. She frequently did not follow through with medical advice. On a routine gynecologic examination, a large pelvic mass was discovered that was diagnosed as advanced ovarian cancer. Her prognosis was poor. To her physician's surprise, Mrs. Samuels became much less anxious, and was grateful for having been provided an explanation for her suffering. Her interpersonal relationships with her husband and the medical community became more mutually satisfying.

INTRODUCTION

The patient–physician relationship* is the cornerstone of medical care. Each relationship that a physician forms with a patient is unique, often intimate, and has characteristics, expectations, and means of communication different from other social interactions. The patient–physician relationship is not simply bedside manner, or an appendage to technologically competent medical care. Rather, the nature of the relationship can have a profound influence on patient well-being (Stewart *et al.*, 1979; Bass *et al.*, 1986a), satisfaction with medical care (Starfield *et al.*, 1981), and outcomes of diseases as diverse as peptic ulcer (Greenfield *et al.*, 1985), diabetes mellitus (Greenfield *et al.*, 1988), and respiratory infections (Bass *et al.*, 1986b). The fundamental goals of the patient–physician relationship are to assist the patient's own healing powers (McWhinney, 1989b), relieve suffering (Cassell, 1982), and foster healthy behaviors. In order to do this, the physician needs to understand the patient, the patient needs to understand her illness, and the patient must know that she has been understood.

In this chapter, I will provide a set of considerations in order to come to a multi-faceted appreciation of this complex social relationship, and general guidelines rather than concrete rules. Most clinicians learn more about the nature of patient–physician relationships from their patients than from teachers and mentors. In my view, the important qualities of a patient–physician relationship are best approached by examining stories of actual patient–physician relationships rather than starting with abstract principles and providing cases to illustrate them. The "messiness" that inevitably occurs when one examines individual stories is part of what makes medicine a human endeavor (McWhinney, 1989b). I will emphasize the importance of meaningful and respectful human relationships, the family and social context, and the need for physicians to develop the capacity for organized self-reflection.

The relief of suffering is a central goal of medicine, and, therefore, of the patient–physician relationship. Eric Cassell (1982) has defined suffering to include an "injury to the integrity of the person," often associated with perceived disassembling of the patient's world as it has been known and requiring adaptations that may not be desired. Health, on the other hand, includes the ability to grow and adapt to change, to rebuild, and to transcend in response to injury. Suffering is ultimately a very personal experience; only

---

*For clarity, and to place emphasis on the centrality of the patient, I will use the term *patient–physician relationship* rather than *doctor–patient relationship* or *physician–patient relationship*.

parts of it can be shared, usually with intimates. Healthcare is concerned with *disease*, an abnormality in the structure or function, as well as *illness*, the experience of being unwell.

Understanding a patient's suffering involves far more than interpreting specific symptoms related to a disease or illness. The biopsychosocial model (Engel, 1977, 1980) emphasizes that it is crucial to understand each patient as a unique person, including past experiences, bodily and emotional memories, and expectations for the future. Each person has relationships with others (including physicians) within which personal experiences are expressed, redefined, and given meaning. The family usually contains the most important set of interpersonal relationships; its members, in turn, have experiences, roles, and expectations (Baird & Doherty, 1990; McDaniel *et al.*, 1990a; Doherty & Campbell, 1988), as well as genetic and historical legacies. Within a particular culture, people are defined by social roles and political power. Aside from beliefs and values, our actions also help to define who we are. All of these factors are involved in suffering, in health, and in the patient–physician relationship.

It is important to remember that suffering can be caused by the illness, the meaning of the illness, the treatment for the illness, or personal and social sequelae of illness. Most importantly, it is very difficult to know all of the sources of a patient's suffering without asking the patient.

The importance of the meaning of an illness is illustrated by an important study by Beecher (1959) during the Second World War. While stationed at a bloody battle in which there were many casualties, Beecher studied the meaning of injuries and requests for pain medications among soldiers wounded in combat. He noted that soldiers wounded in battle required substantially less pain medication and experienced less distress when compared with soldiers with similar injuries not sustained in battle. The difference was explained only by the meaning of the injury to the soldier. The injury in battle means that the soldier would be taken out of danger and his life would be saved; for others, a similar injury might mean prolonged disability, decreased income, and loss of a meaningful activity.

As in Beecher's study, meaning of the illness to the patient described in Case 5-1 played an important part in the experience of and the relief of suffering. Her diagnosis of ovarian cancer validated her suffering and reassured her that she was not crazy. This life-threatening illness carried meanings to the patient and her family that would not have been apparent from casual inquiry. Therefore, it is critical for the physician to understand the illness *from the patient's perspective* (Stewart *et al.*, 1995) in order to understand the patient's response to illness or disability. Furthermore, physicians, by virtue of our ability to make proclamations about a patient's health, can strongly influence the meaning a patient gives to an illness, and, consequently, the patient's experience of illness. Consider, for example, how differently a patient recently diagnosed with cancer might respond if he were told that he has a 70% chance of cure as opposed to being told that he has a 30% chance of dying within 2 years.

The patient–physician relationship is also dependent on experiences with previous relationships, even if they are from different contexts. The most powerful early socialization experiences are usually with our own families of origin (the family in which each of us grew up) (McDaniel & Landau-Stanton, 1991). These experiences have a powerful effect on the nature of relationships that we form throughout the rest of life, especially intimate and emotionally charged relationships. Thus, some physicians are more formal than others, some feel more comfortable with uncertainty, and some are more comfortable caring for dying patients. Some share decision-making easily, and some find it difficult to care for patients who abuse drugs.

Mario Spola is a 45-year-old, mildly mentally retarded, Italian-born man. He acquired HIV infection at least 5 years ago from one of multiple anonymous same-sex partners. He has had no symptoms of HIV disease other than a mild yeast infection in the mouth. He comes to the office regularly, usually every 3 months, to talk, have a brief physical examination, and to have blood tests done. He had several discussions in the past about his sexual behavior with his physician, Dr. Sherrie Newton, but he continued to have sexual relations with men whom he met in public parks and bars. After much encouragement, he began to use condoms, although he was still somewhat reluctant. He had difficulty understanding that, even though he felt healthy, he could transmit a fatal infection to others. He feared being rejected by potential partners if he used condoms; during a frank discussion, he reported that he used condoms only if his partner requested that he do so. He is always cheerful, agreeable, and otherwise follows medical advice. On a recent visit, Dr. Newton told him that his CD4 count, a measure of immune system functioning, has declined further, despite having added a second anti-HIV medication. "But I feel great, doc, really great!" he said with pride, making the point that he is healthy enough to work as a machinist, sometimes 10 hours a day, 6 to 7 days a week. His risk of developing complications is now quite high. He has told no one in his family about his HIV disease, including his ex-wife and teenage children. He is certain that he became infected after they separated.

MODELS OF THE PATIENT–PHYSICIAN RELATIONSHIP

Case 5-2 illustrates several important features of the patient–physician relationship. It is clear that the sharing of illness stories is the basis of the relationships between patients and their physicians. The medical interview is a narrative history involving the transfer of information as well as the development of frames of reference for interpretation of that information. These frames of reference are sometimes shared between physician and patient; often they are *not*. Therefore, the physician must engage the patient in dialogue to uncover the meaning of his distress. Further, the differing interpretations of a single patient's story points to the fact that a physician, a patient, and relevant family members construct the story of the patient's illness together. This is in contrast to the view that the physician is the disinterested collector and processor of objective information.

It is difficult, and probably undesirable, to define an "ideal" patient–physician relationship. However, it is important to understand the principles underlying the relationship. One of the first to do this was Thomas Szasz (Szasz & Hollender, 1956), who described three basic models of the patient–physician relationship: *the activity/passivity model, the guidance/cooperation model,* and *the mutual participation model.* These, along with more recently described models, are presented in Table 5.1.

The activity/passivity model takes as its assumption that physicians are technicians who perform procedures on patients with little or no input from the latter. Stated in its extreme form, it seems repugnant as a model for patient care in general, yet physicians commonly make decisions on a patient's behalf when there is an immediate, life-threatening illness and when the patient is not capable of communicating. Thus, if a patient without prior advance directives suffers a cardiac arrest with no close friends or family

Table 5.1
Models of the Patient–Physician Relationship

Model	Physician's role	Values and assumptions
Activity/ passivity	Does something to the patient without patient involvement	Physician knows best; patient cannot participate in care
Guidance/ cooperation (paternalistic)	Tells patient what to do in order to help patient; uses reassurance rather than explanation	Physician knows how to promote patient's best interest; values are shared between physician and patient
Consumer/ informative	Helps patient to help herself. Physician is a technical expert who informs patient of options; patient chooses	Patient bases decisions on her own values, of which she is aware
Interpretive	Counsels patient to make decisions in keeping with patient's values	Patient needs help from the physician to clarify his values. Physician does not try to change patient's values
Deliberative	Engages patient in discussion to develop values; suggest a course of action	Patient values are malleable; physician's duty is to persuade (not coerce) patient to adopt healthy values
Contractual/ covenantal	Provides a philanthropic, consensual, negotiated, and mutually beneficial relationship with patient	Values are discussed openly. Moral responsibility is shared between physician and patient in the context of acknowledged power differential
Patient-centered	Finds common ground with patient on which to base medical decision-making	Illness must be understood from the patient's perspective as well as the diagnostic perspective. Moral obligation of physician to share power and show a human face
Family systems	Cares for patient in context of family unit. Physician helps patient help herself *and* helps family help the patient	Individual and family values are taken into account. Moral responsibility is shared between physician, patient, and family
Ethnographic	Discovers, with patient, personal and cultural meanings of illness	Cultural values are embedded in illness and must be addressed comprehensively

present, a physician uses the activity/passivity model by default. Similarly, physicians frequently have to make decisions for patients who are delirious, demented, psychotic, or comatose, without input from the patient or the family. Also, physicians and parents are empowered to make decisions on behalf of children.

The guidance/cooperation model has been referred to as a parent–child (Szasz & Hollender, 1956), paternalistic (Spittle, 1992; McKinstry, 1992; Emanuel & Emanuel, 1992), or priestly (Veatch, 1972) relationship. The physician assumes sole responsibility for making decisions that benefit the patient, without doing harm (Veatch, 1972). Until recently, this was the predominant model of medical care, and remains so in many parts of the world. For example, in Italy, it is still common for physicians to withhold the diagnosis of cancer from a patient and prescribe treatment without involvement of the patient in therapeutic decisions (Pellegrino, 1992). From a paternalistic viewpoint, the physician's job is to provide reassurance ("Don't worry, I'll take care of everything") rather than information. Underlying assumptions are that the patient's and the physician's values are identical, obviating a need to explore them further, and that the patient will comply with, and not question, the physician's recommendations. In more homogeneous societies, and in those where the range of possible treatments is small, it is reasonable to see how these assumptions could arise. In North American culture, these assumptions are not useful and may be perilous. However, some patients may want to be relieved of the onerous responsibility of making difficult decisions. Older patients may be accustomed to a paternalistic style and may find invitations for their expanded involvement in medical care initially unsettling. When caring for some children or mentally incapacitated adults, or when insurmountable communication barriers are present, physicians must make paternalistic decisions by default. However, respect must be shown for patients' preferences prior to becoming disabled (if known) and for the preferences of family members.

The mutual participation model's central tenets are patient autonomy, respect for the patient's values and experience, and the fundamental equality of all humans (Szasz & Hollender, 1956). According to Szasz, the physician becomes a participant in a partnership rather than telling the patient what to do. There are several different models developed more recently that are subsumed under Szasz's mutual participation model, such as the *consumer model* (Emanuel & Emanuel, 1992; Lazare *et al.*, 1975), the *ethnographic model* (Katon & Kleinman, 1981; Stoeckle & Barsky, 1981; Kleinman *et al.*, 1978; Kleinman, 1987), the *interpretive model* (Emanuel & Emanuel, 1992), the *deliberative model* (Emanuel & Emanuel, 1992), the *contractual/covenantal model* (Veatch, 1972; Quill, 1983), and the *family systems model* (McDaniel *et al.*, 1990a). The features of each of these, including the physician's role and responsibilities, are summarized in Table 5.1. All of these models assume that a competent adult has the capacity to synthesize information and to articulate values and preferences. They also assume that the physician has sufficient communication skills to elicit the patient's preferences and sufficient self-awareness to know the difference between the patient's preferences and what the physician *imagines* or *assumes* the patient would want.

As an example, consider a seemingly simple situation—and compare the different approaches of four hypothetical physicians.

CASE 5-3

John Matthews, a 23-year-old psychology graduate student, has had a productive cough for 5 days. He was well until a week ago when he began to feel fatigued and feverish. He developed an aching sensation in his joints. The cough has worsened, and he is now coughing up green-brown sputum. He has lost his appetite and has stayed home from work and from school. The cough keeps him and his partner up at night. He has had bronchitis in the past and reported that antibiotics have helped; he inquired whether he could be prescribed an antibiotic. He smokes one pack of cigarettes a day. He looked ill and fatigued. On physical examination, there were some crackles in the right lung base, indicating that he has pneumonia.

To contrast different approaches, consider the following alternative ways of handling this situation, with the same information available:

A paternalistic approach. *Dr. Carol Francis told the patient that this was a "little touch of pneumonia," said not to worry, that the medication would help, and that John should feel better within 3 to 5 days. She wrote prescriptions for amoxicillin and codeine and explained how they were to be used. She advised John to stop smoking and described a method for helping John to quit, including nicotine patches, substitution of noncaloric foods, a smoking cessa-*

tion group, and follow-up visits. She said that her office would call John in 3 days to see how he was doing and that John should call sooner if he became worse.

A consumer approach. *Dr. Dennis Graham informed the patient that this was pneumonia and ascertained that the patient had no drug allergies. Dr. Graham explained the common causes of pneumonia in lay language, indicating that smokers have a much higher incidence of respiratory illnesses. He told the patient that continuing to smoke would shorten his life span; it would be his choice whether he wished to stop. Dr. Graham presented three options to the patient: (1) If John did nothing, most probably his infection would eventually improve; (2) amoxicillin, which is 90% effective, inexpensive, but must be given three times daily for 10 days; or (3) azithromycin, which is more effective and has few side effects, but is five times more expensive than amoxicillin. He asked the patient to make a choice. A similar choice was presented for antitussive medications. After the patient chose amoxicillin and codeine, Dr. Graham asked the patient if his findings and recommendations seemed reasonable. He told the patient to call if there were any further problems.*

A patient-centered, deliberative approach. *Dr. Samuel Harris asked John why he thought he had become ill, and John reported being under considerable stress with graduate studies and a full-time job. Dr. Harris told John that he had pneumonia, that he had some understanding of how stressful graduate studies can be, and that rest and antibiotics are usually helpful. They discussed what the most reasonable plan would be. They agreed that it was wise to take time off from work; however, John felt that he had to try to keep up with readings at school. John felt that he could rest in bed some of the time, but would plan to go to the library to keep up with his reading. John felt that he was under too much stress to stop smoking; besides, his father and grandfather smoked heavily and had no adverse consequences. Dr. Harris asked John about what was important in his life right now. John felt that he needed to get more control of his life and needed to take better care of himself. Based on those values, Dr. Harris asked John what he hoped to do to accomplish those goals. John realized that it was probably in his best interest to do his reading at home rather than the library, so he could rest. Further, Dr. Harris strongly encouraged John to set up an appointment in a week to talk about his smoking. He recognized the patient's reluctance, but emphasized that if John stopped smoking he would regain health faster and would be taking better care of himself. John agreed to talk further about his smoking at a follow-up visit, but did not know if he was interested in quitting. Dr. Harris prescribed amoxicillin and also offered him a prescription for codeine and asked him if his findings and recommendations seemed reasonable.*

A family systems approach. *Dr. Mary Jacobs asked John how the illness has been affecting his life. John reported being under considerable stress with graduate studies and a full-time job. He felt that he could not afford to take time off, that his life was out of control, and that he wanted to take better care of himself. She told him that he had pneumonia and prescribed amoxicillin* *and codeine. Although they agreed that it was wise to take time off from work, John felt that he had to try to keep up with readings at school. Dr. Jacobs also asked John if his partner would be able to help at home for the next few days. John replied that he would and that his partner would be pleased if John were not "hacking away" all night. John also mentioned that both he and his partner had tested HIV-negative 2 months previously and were at no current risk for infection. Dr. Jacobs inquired whether his partner smoked. When John indicated that they both smoked, she invited both of them to come in for a follow-up appointment to discuss how they could help each other take better care of themselves.*

Although these may seem like simplistic caricatures, the four vignettes following Case 5-3 are based on observations of actual patient–physician encounters, all of which took approximately the same amount of time. These same styles of interaction are equally common in other, more "charged" clinical encounters, such as when a patient is informed she has cancer or when discussing major changes in therapy for chronic illness.

In the first vignette, Dr. Francis was practicing within a *paternalistic* (Emanuel & Emanuel, 1992; Spittle, 1992; Neighbour, 1992; May, 1975) model, making choices for the patient and instructing the patient on how to comply with the prescribed treatment. Dr. Francis's care was kind and competent; however, she assumed total responsibility for the patient's care: The patient was not informed of any treatment options, the illness was treated out of context of the patient's life, and the patient's values were never explored. Thus, the physician missed an opportunity to address additional concerns of the patient and did not help the patient to participate in his own care.

By contrast, in the second vignette, Dr. Graham completely informed the patient of his treatment options, and, utilizing a *consumer* model of care (Lazare *et al.*, 1975; Emanuel & Emanuel, 1992), left the choice to the patient. The patient was assumed to have the capacity to synthesize information on his own; conversely, the physician's responsibility was only to provide "value-free" information about the patient's illness. An analogy can be made to the choice of products in a supermarket. The educated consumer reads the well-labeled contents of the product on the side of the box and makes an informed choice about which product to purchase. The patient, willingly or unwillingly, was given total responsibility for his care. This approach, while appropriate for some clinical decisions, often does not address the context of the decision, or the values that the patient brings to the situation, and avoids the positive and negative uses of power in a relationship wherein power is distributed asymmetrically. While giving the illusion of empowering the patient, such an approach is not *patient-centered,* that is, it places importance only on the diagnosis as defined by the physician's medical frame of reference, rather than including the patient's perspective as well. This approach does not call on the physician to help the patient make an informed choice *within the context of the patient's values* and does not place the physician in the position of questioning or attempting to influence the values that underlie the patient's choices.

Dr. Harris, in the third vignette, took a more *patient-centered* (Levenstein *et al.*, 1986; Stewart *et al.*, 1995) approach by exploring the patient's life context, values, and preferences and by offering accurate and appropriate empathy. The physician worked with the patient in a *collaborative* style and gave the patient meaningful choices. Compared with the consumer approach described above, the range of choices of antibiotic was narrower, and there was less deliberation about issues that the physician *imagined* might be important to the patient. Instead, by clarifying and interpreting the patient's values, the physician was able to use the time to address important underlying concerns of the patient—that he learn to care for himself better. By taking this approach, Dr. Harris helped the patient to formulate *his own* solution to a dilemma, a solution John was more likely to follow than had the physician directed the patient to take a similar action. This is in keeping with research that shows that patients who are active participants in their own care have improved medical outcomes and improved satisfaction (Kaplan *et al.*, 1989; Starfield *et al.*, 1981). Dr. Harris went further, by adopting a *deliberative* (Emanuel & Emanuel, 1992) style of interaction. He did not accept at face value John's reluctance to quit smoking, but rather encouraged (but, importantly, did not coerce) John to adopt a different perspective on the problem. While seeming to have elements in common with a paternalistic approach, this approach was different in several important ways. Dr. Harris took into account the patient's values and life context and engaged in dialogue with the patient as an equal, but the physician retained the obligation to advise and to convince the patient to pursue health-promoting actions. This incorporates elements of a *contractual* or *covenantal* model (May, 1975), wherein the moral responsibility is *shared* between physician and patient. It acknowledges that physician and patient have differing expertise and that physician and patient have unequal power in the medical realm.

Dr. Jacobs, in the fourth vignette, incorporated many of the features of a patient-centered, deliberative relationship, but included the patient's *family context* in the information-gathering, problem list, and potential sources of solutions for the patient's concerns. The *family systems model* will be discussed in greater detail in Chapter 6. For now, it is important to consider the family as "not limited to ties of blood, marriage, sexual partnership or adoption, [but to include] any group whose bonds are based on trust, mutual support and common destiny" (World Health Organization, 1994). Dr. Jacobs, on hearing that smoking and HIV risk were concerns affecting John and his partner, enlisted the help of a family member to characterize further and manage John's problems, and, in so doing, defined the *family* as the unit of care. The responsibility for healthcare was shared between physician, patient, and *family*. By considering it a shared rather than individual effort, John was less reluctant to consider a major life-style change.

Finally, an *ethnographic approach* (Stein & Apprey, 1990; Kleinman *et al.*, 1978; Kleinman, 1983, 1987; Good & Good, 1981) would include inquiry not only into the patient's family, but also into the cultural traditions and values that shape the patient's healthcare-seeking behavior, illness experience, and expectations of the physician. In addition to individual attributions about the nature of illness and treatments, there are strongly held cultural beliefs that influence patients and physicians. For example, a patient from an Asian culture where there is a widely held belief that exposure to wind is harmful, may lose trust in a physician who suggests unbundling an infant with a fever. Care must be taken, however, not to infer individual beliefs solely from ethnicity; there are frequently more variations within an ethnic group than between them. These issues are discussed further in Chapter 10.

CASE 5-4

When Dr. David Isaacson first met the patient, Sam Walters, he was a 43-year-old, intermittently homeless man with cirrhosis caused by heavy alcohol use, and infection with hepatitis B and C virus, which in turn were acquired through intravenous cocaine use. He was very jaundiced, gaunt, and wasted. Mr. Walters thought that he did not have much time to live. Tests confirmed recurrent hepatitis and that he was not HIV-infected. His liver disease had resulted in a coagulopathy, portal hypertension with splenomegaly, esophageal varices, and thrombocytopenia.

Dr. Isaacson asked Mr. Walters what he wanted to do with the time he had remaining. He replied that he wished to reunite with his daughters (whom he had not seen in several years) who were then in foster care. He also wanted to live, and would do "anything" to extend his life. At Dr. Isaacson's suggestion, he stopped drinking and remained abstinent. He was referred to a family therapist, who helped him and his daughters heal the wounds of their difficult relationship. He also expressed remorse about several serious crimes he had committed (he had been arrested but never prosecuted). It was a "secret" that he had never told anyone, but could not live with alone any longer. The nature and details of the crimes were kept in confidence; there was no one currently endangered.

After 2 years, he began having severe recurrent right-sided abdominal pain caused by gallstones. Because of his cirrhosis and portal hypertension, his surgical risk was too high to consider cholecystectomy. He refused narcotics for these episodes for fear of becoming addicted again. He came to the office and the emergency room with frequent recurrences of his pain. He had episodes of encephalopathy, and felt progressively worse. He asked if he would likely die of liver failure; Dr. Isaacson's honest affirmative answer changed Mr. Walters's self-concept to that of a dying man.

After another 2 years, his episodes of abdominal pain became more severe, and his liver function deteriorated further during those episodes. His right-sided abdominal pain became constant. He began to feel hopeless, began using IV cocaine, again became homeless, living in "crack houses." He was ashamed to have his daughters see him this way. Despite this relapse, he continued to come to the office for regular appointments and assiduously abstained from alcohol. He continued using cocaine, because "there was no purpose in living anyway." He brought up the possibility of liver transplant. At that time, transplant centers were beginning to accept patients with a recent history of drug use. He was put on the transplant list with the proviso that he be tested periodically to document abstinence.

ATTRIBUTES OF THE PATIENT–PHYSICIAN RELATIONSHIP

Sam Walters' story in Case 5-4 demonstrates that the patient–physician relationship involves far more than the communication that occurs in a single medical encounter. Relationships develop over time (Stewart *et al.*, 1995). Physician and patient grow through life, have crises, share experiences, and develop trust. The nature of the relationship changes with time. As in this case, physicians can, at different times, act solely as a source of technical competence, make contracts, make judgments, act as agent of change, assume an advocacy role, be charitable, and use power in a variety of ways. These roles are listed in Table 5.2. Also fundamental to the patient–physician relationship is the principle of *nonabandonment*. According to Quill and Cassel (1995), this is a "continuous

Table 5.2
Physician Roles

Agent of change
Facilitator of change
Collaborative partner
Advocate on patient's behalf
Contractual partner
Priest/judge
Mentor
Friend

caring partnership between physician and patient" that transcends the multiple challenges that the relationship may face.

It is commonly observed that the *act* of prescribing treatment can be more curative than the pharmacologic value of the medication (Balint, 1957). This may reflect offering hope to the patient in the face of suffering, her participation in a treatment plan, and the psychoneuroimmunologic mechanisms that relate psychological states such as hopefulness and feeling supported with biological phenomena such as improved survival in breast cancer patients (Spiegel *et al.*, 1989). Strategies for facilitating healing in the patient–physician relationship include attending to the patient's need for information, negotiating a treatment plan that is concordant with the patient's values, eliciting and responding to the patient's emotions, offering hope, using touch, involving family members, and activating the patient to take part in her medical care (Novack, 1987; Simpson *et al.*, 1991). The patient–physician relationship can be a way for the patient to create meaning in her suffering, above and beyond the offering of hope (Cassell, 1982). The patient can be helped to find meaningful connections with medical personnel (Suchman & Matthews, 1988), social support networks, and family members (McDaniel *et al.*, 1990a), to help her to reconstruct a world that may seem to have been irreversibly altered by illness (Toombs, 1992). In addition, all of these factors may include the therapeutic aspects of the "placebo effect," which, in part, refers to the use of the patient–physician relationship itself as an important primary therapeutic modality, regardless of whether a drug is prescribed (Brody, 1992).

Physicians are given power by social institutions, by patients, and by their own families (Brody, 1992). Access to knowledge is one of the most potent sources of power (May, 1975). This power is invested in physicians with some direction for its use (see Chapter 12 on ethics), but also with considerable latitude. Some aspects of the power relationship will always be asymmetrical. Physicians have knowledge and skills that, at best, will be shared incompletely with patients.

Physicians can use their power to *empower* a patient by providing information with which a patient can make an informed choice, exploring the patient's values and preferences, respecting the patient's autonomy, and finding means to help the patient achieve a desired behavior change. This does not involve simply a *transfer* of power from physician to patient (as would be the case in the *consumer model* of the patient–physician relationship), but rather a *sharing* of power to the extent possible to achieve a good outcome *as defined by the patient and by the physician*. The physician can be active in identifying patients who may feel powerless and providing them with the means to have more control over their medical care. This has important implications for patient outcomes as well. In a series of studies, Greenfield and Kaplan (Kaplan *et al.*, 1989) have showed that "activated patients," that is, those who are naturally more involved in their care or who are taught how to be more involved in their care, have significantly better medical outcomes. This included better control of diabetes mellitus, fewer chemotherapy-associated symptoms in patients with breast cancer, and improved functional status in patients with peptic ulcer disease. These findings were *independent* of stage of disease and treatment given.

Physicians can act in an advocacy role that directly uses their socially given power. For example, physicians sometimes write letters to the telephone company asking them to provide free telephone service to chronically ill patients who otherwise could not afford a telephone. In some countries, physicians have identified and publicized victims of torture in the hope of preventing future abuses (E. Mishler, 1994, personal communication).

Sometimes the physician must use her power to act in the patient's behalf, but contrary to the patient's wishes. Common examples are initiating involuntary psychiatric hospitalization for a suicidal patient, identifying victims of child abuse, or refusing to authorize a renewal of a driver's license for a patient with poorly controlled epilepsy.

Physicians continue to serve judicial and priestly roles. Physicians make judgments on patients' ability to work and determinations of disability and culpability for injury. There are also more subtle judgments of character that influence the patient–physician relationship. Once a patient is described as "difficult," either verbally or in a written correspondence, this pejorative label is likely to be communicated to future healthcare providers. The "priestly" role also has both positive and negative attributes. Physicians are in a position to use moral persuasion to the patient's benefit (consider the alcoholic who is reluctant to stop drinking). Also, physicians, by virtue of their power, can make *performatives* (Havens, 1986), that is, statements that transform a situation just by having uttered words. An example in everyday life is when a justice says, "I pronounce you husband and wife." A layperson, uttering the same words, clearly would not have the same effect. Similarly, physicians, by uttering words such as, "You have cancer," or "I consider you to be permanently disabled," can also achieve profound (as defined by themselves or by society) changes in patients.

Finally, the patient–physician relationship involves a personal commitment to patients. In long-term caring relationships, as in Case 5-4, feelings and affections form between physician and patient that allow the relationship to withstand tragedy, conflict, and absences. These connections (Suchman & Matthews, 1988; Branch & Suchman, 1990) attend to the spiritual aspect of suffering, which, for many patients, is inseparable from physical or psychological distress. Mutual gift-giving, of objects, time, or attention, often is a manifestation of such strong relationships. In this way, patient–physician relationships often involve *charity*, "giving with love despite the presence or absence of affection for the patient" (McWhinney, 1989a). It is important, however, to emphasize that, in all cases, the patient–physician relationship must first serve the patient's needs, and not primarily the emotional needs of the physician.

CASE 5-5

Frank Rowe is a 77-year-old widowed man who formerly ran a newspaper distribution warehouse. Dr. Laura Cobb knew him for 10 years, but took over his care 3 years ago when his primary physician left the practice. She probably knew him better than any of his prior physicians, because he always seemed to get sick when they were out of town and Dr. Cobb was on call. The first time they met, he had an episode of bronchitis. She mentioned that smoking was probably related to his having developed the illness, and he became annoyed. "Why do you doctors keep lecturing me and why don't you just mind your own business?" He would die when his time came, and had filled out living wills and DNAR (do not attempt resuscitation) papers. The next week he had a cardiac arrest in the parking lot of Dr. Cobb's office. The physicians who came to the scene were not aware of his wishes. Dr. Cobb went outside to see what all the commotion was about, only to discover that he had been "successfully" resuscitated and brought to the hospital. He recovered and went home, but voiced resentment at having been resuscitated against his wishes. He was relatively well for 4 years. The next 4 years brought a sequence of increasingly frequent hospitalizations for heart failure, pneumonia, weakness, and syncopal (fainting) episodes. His wife died, and he was increasingly unable to care for himself. He took medications as he felt he needed them. He was often angry and depressed. He would demand to speak to his physicians in the middle of the night when he knew they were at home sleeping. He frequently expressed fear of dying, and often felt that each exacerbation of his disease would be the last. In the last few months of his life, his congestive heart failure worsened so that he was housebound, on continuous oxygen. He refused nursing home placement, regarding that option as "worse than death." He asked Dr. Cobb if she would prescribe some sleeping pills. She asked him why, and he said, "because I'm too weak to jump off a bridge." They began a discussion about his request, and she offered to discuss it further with him at their next appointment. He died later that week; it was never clear whether the immediate cause of death was the natural progression of his disease, failure to take his medications, or a deliberate suicide.

RESPONSIBILITIES OF THE
PHYSICIAN AND PATIENT

In Case 5-5, Dr. Cobb had a long and complex relationship with Mr. Rowe; several aspects of this pertain to the explicit and implicit responsibilities that physician and patient had toward each other (see Table 5.3). First, physicians are expected to be competent. Competence has been defined by some to consist of a good fund of knowledge, technical skill, clinical judgment, and awareness of limitations (Emanuel & Dubler, 1995). Competence must also include the ability to communicate effectively with patients, their families and colleagues, to elicit and take into account patients' values and experiences (Engel, 1980), to understand and intervene appropriately with the social aspects of illness, and to be empathic (Rudebeck, 1992). These last two features are essential; without understanding the patient's distress, and communicating that understanding to the patient, a physician cannot relieve it. Further, "the doctor's competence is more about accompanying the patient up to her own choice than about giving lots of advice" (Rudebeck, 1992). Part of the competence of a physician is her ability to foster meaningful change.

Moral responsibilities of the physician go beyond the ethical principles of nonmaleficence, beneficence, justice, and autonomy (see Chapter 12 on medical ethics). The physician must not abandon a patient, even when there are difficult decisions to be made and when there are no clear solutions. Mr. Rowe in Case 5-5 would be a demanding patient for most physicians. That made it even more imperative for his physician to listen, to ac-

Table 5.3
Physicians' Responsibilities toward Patients

Being technically competent
Being with the patient
Providing information
Being truthful/trustworthy
Avoiding conflict of interest
Advocating for the patient
Expressing personal commitment to care
Avoiding harm (nonmaleficence)
Acting in the patient's best interest (beneficence)
Maximizing patient autonomy
Negotiating a treatment plan that is concordant with the patient's values

knowledge Mr. Rowe's requests and needs in a nonjudgmental fashion, and to respect him as a person. At the same time, Dr. Cobb had to make explicit her own limitations. She had to make her values known while respecting his. When mistakes occur, addressing them openly often will win a patient's trust more than trying to hide them. In this case, the "mistake" was a lifesaving one, as the patient expressed resentment at having been resuscitated.

Trust is not implicit in any relationship. It is usually won after having faced a challenge together (O'Rourke, 1993). Physicians' honesty and integrity are usually judged by actions, not only words. When patients are ill and emotions are raised, it is difficult not to promise a good outcome. Consider the following story, reported to me thirdhand, and thus probably better considered a parable:

CASE 5-6

Shortly after a young Anglo physician began to work at a clinic on the Navajo reservation, a father brought his daughter into the office. They had traveled a long distance to the clinic. She had had minor upper respiratory symptoms. The physician examined her carefully, shared his findings, prescribed Tylenol for fever, and sent them home.

The next day, the father returned with his mother, a chronically ill-appearing woman with poorly controlled diabetes mellitus and a gangrenous foot. The physician then understood that he had brought in his daughter the previous day in order to "check out" the new physician before trusting him with his mother.

A collaborative approach to care means taking the patient's perspective on an equal footing with the physician's diagnostic perspective (Katon & Kleinman, 1981; Levenstein *et al.*, 1986; Brown *et al.*, 1986). The patient is recruited as an ally in planning further investigation of a problem and in formulating a treatment plan. Patients are given information that will empower them to make important clinical decisions. Information is shared with relevant family members, important social supports, and other healthcare professionals; maintaining a focus on the patient's values, all of these others may make valuable contributions to the patient's care.

In any healthcare system, there is the possibility of physician conflict of interest in caring for patients (Emanuel & Dubler, 1995). Financial conflict of interest in a fee-for-service system is of concern when patients are referred to for-profit, physician-owned diagnostic or treatment facilities. Conversely, in managed care settings, there may be financial incentives to minimize the use of resources. Conflict of interest can be more subtle, and unavoidable; for example, a patient may receive short shrift if a physician is running late and has an important social engagement. Similarly, bias is prevalent in medical settings. For example, it has been shown that women who have the same percentage of excess body weight as men are more likely to be labeled as obese by their physicians (Franks *et al.*, 1982), that black patients are less likely to be screened for hypercholesterolemia than whites (Naumberg *et al.*, 1993), and that Hispanic patients are less likely to receive adequate pain relief compared with non-Hispanic patients in an emergency room setting (Todd *et al.*, 1993). Recognizing, accommodating to, and correcting conflict of interest and systematic bias are part of the physician's responsibility.

In order to accomplish these tasks, physicians need to have a means for organized reflection on their behavior. Commitment to becoming more self-aware will help the physician to reduce miscommunication, recognize the difference between what the patient wishes and what the physician would wish in a similar circumstance, and find more satisfaction with patient care.

Just as physicians have responsibilities in a patient–physician relationship, so do patients. Our notions of what is a "good patient" have changed over the years. Historically, patients have been responsible for accurately reporting symptoms and following physicians' recommendations. A more recent view is that, rather than being passive recipients of healthcare, patients should be more active in their care and take more responsibility for health-promoting activities. However, our language often still suggests that the patient take a passive role in healthcare. For example, the term *compliance* implies that the patient will unquestioningly follow the orders of the physician. Perhaps "adherence to a mutually negotiated plan" comes closer to a more balanced locus of responsibility for health. Still, some questions remain that will need to be answered by each physician who cares for patients. For example, whose responsibility is it to remind patients about screening tests? Does a physician have the responsibility to provide a treatment requested by a patient if she does not believe that it will be helpful? Should the physician initiate inquiry into "personal" issues such as sexual behavior or HIV risk, or should the physician wait for the patient to bring these up? What is the physician's responsibility if a patient does not follow through with a treatment plan? There is little consensus among physicians regarding the answers to these questions.

CASE 5-7

Dr. Carole Sanchez had taken over the care of Ethel Burke 3 months previously because she was dissatisfied with her prior physician. Ethel is a 66-year-old woman with chronic severe unremitting neurogenic shoulder pain resulting from an automobile accident 4 years previously. She also has an anxiety disorder and mild congestive heart failure. After trying several courses of physical therapy, different medication regimens, anesthetic and steroid injections, chiropractic, psychotherapy, acupuncture, and electrical stimulation, the only treatment that offered relief was high-dose oral narcotics. She also had taken diazepam at moderate dose for many years for anxiety.

Dr. Sanchez expressed willingness to maintain her on these medications as long as she used them as prescribed. Two months after she began caring for Mrs.

Burke, the patient requested an urgent refill of her medications 3 days before she was due for a refill. She had gone to the emergency department by ambulance and claimed that the ambulance crew had taken her medication from her and had not returned it. The next month, 2 weeks after having been prescribed a month's supply of medication, she called requesting an urgent refill prescription, claiming that all of her medication was gone. She said that the pharmacy only filled part of her prescription. Dr. Sanchez called the pharmacist, who disconfirmed her allegation. She reported having taken it as prescribed and could not account for the missing medication. She complained of extreme, uncontrolled pain.

On a routine prenatal visit, Mrs. Burke's daughter said that she had something important to tell Dr. Sanchez about her mother. She reported that Mrs. Burke was an addict, unable to control her use of medication, and had been receiving prescriptions for narcotics from several physicians simultaneously.

Dr. Sanchez deliberated whether to discharge the patient from the practice for having been dishonest or try to work with her to control her narcotic use. Not discharging the patient would mean working through a time-consuming process of contacting other physicians, contracting with the patient on use of medications, dispensing supplies of narcotics every 3 days rather than monthly, having the patient evaluated by a drug dependency program, and discussing this plan further in a family meeting. Mrs. Burke and her family came into the office. They negotiated a plan to monitor her narcotic use, and they signed a contract to that effect.

——— TOOLS FOR RELATIONSHIP-BUILDING ———

Case 5-7 illustrates a situation where there were multiple threats to the patient–physician relationship. Caring for Mrs. Burke would be challenging for most experienced physicians. For some physicians, patient dishonesty is a cause for immediate termination of the patient–physician relationship. In my view, direct confrontation about dishonest behavior need not always result in termination of the relationship, but requires careful contracting and rebuilding trust.

Because the patient–physician relationship is a specialized social relationship, no one is born with of all the skills she will need to form effective patient–physician relationships. The noted psychologist Carl Rogers (1961) provided a series of principles for health professionals to consider when forming and developing therapeutic relationships, all of which were useful in caring for Mrs. Burke. These principles are listed in Table 5.4 and are described here:

- *Act in such a way that you will be perceived by the patient as trustworthy, dependable, and consistent.* The emphasis on action implies that trustworthiness must be demonstrated in a way that is understandable to the patient. Patients' interpretations of physicians' actions may be different than the intent of those actions.
- *Communicate clearly and unambiguously.* This includes nonverbal as well as verbal communication. It is important to let the patient take the lead, agree on an agenda, avoid use of medical jargon until you are sure the patient understands, summarize periodically, and check with the patient to make sure you have under-

Table 5.4
Tools for Relationship-Building

Demonstrating unconditional positive regard for the patient as a person
Being dependable and consistent
Being caring and charitable
Understanding the patient's perspective on illness
Eliciting and responding to the patient's emotions
Legitimizing the patient's concerns
Demonstrating respect and support
Offering hope
Using touch
Involving family members
Activating the patient to take part in his medical care
Helping the patient find meaning in suffering
Fostering healthy coping
Activating psychoneuroimmunologic mechanisms (the placebo response)
Respecting boundaries
Being committed to becoming more self-aware
Using self-disclosure judiciously

---

stood him, and that he has understood you (Epstein *et al.*, 1993). When there is hope, let the patient know.

- *In all situations, learn to experience and communicate some positive attitudes toward the patient.* In situations when the patient's life resembles your own, this may be easy. However, it is crucial, in order to sustain a long-term patient–physician relationship, to develop an *unconditional positive regard* for the patient (Rogers, 1961). This does not mean condoning unacceptable behavior, as in Case 5-7, but does mean being capable of understanding the patient's behavior from the *patient's* perspective. This may involve viewing unacceptable behavior as a cry for help or a misguided attempt at healing. It is important to acknowledge and articulate respect for patients' attempts at problem-solving, even if not successful.

- *Enter as fully as possible into the patient's experience of suffering and personal meanings to see these as he does. Then, communicate your understanding to the patient.* Empathy is the basis for therapeutic human relationships, and involves taking a perspective other than our own (Bellet & Maloney, 1991). Physical touch can communicate empathy as well. Once having taken the patient's perspective, it is important to let the patient know that you understand his perspective. *Reflection* ("You clearly were in pain") and *legitimation* ("It is only natural to feel this way facing this situation") are techniques for communicating empathy (Bird & Cohen-Cole, 1990).

- *Be sure to separate* your *needs from those of the patient.* Conflict of interest can be financial, emotional, and logistical. Some emotional needs may not be within the physician's awareness. Because this is a thorny issue, there will be a detailed discussion of boundaries in the next section. When such conflicts do arise, organized self-reflection or a neutral third party can be helpful in resolving them.

- *Act in such a way that the patient does not perceive you as a threat.* An anxious or frightened patient will not be able to listen well or feel empowered to change. If a patient feels that she is being blamed for her illness or humiliated in the course of medical care (Lazare, 1987), she will be less likely to share information and participate in her care. By taking a *nonjudgmental stance,* you will help the patient trust you and help her participate in her care. Mrs. Burke and her family in Case 5-7 were well aware that she might be stigmatized for having a narcotic addiction; only when she and her family felt that Dr. Sanchez would treat her with respect were they able to disclose the extent of her problem.

- *Inquire into and utilize the strengths in the patient's family and cultural background.* Patients' families are intimately involved in the interpretation of symptoms, provision of medical care, and relationships between the identified patient and the healthcare system (Doherty & Baird, 1983; McDaniel *et al.*, 1990a; Epstein *et al.*, 1993). In Case 5-7, Mrs. Burke's family proved invaluable in providing necessary information to understand the patient's problem, developing a therapeutic plan, monitoring her pain control, and driving to the pharmacy every 3 days so that she had lower potential for abusing narcotic medications. Even when the family is not present, inquiry into strengths and attributes of family members is often fruitful. Asking a patient to solicit the assistance of a family member who successfully quit smoking, for example, may reinforce a patient's efforts to quit. Similarly, culture influences significantly the way symptoms are presented to physicians, patients' expectations of care, and patients' explanatory models of illness (Kleinman *et al.*, 1978). These are crucial factors and will be discussed in more detail in Chapters 6 and 10.
- *Demonstrate that you can work together in a partnership.* Make explicit your wish to work on a problem together. Be clear about what you can and cannot do. Follow through with your promises. Don't make promises that you cannot deliver. Describe, and then demonstrate a relationship based on collaboration. With Mrs. Burke, it was critical for Dr. Sanchez to indicate that she would continue to care for her, but would not tolerate her unrestricted use of narcotics.
- *Advocate for the patient in gaining access to healthcare services, social services, and justice.* You can offer *support* ("I will be here with you no matter what happens," or "Mr. Z, the social worker, can help you with that problem; I will give him a call") that is realistic and perceived as helpful by the patient. Also, you can facilitate access to a variety of services that would otherwise be inaccessible to the patient.
- *Communicate your own experience to the patient in a way that will be helpful and meaningful to her.* Be aware of your own experiences, emotional reactions, and prejudices and their sources (Epstein *et al.*, 1993; Weinberg & Mauksch, 1991; Mengel, 1987). With Mrs. Burke, it was helpful to the patient and family to know that Dr. Sanchez had treated patients successfully who had similar difficulties. Judicious use of physician self-disclosure can sometimes be helpful to patients. Take care, however, that disclosure is for the benefit of the patient and not the physician.

CASE 5-8

Dr. Peter Blank lives next door to the Dwyer family. Their 3-year-old daughter is ill with a temperature of 102°F, cough, and nasal congestion. It is Sunday of a 3-day holiday weekend. Mrs. Dwyer calls to see if Dr. Blank will take a look in her daughter's ears to make sure that she does not have an infection. Dr. Blank is not their usual physician, although, as a family physician, he would be competent to diagnose and treat an ear infection. He is not on call, but does have an otoscope at home. He feels somewhat uncomfortable about this because he does not know the child's prior medical history nor would he be able to follow up, but he examines the child, makes a diagnosis of otitis media, and prescribes an antibiotic. He suggests follow-up with the child's family physician.

123

BOUNDARIES OF THE PATIENT–PHYSICIAN RELATIONSHIP

BOUNDARIES OF THE PATIENT–PHYSICIAN RELATIONSHIP

Although diverse, in order to meet complex human needs, the patient–physician relationship is governed by explicit legal regulations, ethical principles, and complex social conventions. The boundaries of the patient–physician relationship protect both physician and patient (Linklater & MacDougall, 1993) so that they can maintain a professional helping relationship that meets the patient's needs. Boundaries define expected and accepted physical, social, and emotional interactions between physicians and patients.

Some examples of blatant boundary violations by physicians include sexual misconduct, abuse of confidential disclosures, inappropriate disclosure of personal information, giving expensive gifts, and seeing patients for medical problems at unusual times and places (Gabbard & Nadelson, 1995). Such violations are common. For example, in a variety of settings, 3–12% of male physicians report having had sexual relations with a patient (Gabbard & Nadelson, 1995). Usually, boundary violations such as these involve misuse of the physician's power, place the physician's interest ahead of the patient's, put patients in a double bind where clinical care depends on continued violations, and involve secrecy (Linklater & MacDougall, 1993).

Patients can also test and violate boundaries. Requesting frequent or "special" appointments, wearing seductive clothing, giving large gifts, sexually harassing their physician (Phillips & Schneider, 1993), being dishonest, and exhibiting threatening or demanding behaviors can all test the integrity of the patient–physician relationship. Family members can test boundaries by requesting access to confidential information about a patient, and third parties can demand information about a patient as a condition of providing benefits.

There are more subtle boundary issues that physicians face on a daily basis. Despite the complexities raised when physicians treat or offer medical advice to family members or friends, as in Case 5-8 (La Puma *et al.*, 1991; Epstein, 1994), sometimes it is unavoidable, such as in the case of physicians in rural areas, or desirable, such as when the physician is the most qualified person to treat the problem. Often physicians seek colleagues whom they know professionally or personally for their own healthcare. The most conservative approach is to avoid such "dual relationships"; however, in certain situations, they can work well if approached with caution. A patient may feel comfortable approaching a physician-friend (or relative) about routine problems, but would not feel comfortable talking about a sexually transmitted disease, diagnosis of terminal illness, or psychiatric problems. Usually, it is best to discuss with the patient-friend how to deal with such situations before they occur. The physician must first reflect on whether she would be able to probe the patient's intimate history, bear bad news, be objective enough to give appropriate care, and recruit the patient-friend's cooperation with care plans. The same questions also should be directed toward the patient. If the friendship is unable to support a therapeutic relationship, then parts or all of the care of the patient should be transferred to another physician (Rourke *et al.*, 1993).

Some rituals help to protect the sanctity of the patient–physician relationship. Physicians use more formal speech and less small talk than that used in typical social conversation. They also use professional attire and the office setting to set therapeutic encounters apart from other social interactions. This context often helps the patient feel safe enough to trust the physician with personal and intimate information. Deviations from established personal practice norms require self-reflection. Even though a patient might offer to come to a physician's home for treatment rather than the physician making a home visit, this is rarely acceptable. Medical consultations should not take place in the supermarket, if physician and patient happen to meet there.

CASE 5-9

Dr. Reuben Marks was caring for Carol Wang, a 71-year-old retired librarian who had multiple medical complaints. Typically, the patient would come into the office having recently seen a television program or read a newspaper article about a new technology or screening procedure. Despite Dr. Marks's explanations that the procedure was not appropriate or necessary, the patient would appear dissatisfied. Sometimes she would seek another physician who would be willing to perform the procedure. Dr. Marks found himself dreading Mrs. Wang's visits, and would feel very frustrated and angry at the end of them.

At one point, Dr. Marks realized that, although he knew that Mrs. Wang had two first-degree relatives who died of colon cancer, he had never ordered a screening colonoscopy. This realization was startling to Dr. Marks, who otherwise was a careful and thoughtful physician. On reflection, he realized that, in many ways, Mrs. Wang's behavior reminded him of his grandmother, who played a prominent part in his childhood. She was never satisfied with anything that he did, was relentlessly demanding, and belittled his accomplishments. For example, when Dr. Marks was accepted at a prominent medical school, she commented that her friend's grandson had been accepted at another prominent school and perhaps Dr. Marks could go there instead. Dr. Marks's response was to avoid contact with his grandmother; he recognized this same pattern of behavior with Mrs. Wang. Having realized that connection, Dr. Marks found it easier to understand his own anger and could become more patient with and attentive to Mrs. Wang's needs, while providing appropriate medical care.

DIFFICULT RELATIONSHIPS

Medical care is emotionally demanding and intense for physicians, patients, and their families. Physicians have a responsibility to care for all patients, regardless of race, sex, personality, and personal values. Physicians face their own limitations when caring for patients with incurable illnesses, ambiguous or vague symptoms, or unsolvable social problems. Environmental barriers, disabilities, cognitive impairment, language barriers, and cultural factors make some relationships intrinsically more difficult (Klein *et al.*, 1982). Also, the stress of illness may bring out more "primitive" or maladaptive aspects of a patient's personality in an attempt to deal with unfamiliar and overwhelming situations.

Table 5.5
Difficult Patient–Physician Relationships

Characteristics of difficult situations
    Problems perceived as unsolvable
        Incurable diseases
        Ambiguous, vague symptoms
        Terminal illness
    Conditions for which patient is perceived as culpable
    Physician feeling helpless or inadequate
    Patient behavior that threatens physician authority
    Violation of physician's personal norms
    Perception of personal risk to physician (e.g., contagion of HIV)
    Specific diagnoses
        Psychopathology—moderate to severe
        Substance abuse
        Obesity
        Chronic pain
        Sexual behavior-related conditions—patient perceived as culpable
        Hypochondriasis
        "Symptom amplification"

Personality characteristics and behaviors of patients that may predispose
        to difficulties
    Expression of anger, hostility, or frustration
    Addiction to or seeking of drugs
    Not following physician's advice
    Expression of seemingly endless needs (overdependency)
    Expression of entitlement for special attention
    Attempts to "manipulate" the physician
    Rejection of help while continuing to complain of symptoms
    Self-destructive behavior

Personality characteristics of physicians that may predispose to difficulties
    Enjoyment of problem-solving and sense of closure
    Satisfaction in being able to help
    Belief in self-sacrifice, stoicism, and hard work
    Belief that science can solve human suffering
    Aversion to risk
    Expectation that patients will share these values

This may result in the patient acting in a hostile or abrasive manner, becoming passive and dependent, appearing manipulative, presenting symptoms in a dramatic way, or avoiding medical care (Groves, 1978). Some patients are dishonest and falsify prescriptions for controlled substances, lie about their drug use, and feign injury to claim disability payments.

When there are difficulties in a patient–physician relationship, most often, it is a combination of factors that contribute to the difficulty. Some of these are listed in Table 5.5.

Just as strong patient–physician relationships have the potential to enhance outcomes, difficulties can lead to patient and physician dissatisfaction because of uncommunicated needs, unmet expectations, and failure of the physician to respond empathically to the patient's suffering (Schwenk & Romano, 1992). There is also a strong relationship between communication failure, increased healthcare utilization (Lin *et al.*, 1991), and more requests for specialty consultation. Breakdown of the patient–physician relationship was identified as a reason for malpractice litigation in 71% of depositions reviewed in a study by Beckman and colleagues (Beckman *et al.*, 1994); specific issues identified by the plaintiffs included being abandoned by the physician, failing to acknowledge the patient's or family's concerns, delivering information poorly, and failing to understand the patient's or family's perspective.

Case 5-9 illustrates some of the effects that a physician's prior experiences can have on his behavior that was outside of his moment-to-moment awareness. Dr. Marks found Mrs. Wang annoying, without quite knowing why, and these feelings affected the quality of care that Mrs. Wang received. In other situations, physician and patient may have difficulty reaching agreement on treatment, physicians can make mistakes (Dimsdale, 1984), or a patient may not take medication as prescribed, without knowing why. Part of understanding these difficulties lies in understanding the concepts of *transference, countertransference,* and *projection.*

Transference refers to the unconscious reactions that patients have to physicians who, in some way, remind them of another important person in their past (usually a close family member). *Countertransference* is the corresponding phenomenon in physicians; as much as physicians may want to consider their relationships with patients "professional," the intimate nature of medical care makes it common for some patients to provoke powerful positive or negative emotions in physicians as in Case 5-9. *Projection* refers to assigning one's own unconscious or conscious feelings or beliefs to another person, often in emotionally charged situations. Case 5-1 is a good example of a situation wherein projection might occur; the physician expected that the patient would become more anxious and afraid based on the meaning that *he* assigned to the illness. Sometimes transference/countertransference and family-of-origin issues can impair a physician's ability to provide optimal medical care (Mengel, 1987). In many cases, however, if the physician can become aware of and utilize her own background, experiences, feelings, and values, she can be more effective in helping patients through difficult times and can reinforce rather than erode therapeutic relationships (McDaniel & Landau-Stanton, 1991; Epstein *et al.*, 1993).

While physicians are diverse, there are some common personality characteristics among physicians that can contribute to difficulties in the patient–physician relationship that may be connected to physicians' choice of career. Physicians describe themselves, and are described, as being hard-working, self-sacrificing, and averse to taking risks (Schwenk *et al.*, 1989; Gerber, 1985). Physicians generally like to solve problems, like a sense of closure, and like to help. Further, physicians expect that their patients will share these values. It is inevitable that some patients may have behaviors or belief systems that violate physicians' personal norms. Consider the physician whose religious beliefs and cultural background have taught her that homosexuality is evil caring for a patient who acquired AIDS through male prostitution, the patient who arrives late for appointments to a physician who values punctuality, and a patient who continues to abuse drugs seeing a physician who values self-control. Other common situations that physicians find frustrating are listed in Table 5.5.

Difficulties in the patient–physician relationship can also involve family members, friends, social contacts, and social agencies. For example, a patient may come into the office reluctantly on the insistence of a spouse, or a patient may become angry because his HMO has denied payment to a psychotherapist whom he has been seeing for a year. A patient may want validation for his symptoms to receive attention and care from family members. Even if the other person or agency is not physically present in the office, the influence is clearly felt. Particularly challenging is when *triangulation* (McDaniel *et al.*, 1989) occurs. In these situations, the physician is invited to take sides in a two-way dispute, often between family members. Consider a situation where the spouse of a diabetic woman reports to a physician that the patient is not as careful with her diet as she reports. On the surface, this may seem like useful information, until the physician looks at the dynamics of the relationship further. The diabetic woman has been criticized by her spouse at home. She insists that she is doing a good enough job of managing her diabetes; she wants the physician to validate this. The spouse wants the physician to make the patient more careful with her diet. Consider what would happen if the physician took either partner's side in the dispute. If the physician were to criticize the patient for her noncompliance, the physician might imperil the relationship with the patient and unknowingly discourage the patient from returning. On the other hand, excluding the spouse from the discussion might escalate his unhelpful criticism at home. In either case, the physician would create a dysfunctional compensatory alliance (Hahn *et al.*, 1988).

When difficulties arise, it is even more important to attend to the principles of relationship-building listed in the previous section. Anxiety tends to make difficult situations more difficult. It is therefore important for the physician to put himself at ease, to attend to his own feelings, and to inquire, in an open-ended way, into the sources of the patient's frustrations. Recognition that there is a problem is usually helpful, along with an offer of help (e.g., "It seems that I haven't addressed all of your concerns. Could you tell me how I could help?"). Explore the meaning of the illness with the patient in a nonjudgmental way. Let the patient know that you have understood his needs, and legitimize the patient's concerns no matter how trivial they may seem to you. Communicate clearly what you can and cannot do for the patient, and do not promise what you cannot deliver. When the patient demands more than you can give, set clear boundaries and be consistent. When a patient has been dishonest, a written behavioral contract is helpful (Quill, 1983). The contract should list specific unacceptable behaviors in observable terms. It should also be spelled out that violations of the contract would initiate a series of measures that might result in termination of the relationship. When problems seem mysterious, expand the focus of your inquiry. Include relevant family members and important social contacts. In family meetings, make sure that everyone's perspective has been articulated and heard; even though you may agree more with some perspectives than others, avoid the temptation to take sides. Often, the physician's job is to facilitate the resolution of conflict by the family, not to provide a solution. Most importantly, recognize your own needs. Not every patient will appreciate your hard work, but a colleague might. For practicing physicians, calling on medical consultants and psychotherapists can be very helpful in providing reassurance and support (Epstein, 1995). Similarly, medical students should be encouraged to make use of mentors, peers, and faculty to discuss cases that are emotionally difficult, and to explore the reasons why. Support groups are another means of dealing with difficult situations, and are increasingly used in medical training (Quill & Williamson, 1990).

Sometimes there are differences between physicians and patients that are irreconcilable. Patients may expect that the physician will be available at all times, prescribe desired medications, order desired laboratory tests, validate disability, or spend exceptional amounts of time in caring for the patient. Often these differences can be negotiated after respectful inquiry and principled discussion about the disagreement. The next step is to inform the patient clearly of the reasons for not complying with her request(s), along with a willingness to work together despite the disagreement (Quill, 1989). When the conflict escalates, and when the issues affect clinical care of the patient, the physician should relinquish care of the patient rather than capitulate to the patient's demands for inappropriate care.

Secrets deserve special mention (Karpel & Strauss, 1983; Newman, 1993). There is a difference between information that is private and that which is secret. Private information has little or no power to harm third parties, and requires little psychological energy to sustain. Secrets, on the other hand, have the potential to be destructive to the patient or to others if disclosed or if not disclosed. It can be especially destructive if the physician is asked to compromise his integrity in order to keep a secret. Bearing private information is part of the burden and privilege of being a physician. Some confidential information must be disclosed if the physician feels that a life is in danger. Suicidal and homicidal intent, child abuse, and elder abuse require prompt evaluation, even if promises of confidentiality have been made. There are many other situations, where there is not universal agreement among the involved parties, when the physician must reflect on his own values and communicate them unambiguously to the patient. Consultation with a trusted colleague can be invaluable in untangling some of these difficult situations. These issues are discussed further in Chapter 12.

CONCLUSIONS

The patient–physician relationship is a complex professional relationship with the goals of relieving suffering, promoting healing, and preventing illness. It is a personal relationship and a social contract that needs to be flexible enough to accommodate to a wide variety of situations, but well defined enough to maintain the primacy of the patient's interest.

The philosophical basis for the patient–physician relationship has evolved considerably during the twentieth century from a predominantly paternalistic model to models that promote patient autonomy. It is critical, though, that the emphasis on patient autonomy not relieve physicians of the obligation to make therapeutic recommendations and to foster behavior modifications in patients who may be reluctant to change. Physicians' wise use of their intimate connections with patients and their socially given power can make them strong advocates for patient well-being.

Earning trust, nonabandonment, continuity, being empathic, and taking a nonjudgmental stance are critical to the development and maintenance of a strong patient–physician relationship. Families and culture have a powerful influence on patient well-being and patient–physician relationships; it is essential to take a family and social perspective on all illness episodes, regardless of whether family members are actually present at the visit.

No aspect of human suffering is excluded from the physician's office. It is a burden and a privilege to bear witness to patients' suffering and to intervene on patients' behalf. You can have a profound impact on a patient's life if you are willing to listen respectfully and accompany her in her suffering. Each patient has a personal language through which she expresses her distress; your task as a physician will be to help the patient interpret her symptoms, to find meaning, and to establish a common purpose. Just as there is a distinction between illness and disease, there is a distinction between curing, caring, and healing. Curing can sometimes be a purely technical matter. Caring involves developing a personal bond with a patient. Only when the patient knows that her suffering has been understood can you heal.

CASES FOR DISCUSSION

CASE 1

Veronica Jones was a 37-year-old woman with advanced AIDS on renal dialysis for HIV-related kidney failure. She was admitted to hospital with respiratory failure and was put on a ventilator in the intensive care unit. Her prognosis was very poor. Dr. John Graham, with whom she had a strong relationship, was out of town; his mother had died suddenly of a stroke. Despite many attempts to discuss end-of-life issues, she would change the topic and make statements that she would later retract. She believed that her family did not know that she had AIDS.

Dr. Tom Rubin was covering for Dr. Graham and knew the patient and her family from a prior hospitalization. Ms. Jones was lethargic and confused. At times she would become more lucid. On one occasion, while on the ventilator, she expressed a wish to die and be disconnected from the ventilator. Dr. Rubin contacted her niece, who was the patient's healthcare proxy listed on an advance directive. However, she could not make decisions on the patient's behalf unless she knew the patient's diagnosis and prognosis.

During a time when Ms. Jones was more lucid, Dr. Rubin strongly advocated that he be permitted to disclose the diagnosis to Ms. Jones's niece, so that she could help make decisions on the patient's behalf. She gave permission; the niece indicated that she was already aware of the AIDS diagnosis, as was most of the family.

Despite the patient's wishes, the niece refused to consider a do-not-resuscitate order. To everyone's surprise, Ms. Jones came off the ventilator and became more lucid. Later in the hospitalization, the patient learned that the niece had been stealing money from her bank account. Dr. Rubin convened a family meeting, at which discussion about end-of-life care provoked heated family conflict, and no resolution was reached.

Dr. Graham returned to town. It was clear to him, and all physicians involved, that the patient, although improved, would likely die in the next few weeks. She required morphine for pain, and she was intermittently sedated and lucid. Ms. Jones asked to go home, but home services could not be arranged because no family member would be available to take 24-hour responsibility for her. During a dialysis session, she asked that the dialysis be stopped. She refused dialysis the next day, consented the following day, but again stopped halfway through the treatment. Dr. Graham asked her if she would like another dialysis treatment, and Ms. Jones replied, "I've had enough." She would not answer whether she would want to be resuscitated in case of now imminent cardiac arrest. Dr. Graham made a decision that resuscitation would be futile, and wrote a DNAR order. The patient remained comfortable on morphine and died quietly 2 days later.

1. *What are the physician's responsibilities in this situation?*
2. *Using your knowledge of models of patient–physician relationships, what approaches were used? Which would you have used in this situation?*
3. *Who should have responsibility for making decisions about the do-not-resuscitate order for this patient?*
4. *What is the physician's role in facing family conflict of this magnitude?*

CASE 2

Joanne Williams is a mentally retarded 48-year-old woman who lives alone in an apartment complex for people with disabilities. She comes to the office frequently for a variety of medical concerns. Many of these concerns are chronic, such as back pain which does not interfere with her activity, or self-limited, such as colds. It is very difficult to keep office visits to their allotted time— the patient continues to ask for more time, and always has additional concerns. Each time that she needs a medication refill for her antiseizure medications, she calls at least three times within an afternoon to make sure that it has been called into the pharmacy. She is on the phone to the office daily with a variety of concerns. She has written many letters to her physician, Dr. Beverly Price, describing how difficult her life has been and how lonely she feels. The patient is on an insurance plan that provided Dr. Price with minimal reimbursement. Dr. Price feels burdened by the patient's unrelenting needs.

1. What is the responsibility of the physician in this situation?
2. What are the boundaries to this relationship?
3. How can the physician care for this patient without becoming overwhelmed?
4. What feelings would you have caring for this patient? How would you approach this relationship?

CASE 3

Mr. Ray Kapsberger is a patient whom Dr. Glenda Lee has seen for many visits for right ankle pain. He fractured his ankle several years ago while intoxicated and recalls nothing of the event. Since then, he has reinjured his ankle on several occasions, mostly while intoxicated. He has a long history of alcoholism, and has been in many alcohol rehabilitation programs, with only a few weeks of abstinence at a time. Mr. Kapsberger frequently comes in complaining of ankle pain. Dr. Lee has referred him to a surgeon who recommended an ankle fusion operation. This is complex surgery that requires a long rehabilitation including physical therapy for 3–4 months following the procedure. The surgeon refuses to operate unless the patient is sober for at least 3 months, as reinjury would be very dangerous during the recuperation period. Also, Dr. Lee is reluctant to prescribe the patient with narcotic pain relievers, given his heavy intermittent binge drinking.

The pain pills take the edge off the pain, but don't get rid of it completely. Mr. Kapsberger is angry. He has several demands: that he be referred to a surgeon who will do the operation regardless, that Dr. Lee fill out a form indicating that he is unable to work, and that he get some narcotics for pain.

1. How should Dr. Lee deal with Mr. Kapsberger's demands?
2. What can Dr. Lee do to create a more satisfactory patient–physician relationship?
3. How can Dr. Lee help the patient to become more active in his care?
4. How would you feel taking care of this patient?

CASE 4

Charles Johnson is a 78-year-old man, a retired professor of psychology. For several weeks he had not been feeling well, with decreased appetite and some mild upper abdominal pain. After several visits to Dr. Sam Green, he had a CT scan and found out that he has unresectable metastatic pancreatic cancer. Since the diagnosis 3 weeks ago, he has consulted a medical oncologist, a surgeon, and a radiologist for the consideration of palliative procedures, including surgery, percutaneous insertion of a stent, and radiation. None of these are possible, as there is too much tumor surrounding the bile ducts. Mr. Johnson was given a prognosis of 4 to 8 weeks at the time of diagnosis. It has now been 4 weeks. He has been getting weaker by the day. He has some upper abdominal pain but does not like to complain about it, especially to his daughter Denise, whom he views as overconcerned and very intrusive. He would like to spend his last days at home in peace and quiet without many visitors. He approaches death with grace but still harbors some fears about what the end will be like, especially as the tumor spreads. Mr. Johnson's wife, Sarah, has been extremely involved and supportive during this time. She has made many calls to the children to update them on his condition, and has passed along his instructions to have them not come to visit.

Because Mr. Johnson previously had been healthy, he has seen Dr. Green rarely until recently. Mr. Johnson is aware that some physicians have prescribed medications for terminally ill patients who wish to end their lives with dignity. While his wife is out one day, Mr. Johnson calls Dr. Green to ask him if he would be willing to prescribe some medicine to end his life before things become intolerable.

1. How would you approach this patient's request?
2. What models of the patient–physician relationship would be appropriate?
3. What are your own feelings about assisted suicide?
4. How would those feelings affect your care of Mr. Johnson?
5. Would you involve Mr. Johnson's family? How?

CASE 5

Frank Roth is a 75-year-old retired schoolteacher in generally good health. Many of his close friends have died, and his two brothers are chronically ill and live far away. He comes into the office to see Dr. Beth Green frequently for concerns that seemed minor to Dr. Green. Once, Mr. Roth had a blood pressure check at a shopping mall screening program; his pressure was 142/88, and he made an appointment to discuss this further. He would call several times a week with mild respiratory symptoms, muscle aches, and other concerns; he would take a long time to describe his symptoms in great detail. He would be easily reassured, and he did not seem to have hypochondriacal preoccupations. The frequent contacts with the office were a social outlet for a patient who led a very lonely life. The patient was not otherwise depressed.

1. How would you approach caring for this patient?
2. What goals would you have for his care?
3. How would you feel about not being able to meet all of Mr. Roth's needs?
4. How could you still remain patient-centered but set appropriate limits?

CASE 6

Muriel Bristol is a 46-year-old woman who has visited Dr. Reginald Bruce occasionally for seasonal allergies and irritable bowel syndrome. Among other concerns at her annual physical exam, she indicated that she would like a series of laboratory tests to check micronutrient levels, immune function, viral titers, and allergy to a wide variety of substances. Although she had generally felt well, she had been advised by an alternative health practitioner that she may have chronic candida syndrome. She presented the physician with articles from the lay press suggesting that a wide variety of symptoms may result from candida, and that intensive nutritional and pharmacologic treatment should be used to eradicate it. Dr. Bruce offered to discuss the patient's concerns, while explaining that these tests are very expensive, often inconclusive, and would likely yield no benefit. Ms. Bristol insisted on testing and accused the physician of being too narrow-minded.

1. Would you be able to care for this patient?
2. How would you maintain a relationship with her given her demands?
3. At what point would you refer her to another physician?
4. What would you do if you did not know a physician who shared her health beliefs?

CASE 7

On a routine physical exam visit, Dr. Carla Long asked Mr. Tom Garcia about sexual risk behaviors for HIV infection. After an uncomfortable silence, Mr. Garcia reported that, while on business trips, *he would occasionally have sexual encounters with men. Often he would meet the men at a bar or health club, and have sex afterwards. None of these encounters has resulted in a long-term relationship. He reported always using condoms for oral sex; he does not engage in anal sex. Mr. Garcia is married and has three teenage children. He reports that his marriage has been generally good, and feels that disclosure of his bisexuality to his wife would be devastating. The results of an HIV test a year ago at the county health department were negative. His wife has not been tested, as far as Dr. Long knows. His wife is also a patient of Dr. Long. Dr. Long felt uncomfortable harboring this secret from the patient's wife, even though her risk for HIV is very low. On the other hand, she would not tell the patient's wife without Mr. Garcia's permission. Dr. Long found this situation very troubling also because of her own religious beliefs: As a fundamentalist Christian, she believed that homosexuality was an abomination and that Mr. Garcia should abandon his current sexual practices.*

1. *Should Dr. Long care for Mr. Garcia?*
2. *What principles should she use in approaching his care?*
3. *How would you advise her to deal with her own feelings about Mr. Garcia's sexual orientation and behaviors?*
4. *How should Dr. Long handle the secret that Mr. Garcia is keeping from his wife?*

ACKNOWLEDGMENTS. I have learned the most about patient–physician relationships from my patients, to whom I am greatly indebted. Drs. Cecile Carson, Dan Duffy, George Engel, Leston Havens, Ian McWhinney, Susan McDaniel, Tim Quill, Peter Reich, and Charles Solky provided guidance and inspiration at critical points. My children, Eli and Malka, taught me how to listen with both ears.

RECOMMENDED READINGS

Cassell EJ: The nature of suffering and the goals of medicine. *N Engl J Med* 306:639–645, 1982.

> This is an eloquent exposition of the need for physicians to understand the totality of patients' experiences and to communicate empathy. It provides guidelines on a clinical approach based on understanding the patient as person.

Emanuel EJ, Emanuel LL: Four models of the physician–patient relationship. *JAMA* 267:2221–2226, 1992; May WF: Code, covenant, contract, or philanthropy? *Hastings Cent Rep* 5:29–38, 1975; Szasz TS, Hollender MH: The basic models of the doctor–patient relationship. *Arch Intern Med* 97:585–592, 1956.

> These three articles are all excellent descriptions of models of the patient–physician relationship. Each takes a different perspective on patient autonomy and the role of the physician.

Stewart M, Brown JB, Weston WW, McWhinney IR, McWilliam CL, Freeman TR: *Patient-Centered Medicine: Transforming the Clinical Method.* Beverly Hills, CA, Sage Publications, 1995.

> This book examines the practice of medicine, from theoretical models to the provision of care, from a patient-centered perspective that takes the patient's experience of illness on equal ground with the physician's diagnostic perspective.

CHAPTER 6

A. Relationships

The Family System

Thomas L. Campbell, Susan H. McDaniel, and David B. Seaburn

CASE 6-1

When Bill Guyer, a 52-year-old accountant, arrived at the emergency room, it was obvious to the staff that he was having a heart attack. Pale and sweating, he looked terrified as he clutched his chest. He was accompanied by his new wife Cathy, a 38-year-old nurse whom he had married shortly after his divorce, 1 year ago. Distressed, Cathy shouted continually at the ambulance and ER staff that they were doing something wrong or not working quickly enough. Finally, two of the nurses were able to escort her into the ER waiting room, while her husband was being treated.

Several minutes later, Bill's ex-wife Martha arrived in the waiting room demanding to know what had happened. Apparently, Bill had developed chest pain in the midst of a heated argument with his 17-year-old daughter Jane after she returned home drunk at 2 AM. When the ambulance took her father to the hospital (Cathy, her stepmother, had not allowed Jane to come), Jane called her mother and explained that she had caused her father's heart attack.

──────── INTRODUCTION ────────

The family remains the most important social unit in our culture and plays an essential role in all aspects of health, illness, and medical care. As illustrated in Case 6-1, family relationships have a powerful impact on health, and illness strongly influences the family (Campbell, 1986; Doherty & Campbell, 1988). In clinical practice, family members may act as informants, customers for treatment, part of the problem, or members of the treatment team (McDaniel *et al.*, 1990a). Whether in primary care or a subspecialty, the physician must have some understanding of the patient's family system and how the family context influences the patient's health and vice versa.

This chapter will present a basic approach to understanding and working with the family in medical practice. Using examples and research data, we will demonstrate how the family is an important source of stress, social support, health beliefs, and health behaviors. We will discuss the basic principles of a family systems approach to healthcare, including how to understand the family context of presenting symptoms, the use of genograms, the value of meeting with families and convening family conferences, and the importance of working collaboratively with mental health professionals.

THE FAMILY SYSTEM

DEFINITION

Despite rapid changes in the demographics of U.S. families, most Americans live with other family members. The traditional or stereotypical U.S. family, however, which included father as breadwinner, mother as homemaker, and one or more children, has become a shrinking minority of U.S. households. Today, families are couples, two parents and children, blended families, single-parent households, and nonfamily households. As the U.S. family evolves, we need to adapt our understanding and definitions of family to capture its diversity.

We define "family" as "any group of people related either biologically, emotionally, or legally" (McDaniel *et al.*, 1990a). The World Health Organization has a broader definition:

> The concept of family need not be limited to ties of blood, marriage, sexual partnership or adoption. Any group whose bonds are based upon trust, mutual support and a common destiny may be regarded as family. (World Health Organization, 1994)

The relevant family context may include family members who live a distance from the patient, although physicians are most often involved with family members who live in the same household. In caring for Bill Guyer in Case 6-1, the relevant family included three generations of this remarried and blended family.

A biopsychosocial approach to healthcare is central to working effectively with families. The biopsychosocial model, first described by George Engel (Engel, 1977), is more than the addition of psychosocial data to biomedical data. It is based on a *systems* approach to healthcare that emphasizes the interdependency and interplay among the different levels of any system, whether it is the cardiovascular system, the individual, family members, or the community. In Case 6-1, Bill Guyer's health is affected not only by the complex interrelationships of his organ systems, particularly his cardiovascular and nervous system, but also by the complex relationships within his own extended family system. The Guyer family system is in turn influenced by larger community and social forces, such as the changing roles of women in society, increasing rates of divorce, and drug and alcohol problems in our schools and community.

The family is a system, like the cardiovascular system, in which the whole is greater than the sum of its parts, and its component parts (family members) reciprocally influence each other. The relationships between family members are as important as individual characteristics of family members. One useful analogy to the family system is the solar system, in which one cannot understand the behavior or movements of a single planet without considering the movements and gravitational influence of other planets. Thus, we cannot fully understand a patient's behavior or health without considering the influence of the family and other larger systems, including work, community, and culture.

Numerous studies have shown that an individual's physical health and longevity are influenced by the quality and quantity of her social relationships, especially within the family (Doherty & Campbell, 1988). In a review of the research on social relationships and health, sociologist James House concludes:

> The evidence regarding social relationships and health increasingly approximates the evidence in the 1964 Surgeon General's report that established cigarette smoking as a cause or risk factor for mortality and morbidity from a range of diseases. The age-adjusted relative risk ratios are stronger than the relative risks for all cause mortality for cigarette smoking. (House *et al.*, 1988)

The marital relationship seems to have a particularly strong influence on health. Men and women who are in unhappy marriages have been shown to have poorer health status and immune functioning (Kiecolt-Glaser *et al.*, 1987). The adverse effects of the two most stressful life events, the death of a spouse and divorce, are well documented (Campbell, 1986; Doherty & Campbell, 1988). The family is the primary social context in which health promotion and disease prevention takes place. The World Health Organization has characterized the family as the "primary social agent in the promotion of health and well-being" (World Health Organization, 1976). A healthy life-style is usually developed, maintained, or changed within the family setting. Behavioral risk factors tend to cluster within families, as family members share similar diets, physical activities, and tobacco and alcohol use. In a 1985 Gallup survey of health-related behaviors, over 1000 adults reported that their spouse or significant other was more likely to influence their health habits than anyone else, including their family physician (Gallup Poll, 1985).

A number of studies have demonstrated the effectiveness of couple and family interventions for physical health problems (Campbell & Patterson, 1995). Family-oriented cardiovascular risk reduction programs are more effective and cost-effective than individually oriented programs. Couples-based weight reduction programs result in greater maintenance of weight loss. Family therapy and psychoeducation for childhood illnesses seem to be particularly effective. Interventions for family caregivers of dementia and stroke patients reduce caregiver burden and depression and can delay institutionalization of these patients.

CASE 6-1 *continued*

As their family physician, Dr. C. knew the Guyer family quite well. He had delivered their second child, Mike, who was now 14 and had insulin-dependent diabetes mellitus. He had treated Martha for depression, which developed at the time of their stormy divorce. He had rarely seen Bill in the office, despite years of efforts by Martha and more recently Cathy encouraging him to visit their physician. Dr. C. knew that Bill was overweight and smoked, despite having a strong family history of heart disease. The few times Dr. C. saw Bill, he was fatalistic about his health, stating that if heart disease was in his genes, there was nothing he could do about it. Dr. C. also knew that his daughter Jane was having serious problems at school and had been suspended several times over the past year. In addition, he was the physician for Martha's father, who had moderately severe Alzheimer's disease and had moved into the family's home 2 years before. With

*all of these issues occurring over the past several years, Dr. C. knew that this
illness episode would be a challenge.*

——— THE BIOPSYCHOSOCIAL APPROACH ———

To implement a family systems approach, the physician must not split biomedical
from psychosocial issues during patient care. Using an integrated, biopsychosocial approach is a challenging task: Our culture and medical training encourages diagnosing
problems as either physical or emotional and often focuses exclusively on one aspect of
the problem. This mind–body split causes particular difficulties when caring for patients
who present with physical symptoms for which no biomedical cause can be found or for
which the psychosocial factors are significant. The challenge for physicians is to evaluate
the biomedical and psychosocial aspects of the problem simultaneously and to decide at
which level of the biopsychosocial model one should intervene. Occasionally, when faced
with urgent problems or emergency medical problems, as in this case, the biomedical
issues must be addressed first, without forgetting to address the psychosocial issues as
soon as possible.

Because Dr. C has a long-standing relationship with the Guyer family in Case 6-1, he
has a good understanding of the family context and some hypotheses about what family
stresses may have contributed to the patient's heart disease. However, initially Dr. C.
needed to address the family's urgent need for information and reassurance and begin to
assess the circumstances surrounding the onset of symptoms.

CASE 6-1 *(continued)*

*Shortly after Bill stabilized in the intensive care unit, Dr. C. met with Bill's wife
Cathy, explained what had happened and the treatment her husband was receiving, and reassured her about his prognosis. Then, he gathered more history of the
events surrounding his heart attack.*

*Dr. C. learned that Cathy had been concerned about Bill's health ever since
they had met 2 years earlier. As a nurse, she knew he was at high risk for heart
disease, because of his family history, smoking, poor nutrition, and lack of exercise. Since being married, she had completely changed his diet, serving him only
low-fat meals. However, she knew that he went regularly to McDonald's for lunch
and brought home pints of Ben and Jerry's ice cream for late-night snacks. She
occasionally fought with him about his smoking and would hide or throw out any
cigarettes she could find. He refused to join her aerobics classes at the local
YMCA. Cathy thought that he might have been having episodes of angina over the
past few months, but he always denied it and refused to see a physician.*

*Cathy also described the increasingly conflictual relationship between Bill
and his daughter Jane. Jane blamed her father for the divorce and had become
openly rebellious. She was failing in high school, drinking alcohol regularly, and
dating a college junior whom neither Bill nor Cathy liked or trusted. They were
also worried that she was using drugs.*

THE FAMILY CONTEXT OF THE PRESENTING PROBLEM

Most illnesses are influenced by or influence the family, so it is helpful for the
physician to have some understanding of the family context of every presenting problem.

This may involve knowing who is in the household, what treatments other family members have recommended, or who is the primary caretaker of the patient. Patients often present with physical symptoms that are related to family stress or family problems. These somatic symptoms may represent a stress-related illness, an exacerbation of an underlying chronic illness, or some type of somatization for which no physiological abnormalities can be found. Physicians should be aware of "red flags" that alert them that a more complete exploration of the context is indicated. These "red flags" may include stress-related symptoms, such as chronic headaches, unexplained or inconsistent physical symptoms, abnormal mood, or who accompanies the patient to the visit (Doherty & Baird, 1983). In these situations, more detailed information about the family should be obtained. In Case 6-1, the history of Bill's presenting complaint makes it obvious that family stresses and conflict are contributing to his health problems. The arrival of both his wife and ex-wife to the emergency room suggests that there may be more complex issues.

A few simple questions can be used to assess the family context quickly. Asking "Who is at home?" provides information about the family structure. Knowing the ages of family members allows one to hypothesize what developmental issues the family may be handling at the moment. Other useful questions include:

- How has this problem affected you and your family?
- Has anyone else in your family ever had this problem?
- Who knows about this problem?
- What does your family think about the problem you are having?
- What suggestions has your family made?
- Have there been any recent changes or stresses at home that you have had to deal with?

A family systems approach provides a way to understand the patient and his problem in a larger context of meaningful relationships. It does not mean the physician meets with the family at every visit. Most of the time, physicians meet with individual patients. But by being alert to "red flags" and asking a few routine family questions, the physician can make an initial assessment of the family context as it relates to the presenting problem. If that initial assessment suggests that family issues play an important role in the patient's health problem, more detailed information about the family needs to be obtained.

CASE 6-1 *(continued)*

Dr. C. reviewed the genogram that he had constructed over many visits with different members of the Guyer family (Fig. 6.1). He had been very involved in the care of the son, Mike, who developed insulin-dependent diabetes mellitus at the age of 6. During the first few years of his illness, Mike was in and out of the hospital with frequent episodes of diabetic ketoacidosis. Mike's illness had been very stressful on his parents and their relationship. Bill felt that Martha "smothered" their son and was overprotective, not letting him become as involved in sports as Bill felt he could. Though Mike's illness stabilized, the conflict between his parents had escalated.

Dr. C. knew that Bill was an only child and that his parents had divorced when Bill was 16. A few years after the divorce, Bill's father died suddenly from a heart attack. His father had been alcoholic and his relationship with his son had been conflictual. Bill did not have any contact with his father after his parent's divorce and refused to attend his father's funeral. On the other hand, Bill remained close to his mother until she died from ovarian cancer in her late 60s.

USE OF THE GENOGRAM FOR FAMILY ASSESSMENT

The family tree or genogram is one of the most basic and useful family systems tools. It allows the physician to obtain and record basic family information and provides a visual record of the family (McGoldrick & Gerson, 1986). Although similar to the family trees used to record genetic diseases, the genogram also provides information about family structure, developmental issues, relationship patterns, life cycle stages, and stressful life events. By reviewing the Guyer genogram (Fig. 6.1) before seeing Bill, Dr. C. has a snapshot of the family context and is alerted to the relevant individual and family issues.

During a patient's initial visit or physical examination, a brief, skeletal genogram can be obtained in less than 5 minutes as part of the family and social history. Patients are usually comfortable helping to construct the family tree. The genogram communicates to the patient that the physician is interested in all aspects of the patient's life. When the genogram is obtained in a nonthreatening manner, as a part of routine practice, patients are more likely to reveal sensitive and important family issues, such as substance abuse or domestic violence.

The genogram is particularly important when caring for divorced, remarried, or blended families, such as the Guyer family. In these families, adults and children often have different last names. It is essential to know which children belong to which parents, and who lives in which household. For example, if one falsely assumed that Cathy Guyer was Jane's mother and that Jane lived full time in their household, it would have caused major difficulties in treatment. With a genogram, the physician can see immediately what the relationships are between family members.

When the physician cares for more than one member of a family, as with the Guyer family, it is also helpful to organize these individual charts into a family folder (Farley, 1990). The family's genogram can be included in the folder and added to during any family members' visits. With a family folder, the provider has access to other family members' charts during a patient's visit.

CASE 6-1 *(continued)*

Dr. C. was aware that the Guyer family was facing numerous developmental stresses. The most immediate concern was Bill's health and whether he would recover completely and be able to return to work. Bill and Martha's bitter divorce and Bill's remarriage was the greatest challenge that the family had confronted. Occurring at a time when their daughter Jane was beginning plans for college and leaving home, she was having the most difficulty coping with the divorce. Protective of her mother, she blamed her father and rarely visited him since he remarried. Her grades in school plummeted, and her prospects for college looked poor. Martha was essentially a single parent while also caring for her demented father. She had been forced to quit her job, which she enjoyed, to be home with her father. Over the past year, she had gone through early menopause and began treatment for her depression.

THE FAMILY LIFE CYCLE

By knowing the ages of the family members and examining the genogram, the physician can assess what developmental issues may be affecting the family and whether

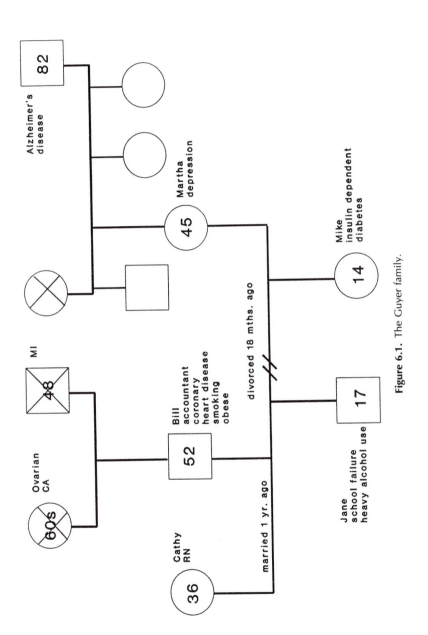

Figure 6.1. The Guyer family.

these normative stresses are affecting the presenting health concerns. The family life cycle is a useful conceptual framework for understanding family development (Carter & McGoldrick, 1988a) (see Chapter 2). Similar to the individual life cycle, the family life cycle assumes that families go through different stages for which there are specific developmental tasks to be accomplished. Families who do not accomplish these developmental tasks at one stage may develop difficulties with subsequent family development.

Many normative family life transitions can be very stressful and can precipitate or exacerbate health problems. Many women, like Martha Guyer, and some men in their 40s are faced with the demands of caring for elderly and disabled parents while they are simultaneously raising young children. As in the Guyer family, an increasing number of families are coping with the stress of divorce. Since one-half of all couples will eventually divorce, divorce and remarriage is a common developmental stressor for many families (Carter & McGoldrick, 1988a). As a result, physicians are caring for more divorced and remarried families. In these families, there are often unresolved conflicts that physicians can unwittingly be pulled into.

CASE 6-1 (continued)

Dr. C. realized that the stress of Bill's heart attack and the circumstances around which it developed were contributing to the problems and conflicts that already existed in the family. Shortly after Bill's admission to the MICU, Dr. C. met briefly with Cathy and Martha together in the waiting room. After answering their questions about Bill, he asked how they were both doing. Cathy expressed her fears about Bill and Martha talked about her worries about Jane, who felt responsible for what had happened. This provoked an argument between Cathy and Martha, which Dr. C. quickly interrupted.

Dr. C.: "Excuse me. I need to interrupt this discussion. I realize that some of your family's relationships have become quite conflictual since the divorce and that Bill's illness has only added to the enormous stress that both of you are experiencing right now. I really think some of the problems will need to be dealt with, but not now. While Bill is in the hospital, it is very important for his health and for the kids' well-being that both of you put aside your conflicts as much as possible and help Bill recover and the kids to cope with their father's illness. Do you think you can do that?"

THE THERAPEUTIC TRIANGLE

Another principle of a family systems approach is that medical visits are not just between physician and patient but involve the family, even when they are not in the exam room. Doherty and Baird (1987) have called this physician–patient–family interaction the therapeutic triangle in medicine (Fig. 6.2). The triangle emphasizes the important role of the family in every encounter and how the family affects the patient and vice versa, as well as how family members can influence the physician–patient relationship. By giving their opinions about the care the patient is receiving, family members can undermine or support the physician–patient relationship. When there is a poor medical outcome, the family often decides whether the physician was at fault and should be sued.

Whenever two people are in conflict, one person is likely to involve or triangulate a third person into the relationship to reduce the tension, anxiety, and seek an ally. Most

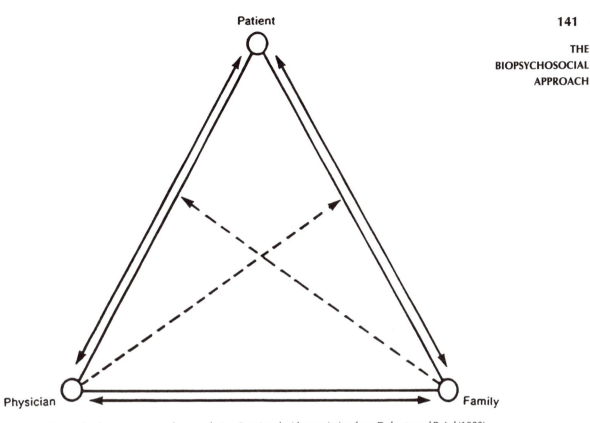

Figure 6.2. The therapeutic triangle in medicine. Reprinted with permission from Doherty and Baird (1983).

people prefer to complain to a third person about the problems one is having with a spouse, friend, or co-worker than it is to confront the offending person directly about the problem. When a patient comes to the physician with a complaint related to an interpersonal problem, he will often try to get the physician to take his side. Depressed or anxious patients may complain to the physician about another family member, such as "My husband drinks too much," "I think my wife is having an affair," or "Our son won't listen to us anymore." Physicians will often support and empathize with the patient, inadvertently taking sides in the conflict.

The difficult task for the physician is to develop and maintain a positive relationship with each family member and avoid taking sides in any conflict. The physician should not take sides or blame other family members. To listen repeatedly to a patient complain about another family member is similar to only prescribing pain medication for a peptic ulcer: It may make the patient feel better acutely while the underlying problem gets worse.

In Case 6-1, there are multiple triangles into which Dr. C. may be pulled, being pressured to take sides. The most obvious and conflictual is between the divorced parents. In conflictual divorced families, parents and stepparents may try to get the physician to take sides with them, particularly with regard to the children. For example, one parent may bring his child for an acute visit to a physician and try to get the physician to agree that the health problem is somehow the result of what the ex-wife did, sometimes without even letting the physician know that the parents are divorced. In extreme cases, warring parents may take their children to different physicians and then try to pull these physicians into the divorce conflict.

The conflict between Jane and her parents is another common situation into which physicians can be pulled. One parent may try to get the physician to convince their teenager not to be sexually active or not to smoke. In another triangle, Cathy might ask Dr. C. to reinforce her message that Bill should eat better and exercise. While the physician will always advocate for a healthy life-style, if she takes sides in family conflicts, she usually loses effectiveness in working with the family member who is being sided against. When there is family conflict, the challenge is to remain allied with each member of the conflict and not take sides, while still being clear about what good healthcare warrants. Often, this can be done most effectively by meeting with the entire family.

CASE 6-1 *(continued)*

On the day prior to discharge from the hospital, Dr. C. met with Bill, Cathy, and the children. During the hospitalization, Cathy had agreed to participate in Bill's cardiac rehabilitation program and had attended informational classes on exercise and nutrition. She was relieved to see how much exercise he was allowed to do prior to his discharge. Dr. C. met separately with Bill and Cathy to discuss medication and resumption of sexual activity.

During the family meeting, Dr. C. reviewed Bill's hospital course and the plans for rehabilitation as an outpatient. He answered several of the children's questions about what had caused their father's heart attack and in what activities he could participate. He asked them all how they were feeling about what had happened and what fears they had.

THE FAMILY CONFERENCE

Although a family systems approach is often used with individual patients, meeting with the family is frequently useful and sometimes necessary. Physicians often meet other family members at regular office visits, during hospital rounds, or for more extended family conferences. Family members often accompany patients to the physician's office and may be invited in from the waiting room. Examination and consultation rooms should have a second chair for family members, so that they do not have to stand or sit on the exam table. Seeing elderly couples together for joint appointments acknowledges their interdependency, especially about health concerns.

A family meeting or conference can be particularly helpful in certain circumstances (McDaniel *et al.*, 1990a). It is generally useful to meet with the family at least twice during a hospitalization, at the time of admission and shortly before discharge. Family members always want information about the patient's medical condition and can often provide valuable information about events leading up to the admission. At the time of hospital discharge the family usually takes over the care of the patient. Before discharge, the physician should meet with the family to review the hospital course and ongoing treatment plans and elicit any family concerns about the patient returning home. Patients should receive "bad news" when they have the support of their families. In a family meeting, the physician can assess how well the family is coping with the illness and how to assist them.

It is particularly important to meet with the family when the diagnosis of a terminal illness is made or when a patient dies. Often, family members are in a state of shock and need information and support. Because of the strong emotions surrounding death in a family, there is often a high degree of denial that can interfere with effective communication and the sharing of feelings. Death is often viewed as a failure by physicians who then feel guilty. This guilt may result in the physician avoiding the family when it is most important for both parties to meet.

Family members are usually willing to accompany the patient to a physician's appointment or a family meeting. However, if there are serious family conflicts such as in the Guyer family, some family members may be reluctant to attend, fearing they will be blamed for the problem.

CASE 6-1 *(continued)*

In discussing their fears, both children said they were worried that a family argument might precipitate another heart attack. Dr. C. explained that Bill's heart attack was not caused by the argument with Jane prior to his admission. His heart disease resulted from a combination of genetics, poor diet and exercise, and smoking. Dr. C. added that he would be working with Bill to help him deal with family stresses in a healthier manner, and that the family needed to find better ways of resolving their conflicts.

This comment led to a broader discussion by the family of some of their conflicts. Dr. C. mostly listened, occasionally interrupting when arguments seemed to be escalating. Collectively, the family agreed that for the sake of Bill's health, they needed to work together to resolve some of their difficulties.

———— LEVELS OF WORKING WITH FAMILIES ————

When using a family systems approach, it is important to assess continuously what level of involvement the physician wishes to have with the families in her practice. As with other areas in medicine, she needs to decide what level of skills and knowledge she has or wishes to have in a particular area. For example, when treating cardiac patients, she must decide whether she has the skills to treat complicated post MI patients in the intensive care unit, or refer them to a cardiologist.

Based on the physician's knowledge, personal development, and skills, Doherty and Baird (1987) have outlined five levels of physicians' involvement with families (Table 6.1). They developed these levels to emphasize that all physicians work with families at some level and that some problems require the expertise of a trained family therapist. Some physicians only deal with families when it is necessary for medical–legal reasons, Level One.

Most physicians usually work at Level Two, providing ongoing medical information and advice to families. For the Guyer family, this involved assembling the family before hospital discharge and providing detailed information about the illness and treatment plans. If this kind of information is only provided to the individual patient, it can create confusion and conflict as the family tries to decide what activities are safe for the patient.

Working at Level Three involves eliciting feelings and providing support to families and can be very therapeutic for patients and families. Many families never share their

Table 6.1

Levels of Physician Involvement with Families

Level One: Minimal Emphasis on Family	*Level Two: Ongoing Medical Information and Advice* / *Level Three: Feelings and Support*	*Level Four: Systematic Assessment and Planned Intervention*	*Level Five: Family Therapy*
This baseline level of involvement consists of dealing with families only as necessary for practical and medical legal reasons, but not viewing communicating with families as integral to the physician's role or as involving skills for the physician to develop. This level presumably characterizes most medical school training where biomedical issues are the sole conscious focus of patient care.	**Level Two: Ongoing Medical Information and Advice** Knowledge Base: **Primarily medical**, plus awareness of the triangular dimension of the physician–patient relationship. Personal Development: Openness to engage patients and families in a collaborative way. Skills: 1. Regularly and clearly communicating medical findings and treatment options to family members. 2. Asking family members questions that elicit relevant diagnostic and treatment information. 3. Attentively listening to family members' questions and concerns. 4. Advising families about how to handle the medical and rehabilitation needs of the patient. 5. For large or demanding families, knowing how to channel communication through one or two key members. 6. Identifying gross family dysfunction that interferes with medical treatment and referring the family to a therapist. **Level Three: Feelings and Support** Knowledge Base: Normal family development and reactions to stress. Personal Development: Awareness of one's own feelings in relationship to the patient and family. Skills: 1. Asking questions that elicit family members' expressions of concerns and feelings related to the patient's condition and its effect on the family. 2. Empathetically listening to family members' concerns and feelings and normalizing them where appropriate. 3. Forming a preliminary assessment of the family's level of functioning as it relates to the patient's problem. 4. Encouraging family members in their efforts to cope as a family with their situation. 5. Tailoring medical advice to the unique needs, conerns, and feelings of the family. 6. Identifying family dysfunction and fitting a referral recommendation to the unique situation of the family.	Knowledge Base: Family systems. Personal Development: Awareness of one's own participation in systems, including the therapeutic triangle, the medical system, one's own family system, and larger community systems. Skills: 1. Engaging family members, including reluctant ones, in a planned family conference or a series of conferences. 2. Structuring a conference with even a poorly communicating family in such a way that all members have a chance to express themselves. 3. Systematically assessing the family's level of functioning. 4. Supporting individual members while avoiding coalitions. 5. Reframing the family's definition of their problem in a way that makes problem solving more achievable. 6. Helping the family members view their difficulty as requiring new forms of collaborative efforts. 7. Helping family members generate alternative, mutually acceptable ways to cope with their difficulty. 8. Helping the family balance their coping efforts by calibrating their various roles in a way that allows support without sacrificing anyone's autonomy. 9. Identifying family dysfunction that lies beyond primary care treatment and orchestrating a referral by educating the family and the therapist about what to expect from one another.	Knowledge Base: Family systems and patterns whereby dysfunctional families interact with professionals and other health-care systems. Personal Development: Ability to handle intense emotions in families and self and to maintain neutrality in the face of strong pressure from family members or other professionals. Skills: The following is not an exhaustive list of family therapy skills but rather a list of several key skills that distinguish Level Five involvement from primary care involvement with families: 1. Interviewing families or family members who are quite difficult to engage. 2. Efficiently generating and testing hypotheses about the family's difficulties and interaction patterns. 3. Escalating conflict in the family in order to break a family impasse. 4. Temporarily siding with one family member against another. 5. Constructively dealing with a family's strong resistance to change. 6. Negotiating collaborative relationships with other professionals and other systems who are working with the family, even when these groups are at odds with one another.

worries and fears about a family member's illness unless encouraged to do so in a family meeting. These families often have the belief that expressing their feelings will upset the patient and worsen his illness. Level Three requires the physician to be comfortable eliciting, attending to, and normalizing strong emotions. As in the Guyer family, simply asking how they are feeling about the illness or what has happened usually elicits family members' feelings.

Level Four, Systematic Assessment and Planned Intervention, requires additional training in family systems theory and its application. At this level, physicians provide brief and focused family counseling for uncomplicated family problems. This involves getting family members to talk with each other, intervening to change communication patterns, but not engaging in therapy to address ongoing relationship problems. More complex and chronic family problems need family therapy, Level Five, a specialty service that requires 3 to 5 years of postgraduate training and supervision and is beyond the interest and training of most physicians. Since physicians often see these types of problems in their practice, they need to work collaboratively with family therapists so effective referrals can occur.

CASE 6-1 (continued)

Because Dr. C. had a long-standing relationship with the family and they trusted him, they asked him if he would help them with some of their conflicts. Although flattered and initially tempted to take on the challenge, Dr. C. recognized that he was over his head and that the Guyers' difficulties were beyond the training in family counseling that he had received in residency.

Dr. C. expressed his desire to help the family with these problems, but said they needed and deserved a specialist who has special expertise dealing with family problems. He made the analogy to Bill's need to see a cardiologist to do a cardiac catheterization and help decide on further treatment. Dr. C. explained that he would remain involved in their care and work closely with the family therapist he recommended. Dr. C. recommended that they contact Dr. M., a family therapist with whom he has worked closely. He agreed to join the family at the first visit with Dr. M.

COLLABORATION WITH A MENTAL HEALTH PROVIDER

Using a biopsychosocial and family systems approach to medical care requires the physician to assess problems at multiple levels and to decide at what level or levels to intervene. In Case 6-1, it was important to intervene at the cardiovascular system level (cardiac catheterization and medication), the individual level (change in diet, exercise, and smoking), and the family system (family therapy). However, it is crucial for the physician to know what the limits of his expertise and skills are and when to consult or refer to a specialist. Most physicians have learned to do this quite skillfully for medical problems.

Many psychosocial problems can be handled by primary care family counseling (Level Four) by physicians who have the time, interest, and skill to do such counseling. Table 6.2 lists the common types of problems amenable to family counseling, as well as

Table 6.2
When to Treat and When to Refer Problems Seen in Primary Care

Problems commonly seen in primary care counseling	Problems commonly referred on to a mental health specialist
Adjustment to the diagnosis of a new illness	Suicidal or homicidal ideation, intent, or behavior
Other adjustment or situational disorders	Psychotic behavior
Crises of limited severity or duration	Sexual or physical abuse
Behavior problems	Substance abuse
Mild depressive reactions	Somatic fixation
Mild anxiety reactions	Moderate–severe marital and sexual problems
Uncomplicated grief reactions	Multi-problem family situations
	Problems resistant to change in primary care counseling

Reprinted with permission from McDaniel *et al.* (1990).

those that usually need referral to a mental health provider. Factors that influence whether a problem should be referred to a therapist include the severity of the problem, its chronicity, and previous attempts to treat the problem. The more severe and chronic problems that have failed previous treatments require referral. Sometimes the patient or family may request a referral to a mental health provider, either because they recognize the severity of the problem or because they prefer to discuss a sensitive topic with someone other than their physician who they see regularly (McDaniel *et al.*, 1992). Finally, the physician may decide that the issues that the family is dealing with are too close to unresolved issues in the physician's own life.

CASE 6-1 *(continued)*

Dr. C. had recently gone through his own painful and sometimes conflictual divorce. As a result of his experience, he knew how important it was to buffer the children from the effects of the divorce, by keeping them out of conflicts between ex-spouses, by reducing these conflicts, and by developing as smooth a working relationship as possible. He also knew that his divorce was still fresh and that there were many issues that he had not yet resolved. As a result, he was very cautious about advising or counseling the family about how they should deal with their postdivorce conflicts. He was tempted to suggest the best custody arrangements and how to communicate between ex-spouses, but realized that part of his desire resulted from his need to convince himself that what he had done was the best approach.

Dr. C. also had some struggles with his teenage son, who was at a rebellious stage. He used his own experience to empathize with Bill about the difficulties of raising teenagers, but realized that he did not have any expertise in how to deal with these problems.

PHYSICIAN SELF-AWARENESS AND FAMILY OF ORIGIN

A physician's past and current personal issues can be either a major resource or a profound hindrance in the physician–patient relationship. Styles of caretaking and authority as well as tolerance for affect are all learned in our families of origin. Many physicians are able to use their past experiences to enhance their empathy and their credibility with patients. However, current problems or unresolved struggles from the past can cloud or distort our perceptions of patients and their families. Utilizing personal issues as a resource depends on being able to recognize these issues when they occur in our work. When the physician recognizes that a patient or family is stimulating an important personal issue, the physician then has the opportunity to decide whether to treat, collaborate with a colleague, or refer. Physicians can benefit their own practice by regularly consulting with colleagues or, in some instances, seeking personal psychotherapy. Difficult or "problem" patients often elicit strong reactions in their physicians and may result in "stuck" interactions where the physician is spending a great deal of time with little change in the patient or relationship. These problematic relationships often result from experiences in the physician's own family of origin. The patient's family may mirror some of the same relationships or issues in the physician's own family.

CASE 6-1 *(continued)*

The Guyer family met with the family therapist, Dr. M., for ten visits over the following 6 months. Dr. C. joined the family for the first session and shared his concerns about the conflict in the family and how it was affecting each family member. He stressed how he thought Dr. M. could be helpful to the family.

Dr. M. met with the entire family for several sessions and helped them to address the conflicts and loyalties that had developed because of the divorce. Bill, Martha, and Cathy met separately with Dr. M. to address parenting issues and how to help and support their daughter Jane. Dr. M. also held separate sessions for Bill and Cathy to deal with stresses that had developed in their marriage and the impact of Bill's MI, and with Martha to help her decide what to do about her demented father.

CONCLUSION: COLLABORATIVE FAMILY HEALTHCARE

Because of the complex nature of patients' problems, the increasing age of the general population, and the growing emphasis of primary care, it will be important for physicians to develop effective partnerships with families and mental health professionals (Seaburn *et al.*, 1996). Applying a family systems approach to healthcare provides helpful information for diagnosis and opens new options for treatment of patients and their families. This approach is based on the biopsychosocial model, but puts special emphasis on the role of the family in healthcare. It can be implemented in daily practice by considering the family context of all presenting health problems, including the developmental phase of patients and their families, through the regular use of genograms. It does not require seeing family members at every visit.

In addition, some physicians may obtain additional training in order to counsel families in their practices (Level Four). However, many family problems will require referral to a mental health professional, usually a family therapist (McDaniel *et al.*, 1992; Seaburn *et al.*, 1996). Collaborative family healthcare, working collaboratively with families and mental health providers, helps physicians to practice a fully integrated biopsychosocial approach and provides comprehensive and effective care for a broad spectrum of health problems (Dym, 1994).

CASES FOR DISCUSSION

CASE 1

J. P. is a 35-year-old woman who has a partner of 6 years and a daughter, aged 4. This medical visit is the second one regarding low back pain, leg pain, and headaches. The patient is very anxious about these symptoms: They have persisted for many years but have worsened in the last 3 months. The patient has not been able to work for over a month. She presents her symptoms in an anxious manner, moving quickly from one symptom to the next. Unknown to the physician, the patient's mother had similar problems. The mother feels that her daughter has "something serious," maybe cancer.

The patient's partner is unconcerned and not supportive. He has a drinking problem. The patient is worried about their relationship. Her father has told her to leave him. The patient's daughter worries about her and tries to take care of her. As a child the patient was sexually abused by an uncle. She is seeing a therapist about this, but the physician is unaware of the abuse or the therapy.

1. *How might the patient's family be influencing her presenting symptoms? What role might her history of sexual abuse play in her current problems?*
2. *How would you involve this patient's family in her care? How would you work with her partner, daughter, and parents?*
3. *How would you work with the therapist who is seeing the patient?*

CASE 2

M. S. is a 65-year-old mother of ten who presented to the hospital 3 days after a myocardial infarction. She had experienced chest pain and shortness of breath at home where she lived with her son, but refused to go to the hospital or to see a physician. When her children finally prevailed on her to go to the hospital, she was very argumentative with the residents on the floor. It took several days for them to convince her to have the appropriate tests and begin medical treatment for her cardiac disease. The patient felt frustrated that her children were "smothering me," and the adult children were upset that their mother was not receiving the care she needed.

1. *Why do you think the patient is not seeking timely medical care for her health problems? How might her family be affecting her behavior?*
2. *How would you help this patient and her family? How might a family meeting be helpful? What additional information would you want to obtain from the patient and her family?*

CASE 3

H. M. is a 48-year-old businessman who rarely seeks medical care. The morning before his scheduled routine physical examination, his wife calls the office to tell you that he has a serious drinking problem and asks, "Could you talk with him about it?"

1. *What do you tell the wife on the telephone? How would you address her concerns? If you ask the wife to join him at his visit and she refuses, what do you say?*

CASE 4

G. R. is a 70-year-old man with a long smoking history who is brought to your office by his daughter who is his primary caretaker. He has had some difficulty urinating and has passed some blood. On rectal exam, you feel a hard nodule in his prostate. You order blood work and refer him to a urologist for a biopsy.

As they are leaving the office, his daughter pulls you aside and says that if he has cancer, she does not want him to be told. She says that she knows her father very well, that he has always been terrified of cancer, and that he cannot deal with the diagnosis.

1. *How do you respond to her request? What further information would you want from her?*
2. *The nodule is malignant, and you decide to meet with the patient and his daughter. How would you deal with his new diagnosis and his daughter's concerns?*

RECOMMENDED READINGS

Campbell TL: *Family's Impact on Health: A Critical Review and Annotated Bibliography.* NIMH Series DN, No. 6, DHHS Publ. No. (ADM) 86-1461, 1986. Also published in *Fam Sys Med* 4(2&3):135–328, 1986.

This monograph and special issue of *Family Systems Medicine* review the research literature on how family factors, especially family relationships, influence health. It also includes an annotated bibliography of the reviewed studies.

Doherty WJ, Baird MA: *Family Therapy and Family Medicine.* New York, Guilford Press, 1983.

This landmark book outlines the theory and practice of a family systems approach to healthcare. It has excellent chapters on how to assess, refer, and counsel families in primary care.

Doherty WJ, Baird MA (eds): *Family-Centered Medical Care: A Clinical Casebook.* New York, Guilford Press, 1987.

Family physicians and collaborating therapists describe 71 cases of working with families in clinical practice. The cases are organized around the editors' Levels of Working with Families and include commentaries by the editors.

Doherty WJ, Campbell TL: *Families and Health.* Beverly Hills, CA, Sage Publications, 1988.

This book is part of the Sage Family Studies literature and is written for family professionals as well as medical providers. It reviews the literature on families and health and its implications for health professionals. It is organized around the Family Health and Illness Cycle.

McDaniel SH, Campbell TL, Seaburn DB: *Family-Oriented Primary Care: A Manual for Medical Providers.* Berlin, Springer-Verlag, 1990.

This practical guide to implementing a family-oriented approach in primary care has chapters on how to convene a family conference, conduct a family interview, and specific practical guidelines for dealing with numerous life-cycle and health-related issues.

CHAPTER 7

A. Relationships

The Community

Elisabeth D. Babcock and Laura B. Frankenstein

CASE 7-1

Mrs. Josephs was an 81-year-old woman living on her own in a third-floor tenement apartment in a crowded urban area. She had no family and was in very frail health. Despite repeated urging by her regular physician, she had refused to enter a nursing home.

During a 3-day period of 90-degree weather, Mrs. Josephs was discovered by her home health aid hyperthermic and dehydrated. The aid called an ambulance and Mrs. Josephs was rushed to the local emergency room.

At the hospital, Mrs. Josephs's physician in conjunction with the hospital social worker stressed to her that she could not continue living at home without greater support. They suggested she either enter a nursing home or join a new managed care program designed to provide extensive support to very frail elders who wished to remain in their homes.

INTRODUCTION

Just as it is impossible to understand and therefore treat patients without understanding the dynamics of the families within which they live, it is equally important to understand their communities. The community will often house clues to the causes of patients' diseases as well as the resources with which to treat them. A recent study by the Province of Ontario, Canada, Department of Public Health, showed that the entire healthcare system of Ontario accounted for only 11% of the total variation in patient outcome; the balance of 89% was controlled by factors outside of the healthcare system such as level of education, poverty, housing, and ethnicity (Society for Ambulatory Care Professionals, 1993).

Carefully defining the factors within a community that create barriers to good health as well as barriers to care, and then seeking to remedy those barriers, can often yield far-reaching and cost-effective improvements in patient outcome. This approach to understanding and caring for patients through understanding and caring for their communities is called community-oriented primary care (COPC). COPC gives the clinician tools for more rapid diagnosis of patients, better mechanisms for devising treatment plans, and the opportunity to provide new programs of care within communities which benefit not only the patients that the clinician treats directly, but also patients the clinician might never see.

As Case 7-1 demonstrates, patients often present with a host of obstacles to receiving good care within the limitations of the traditional medical system. To adequately treat such patients, the clinician may have to devise new programs to bridge barriers to care. The patient in Case 7-1 was fortunate that she could participate in a new program of managed care for the frail elderly within her community called PACE (Program of All inclusive Care for the Elderly). Her medical care would then be provided by a clinic that had observed many of the frail elderly of the community going into nursing homes due to lack of resources to care for them in their homes. Many of these patients did not wish to be admitted to the nursing home and once admitted had significant diminution in health status including mental decompensation and death.

To address this problem, the clinic joined with the local elder services agency to seek ways to provide better supports for frail elders to remain in their homes. The clinic and the leader service agency successfully applied for a Robert Wood Johnson Program grant to begin a PACE program in their community. The program provided special capitation rates from Medicaid and Medicare that paid the clinic a monthly stipend in place of the traditional system of billing for medical services rendered. Under this new PACE program, funds paid by Medicaid and Medicare could be used for anything that clinicians determined would lead to healthy patient outcomes and prevent unwanted nursing home admissions. Therefore, instead of entering a nursing home, the patient in Case 7-1 received an air conditioner from her PACE program. She thus remained happily in her own apartment and her health status was restored. Needless to say, the cost to the healthcare system of an air conditioner was far less than the cost of nursing home admission. By looking at patient needs within the context of the community and devising community-based solutions, the outcome of the patient in Case 7-1 was improved and a new cost-effective tool for patient care was added to the clinicians' armamentarium.

This chapter offers clinicians a framework for learning about their patients' communities and ideas as to how such knowledge can improve the diagnosis and treatment of patients as well as the development of new resources for patient care.

CASE 7-2

Dr. Jenkins was the medical director of a 230-bed hospital that served the population of an aging factory town. Over the years, as the factories closed and jobs had been lost, the old corps of general practitioners who had provided most of the town's primary care had retired and Dr. Jenkins had found it increasingly difficult to attract new physicians to the community.

During this period, Dr. Jenkins also began to observe significant increases in the numbers of patients seeking emergency care at the hospital for diabetes mellitus, asthma, and bacterial pneumonia. He wondered what conditions in the community might be contributing to the sharp increase in the incidence of these diseases and what he could do to prevent their occurrence.

153

PRIMARY CARE
SHORTAGES

——————— PRIMARY CARE SHORTAGES ———————

The U.S. healthcare system is specialty dominated. Unlike many European countries, which have at least two primary care physicians for each specialty physician, the United States has almost the exact opposite (Council on Graduate Medical Education, 1992). There are 2.07 active generalist physicians per 1000 U.S. citizens; ratios should be twice that number per thousand (Whitcomb, 1995). When health insurance was predominantly indemnity based and patients could freely gain access to specialists, this specialty-dominated model did not pose a barrier to access. Now that less than 5% of patients are insured by indemnity plans and the rest must seek the care of a primary care physician who in turn controls access to specialty physicians, many areas of the nation are experiencing shortages of primary care physicians (Bindman *et al.*, 1995).

These shortages are especially severe in areas of the country where there are high concentrations of the most vulnerable patients, such as communities of urban or rural poor. Competition for primary care physicians is so extreme that most physicians settle in the more affluent communities where salaries and benefits are highest. Communities with high numbers of uninsured or publicly insured residents are often unable to attract and keep the physicians they need to maintain basic health. Such communities are termed "medically underserved."

If the community has one or more of the following characteristics, it may be medically underserved:

- It is designated by the federal government as a Medically Underserved Area (MUA).
- It has ratios of 3000 residents or more per primary care physician [Bureau of Health Care Delivery and Assessment (BCHDA), 1990].
- It has more than 1.3 emergency room visits per 10 residents per year (Health Employer Data Information Set, 1994).
- It has preventable hospitalization rates for asthma higher than 2 per 1000 residents per year (Massachusetts Rate Setting Commission, 1995). Preventable hospitalizations are admissions for diagnoses that are normally successfully treated on an outpatient basis when a patient has ready access to a physician. Such diagnoses include asthma, diabetes mellitus, and bacterial pneumonia.
- Average waits for a normal complete physical examination are more than 6 weeks.

Like Dr. Jenkins in Case 7-2, clinicians may first suspect that they are delivering care in a medically underserved community when they find themselves delivering care to patients who they feel should have received earlier intervention. Often patients in such communities are able to access physicians only when they are ill or in the later stages of disease. Patients may lack a history of preventive care such as good immunization compliance or comprehensive perinatal follow-up. There may be significant discontinuity of care such as problems with coordination of medications or posthospitalization follow-up.

There may also be difficulties in obtaining accurate patient histories; patients in medically underserved communities often do not know the name of their previous physician or what their instructions for care were.

Providing care to patients in such communities is often frustrating and substandard. Although clinicians in such communities may attempt to provide good care, the dynamics of provider availability will often undermine the best-laid treatment plans.

The best long-term treatment plan may be to treat the underlying problem of physician shortages. Areas of the country federally designated as MUAs qualify for special programs to expand physician availability.

The federal Public Health Service within the Department of Health and Human Services provides two loan repayment programs for clinicians who are willing to locate within an MUA. The first program is the National Health Service Corps (NHSC) Scholarship Program. Under this program, students pursuing medical degrees agree to place within an underserved area at the completion of their training. In exchange for this commitment, the federal government pays for most or all of the cost of their training.

In the 1980s, over 6000 medical graduates per year were NHSC scholars, but in recent years, because of funding cuts and high default rates by the scholars, the number of annual graduates has dropped to 50 (Hanley, 1993).

Under the program, clinicians are given three choices of where to serve at the time they complete their education. They must choose one of the three locations, no matter how remote or undesirable the locations might be.

Because many complained about the lack of choices in the NHSC Scholarship Program, the federal government developed a second program called the National Health Services Corps Loan Repayment Program. Under this program, healthcare organizations located within an MUA may apply to be designated as eligible to hire a NHSC Loan Repayment Clinician. Once deemed eligible, the organization may offer federal loan repayment to the next clinician they hire. Under the loan repayment program, the federal government then assumes the debts incurred for previous medical training of the new clinician. The normal maximum obligation of the program is repayment of $25,000 in school debts per year of service for 3 years.

The NHSC program allows clinicians to match with any site that is deemed eligible for loan repayment and therefore provides a wider range of placement opportunities than the NHSC Scholarship Program. The wide selection of placement opportunities has made the NHSC Loan Repayment Program much more successful; its default rates are practically zero.

Many states and some local governments also offer various loan repayment and education incentives to attract providers to underserved areas. These programs range from formal programs such as grants to medical and nursing schools that provide care in underserved areas and state loan repayment programs, to less formal initiatives such as local community sponsorship of an individual clinician's training.

CASE 7-3

Maria Contreras had come with her parents and four siblings to the United States from her native Dominican Republic in search of a better life. What the 17-year-old woman had found was that with no high school education and only limited ability to speak English, she and most of the other members of her family could not find work. Because of this, they all shared a two-bedroom apartment with an aunt and uncle who had work cleaning office buildings.

When Maria became pregnant, she would not consider having an abortion or giving the child up for adoption. She had her baby and she then qualified for welfare, but the waiting list for permanent housing was so long that she had no hope of getting her own apartment for at least 2 years. Her medical providers had strongly urged Maria to breast-feed her child, but the infant was fussy and Maria gave up trying to nurse because she was exhausted from trying to keep the baby quiet in the overcrowded apartment and a girlfriend had told her that the baby would sleep better on formula. However, Maria had no space to refrigerate or store all of her baby's bottles. Her child had repeated problems with the formula and started to lose weight. The infant did not sleep and neither did other household members.

On the sporadic visits when Maria brought her child to a clinic, the child was not well dressed for cold weather and had upper respiratory and ear infections, as well as symptoms of failure to thrive. Maria was usually exhausted and seemed totally unable to cope.

POVERTY

In 1990, 13.1% of all Americans were living below the poverty level (Census, 1993). The poverty level is defined as $15,150 for a family of four (U.S. *Federal Register*, 1993). When treating patients with such a lack of resources, even the simplest treatment plan may be virtually impossible for a patient to follow.

In Case 7-3, we see the results of poverty: overcrowding, limited education, and stress on the provision of basic care to a newborn. In these circumstances, the provider would certainly advise the patient to move into her own apartment where she could get more sleep and where her baby would not be exposed to so many infections. She would also be advised to pay more attention to her diet and that of her child. She obviously needs help with her parenting skills.

Patients such as Maria have needs that extend far beyond the capacity of the medical system to satisfy. There is no simple prescription for this patient. The thoughtful clinician will often have to seek resources beyond the healthcare system in order to care adequately for patients such as Maria and her child.

Indicators of extensive poverty within communities include:

- 20% or more of the population living below the federal poverty line (BHCDA, 1990)
- High infant mortality rates (greater than 9 deaths per 1000 live births) (BHCDA, 1990)
- Higher than average unemployment rates (average U.S. unemployment for 11/1/94–10/31/95 was 5.6%) (Massachusetts Bureau of Labor Statistics, 1995)
- Unaffordability of housing (median rent greater than 30% of median income) (Apgar, 1991)
- Extreme overcrowding of living conditions (average census report numbers of residents per room greater than 1.5) (Census, 1993)

- High rates of crime (total crime rates higher than 50 crimes per 1000 residents per year; violent crimes greater than 8.5 crimes per 1000 residents per year) (Massachusetts Office of Public Safety, 1993)
- High rates of uninsured (greater than 12% of the population) (BHCDA, 1994)

Clinicians who provide care in impoverished communities will often encounter patients who have histories of episodic illness and care, and who often delay seeking care until they are in the advanced stages of an illness.

The lack of financial resources will also cause patients not to follow through on recommended treatment plans including the purchase of necessary medications. Patients with chronic conditions such as hypertension and diabetes mellitus who could remain very healthy with appropriate use of medications will often be unable to afford those medications or, if they can occasionally afford them, will take them only when their budgets permit. They may take the medications at only half the recommended dosages or intervals. Similarly, when told to reduce work levels, or to change dressings regularly, poor patients may fail to comply because they simply cannot afford to do so.

The overcrowded living circumstances of patients in these communities often lead to high rates of infectious diseases such as tuberculosis, hepatitis, and upper respiratory infections. Such living conditions and the poverty that causes them also lead to increased stress, higher rates of domestic violence, and mental health problems. Finally, clinicians like those who treated Maria in Case 7-3 will often find higher rates of malnutrition and failure to thrive in poor communities.

Obviously clinicians cannot cure all of the social ills that cause their patients' disease, but many communities do have social supports that may benefit patients living in poverty. Community Action Programs (the so-called CAP Agencies) help patients obtain subsidized housing, temporary shelter, fuel assistance, and day care. Early Intervention Programs and Head Start are federally and state-supported programs that provide early stimulation and education to children at risk. They also occasionally provide training in parenting skills.

Children from low-income families qualify for federally and state-financed Medicaid Early Periodic Screening and Treatment of Disease (EPSTD) care. Such care guarantees payment to clinicians providing primary care and specialty services such as hearing and vision screening, occupational, physical, and speech therapy, and mental health treatment, when any of the aforementioned care is necessary for normal development of children and readiness to learn in school.

The Women, Infants, and Children (WIC) Program of the federal government provides nutritional counseling and food supplementation to women and children living below 185% of the federal poverty limit ($28,028 for a family of four) (Massachusetts Department of Public Health, 1995c). This federal program, which began during the War on Poverty era of the Johnson Administration, provides pregnant and breast-feeding women and their children up to the age of 5 with vouchers for food "prescribed" by a nutritionist. Prescribed food items are those that will provide the greatest health outcome and cannot be substituted for others. Pregnant and breast-feeding mothers are given food vouchers for milk and other high-protein items; infants whose mothers are not breast-feeding will have an appropriate formula prescribed. Clients in the program have their weights and hematocrits checked regularly to assure good outcomes. The federal government estimates that for every dollar spent on WIC, three dollars is saved in medical costs as a result of prevention of premature birth, failure to thrive, and other health complications (Massachusetts Department of Public Health, 1995c).

It is very important for a clinician who is caring for poor patients to also know the services provided by the various public agencies run by that state. Most states will have local welfare, social service, youth service, public health, mental health, and public housing departments that provide an array of services helpful to the impoverished patient. Although it is often difficult to know exactly which services are provided by such public agencies, many social service departments of hospitals will have printed lists of agencies with a guide to the services they provide.

Although the services of the agencies mentioned here may help ameliorate the environmental conditions in which a patient lives, they usually do not improve the problems the poor and uninsured patient encounters when trying to obtain care within the medical system. It can be very difficult if not impossible to get patients the care they require when they are poor and uninsured. When trying to obtain emergency care for uninsured patients, providers may refer them to Hill-Burton-funded emergency rooms, which under federal law are required to treat any patient with a life-threatening condition and to provide care until the patient is stable. The Hill-Burton program was a federally funded program providing funds for the construction of hospitals under the proviso that the hospitals would agree to provide emergency services regardless of ability to pay.

Increasingly, the offices of the attorneys general of many states are also producing guidelines for the community services required to be rendered by nonprofit hospitals. Nonprofit hospitals are exempt as charities from state and federal taxes and are therefore required to provide charitable services in exchange for this exemption. State guidelines for the services required to be provided by the hospital usually include, at a minimum, free emergency care for patients with life-threatening illnesses. A description of the other services required of nonprofit hospitals to their communities may usually be found at the attorney general's office of the respective states.

Because of the high cost of insurance and declines in trade unions, the number of uninsured in the United States has been increasing at a rate of 100,000 per month since 1993 ("Shaky Statistic . . . ", *Wall Street Journal*, 1993). In that year, 16.1% of the population was uninsured, compared with 14.3% in 1989 (Employee Benefit Research Institute, 1995). Because of this alarming rate, and because the federal government has failed to institute any program to deal with it, many states have formulated their own programs for the uninsured. These programs range from virtual statewide entitlement to care in such states as Hawaii and Oregon, to pilot programs such as the free-care pools of Massachusetts and Florida. Many states have liberalized the eligibility requirements for Medicaid beyond those promulgated by the federal government. Providers should familiarize themselves with the programs that provide a "safety net" to the uninsured in their states.

The only federal program that provides primary care services to the uninsured is the Community Health Center Program (defined under Sections 329, 330, and 340 of the Public Health Service Act). Community Health Centers (CHCs) are outpatient primary care organizations specifically designed to provide care to underserved communities. CHCs were started in 1965 by the Office of Economic Opportunity of the federal government to provide care for patients who lacked access to providers because of poverty or living in an underserved area. CHCs are supported by federal, state, and local grants as well as patient revenues and provide the single largest source of care to underserved patients in MUAs.

CHCs must provide care to patients without regard to their ability to pay or insurance status. These centers are designed to treat patients with barriers to care in the traditional medical system and frequently have bilingual staff, special transportation programs, and health education and disease prevention programs tailored to their communities. Most CHCs are independent charitable organizations run by community-based boards of directors and are therefore very familiar with the needs of the communities they serve. Over 850 CHCs provide care from more than 2000 locations to 8.8 million patients per year (National Association of Community Health Centers, 1995). They are essential resources for communities with high numbers of uninsured citizens.

CASE 7-4

A Bus Stop in Every Differential
—by Laura Frankenstein, M.D.

It Left as we watched
Muddy, defaced, wounded by
Bullets
But it was ours, and had been for decades.

Abducted on a flatbed truck,
Yanked from the hard earth so near
Our door
Without notice, without alternative.

Now, if they came, they descended
Bus stops six blocks from our clinic's chaos.
Unfamiliar
Scary blocks, wet, cold, or searing hot, often dark blocks.

Inside the clinic we continued to care for people.
Or did we? Why did he miss his visit? Why did she
Stay at home
With her febrile infant's swollen red eyelid?

The day they took it
They said it was a mistake, changed the route,
"Forgot"
The stop served a clinic for the medically indigent.

Didn't mean to abandon the elderly, the frail, the addicted,
The wounded, the ill, the newborn of all colors, really.
But
Can't change a route for a year. "Takes that long."

"Takes that long" to alter a bus route, but
At least it might happen before a generation slips by.
How long
Before we value people, especially those unlike ourselves?

Together we scrambled, using mighty phone and
Pen, tried a few connections, and waited
Longer
Than a full-term pregnancy.

They heard our noise about the bus stop, but not our
Outrage about insidious sanctions that allow poverty to fester,
To flourish,
That make it OK to shove away the undesirables.

We were students, residents, patients, members of staff
And board, determined to be heard.
We got it
Back, just outside our rusty door, and people came again.

(Reprinted with the permission of the Journal of Family Practice)

TRANSPORTATION BARRIERS

The above poem was written by a physician at a CHC after learning a lesson that had been omitted from her medical school residency training. Many patients are logistically barred from a regular source of primary care, and as Case 7-4 indicates, the lack of transportation can be an enormous barrier to effective patient care.

When patients live in a high-poverty area and there is no regular source of affordable public transportation or the average travel time to an affordable source of primary care exceeds 30 minutes, clinicians will begin to observe the effects of logistical barriers to care. These effects will usually include increased patient "no-show" rates for appointments and difficulties with patient compliance with follow-up treatment plans such as referrals, pediatric prevention visits and immunizations, as well as failure of some patients to obtain prescribed medications.

As Case 7-4 suggests, sometimes the provider needs to advocate for transportation necessary for adequate patient care. Other options open to the provider include working with Medicaid to provide transportation vouchers for deserving patients. Transportation programs also are occasionally provided by certain philanthropic organizations. For example, local chapters of the American Cancer Society often provide volunteers who will drive patients for visits necessary for diagnosis and treatment of cancer. Also, CHCs, which receive funding from the federal government, are required to provide funding for transportation of their patients to necessary medical services.

If a clinician suspects that a patient may not receive necessary medical treatment because of the lack of transportation, the provider should broach the subject of transportation problems with the patient and recommend one of the alternatives just mentioned.

CASE 7-5

Mr. and Mrs. Ieng had only resided in the United States for 18 months when Mrs. Ieng discovered that she was pregnant. They spoke no English and worked in a Cambodian market. Mrs. Ieng had very little knowledge of our medical system and did not seek any prenatal healthcare. She went to her local hospital when she realized that she was in labor. She was very frightened both because she guessed that her baby was coming too soon and because she did not know anyone at the hospital and none of the hospital staff spoke Khmer.

Mrs. Ieng soon delivered twin sons who weighed 3 pounds each and had to be transferred to a tertiary care facility at the next largest city more than 30 miles away. When Mrs. Ieng was discharged, she was told by the telephone translation service used by the local hospital that her babies had been sent to another hospital, but she was never told the hospital address or that she was allowed to visit her babies. She was given the hospital address and visiting hours written in Khmer on a printed sheet that the hospital used for directing patients to the tertiary care facility. However, like many Cambodian patients, the Iengs were not literate in Khmer and therefore could not read the directions.

Days went by, and when the parents of the twins did not attempt to visit them in the tertiary care hospital, the hospital social workers tried to contact the Iengs, but they had no telephone. As the twins improved, the social workers moved to have the children placed in foster care, feeling that the parents had abandoned them. It was only when, in a final effort to contact the parents, they called the CHC in the Iengs' hometown that they were finally able to reach the Iengs. As luck would have it, the Iengs had received their immigration physicals at the CHC and were known to one of the Cambodian caseworkers there. The caseworker went to the Iengs' market and found them totally distraught, having thought, when no one returned their children, that their babies had died or were severely ill.

Without the help of the health center staff who assisted the Iengs' at the custody hearing for their children, the children would have been placed in foster care.

LANGUAGE, LITERACY, AND CULTURAL BARRIERS

As Case 7-5 illustrates, language and cultural barriers, coupled with illiteracy, can have tragic consequences. The family in that case almost lost their children as a result of the inability of the medical system to cope with those barriers.

Over 1.1 million individuals immigrated to the United States in 1993: 700,000 permanent residents, 100,000–150,000 refugees, and 300,000 undocumented immigrants (U.S. Department of Justice, 1994). Many of them are not even literate in their own first languages. Often these newcomers have little or no knowledge of Western medicine and bring their own deeply ingrained beliefs and methods of healing.

In order to provide adequate care to patients from communities where there are significant numbers of residents who are not native to the United States, do not speak English, or who cannot read, it is extremely important to know the degree to which these problems exist. If any of the following conditions prevail in a given community, then that community has higher than average language, literacy, or cultural barriers to care:

- Greater than 10% of the school enrollments are in bilingual classes (Massachusetts Department of Education, 1990).
- Greater than 10% of the community census is non-English-speaking (Census, 1993).
- Community school dropout rates are 5% or higher (Massachusetts Department of Education, 1990).
- Less than 80% of the residents have a high school education (Census, 1990).

When conditions such as the above prevail, patients will often have difficulty with written instructions, even when those instructions are written in their own language. Many times, patients will not readily admit that they cannot read and the clinician will have to reiterate instructions verbally and have patients repeat them back to ensure understanding.

With patients who are newcomers to this country, there may be higher rates of atypical infectious microbial and parasitic diseases, and higher rates of preexisting conditions. One CHC with considerable numbers of newcomers diagnosed within a 6-month span both preexisting tumors in one child who had lived close to the Chernobyl nuclear plant and tuberculosis of the bone in a Hispanic child. These conditions would be highly unusual in children native to the United States.

Newcomer populations may have strongly held healing traditions native to their own countries and very limited knowledge of or appreciation for Western medicine. A lack of trust of providers who do not know or respect the cultural roots of their patients is not uncommon regarding patients from other countries. It is very important that providers become familiarized with the cultures and traditions of the predominant patient populations they treat (see Chapter 10 for additional information). Without such knowledge, treatment can be impossible.

For example, if a clinician is treating a primarily Chinese-born population and decides to give the clinic a touch-up coat of paint, she might be very surprised when no prenatal patients come to the clinic. One might think that a simple "Caution! Wet Paint" sign would suffice to make patients comfortable. However, many Chinese people believe that if a pregnant woman inhales paint fumes, her baby will have birthmarks. Such unique beliefs can be found in all cultures, and must be known as well as respected if the provider is to forge a bond of mutual trust with newcomer patients.

Providing care to newcomer populations obviously poses some unique problems. Local cultural organizations that usually exist in areas with large populations of non-English-speaking immigrants can provide great resources in training caregivers about prevailing customs and perspectives on disease and treatment. Organizing presentations by such groups for clinical staff can not only serve to familiarize staff with such customs, but can also make members of the community aware that the providers are trying to become knowledgeable and want to be respectful of the traditional beliefs and customs of their patients.

Language barriers are also difficult for the provider. However, failure to bridge such language barriers can have drastic consequences, including impaired information flow from physician to patient that may result in inaccurate assessment of symptoms and misdiagnosis, increased dependency on testing with resulting increased inconvenience to patients, higher costs of care, and higher risks of false-positive results, problems with informed consent for procedures, and decreased medical compliance (Woloshin et al., 1995).

Although translation services provided by the telephone company for a fee exist in most areas and are available in most languages, such services provide a very poor alternative to communicating directly with the patient in the patient's own language. Hiring bilingual office and medical assisting staff is a very good intermediate step to this problem. Where bilingual education programs exist, courses in the patient's native tongue are also often available. Many Community Action Programs, public schools, and colleges offer such foreign language programs. Also, large teaching hospitals in areas of high concentrations of foreign-born patients often offer medical foreign language programs. These programs are usually available at little or no cost.

If the clinician is consistently seeing patients who speak a language other than English, it is surprising how relatively little training in a foreign language is necessary in order to become proficient in basic communication with patients. Clearly one should not rely on limited foreign language skills alone when treating patients, but as a bridge between the patient and translation of some kind, even limited language skills are greatly appreciated by patients and help gain their trust.

Occasionally state or local philanthropic grants are available to organizations trying to hire bilingual staff, train existing staff, or in other ways make themselves more accessible to non-English-speaking minorities. Additionally, areas that have CHCs have fine resources for multilingual, culturally competent care, because CHCs specialize in providing such services to linguistically and culturally barred populations.

CASE 7-6

Joseph Connolly was a 45-year-old Caucasian postal worker who had been employed by the post office for 10 years in the city where he had been born. He liked the work because it gave him a chance to exercise regularly and to be outside daily. Over the years, Joe found himself becoming dizzy and short of breath when he hiked around his route. He also started getting sharp pains down both legs and he became increasingly worried that there was something seriously wrong with his health. However, even though his symptoms persisted and even worsened over the course of several months, his diagnosis of severe hypertension and sciatica was not made until Joe was forced to see a physician in order to obtain a premarital blood test.

PROVIDER DISCRIMINATION

It may well be a puzzle that the patient in Case 7-6 had worked around the corner from a large group practice and even though he had insurance and had worried about his symptoms, he had not sought medical care. However, the physician he sought for his blood test gradually uncovered a previous history of severe alcoholism that had left the patient destitute, without family, and living on the streets. In the past, when he had sought care, he had been so shabbily treated by his medical providers that he had decided to never seek care again unless he absolutely had to.

No one should make light of the fact that treating patients who are substance abusers, seriously mentally ill, homeless, or have personal beliefs that differ strongly from the caregiver's is not an easy matter. However, discrimination against such patients prevents adequate caregiving and can cause patients to refuse to seek or accept treatment. For these reasons, providers who work in communities with high numbers of complex and vulnerable patients need to be aware of the problems that exist within their communities and aware of the resources available to help such vulnerable patients.

Characteristics of communities with high concentrations of patients with complex needs include:

- Total reported violent crime greater than 746 per 100,000 population (U.S. FBI, 1994)
- Drug arrest rates higher than 400 per 100,000 (U.S. FBI, 1994)
- Driving while intoxicated arrest rates greater than 120 per 100,000 (U.S. FBI, 1994)
- Alcohol- or drug-related hospital discharge rates higher than 600 per 100,000 (Massachusetts Department of Public Health, 1995a)

- HIV positivity rates greater than 4 per 1000 (Massachusetts Department of Public Health, 1995b)
- AIDS rates greater than 1.8 per 1000 (Massachusetts Department of Public Health, 1995b)

When a provider is working in a community with significant problems such as those listed above, caregiving can become complicated. Often patients in such communities display the lack of trust shown by the mail carrier in Case 7-6. They may also have difficulty in providing an adequate history of past treatment because of discontinuity of care or memory lapses.

Patients with alcoholism, substance abuse, or mental health problems may have multiple primary diagnoses coupled with their history of poor prior treatment. They may also show considerable lack of willingness to work with the provider to treat underlying medical problems and may only integrate into the medical system as long as it takes to alleviate the symptoms that brought the patient to the provider in the first place. Providers of complex patients such as these may feel "used", thinking that the patient is only trying to "get something from them" and that they can't trust the reliability of their patients' reporting. The important thing is to render the best care that one can in a nonjudgmental way, thus leaving the door open to future patient contact should the patient desire it.

Most areas have free substance abuse treatment programs supported by the federal government. These federal Office of Substance Abuse Prevention (OSAP) programs provide outpatient as well as inpatient treatment for patients with substance abuse problems. Sometimes the waiting lists for such programs are long. However, there are no waiting lists for 12-step programs such as Alcoholics Anonymous or Narcotics Anonymous available in most communities. Although the 12-step programs do not take the place of comprehensive OSAP programs, they can help maintain patients' sobriety and provide a supportive environment for patients.

Additionally, many states offer mental health programs through Medicaid, disability and general relief status, or through Departments of Mental and Public Health, which provide clinical support to those with substance abuse or mental health problems. Once a patient has a mental health provider, that provider can often bypass waiting lists for programs such as OSAP and can get patients much-needed treatment more efficiently.

CONCLUSION

Patients come into their caregivers' offices encumbered with many and varied obstacles to care related to their environments and social circumstances. Adequate treatment of patients depends on the ability of the provider to diagnose not only the patient, but also the community from which the patient comes. Only then will the provider have the correct context in which to make assumptions about the likely diagnosis and prognosis of the patient's disease; only then will the provider know the treatment plan most likely to effect a satisfactory outcome; only then will the provider know the most efficient and effective resources to bring to bear on the patient's problem.

When patients repeatedly seek care for the same problem and obstacles to effective treatment exist in the community, the most efficient and comprehensive treatment plan the provider can effectuate may be a change within the environment itself. We have seen that when environmental resources fall short in the treatment of disease, sometimes the caring provider can help create them. At a minimum, he can make others aware of the barriers to care that exist within the community and, through advocacy, can remove them.

CASES FOR DISCUSSION

CASE 1

The local elder service agency has called you to make a home visit to assess the status of an 81-year-old woman who is allegedly a victim of abuse by her daughter and son-in-law with whom she lives. On reviewing her records from the VNA, you find that she is status-post two hip fractures and has Parkinson's disease, chronic obstructive pulmonary disease, and a seizure disorder. Your examination reveals that she has severe rheumatoid arthritis and angina pectoris, as well as failure to thrive. You suspect that both the daughter and the son-in-law with whom she lives are schizophrenic and labile. You also suspect that they may be substance-dependent and may be stealing your patient's Social Security checks.

The patient is reluctant to leave the home because she is very attached to her two granddaughters, aged 7 and 13, who also live with her.

    1. How do you best stabilize and treat this patient?

    2. What are the implications of supporting the elder service agency's recommendation to file a protective court order which would have her removed from the home and placed in a safe environment?

    3. Are there other options for the protection and care of this patient?

CASE 2

Your patient is a Hispanic woman with advanced AIDS (CD4 count = 15). Even though you had told her many times to call you if she had any problems, one night when she couldn't breathe, had a temperature of 102°F, and was very frightened, she drove herself to the nearest emergency room and was admitted with a diagnosis of histoplasmosis. You did not have staff privileges at the hospital where she was admitted, and that hospital was not used to treating patients with AIDS.

Her care during her hospitalization was uncoordinated. Even though you discussed her case over the telephone with her attending physician, an open lung biopsy was performed instead of the bronchoscopy you recommended. Staff at the hospital shared her AIDS diagnosis with family members without the patient's permission.

    1. How can you best help to care for your patient under these circumstances?

    2. The Hispanic social worker from your clinic is very concerned about the patient's two children who are staying with an aunt. The social worker says that the aunt cannot care for the children much longer and they will be placed in foster care if something is not done.

    3. Finally the patient is stable and discharged. You want to prevent this type of occurrence again, but you realize that the hospital where she was admitted is the closest one to her home. What should you do to help your patient in future care?

CASE 3

The triage nurse in your clinic calls you requesting that you see a walk-in patient who has never been treated at your clinic before. The patient is highly agitated, disheveled, and confused. She tells you that she thinks she has "bugs" and that her dog has them too, whereupon she opens a large shoulder bag she is carrying and her dog scampers out into your exam room. She says that she can't take the itching anymore and that she will kill herself if you can't help her. She states that she has already "chopped" her own hair and she will chop herself next.

    1. How should you begin to assess this patient? She has no self-reported history of primary care or mental health treatment. In fact, she says that physicians "give her the creeps."

2. Should you attempt to begin a primary care relationship with this patient, and if so, how do you do so?
3. The patient tells you that she wants you to help her dog and her boyfriend too because she knows that they have the "bugs too" and she'll just get them back. How do you respond to her?

CASE 4

A 19-month-old child is brought to your clinic with a temperature of 102°F and tugging at his ear. You quickly diagnose otitis media, but on reading his chart you realize that he is long overdue for a history and physical examination. His last immunizations were at 6 months of age.

1. How do you best care for the child?
2. When you ask the mother why she has missed so many appointments, she states that she "just forgot" and that she also has changed addresses twice since the last visit and she has no car. How do you help her and reinforce the importance of the child's regular primary care?

CASE 5

A 50-year-old black Haitian-American male who speaks only French Creole comes to your office with his wife. His wife speaks enough English to serve as the translator and when you request the patient's chief complaint, the patient seems to gesture and say that he has chest pains. His wife adds that the chest pains come from an evil spirit placed on the husband because he had an affair with the woman next door. She states that the only way the husband will get any better is if he goes to her French Pentecostal church, confesses his sin, and is exorcised. The wife appears to you to be attending the patient's appointment grudgingly and with great hostility. You are not convinced that she is providing a word-for-word translation of your dialogue with the patient.

1. What is the best way to begin to treat this patient?
2. Should you continue to use his wife as the translator for his care?
3. You have in your office a young nursing student who is fluent in French and says that she understands some Creole. Should you use her as a translator instead?

CASE 6

You work in a clinic in an impoverished inner-city area. The wait for an appointment for a physical examination of a new patient is 12 weeks, and a regular patient of the clinic must wait at least 8 weeks. Your patients call all the time needing immediate physical examinations for entry into school, Head Start, summer camp, or to get jobs. Without these exams, you know that your patients will suffer.

1. How do you handle your patients' requests?
2. In the long run, how should you begin to deal with this problem?

——————— RECOMMENDED READINGS ———————

Aday LA: *At Risk in America. The Health and Health Care Needs of Vulnerable Populations in the United States.* San Francisco, Jossey–Bass Publishers, 1993.

A comprehensive examination of vulnerable patient populations as well as a description of approaches to their care.

Birrer RB: *Urban Family Medicine.* Berlin, Springer-Verlag, 1987.

A practical guide to physician practice within the community.

Nutting PA: *Community Oriented Primary Care: From Principle to Practice.* Albuquerque, University of New Mexico Press, 1990.

A thorough examination of the COPC approach to defining and then preventing and treating disease within a community.

Sardell A: *The U.S. Experiment in Social Medicine. The Community Health Center Program, 1965–1986.* Pittsburgh, PA, University of Pittsburgh Press, 1988.

An interesting exploration of the history of community health centers and the role they play in today's medical system.

CHAPTER 8

A. Relationships

The Workplace

Annette M. David and Mark R. Cullen

Mr. A. K. is a 43-year-old man who was seen at the Primary Care Clinic with a chief complaint of "fatigue." He stated that he had been feeling "crummy" for over a month and was concerned about his health. The physician was unable to elicit a coherent history of any illness. However, the review of systems was replete with nonspecific symptoms such as joint aches and several episodes of crampy abdominal pain which Mr. A. K. attributed to "dyspepsia." The physical examination was unremarkable.

At this point, the physician began to suspect a nonorganic etiology for Mr. A. K.'s symptoms. Still, because the patient insisted on it, blood was drawn for a CBC. This revealed a low hemoglobin and hematocrit, results that surprised the clinician. Red blood cell indices were indicative of a normocytic, normochromic anemia. He called Mr. A. K. back for a follow-up visit, during which a second blood draw was done for a reticulocyte count, which proved to be elevated.

Called back for his third clinic visit, Mr. A. K. was questioned extensively about a family history of hemolytic anemia, which he denied. There was no previous history of sickle cell trait, G6PD deficiency, or the presence of an intravascular prosthesis. However, Mr. A. K. did mention that his symptoms began shortly after he started restoration work on a 150-year-old farmhouse. Intrigued, the physician asked Mr. A. K. what his job entailed. "I'm a painter," replied Mr. A. K. Properly enlightened, the physician did a third blood draw, which indicated a marked elevation in blood lead level and zinc protoporphyrin. The diagnosis: acute lead poisoning.

167

INTRODUCTION

The Bureau of Labor Statistics of the U.S. Department of Labor estimates that in 1993 there were close to 92 million people employed in private industry (Deptartment of Labor Bureau of Labor Statistics, 1995). Not included in that figure are the self-employed as well as the numerous employees of federal and state agencies. Altogether, the total number of workers in the United States comprises the majority of the adult population.

Physicians and public health officials are becoming more cognizant of the impact of the workplace on the health of workers. On one hand, the workplace is being targeted for interventions to promote health and to prevent disease. On the other hand, we continue to discover many potentially damaging effects of workplace exposures. Clearly, the workplace is an arena that must be of interest to all practitioners of medicine caring for adults.

Most working men and women obtain their healthcare not from occupational or worksite-based clinics but from primary care providers: internists, family practitioners, physician's assistants, and nurse practitioners. Mr. A. K. in Case 8-1, for example, sought help from a physician at a primary care clinic. Whether they are conscious of it, these clinicians are engaged in the practice of occupational medicine and should be knowledgeable about the basic principles of occupational disease.

Unfortunately, occupational medicine training remains outside the mainstream of U.S. medical education and training. For instance, in 1985, a survey showed that only 50% of U.S. medical schools included occupational and environmental health in their curricula; the average time spent on occupational medicine during 4 years was 4 hours (Levy, 1985). By 1992, not much improvement was noted, with 66% of schools devoting an average of 6 hours to occupational and environmental medicine (Burstein & Levy, 1994). Residency training in the primary care specialties offers little as well (Cullen & Rosenstock, 1988).

WORK-RELATED MEDICAL VISITS

How many medical encounters involve work-related problems? Definitive data to answer this question do not exist. However, experienced primary care providers would agree that a significant portion of their patient encounters are generated by health concerns that are directly related to workplace issues. There are straightforward "industrial medicine" visits that require healthcare providers to evaluate individuals for work fitness. Preplacement physicals and respiratory fitness evaluations are good examples. In addition, many corporations are downsizing their medical departments for economic reasons and utilizing community primary care facilities to do urgent care for their employees who suffer from on-the-job accidents and injuries. Because of recent federal mandates on drug and alcohol testing in the workplace, physicians are being asked to serve as medical review officers by both government and private sector companies.

Increasingly, third-party payers are expecting primary care practitioners to provide information regarding disability and work restrictions. Such requests also come from lawyers involved in workers' compensation cases or class action suits related to workplace exposures. Patients themselves may present to their healthcare providers for a variety of reasons. Some may request an evaluation and a letter to excuse themselves from absence at work because of an illness—the sickness excuse. Others have illnesses that they suspect may be attributed to their work. Most importantly, patients with symptoms that were not initially ascribed to a workplace exposure may turn out to have an occupational disease. The case of Mr. A. K. presented at the beginning of this chapter is a good example.

WORK AND DISEASE CAUSATION

Where does the workplace fit in disease causation? Medicine has traditionally focused on the infectious disease model that emphasizes the host–agent interaction, almost to the exclusion of the environment within which this interaction occurs and of the patient's activities in that setting. Occupational medicine broadens that view, with agent, environment, and activity all assuming major roles in disease causation. Most working people spend an average of 8 hours at work per day, which translates into at least a quarter of one's entire life spent at the workplace. It should be apparent that the work environment may have a substantial impact on an individual's state of health. A good physician must spend some time understanding what the work environment entails to better understand the nature of the work-related health problem.

In the infectious disease model, the infectious agent and the host assume paramount importance. Measures to prevent or control disease can be targeted toward either the agent causing disease or the susceptible host. For example, if the virus causing an infection can be identified, an antiviral agent can be developed against that virus. Antibiotics can be manufactured to combat specific bacteria. The host can be immunized or prevented from coming into contact with agents of disease. Occupational health extends this concept one step further by taking the broader workplace environment as a third potential target for interventions designed to prevent or cure disease. Thus, engineering and administrative controls can be instituted to reduce harmful exposures. Work processes can be changed to alter their impact on disease. And when necessary, protective devices can be used to further control risks.

How can work cause disease? There are certain health hazards that exist because of harmful agents in an individual's work. The miner exposed to silica, the firefighter exposed to carbon monoxide, the medical intern exposed to *Mycobacterium tuberculosis*, the pathology technician who uses formalin (formalin can contain up to 50% formaldehyde by weight), and the house painter exposed to lead in paint are good examples.

In other cases, the work itself is the hazard. The movie stuntman is constantly at risk of losing life and limb. A data entry clerk who uses a keyboard 8 hours a day can eventually develop cumulative trauma to her wrists and hands. Outdoor workers must contend with markedly enhanced ultraviolet radiation exposure and hazards associated with the elements.

Preexisting health conditions can be aggravated by work. The asthmatic laborer in a dusty factory and the diabetic with neuropathy who works with solvents are both at risk of worsening their preexisting health problems.

Psychological and social stresses at work can also affect an individual's sense of well-being. In today's economic climate, the constant threat of unemployment is a real fear for many people. In addition, in this technological age, workers have to grapple with uncertainty about the future as automation replaces skilled craftsworkers and laborers. Persons employed in factory lines and large office pools have to come to terms with the drudgery of their work. For the sake of efficiency, their workplaces have been dehumanized, their tasks reduced to often meaningless, repetitive motions. An increasing number of working adults no longer obtain a sense of satisfaction and personal identity from what they do. Instead, work to them is a chore, something that must be done in order to survive, nothing more than a distasteful necessity to be gotten over with each day as quickly as possible. The anxiety and resentment that this situation generates often spill over into the personal lives of these individuals. Indeed, the complex interplay of work, health, and personal and family life is a reality that healthcare providers need to recognize, assess, and be able to address.

WORK AND HEALTH

While acknowledging that the work environment is an integral component of disease causation, an experienced physician also recognizes the positive effects of work on health. Work can be defined as any activity that is expended to support the basic needs of the individual and of society. From an individual perspective, work is the means by which people procure the ability to provide for their desires and needs. By working, one also makes a contribution to society and establishes a social identity. A successful worker is a successful person. Work achievement becomes a measure of adult functional capacity and is therefore an affirmation of health (Deubner, 1987b). Occupational medicine is as committed to supporting well-being and excellent function in the healthy worker as it is to uncovering work-related illness and preventing disease *per se.*

ETHICAL DILEMMAS IN THE OCCUPATIONAL MEDICINE ENCOUNTER

By its nature, dealing with occupational health problems often gives rise to ethical dilemmas. When the referral source is other than the individual patient, the issue of loyalty or allegiance arises. Can the healthcare provider function in an unbiased, objective manner toward the worker when the paycheck comes from the company or third-party payer? On the other hand, will the provider be fair to the employer when the individual worker or his labor union is footing the bill? Where should the provider's loyalty lie? Another area of conflict in the occupational setting is that of patient confidentiality. To what extent do employers and third-party payers have a right to know about individual employees' health histories? If a provider is aware of a condition in an individual worker that could pose a potential risk to that individual, his co-workers, or that segment of the public whom he serves (e.g., a school bus driver who has a substance abuse problem), can the provider break confidentiality? Sometimes, a provider's health concerns may be in direct conflict with the patient's economic security. When removal from a workplace exposure is the safest means to control an occupational illness, what do you do when the patient has no other source of income? Although ethical guidelines exist, there is no consensus as to how to respond to these dilemmas. The primary care provider must be sensitized to these issues and should have a sound ethical framework within which to resolve the ethical dilemmas she may encounter (Rest & Patterson, 1986; Deubner, 1987a; American College of Occupational and Environmental Medicine, 1994).

The following sections of this chapter revolve around some of the key issues in the practice of occupational medicine. Special considerations in the diagnosis and management of work-related disease are emphasized. The last few pages introduce the reader to the concepts pertinent to disability and impairment evaluation and to the federal agencies involved in workplace regulation.

A previously healthy 40-year-old Hispanic man presented to the emergency room of a tertiary care teaching hospital with chief complaints of headache, abdominal pain, and nausea. He reported that his symptoms appeared shortly after he began work as a machine operator coating fabrics with a plastic compound. On further questioning, he stated that other coworkers suffered similar symptoms. Liver function tests showed an elevated aspartate aminotransferase level with normal alkaline phosphatase and bilirubin levels, consistent with hepatocellular injury. Results of the hepatitis screen were negative. There was no history of alcohol or drug abuse, or of previous blood transfusions. The emergency room physician, suspecting a possible occupational cause of the man's hepatitis, consulted the occupational medicine specialist. The man was temporarily removed from work.

In the meantime, the occupational medicine physician consulted an industrial hygienist. Together, they went to the man's workplace and evaluated the potential exposures. They noted the presence of numerous solvents that were mixed into the polyurethane compound used to coat fabrics; a number of these were known or suspected hepatotoxins. The index patient's coworkers were evaluated for subclinical liver disease; several of them turned out to have abnormal elevations in their liver transaminases. An epidemiological investigation pointed toward one particular hepatotoxic solvent, dimethylformamide, as the most likely culprit. The employers, aware of the possible legal and health consequences of the problem, stopped production and installed an improved ventilation system. The company substituted a less toxic agent for the dimethylformamide and returned to full production. The index patient eventually recovered normal liver function. At the urging of the labor union, a medical screening program was instituted for the workers. Those employees who chose to leave the company were referred to an experienced social worker for counseling and assistance with job placement (Redlich et al., 1988).

THE FIELD OF OCCUPATIONAL MEDICINE

Unlike other medical specialties that delineate themselves on the basis of organ systems (e.g., cardiology, neurology) or medical procedures and technology (e.g., nuclear medicine, radiology, or surgery), occupational medicine is defined by the environment in which work-related health and illness occur. The workplace is usually an easily identifiable entity and in many cases its structure is conducive to developing a healthcare delivery system specific to it. The design of an occupational medicine healthcare delivery system and the players involved differ from the more traditional medical specialties.

Occupational medicine is an established specialty of medicine that seeks to identify, treat, and prevent disorders related to hazards and exposures in the workplace as well as to institute measures designed to promote the health and fitness of workers. The practice of occupational medicine goes beyond the care of the individual patient; public health and prevention are of paramount importance. Diagnostic and therapeutic interventions are targeted toward the work environment as well as toward the individual patient. Finally, social, legal, and economic factors are incorporated into the occupational health provider's decision-making strategies to a much larger extent than in other fields of clinical medicine. It is a dynamic, rapidly evolving medical specialty that requires energy, ingenuity, and the ability to grasp intuitively the "big picture."

Although several models of occupational medicine practice exist, the composition of the occupational health team always requires certain key components. The primary provider is a physician, nurse practitioner, or physician's assistant who is well grounded in the principles of general medicine and in addition has specialized knowledge about work requirements, workplace hazards, and legal issues relating to the workplace. This individual is responsible for the diagnosis, treatment, and determination of the work-relatedness of illness or injury in the working population being served. The primary provider works in coordination with an industrial hygienist whose role is to evaluate the workplace for chemical, physical, and biologic hazards and to recommend measures designed to minimize or control them. Ideally, the primary provider also has access to a social worker or counselor who is well versed in social and legal issues affecting the workplace. Patients often need such assistance if work disability occurs, when considering a job change for health reasons or when negotiating the tangled path of worker's compensation. These professionals form the core of the occupational health team.

Case 8-2 demonstrates the "team approach" that is so crucial to the successful resolution of work-related problems. The physician of first contact in the emergency room, suspecting an occupational cause for the patient's problem, called in an internist who was trained in occupational medicine. She, in turn, consulted with an industrial hygienist during the process of evaluating the worksite. While the occupational medicine physician managed the medical problems of the patient and his affected coworkers and the industrial hygienist addressed the engineering requirements of the workplace, the social dilemmas were resolved with the assistance of a social worker. An occupational physician working alone would not have been able to address the various facets of this case so thoroughly.

In general medicine, the therapeutic relationship used to have only two parties, the provider and the patient. Increasingly, "payers" are becoming third parties to be coped with. Unique to occupational medicine is the addition of yet other parties to the therapeutic relationship, including employers, labor unions, and lawyers. A significant proportion of patient referrals to occupational medicine providers may come from these parties. The special interests of these groups may parallel or conflict with those of the patient. Although the actual diagnosis and assessment of workplace risk remains unchanged, the provider needs to be aware of the forces that motivate each party. In Case 8-2, for example, the employers wanted to avoid legal repercussions while maintaining productivity. The labor union wanted to ensure the safety of all of its members by securing adequate medical care and surveillance as well as engineering controls such as improved ventilation. The individual workers were anxious to keep their jobs but were concerned about their personal health at the same time. The different agendas of these parties and of the patient can affect access to information and can limit the range of therapeutic options available. While the provider needs to maintain her objectivity, she must also constantly attempt to see the situation in its entirety to make effective diagnoses and therapeutic recommendations. This is one aspect of the field that constantly challenges physicians dealing with occupational health problems. It is a good reason for consulting an occupational medicine specialist.

CASE 8-3

Mrs. G. B., a 48-year-old previously healthy nonsmoker, consulted her family physician because of periodic shortness of breath. About 2 months ago, she started having dyspnea at night, accompanied by wheezing. She experienced no chest pain, orthopnea, paroxysmal nocturnal dyspnea, or symptoms of gastro-esophageal reflux. On further questioning, she recognized that her symptoms seemed to be worse during midweek. In the past 2 months, the only time she was asymptomatic was when she went on vacation to Bermuda. Results of her physical examination were unremarkable. Spirometry revealed a pattern of mild airway obstruction.

Asthma was diagnosed, but the physician could not find the trigger factor. She then reviewed the original screening questionnaire that Mrs. G. B. filled out during her first clinic visit 6 months ago. On that questionnaire, she noted that her patient was a furniture maker who had just started working with Western red cedar. She did a Medline search and discovered that Western red cedar is a known precipitant of occupational asthma and that the pattern of airway dysfunction may be of the delayed type, that is, symptoms may occur several hours after exposure, consistent with Mrs. G. B.'s nocturnal episodes. Mrs. G. B.'s symptoms were relatively well controlled by standard bronchodilator therapy, but only after she stopped using Western red cedar did the symptoms abate completely.

HAZARDS IN THE WORKPLACE

Every healthcare provider will encounter cases in his practice that involve unfamiliar hazards or activities, leading to difficulty in recognizing and diagnosing occupational disease. General principles that can be applied to all work-induced disorders exist. These principles can provide a conceptual framework to aid providers in approaching work-related illness, especially when specific knowledge of toxicity is limited (Rosenstock & Cullen, 1994).

Principle No. 1: The clinical and pathologic expressions of most occupational diseases are indistinguishable from those of nonoccupational diseases. To be diagnosed, occupational disease must first be recognized. Many healthcare providers imagine that the patterns of illness produced by hazards in the workplace are somehow unique and that the clinical presentation of occupational diseases will distinguish them from non-work-related disorders. In reality, occupational diseases present in much the same way as common disorders of nonoccupational origin. Usually, there is nothing in the clinical presentation of a disease that will indicate a work-related etiology.

Consider Mrs. G. B. in Case 8-3. Although she was ultimately diagnosed with occupational asthma, her presenting symptoms were indistinguishable from those of "garden-variety" asthma that is unrelated to workplace exposures.

Principle No. 2: More often than not, it is the history of the illness in relation to work activities and exposures that will provide clues pointing toward a work-related cause. The occupational health history is fundamental to the assessment of the work-relatedness of a health problem. It must be incorporated into the routine health history obtained from every patient. This point cannot be overemphasized.

The occupational history has several purposes. These include increasing patient awareness of occupational and environmental factors, making accurate diagnoses, preventing the development of occupational disease, preventing the aggravation of underlying medical conditions by workplace factors, identifying potential workplace hazards, detecting new associations between exposure and disease, and establishing the basis for compensation of work-related disease.

Table 8.1
Principles of Occupational Disease[a]

1. The clinical and pathologic expressions of most occupational diseases are indistinguishable from those of nonoccupational diseases
2. More often than not, it is the history of the illness that will provide clues pointing toward a work-related cause
3. Nonoccupational factors can contribute to the development of work-related disease
4. There is a biologically predictable latency period between occupational exposure and overt disease
5. A dose–response relationship typically holds true for occupational exposures
6. Individuals vary in their clinical response to workplace hazards

[a]Modified from Rosenstock & Cullen (1994).

The two major components of the occupational history are the work and exposure history and the general health history. In the work and exposure history, information about current and previous jobs and other nonoccupational environmental exposures should be obtained. This portion of the history should contain not only the patient's job title but also information regarding the nature of her work and a description of the actual tasks performed. The job title alone often is insufficient to provide clues as to what the significant exposures are. For example, a painter involved in new construction does not have the same risk of lead exposure as Mr. A. K. in Case 8-1, who had to scrape and burn lead-based paint on the 150-year-old farmhouse that he was refurbishing.

Potential work exposures should be sought and enumerated. If the worker is well informed about his specific workplace exposures, the information that he provides may be sufficient. By law, employers must make exposure information available to their workers in the form of Manufacturers' Safety Data Sheets (MSDSs). MSDSs can be a rich source of data; the worker has the right of access to them and should be encouraged to exercise this right. Occasionally, hazardous exposures are identified during an industrial hygienist's worksite evaluation, which is what happened in the case of the solvent-exposed factory worker in Case 8-2.

Nonoccupational exposures need to be pinpointed. The patient should be asked about hobbies, recreational activities, and the home environment. Some extremely toxic chemicals are available for home use, e.g., caustic substances in household cleaners and pesticides for use in gardening. Tobacco and alcohol use should be investigated, since these environmental exposures may interact with or aggravate occupational exposures. If the factory worker in Case 8-2 also happened to be an alcoholic, the extent of his liver injury would probably have been much worse because of the combined hepatotoxicity of dimethylformamide and alcohol. Had Mrs. G. B. in Case 8-3 been a heavy smoker, her asthmatic reaction to Western red cedar would likely have been more severe.

Finally, an inquiry about habits as they relate to hygiene at work should be made. In Case 8-1, the house painter's body burden of lead would have increased significantly from hand-to-mouth contact if he ate or smoked in the workplace.

Information regarding health problems and symptoms as they relate to work should be elicited in the general health history. The temporal relationship of these symptoms with the work day or work shift may be crucial to the diagnosis and should not be overlooked. Some work-related conditions will have a strong relationship to time spent at work. Airway irritation with cough and bronchial spasm from high levels of formaldehyde occurs within a short time of exposure and resolves within hours to days from cessation of exposure. Occupational asthma from red cedar, on the other hand, is of the delayed-onset type, with nocturnal wheezing as the first manifestation. Hence, the timing of Mrs. G. B.'s wheezing and dyspnea together with her workplace exposure were crucial in making the diagnosis in Case 8-3. Finally, a number of chronic work-related conditions may exhibit no particular variation with work exposure; most conditions with long latency have this character.

Information can be obtained by interview or by a self-administered questionnaire. Studies affirmed the validity of self-reported data for occupational and environmental exposures (Rosenstock *et al.*, 1984). Of course, whenever possible, other sources of supplemental information should be sought. These include prior medical records of the affected worker, exposure information from the employer (e.g., MSDSs), results of prior inspections of the workplace by a regulatory agency such as the Occupational Safety and Health Administration (OSHA) or the local Department of Health, and direct exposure assessment from a site visit. Substantial amounts of information, often of good quality, can sometimes be obtained from labor unions and community groups concerned about potentially hazardous exposures.

Principle No. 3: Nonoccupational factors can contribute to the development of work-related disease. Most occupational illnesses have a multifactorial etiology. For example, the risk of developing lung cancer is much higher in asbestos workers who also smoke. Clinicians must recognize that identifying a nonoccupational cause of a disease does not eliminate the possibility of a second work-related factor. Even if Mrs. G. B. in the preceding case example were a heavy smoker, the occupational exposure to Western red cedar remains the primary etiologic agent of her asthma. The potential role of a workplace hazard should not be overlooked just because another nonoccupational hazard exists.

Principle No. 4: There is a biologically predictable latency period between occupational exposure and overt disease. This fact is crucial in correctly attributing a disease to an occupational exposure. Certain illnesses may manifest long after the original exposure. Mesothelioma, for example, has a mean latency period of about 35 years from the initial asbestos exposure. On the other hand, a number of irritants and toxins are unlikely to cause delayed reactions. For example, acute upper airway irritation cannot be ascribed to an ammonia exposure that occurred uneventfully 5 weeks earlier.

Principle No. 5: The dose–response relationships are important for the diagnosis of occupational diseases. The dose of an exposure to a workplace hazard is a strong predictor of the type and intensity of the response. For example, acute silicosis, an aggressive disease characterized histologically by alveolar proteinosis, is unlikely unless an overwhelming exposure to freshly fractured silica occurred. On the other hand, once sensitized, even a very small exposure to Western red cedar can trigger an asthmatic attack in someone like Mrs. G. B. from Case 8-3. The clinician's ability to make a reasonably accurate assessment of previous and current exposure dose will determine to a large extent the successful evaluation and management of a patient suspected of having an occupational disease.

Principle No. 6: Individuals vary in their clinical response to workplace hazards. Persons respond differently to the same type of exposure. In Case 8-3, for example, there were three other furniture makers who were not susceptible to the sensitizing effects of Western red cedar and who never developed respiratory symptoms. The response to solvent exposure in Case 8-2 ranged from no response to subclinical liver enzyme abnormalities to overt hepatitis. This variation may cause a provider to underestimate the relationship between a workplace hazard and a disease. Astute clinicians will acknowledge that this variability in response may be a function of variability between individuals and not necessarily proof that the occupational exposure is unrelated to the health outcome.

If, after evaluating the patient with a thorough history and physical examination, the possibility of an occupational disease is seriously considered, the ideal next step is to do an assessment of the workplace.

The usual concept of "the workplace" is that of a physical entity that is geographically defined. A factory in the suburbs, a city office, and a mine in West Virginia are good examples. However, there may be instances when "the workplace" is not confined to one location. Consider Mr. A. K., the painter in Case 8-1. His workplace, rightfully defined, is wherever he is currently working. It could be a bridge, an old building, or a construction site. It could be one construction site today and a different one tomorrow. Some workplaces may not conform with the conventional image of a worksite. Think of the airline pilot. A housekeeper's place of work is another person's home. With the advent of computer technology, more and more people are opting to work in their own homes. The point is that "the workplace" is not always defined by structure.

An essential prerequisite to a worksite evaluation is familiarity with the work itself. By knowing what a specific job entails, what materials are handled, what processes/tasks are carried out, and what products are generated, hazard recognition is facilitated. In Case 8-3, for example, knowing that Mrs. G. B. was a furniture maker who worked with Western red cedar was crucial in establishing the deleterious exposure. Although patients may not know much about specific chemicals, they can almost always provide good information about the major products and materials and the kinds of activities that they and others do.

DIAGNOSTIC DECISION-MAKING

The principles of medical diagnostic decision-making also apply to occupational disease (Rosenstock & Cullen, 1986). The clinical presentation should be consistent with the nature of the illness. The interval between onset of disease and exposure should conform to the known latency of the suspected causal agent. The intensity of the exposure should be appropriate for the magnitude of the disease, given the known dose–response characteristic of the suspected workplace hazard. The hazard itself should be verified and the dose range established to the fullest extent possible. Supplemental information should be obtained from other sources, such as employers, labor unions, other physicians, manufacturers, and even regulatory agencies if required. The final step is processing all of this information and deciding the likelihood that the disease is work-related.

In practice, the information available to the healthcare provider will often be insufficient to establish with absolute certainty that a disease is occupational. Commonly, the decision regarding the work-relatedness of a disease will require a judgment. Such a decision merits careful thought because, unlike general medicine, the consequences of that decision go beyond medical concerns. There are economic, social, and legal ramifications in making the diagnosis of an occupational disease and dreadful personal and public health consequences of not making the diagnosis. All of these factors must be taken into consideration so that the probable outcome is in the patient's best interest. For example, from a purely medical perspective, Mrs. G. B. in Case 8-3 should have been removed from further exposure to Western red cedar. However, quitting her job would have a considerable impact on her life, especially since she is a widow with two young children. Fortunately, her employer assigned her to work with less allergenic hardwoods and provided her with the appropriate respirator. On the other hand, if the diagnosis was missed and the exposure to Western red cedar continued, Mrs. G. B.'s asthma very likely would have progressed, perhaps to the point of incapacitating her.

177

HAZARDS IN THE WORKPLACE

MANAGING A WORK-RELATED ILLNESS

Once a diagnosis is established, the clinician can then proceed to formulate a treatment plan. Depending on the circumstances, this plan can operate on two levels: The first is tailored toward the individual patient, and the second addresses the public health dimension of the problem.

The portion of the treatment plan that concerns itself with the individual patient needs to take into account not only medical concerns but also the various economic, social, and legal factors that may be pertinent to the case. One text puts this succinctly: "Although one choice or another may seem preferable from a strictly medical perspective, it cannot be presumed that this choice satisfies the needs of the patient, or that it is included among the options offered by the employer or other relevant parties" (Rosenstock & Cullen, 1994). This is the point in the encounter when a thoughtful consideration of the various agendas of the patient and other parties is crucial. Options need to be explored and alternatives considered, with the main goal of optimizing benefit for the patient. It is also at this point when the services of a social worker may be required.

Responsibility may not end with the conclusion of care of the individual patient. When a workplace hazard is identified and other workers may be at risk of exposure, the provider should consider acting on the public health implications of the situation. At the very least, the opinion that others may be at risk should be documented and reported to local health authorities. In some instances, hazardous workplaces will be recognized about which little can be done, though often employers will respond directly to such concerns. The clinician may have additional recourse through a regulatory agency such as OSHA or through a labor union so that employees may be informed of their potential risk. In addition, it is vital that the employer or whoever has ultimate responsibility for the workplace be made aware whenever safety concerns have been raised.

CASE 8-4

Mr. D. L. is a right-handed 27-year-old mechanic who was working on a car engine when an accident occurred. The rod holding the car's hood open buckled and the car hood came down onto his left hand. His left thumb had to be amputated from the metacarpophalangeal joint. He was evaluated to have a 100% percent loss of the left thumb, which translated into a 40% impairment of the upper extremity. With appropriate occupational rehabilitation, he was able to return to his job in 3 months.

CASE 8-5

Ms. M. F. is a 53-year-old data entry clerk for a large corporation. She joined the company in 1980 and has been doing data entry for 15 years. Over the past year, she noticed the onset of bilateral forearm pain. The pain progressively worsened over time. Eventually, she was unable to perform activities of daily living because of the severe pain. Results of repeated physical examinations including neurologic testing were inconsistent with carpal tunnel syndrome or other well-characterized clinical entities. She underwent various radiographic and electrophysiologic tests under the supervision of a hand surgeon. Although a mild nerve conduction abnormality was noted bilaterally, it was insufficient to explain her degree of dysfunction. A psychiatric evaluation was not helpful. She was diagnosed with repetitive stress disorder. Despite physical therapy and active participation in a pain management program, she was unable to regain function in both arms. Although impairment could not be documented, she was awarded permanent partial disability after a year of treatment, but she was never able to return to her job and suffered enormous economic and personal loss.

EVALUATING DISABILITY, IMPAIRMENT, AND WORK-RELATEDNESS

Disability problems are the most common reasons that persons with work-induced illnesses are evaluated by primary care providers. Often the referral source is a third party, usually an employer or insurance agency. The task for the provider is to determine the extent and permanency of functional loss, what residual work capacity is left, what work restrictions should apply, and what degree of impairment or disability should be awarded for purposes of worker's compensation or disability benefit allocation.

Certain terms need to be defined. Impairment, as defined in the American Medical Association's *Guides to the Evaluation of Permanent Impairment*, is "an alteration of an individual's health status that is assessed by medical means" (American Medical Association, 1988). It refers to the objective loss of the function of an organ or part of the body as compared with a preexisting baseline. Because it is an objective finding, it can generally be demonstrated by clinical maneuvers and quantified. It is independent of the patient's functional status. Disability, on the other hand, is defined as "an alteration of an individual's capacity to meet personal, social, or occupational demands, or to meet statutory or regulatory requirements" (American Medical Association, 1988). Disability is assessed by nonmedical means; the patient's functional status and occupational and social circumstances need to be taken into account. Disability may be temporary or permanent. Permanent disability is usually determined after a period during which maximum medical improvement can be expected to occur. Note that an impaired individual is not necessarily disabled. The mechanic in Case 8-4 is impaired because he lost his left thumb. However, he was able to return to his job after a period of rehabilitation; hence, he is not, by definition, disabled. In contrast, the woman in Case 8-5 exhibits significant disability in the absence of measurable impairment.

A component of most disability evaluations is the determination of the work-relatedness of an injury or illness. Simply put, an injury or illness is work-related if it resulted from some activity or exposure at work. Although the work-related nature of most on-the-job accidents is evident, the situation with chronic illnesses is more complicated. Because of the multifactorial nature of most chronic diseases, it is often difficult to ascertain the cause of a particular disorder with certainty. The legal standard is less rigorous than the medical one, and benefits are based on the legal standard. Therefore, it is the more important one for this decision, a fact that makes many physicians uneasy. Cause is established from a legal perspective if it is more likely than not that a workplace exposure caused or aggravated the disease. In numerical terms, if the probability that an occupational factor resulted in disease is greater than 50%, then sufficient cause exists.

A more detailed discussion of this topic is beyond the scope of this chapter. Because it puts a different slant to the traditional role of the provider as patient advocate, however, certain guidelines need to be mentioned.

First, to be effective, the provider who is doing the evaluation needs to distance herself from personal feelings regarding the appropriateness of the benefit system. For example, a provider may believe on a personal level that any person who seeks disability insurance is "out to milk the system." If she is unable to prevent that personal belief from influencing her professional judgment, her ability to assess the patient objectively is questionable. In order to do a credible job, the provider as evaluator must be unbiased. Second, both provider and patient need to understand that the traditional clinician–patient relationship is modified when disability is being evaluated. If the provider is doing an evaluation on an individual who also happens to be a patient whose medical care she oversees, then she needs to be able to distinguish her role as evaluator from that of medical caregiver. It may be appropriate in this situation to refer the patient to another provider, a social worker or some other professional who can take over the role of patient advocate. Third, if the provider is uncertain about the disability and its cause, she should consider obtaining a second opinion early on during the course of the evaluation. The evaluator's opinion should always be communicated in an unequivocal fashion to the patient as well as to the referral source in writing. Finally, the decision to remove a patient from his job should be done only after a thoughtful consideration of the consequences, both financial and psychological, that such an action could have.

179

EVALUATING
DISABILITY,
IMPAIRMENT,
AND WORK-
RELATEDNESS

WORKER'S COMPENSATION

A significant number of disability and work-relatedness evaluations are performed for worker's compensation purposes. Worker's compensation is a system defined by a set of federal and state laws instituted to provide income replacement, medical expense benefits, and rehabilitation services to workers disabled by work-related injury or illness. In essence, it is a form of insurance against occupational disease or injury that is paid for by the employer. In return, it operates on a "no-fault" assumption that precludes the worker from suing the employer. Any injury or illness that fulfills the legal standard for work-relatedness is compensable regardless of who was at fault. The worker bears the burden of proof of the work-relatedness of his health condition. Claims are paid for either directly by the employer or indirectly by an insurance company contracted by the employer. Claims have to be filed in a timely manner with the state agency that administers the worker's compensation system. Claimants do not become eligible for benefits until after a waiting period in which claims can be, and often are, contested. When this happens, they undergo review by either an administrative or a judicial agency.

The benefits received by a disabled worker from the worker's compensation fund may be insufficient to meet his needs. There are other sources of benefits available to him. Social Security Disability Insurance (SSDI) supplements worker's compensation with monthly benefits for qualified workers. Income from SSDI is paid in coordination with worker's compensation provided the sum of the combined benefits does not exceed 80%

of the worker's current average earnings. The Social Security benefits would be reduced, not the worker's compensation, in order to meet the 80% limit.

To qualify for Social Security disability benefits, the injured worker must meet several criteria. First, he must be totally disabled, that is, he must be unable to do any substantial gainful work. Second, the disability must be expected to last for at least 12 months or result in premature death. Finally, the worker must have worked long enough and recently enough and paid the required number of quarters into Social Security to be insured. SSDI begins to provide benefits to the worker 6 months after the onset of total disability (Division of Worker Education, Workers' Compensation Commission, 1989).

A worker, however, may be ineligible for SSDI benefits because he has not worked long enough to qualify. This individual can apply for benefits under the Supplemental Security Income (SSI) program. SSI is designed to assist the disabled with limited income and few resources. Unlike SSDI, a person does not need to have worked to qualify. Economic need is the basis for determining SSI eligibility. Monthly payments begin once eligibility criteria are met.

Although worker's compensation pays for all medical bills from an on-the-job injury or illness, a disabled worker who is unemployed or waiting for worker's compensation may need some basic health insurance. If this individual qualified for Social Security disability (SSDI) benefits and has been receiving these for 2 consecutive years, then she is eligible for Medicare Part A coverage. On the other hand, a worker who did not qualify for SSDI but who instead obtained SSI benefits is covered by Medicaid. Medicaid is a state-administered public assistance program for persons who cannot meet the cost of the medical care that they need. Individuals who receive SSI benefits are automatically entitled to Medicaid since they have already proved disability and economic need (Goldenson *et al.*, 1978).

The physician's role in worker's compensation, SSDI, and SSI centers on the determination of impairment, disability, and work-relatedness. Medical certification of the extent of disability is required to establish eligibility for these benefits (Herrington & Morse, 1995). To do a credible job, clinicians need to be knowledgeable about the different benefits systems and the various medical, social, and legal issues involved.

CASE 8-6

When E. L., a 34-year-old factory worker, was diagnosed with noise-induced hearing loss, his physician suspected an occupational cause. E. L. had no other risk factors such as the use of guns or noisy equipment at home, and he disliked loud music. E. L. told his physician that the grinder he operated at work seemed excessively noisy. E. L. further stated that hearing protection was not provided by his employer. As far as he knew, noise levels had never been monitored at the factory.

Concerned, the physician called E. L.'s employers. He explained the problem and offered to do a workplace evaluation together with an industrial hygienist. The factory owners refused. Several other attempts to obtain their consent were unsuccessful. Frustrated by his employers' lack of cooperation, E. L. called the nearest OSHA office and explained the problem. An OSHA inspector appeared at the factory 2 weeks later for an inspection. The factory noise levels were found to be in excess of the noise standard. The factory owners were cited and fined a considerable sum. They were required to institute a hearing protection program for their employees. During the initial screening, four other cases of noise-induced hearing loss were identified.

181

REGULATION IN
THE WORKPLACE

REGULATION IN THE WORKPLACE

Case 8-6 illustrates the important role that government agencies such as OSHA play in regulating workplace safety. Sometimes, the efforts of the individual worker and her private physician may be insufficient to generate the necessary action to improve the conditions at a particular worksite. Knowledge about the various entities involved in workplace regulation and of the various laws enacted to safeguard worker safety is helpful to clinicians who encounter work-related problems in their medical practice.

In 1970, the Occupational Health and Safety Act was passed with the objective of reducing the risk of injury and illness to workers in the workplace. It mandated the creation of the Occupational Safety and Health Administration (OSHA), housed under the Department of Labor. The legislation envisioned controlling workplace hazards by promulgating safety standards that are enforceable by safety inspectors. Compliance with these standards is monitored by complaint, by set priorities, by random inspections, or after a major disaster. Written into the Act was the option for individual states to take over part or all of the role of federal OSHA if they proved to be as effective as the federal agency. Standards relate to plant operations and physical setups. Inspections are conducted either according to priority or in response to complaints by employees, healthcare providers, labor representatives, or other concerned parties. Citations are issued for failure to maintain specific standards. Violators are fined and violations must be corrected within a stipulated time period.

The National Institute for Occupational Safety and Health (NIOSH) is a component of the Centers for Disease Control (CDC). Its major tasks are to support education and research in the field of occupational health and to establish new workplace standards. NIOSH has a branch that conducts Health Hazard Evaluations (HHEs) at the request of private industry, labor unions, or other employee groups. Unlike OSHA inspections, which focus primarily on the industrial hygiene aspects of a workplace, HHEs include health evaluations in their investigations. NIOSH is not limited to evaluating only those substances for which standards already exist. However, it has no capacity to enforce its recommendations.

Other laws exist for specific industries in the United States. The Mine Safety and Health Act, the Clean Air Act, the Clean Water and Safe Drinking Water Acts, the Federal Insecticide, Fungicide and Rodenticide Act, and the Federal Food, Drug and Cosmetic Act are examples of legislation that affects the safety of the workplace. The Mine Safety and Health Act, for example, created the Mine Safety and Health Administration (MSHA) in the Department of Labor to deal with health and safety risks to all surface and underground miners. The Federal Insecticide, Fungicide and Rodenticide Act gave authority to the Environmental Protection Agency (EPA) to protect both consumers and workers who handle pesticides.

Despite their number, these laws remain insufficient to guarantee workplace safety for every worker. At best, they provide standards to reduce risk at work. The regulatory process traditionally is slow to react to crises in the workplace. Economic interests often conflict with safety concerns, further complicating the picture. Vigilance and commitment to the highest level of worker safety will therefore remain the responsibility of employers, workers, and the healthcare providers of workers.

CONCLUSIONS

This chapter has focused on some of the issues that pertain to health and the workplace that are important for practitioners of medicine. Occupational factors play a role in numerous general medical encounters. Because there are no clinical markers to distinguish occupational disease from non-work-related disorders, it is imperative that a good occupational history be included in any health evaluation. Providers need to be sensitized to the various issues involved in work-related illness. An environmental perspective and coordination with other professionals involved in workplace issues is crucial to the successful control of work-related medical problems.

Clinicians should use the general principles in the diagnosis of occupational disease presented in this chapter as guidelines when confronted with a potentially work-related clinical problem. Concurrent diagnostic evaluation of the workplace, a key difference from the traditional medical encounter, and familiarity with the work itself are necessary components of a thorough occupational evaluation. Management of occupational disease requires a careful consideration of the medical, social, legal, psychological, and economic consequences of each therapeutic option. Care does not end with the resolution of the individual patient's problem; prevention of further disease in other workers and the protection of the general public from potential environmental hazards must be considered.

A brief discussion of the issues related to the evaluation of impairment, disability, and work-relatedness is provided since this type of evaluation is commonly encountered in a primary care practice. The chapter ends with an overview of the various government agencies and legislation that seek to regulate the workplace. However, these are inadequate to safeguard the safety of every worker. Clinicians have the responsibility to advocate for safety in the workplace for as long as they continue to provide services to the working population.

CASES FOR DISCUSSION

CASE 1

Mr. E. F. is a 52-year-old firefighter. During a fire, he was noted to be pale and clammy by his colleagues, who measured his blood pressure at 200/110 mm Hg. A physician diagnosed his problem as new-onset hypertension. E. F.'s father, who died of a heart attack at the age of 42, also had hypertension. The insurance carrier for the Firemen's Disability Board referred Mr. E. F. to you. During the initial interview, you discover that Mr. E. F.'s favorite snack food is salted peanuts. Physical examination revealed a 28-lb excess over ideal body weight. The fundi were normal.

1. *Is Mr. E. F.'s hypertension job-related? Why or why not?*
2. *What, if any, work restrictions would you recommend?*
3. *What do you think was the underlying agenda of the insurance carrier in referring Mr. E. F. to you? Mr. E. F.'s supervisor strongly encouraged him to keep the appointment with you. What could his agenda be? What of Mr. E. F. himself? How do you take all of these different agendas into account when making your recommendations?*

S. D., a 26-year-old secretary, comes to your office because she needs a letter from you excusing her from the previous week's absence from work. She tells you that she had a "stomach virus" and was too sick to work. Results of her physical examination are completely normal.

1. *Do you accede to her request?*
2. *What ethical guidelines can you think of to help you whenever you are confronted with a similar situation?*

CASE 3

The director of human resources of a large company refers one of their employees to your medical practice for a health evaluation because of recurrent absenteeism. During your encounter with the patient, you learn that he is in the midst of divorce proceedings. To help cope, he has started smoking again, after having quit for 3 years, and is taking an average of six to eight alcoholic drinks daily. His appearance is unkempt, he has trouble sleeping, and his appetite is poor. He works as a forklift operator.

1. *What ethical dilemmas can you identify? How would you address them?*
2. *How much information do you provide the human resources director who referred the patient to you?*
3. *What recommendations would you give the patient? Would you refer him to anyone else?*
4. *Would you remove him from his job? If yes, how would this potentially affect your patient's situation?*

CASE 4

You work at an urgent care clinic. A 30-year-old woman is brought in for evaluation. She had fainted while at work. Shortly after she is brought into your clinic, she wakes up. She describes feeling dizzy and nauseous just before passing out. She works in a company that manufactures formica cabinets. In the past month, four other coworkers were brought into your clinic for similar complaints. Unfortunately, the patient doesn't know the names of the chemicals she is using.

1. *Could your patient's fainting spell be work-related? How would you go about investigating the possible work-relatedness of the problem?*
2. *You decide to call the factory owner to obtain additional information. He tells you to mind your own business. What other options do you have to learn more about the workplace?*
3. *The employees finally complain to OSHA. During the inspection, the air levels of a number of organic solvents were found to exceed the Permissible Exposure Limits (PELs). The factory owner is fined and given 3 months to install a ventilation system capable of reducing the solvent air levels. Two weeks later, you receive a phone call from attorney X. He wants to know if the young lady with the fainting spell, whom he now represents, had acute solvent intoxication, because if so, she will be filing a worker's compensation case. In the meantime, the results of the beta-HCG test that you did when the patient came to your clinic come back positive; your patient is pregnant. What is your opinion now? Does the case meet the legal standard for causation? Does it meet the medical standard with the same degree of certainty? If you feel there is a conflict here, how do you resolve it?*

CASE 5

D. V., a 60-year-old plumber, is referred to you by the local plumber's union for a screening evaluation. D. V. tells you that he started working as an apprentice plumber at the age of 17. He intends to retire in 5 years. During your review of systems, you elicit a history of exertional dyspnea that started about 3 years ago. Results of the physical examination were unremarkable. However, the chest X ray showed extensive pleural disease from asbestos exposure and a suspicious-looking nodule in the right upper lung zone. After a diagnostic workup, adenocarcinoma is diagnosed. D. V. is a heavy smoker with a 75-pack per year smoking history. His father and uncle, both heavy smokers, also died of lung cancer.

1. *What questions would you ask in the occupational history to help you assess the amount of asbestos exposure of this patient?*
2. *Is D. V.'s lung cancer work-related? What elements in the history would support a diagnosis of asbestos-related lung cancer?*
3. *How would you explain the role of D. V.'s smoking and family history? Do they go against the diagnosis of a work-related cancer?*
4. *D. V.'s lawyer contacts you and asks if you believe the legal standard is met for a diagnosis of asbestos-related lung cancer, because if so, D. V. will apply for worker's compensation benefits. What is your reply? How do you feel about becoming involved in the process of applying for compensation?*

——————— RECOMMENDED READINGS ———————

Goldman RH, Peters JM: The occupational and environmental health history. *JAMA* 246:2831–2836, 1981.

> In this journal article, the authors discuss the elements of good history-taking in the occupational setting. Key points in eliciting a thorough exposure history are stressed.

Hadler NM: Occupational illness: The issue of causality. *J Occup Med* 26:587–593, 1984.

> This article focuses on the legal issues surrounding causality as it applies to disability benefits and worker's compensation claims.

Rest KM, Patterson WB: Ethics and moral reasoning in occupational health. *Semin Occup Med* 1:49–57, 1986.

> A thoughtful, well-written essay that explores the ethical dilemmas often encountered in the practice of occupational health.

Rosenstock L, Cullen MR: *Clinical Occupational Medicine.* Philadelphia, WB Saunders Co, 1986.

> Paper-cover volume that provides the essential information that general practitioners and occupational health providers require when faced with patients with possible work-related illness.

Rosenstock L, Cullen MR: *Textbook of Clinical Occupational and Environmental Medicine.* Philadelphia, WB Saunders Co, 1994.

> A reference textbook that covers the entire range of occupational medicine issues with depth and clarity.

CHAPTER 9

A. Relationships

Public Health and the Environment

James N. Hyde and Barry S. Levy

Bill Small had a successful and growing primary care practice in a medium-sized city of 100,000 in the Midwest. Among the things he enjoyed most was the new role he had begun as physician consultant to the city's largest nursing home facility. He looked forward to his regular visits to the facility both for the opportunity to visit his own patients as well as the chance to talk to a wide variety of others. This nursing home facility was one that was modern, well run, and provided excellent care.

He was surprised, therefore, when he arrived at the nursing home one day and learned that two of his six patients were seriously ill with diarrhea and severe gastrointestinal symptoms. Both were started immediately on symptomatic medication and appropriate tests were ordered. He was relieved to find that his other patients were apparently not sick.

In discussions with the nursing staff, however, Dr. Small learned to his dismay that there were several other patients at the nursing home who were experiencing similar symptoms, suggesting the possibility of a common-source outbreak of diarrheal illness.

As a precaution, Dr. Small ordered that stool samples be taken on all of the patients, that they be carefully monitored for GI symptoms, and that the staff be reminded about the critical importance of maintaining a high level of sanitation. He also advised the nursing home administrator that he intended to report the existence of a probable outbreak of diarrheal illness to the chief epidemiologist at the state health department. While not happy about the prospects of potentially adverse publicity, the administrator was well aware of the mandate under the state's licensure laws to report the existence of a potential disease outbreak.

The chief epidemiologist expressed gratitude to Dr. Small when he called to report on the situation. She concurred with the steps that had been initiated but on a hunch requested that all stool samples be sent to the state laboratory for analysis.

A few days later the report came back from the state laboratory indicating that 10 of the 12 patients with symptoms were positive for Cryptosporidium parvum. *In reporting this finding to Dr. Small, the state epidemiologist explained that* C. parvum *has been recognized as a serious human pathogen only since 1976 (CDC, 1995). Prior to the AIDS epidemic, it was reported only sporadically and then in cases of persons who were immunocompromised. With the development of new highly sophisticated laboratory techniques, the organism began to be identified among immunocompetent individuals as well, particularly the elderly.*

She went on to explain that Cryptosporidium *is a protozoan parasite that is transmitted by the ingestion of oocysts excreted by infected animals or humans. Transmission can take place through person-to-person contact, animal-to-person contact, or the ingestion of fecally contaminated food or water. Of particular concern is the demonstrated resilience of the organism to removal from the water supply, the prevalence of oocysts in 65–97% of all surface waters tested in the United States, and the ineffectiveness of chemical disinfection in eliminating the organism. Water filtration does appear to reduce the risk of infection, but many localities do not use filtration as part of their water treatment process.*

Particularly troublesome, she said, was the potential for waterborne outbreaks, several of which had occurred in the United States since 1984. The most serious of these occurred in Milwaukee, Wisconsin, in 1993 involving an estimated 400,000 people, 4000 of whom required hospitalization (MacKenzie et al., 1994). Equally worrisome was the fact that all of these outbreaks occurred in municipalities that either met or exceeded state and federal drinking water quality standards (CDC, 1995).

The search was on for the source of the infection.

INTRODUCTION

We live in a world of increasing complexity with the constant threat of a myriad of unanticipated environmental exposures. Among such exposures are: infectious agents as in Case 9-1, pesticides and other toxic substances, microcontaminants, ionizing and non-ionizing radiation, ambient air pollutants, and indoor air contaminants.

Consider the following clinical scenarios:

A 45-year-old fisherman is diagnosed by his primary care physician with malignant melanoma. Does his cancer result from degradation of the ozone layer or an excess exposure to UV light as a result of the patient's occupation? What might a physician do to prevent this event? Counsel on the use of sunscreen? Fight for the elimination of fluorocarbon propellants? Advocate for the establishment of education programs for all commercial fishermen?

A young mother, one of whose children has leukemia, calls her primary care physician's office after the neighbors next door contract with a lawn service company to care for their yard. She is concerned that her family may be inadvertently exposed to toxic chemicals and agents. How can her physician appropriately counsel her about the risks? What is the role of the state, county, and local regulatory agencies to ensure that the agents that are used are "safe" and that those applying them have been adequately instructed in their application and disposal?

A 30-year-old father of two young children calls for your advice on whether or not to buy an otherwise perfect house that he and his wife have found after a lengthy search. His concern is that the house is located within 100 yards of an electric company substation. He has heard about the possible association of electromagnetic fields with cancer. How does the physician help this patient place this risk in perspective? How can a patient's concerns and worries be channeled into positive or constructive directions?

Case 9-1 and these vignettes illustrate the breadth and range of environmental issues and concerns that are increasingly confronting physicians in practice. The effective management of these situations requires careful attention to developing and maintaining clinical skills, particularly taking an exposure history and conducting a thorough physical examination, skills in effectively discussing and communicating to patients about risk, knowledge of the physician's reporting responsibility to alert public health authorities about possible adverse environmental exposures, and a willingness to take on and play a larger role as an advocate for patients and the community.

While medical education tends to emphasize one-on-one clinical skills, the training and skills required to equip physicians to play roles as population physicians receive far less attention. It is critical for the practicing clinician to be aware of the basic principles and concepts that underlie the science and practice of public health. The purpose of this chapter is to acquaint readers with these principles and concepts and to illustrate and explore some of the conflicts and dilemmas that they pose.

CASE 9-2

Late in January, 21-year-old Hortensia Valasquez was taken by ambulance to the hospital emergency department 1 hour after being found unconscious in her mobile home. She had been intubated by the Fire Department Rescue Squad and had received 100% oxygen while en route to the hospital. Hortensia's husband, Carlos, was also found at the scene and brought to the hospital. Although disoriented, he was lucid at the time of arrival at the emergency department.

From the history given it was determined that the couple's gas heater had broken. They were using a portable propane construction heater to heat their unventilated home. Carlos also revealed that his wife was pregnant.

Dr. Katherine Woolesy, their primary care physician, happened to be in the hospital at the time of admission. During her physical examination she noted that the patient was combative and confused, her carboxyhemoglobin level was 7%, and abdominal examination results were consistent with a 28-week intrauterine pregnancy, although no fetal movement could be detected. The patient was being treated with oxygen continuously.

On the second day following admission, Hortensia went into labor sponta-
neously and delivered an 1100-g stillborn female fetus of approximately 27 weeks
gestation. The gross autopsy findings were unremarkable except for bright red
discoloration of the skin and visceral organs.

Hortensia continued to recover slowly postdelivery and was discharged on
the ninth day postadmission. Dr. Woolesy and her colleagues agreed that the loss
of the Valasquez child was almost certainly the result of carbon monoxide expo-
sure from the use of a propane construction heater in an unventilated mobile
home (Adapted from: Farrow et al., 1990).

EPIDEMIOLOGY AND PUBLIC HEALTH PRACTICE

Epidemiology is the basic science of public health. Although there are many good definitions of epidemiology, we would propose the following: *Epidemiology is the study of the patterns, distribution, antecedents, and determinants of illness and health-related events in human populations and the application of that study to the prevention and control of disease.* There are several important conceptual notions inherent in this definition that have an important bearing on how epidemiologists and public health practitioners function and how they view the world.

The first is that epidemiology is an applied science. It is concerned with the prevention and control of disease and not with the acquisition of knowledge for its own sake. Efforts to study HIV infection, Legionnaires' disease, breast cancer, traffic fatalities, and carbon monoxide poisoning are all predicated on the desire to reduce the incidence of morbidity and mortality from these events, not to study them for the sake of satisfying idle intellectual curiosity.

Second, epidemiology is concerned with understanding etiology. While it is not always necessary to understand the etiologic mechanism of disease in order to reduce its incidence, understanding causes is usually an important step in devising plans that ultimately lead to their elimination. Conversely, it should be noted that understanding causes is not always synonymous with prevention of morbidity and mortality. Case 9-2 illustrates this quite dramatically.

Third, epidemiology is concerned with understanding the patterns and distribution of disease in human populations. Most often this is addressed in terms of trying to identify common characteristics of the individuals who are affected. The epidemiologist looks for common characteristics of the *persons* affected, e.g., their age, sex, occupation, education. Also of interest is the *place* where these events have occurred, e.g., on one floor of a nursing home (Case 9-1) or in one part of the city. Finally, the epidemiologist checks to see if there are certain patterns or characteristics in the *timing* of these events. Figure 9.1, which shows deaths in the United States from carbon monoxide poisoning over a 10-year interval, illustrates this point.

A knowledge and understanding of the characteristics and antecedent events associated with an outbreak are very often essential ingredients in constructing a strategy of prevention and control. Carbon monoxide poisoning associated with incomplete or unventilated combustion is most prominent during certain times of the year, i.e., late fall and winter, and is most often associated with persons in lower socioeconomic settings where the costs of central heating are prohibitively expensive, forcing them to use gas heaters,

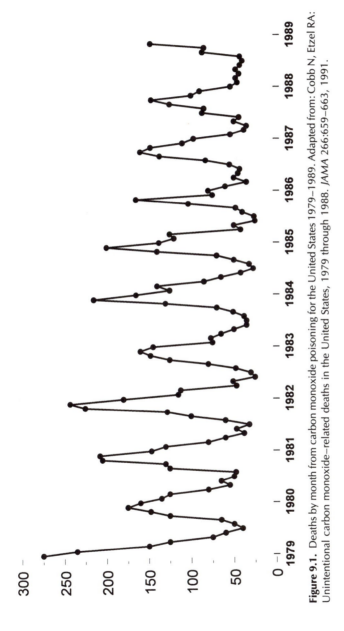

Figure 9.1. Deaths by month from carbon monoxide poisoning for the United States 1979–1989. Adapted from: Cobb N, Etzel RA: Unintentional carbon monoxide–related deaths in the United States, 1979 through 1988. *JAMA* 266:659–663, 1991.

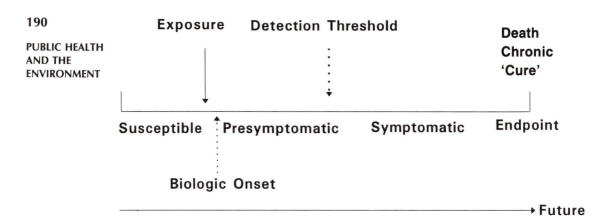

Figure 9.2. Phases in the natural history of disease and illness.

stoves, or even barbecue grills. Understanding the characteristics of CO poisoning victims leads quite naturally to certain decisions about how to target educational or regulatory efforts.

Fourth, epidemiology seeks knowledge of antecedent events associated with those who become ill, since such information may provide clues to causes or may allow the development of profiles of people who are at greatest risk of developing a given illness, e.g., childhood aspirin use and its association with Reyes' syndrome.

One important concept that implicitly underlies the epidemiologist's view of the world but is not explicitly contained in the definition given is the concept of the natural history of disease. Figure 9.2 provides a schematic representation of what is meant by natural history.

Every clinician knows that in treating otitis media, Type II diabetes mellitus, or a urinary tract infection, the progression of events will generally fall into one or another pattern. In public health, the epidemiologist sees these same patterns, with each disease having a unique signature in the absence of any outside intervention. The stages or phases through which disease is seen to progress include preexposure, a period of susceptibility, the exposure phase, biologic onset, a symptomatic phase, and then certain end points—either cure, a chronic symptomatic phase, or death.

A critical feature of the natural history is the length of time that it takes for an individual to progress from a susceptible phase to a symptomatic phase or end point. The longer this latency period, the better are the prospects for prevention. In the case of infectious diseases this period is very short, i.e., days or weeks. In the case of chronic disease, such as coronary heart disease and cancer, this period may be quite long. A characteristic of environmentally induced illnesses is that this latency period can be either very lengthy, e.g., UV exposure and melanoma, or incredibly short, as was the outcome in the case of Hortensia Valasquez's stillborn child.

CASE 9-3

Six adults and three children present to the emergency department of a hospital in a small town in the South. All complain of fever, nausea and vomiting, abdominal pain, and other symptoms. Each of them ate the day before at a church picnic that had been catered by a local restaurant in town. There are indirect reports that other people have been similarly affected.

The local health officer closes the restaurant as a precaution and asks local physicians and community residents to report any additional cases. She asks local physicians to also advise their affected patients about precautions to prevent secondary spread of this likely infectious disease within households. She finally asks for assistance from the state health department in investigating the outbreak.

The state epidemiologist, with the assistance of local public health nurses and sanitarians, conducts a questionnaire survey of people who had eaten at the church picnic, specifically focusing on what food items they had eaten and which symptoms they had that might be related to the outbreak. Local physicians reported 46 additional cases that are suspected to be part of the outbreak. The food preparation area in the restaurant is inspected, food service workers are interviewed about symptoms before and during the outbreak, and stool samples are obtained from several of those affected as well as all food handlers.

The investigators develop a working definition of illness in this outbreak. Analysis of questionnaire data involves calculating attack rates of illness for those who had eaten each food item. This analysis reveals that those affected had eaten potato salad more frequently ($p < 0.05$*).* **Salmonella typhimurium** *bacteria are grown in cultures of stool from several of those affected and one of the food handlers as well. Further investigation finds opportunities where this food handler may have contaminated the potato salad during its preparation. In addition, it is found that the potato salad had been kept at room temperature overnight (for 12 hours), allowing* **Salmonella** *bacteria in it to multiply.*

After training food handlers at the restaurant in safe food handling techniques and removing the infected food handler from work (until his stool cultures became negative), the restaurant is allowed to reopen. Those who became ill during the outbreak all recover within 1 week.

THE EPIDEMIOLOGIC INVESTIGATION: AN OVERVIEW

The outbreak in Case 9-3 is typical of the approximately 500 foodborne disease outbreaks reported each year in the United States. However, these reported outbreaks are just the tip of the iceberg. Were it not for all of those affected in this particular outbreak having eaten a catered meal, the outbreak might not have been detected or reported.

Foodborne illness accounts for much of the morbidity and some mortality in the United States and abroad. Many types of agents account for these disorders (see Table 9.1).

Large-scale, centralized food production and processing and substantial imports of fresh produce and other food items from other countries may be increasing the risk of foodborne illnesses in the United States today.

Prevention of foodborne illness depends on epidemiologic and laboratory surveillance of gastrointestinal illness and pathogenic organisms responsible for foodborne disease, investigation of outbreaks, the institution of control measures, education of food service workers, inspection of food service establishments, and other measures. Costs of preventive measures like these are substantially lower than the costs of foodborne illness.

Table 9.1
Classification of Foodborne Disease, with Illustrative Examples[a]

Category	Examples
Bacterial infection	*Salmonella* and *Clostridium perfringens* infections
Bacterial poison	Staphylococcal and botulinal toxins
Viral infection	Hepatitis A
Parasitic infection	Trichinosis
Chemical poison	Poisoning caused by salts and oxides of arsenic, antimony, copper, and lead
Plant or fungal poison	Mushroom poisoning
Animal (including marine)	Ciguatera and scombroid poisoning
Radionuclides	Strontium-90 poisoning

[a]Adapted from Werner SB: Food poisoning, in Last JM, Wallace RB (eds): *Maxcy–Rosenau–Last Public Health & Preventive Medicine*, ed 13. Norwalk, Conn, Appleton & Lange, 1992, p 193.

Clinicians play important roles in diagnosing, treating, and reporting to public health authorities cases of suspected foodborne disease. In addition to alerting public health authorities to the possible existence of an outbreak such as in Cases 9-1 and 9-3, physicians may be asked to cooperate in an investigation of a disease outbreak or participate in the screening of food handlers. It is important, therefore, to have some understanding of how these investigations are conducted. While the example we have chosen relates to a foodborne illness, the steps that are followed in the investigation are quite similar to those that might be followed in the field investigation of any type of exposure.

Steps in an epidemiologic investigation are:

1. *Collect information.* The first step in undertaking the investigation of any disease outbreak is to collect all available data about the cases of interest. Basic descriptive epidemiologic measures are used to characterize those affected, and those not affected, in terms of person, place, and time. This involves interviewing persons who are ill as well as those who may have recovered, collecting data on the time of onset and duration of illness, gathering information on demographics, and other important antecedent events.

2. *Formulate a hypothesis.* At this stage investigators often develop a working hypothesis based on data gathered in the field, e.g., the culprit is the potato salad, the mayonnaise, or the baked ham. The working hypothesis is tested in a subsequent analytic study.

3. *Choose an appropriate study design.* Most often the investigation of an outbreak will employ a retrospective case–control methodology. Persons who are ill will be ascertained and are matched with persons who are not ill but have similar demographic characteristics. Data collection will focus on possible exposures. In the case of a foodborne illness, information about the types of food, frequency, and amount consumed are gathered for both cases and controls.

4. *Develop a good "working" case definition.* Without a tight operational definition of what constitutes a "case," it is not possible to mount a thorough and rigorous investigation. One might decide to employ a strict case definition, in which event only the most severely affected individuals would be included. Alternatively, a loose case definition would include more cases, but might, as a consequence, include some individuals without the illness under investigation.

5. *Case identification.* Ascertain all of the cases possible that meet the case definition

during a prescribed time interval and area. Failure to ascertain all cases during an illness investigation may bias the outcome of the investigation.

6. *Instrument construction.* Develop and, if possible, pretest, refine, and retest instruments (questionnaires, interview instruments, data-abstracting forms) in order to gather data on subject characteristics, e.g., person, place, and time, symptoms, and exposure history. The single weakest link in field epidemiologic investigations is often the quality of the data that are gathered. There are inherent weaknesses in relying on self-reported information. The epidemiologist tries to obtain information from multiple sources wherever possible, in addition to self-reported data such as medical records and employment records. Using alternative sources to augment self-reports often provides a mechanism for validating the data collected in the field.

7. *Analyze the data.* The analytic approach in examining the results of a case–control study proceeds from the premise that a putative causal exposure will be reported more frequently among the cases than among the controls. Hence, the investigator looks for a higher proportion of potato salad eaters among the cases than the controls. The term that epidemiologists use in describing the association between an exposure and an outcome is *relative risk.* Crudely stated, the relative risk is simply a statement of how much more likely an outcome is given a particular exposure. For example, given that one eats a portion of potato salad, one has a 4.0 times greater chance of reporting gastrointestinal illness. (These concepts have been simplified for the purposes of this discussion. In fact, in a case–control study, one often must estimate the relative risk using another measure called an *odds ratio.*)

In addition to sloppiness and carelessness in the design and execution of any investigation, sampling variability and chance are always possible explanations for the results that are observed. An estimate of relative risk of 4.0 for potato salad eaters versus noneaters could well be a chance finding and not in fact reflect a valid association. To determine whether an association is a chance finding, the epidemiologist employs inferential statistics. Statistical procedures permit the epidemiologist to assess the likelihood that chance accounts for a particular finding. It is these procedures, called *statistical tests*, that produce the much discussed "p value." The p value is merely a statement of the probability that chance accounts for the finding observed. Hence, in Case 9-3, the statement that "those affected had eaten potato salad more frequently ($p < 0.05$)" may be interpreted as meaning that there is a less than 5 in 100 (5%) chance that the observed association between potato salad and the illness is a chance finding. In the language of the statistician we say that the finding is statistically significant at the 0.05 level. Conversely, there is always a chance, less than 5 in 100, that we are wrong in making such an assertion. The power and promise of inferential statistics is that it allows the epidemiologist/researcher to make inferences from samples of subjects when it is impractical or impossible to study everyone.

8. *Examine the results in the light of consistency with previous studies and biologic plausibility.* Epidemiology is a fusion of many different disciplines: the basic biological sciences, clinical medicine, laboratory sciences, and the science of statistics. It is always more impressive in examining the results of an epidemiologic investigation to find that the results observed are not only unlikely due to chance but are also consistent with what we know and what previous investigators have observed and reported. The epidemiologist always looks for indirect corroboration of a hypothesis before arriving at a conclusion.

9. *Formulate a conclusion.* The conclusion of this analytic process is often an action that will likely have an important programmatic or policy impact, e.g., closing a restaurant (Case 9-3), closing a reservoir (Case 9-1), or regulating the use of space heaters (Case

9-2). Such conclusions are often the last act of the process, but because these conclusions may have sweeping implications, they must be carefully considered by the epidemiologist, the public health official, and the government policymaker.

CASE 9-4

Maria is a 3-year-old who has just been brought into the community health center. Maria is accompanied by her mother, Dorothy (aged 28), and two other children, Kenneth (7) and Susan (5). Maria's father, Frank (29), reportedly works for West Bridge Construction Company. Frank had been working at various odd jobs in rural Maine until 6 months ago, when the family moved to the city. Frank found part-time work with West Bridge Construction Company, where he has been working on the maintenance and reconstruction of highway bridges across the state. The family has no source of health insurance, since Frank's company only provides insurance for full-time employees. The family is currently living on the top floor of a three-family "triple-decker" where they pay $650 a month for rent.

Maria's mother reports that the child was in generally good health until a few weeks ago when she began to notice a loss of appetite. Dorothy described Maria as an easygoing child although recently she has become more and more irritable and difficult to control. She decided to bring Maria to the health center after Maria stopped eating completely. The other two children appear to be in good health although Kenneth has been having behavioral problems at school. Dorothy thinks that is because Kenneth is having difficulty adjusting to a new school and finding new friends. Dorothy says she is very concerned about how she is going to be able to afford the cost of the health center visit.

The physical exam revealed that Maria was of normal height although she was below the 5th percentile for weight, perhaps as a result of her loss of appetite. Her vital signs were all within normal limits. She had a hematocrit of 31% and a serum blood lead level of 28 fg/dl.

—— THE MULTIFACTORIAL NATURE OF DISEASE ——

The adverse health effects of high levels of lead exposure have been known since Roman times, although it has only been in the past 15 years that the adverse effects of low-level lead exposure have become increasingly well understood (DHHS, 1991). As is evident from Fig. 9.3, lead affects virtually every system of the body, causing encephalopathy, nephropathy, and even death at levels around 100 μg/dl.

Subtler neurological effects, such as slowed nerve conduction and subtle developmental effects at levels of 10–20 μg/dl, exact a terrible toll on our nation's children. Those at highest risk are children living in pre-1970s' housing, which was built before lead had been banned as a color stabilizer in paint, and adults working in industries or occupations that use some form of lead in the manufacturing process (see Table 9.2).

As the more subtle neurological, behavioral, and developmental effects of lead have become increasingly well understood, expert groups ranging from the American Academy of Pediatrics to the U.S. Centers for Disease Control and Prevention (CDC) have continued to lower the criteria for blood lead levels that require immediate action. The CDC currently recommends that children with blood lead levels greater than 10 μg/dl be retested and closely monitored (see Fig. 9.4).

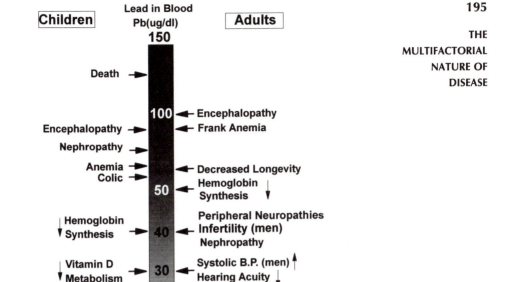

Adapted from: U.S. Department of Health and Human Services, Public Health Service, Centers for Disease
Control and Prevention.Preventing Lead Poisoning in Young Children: A Statement by the Centers for
Disease Control, October 1991, p 8.

Figure 9.3. Effects of inorganic lead on children and adults: lowest observable adverse effect levels.
Adapted from DHHS (1991, p. 8).

With the knowledge that blood lead levels once considered "safe" may indeed constitute a threat to a child's normal growth and development, a greater and greater appreciation of the diversity of sources of lead in the environment and the importance of a multiplicity of different exposure routes has also developed. While flaking and peeling paint chips and dust from lead paint generated by friction surfaces or removal in the home constitute the principal source of exposure for children, it is clear that lead in soils, in drinking water from soldered pipes, and from work environments (e.g., bridge maintenance and construction) constitute additional important sources of exposure.

Lead has been used without restriction for many generations in industrial manufacturing (solder, car batteries), as an additive (tetraethyl lead in gasoline banned in 1976 in the United States), in construction (flashing, pipes), in home products (paint lead used as a color enhancer), by hobbyists (pottery as a glaze), and in recreation (fishing weights and lures). Pathways or sources of childhood exposure are varied and include paint, dust, soil, drinking water, air, and food. Because lead is extremely stable and persistent, millions of tons of lead that are already in the environment will not soon disappear and will remain a threat to human health whenever it is dislodged or disturbed.

Table 9.2
Sources of Lead Exposure[a]

Occupational	Environmental	Hobbies and related activities	Substance use
Plumbers, pipe fitters	Lead-containing paint	Glazed pottery making	Folk remedies
Lead miners	Soil/dust near lead in-	Target shooting at fir-	"Health foods"
Auto repairers	dustries, roadways,	ing ranges	Cosmetics
Glass manufacturers	lead-painted homes	Lead soldering (e.g.,	Moonshine whiskey
Shipbuilders	Plumbing leachate	electronics)	Gasoline "huffing"
Printers	Ceramicware	Painting	
Plastic manufacturers	Leaded gasoline[b]	Preparing lead shot,	
Lead smelters and refiners		fishing sinkers	
Police officers		Stained-glass making	
Steel welders or cutters		Car or boat repair	
Construction workers		Home remodeling	
Rubber product manufacturers			
Battery manufacturers			
Bridge reconstruction workers			
Firing range instructors			

[a]Adapted from Needleman HL (ed): Case studies in environmental medicine: Lead toxicity, in *Environmental Medicine*, U.S. Department of Health and Human Services, Public Health Service, Agency for Toxic Substances and Disease Registry, Institute of Medicine. Washington, DC, National Academy Press, 1995, p. 415.
[b]In countries where lead is not banned.

In many ways lead presents a paradigm for many of the environmental exposures that society faces: It is pervasive, it is persistent, and its effects range from subtle neurological and developmental effects, which are nonspecific and often easily confused with other causes, at low levels to life-threatening effects at the higher levels of exposure.

Case 9-4 presents the physician with multiple challenges: (1) the need to manage the

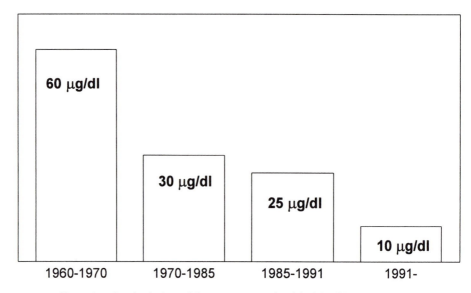

Figure 9.4. Steady decline of the CDC's action level for blood lead in children.

patient's clinical care, (2) the need to follow up the other two children, making certain they are screened and treated if necessary, (3) the need to explore other possible sources of lead exposure, e.g., through Frank's employment and through dirt in the children's playground, (4) the need to alert the appropriate authorities so that an environmental assessment can be conducted, and (5) the need to advise the landlord so that remedial action can be taken to protect the family from further exposure and insult. Each of these steps needs to be done without threatening Frank's employment status, without creating higher exposure levels than already exist, i.e., by having the family attempt to de-lead their apartment themselves, and without adequate medical insurance coverage. Maria's physician also has a responsibility to the families and children who live in the two other units in their "tripledecker" and to the other children and families in the city for whom protection from this environmental exposure is vital to their health and well-being.

Were the clinical management of Maria's low-level lead exposure the only goal of clinical practice, the next steps would be reasonably straightforward: Identify the source of lead, erect barriers to it or protect Maria from it, monitor her blood lead levels carefully, assess her nutritional status, and monitor her neurological and developmental milestones frequently to ensure that they were not compromised in any way. However, managing the physician's larger role is not as simple. Where does one intervene? What are the factors that will likely affect the problem? Who to contact? It is in this context that the basic tools and science of epidemiology are so valuable.

Epidemiology, as has been seen, focuses in part on studying the patterns and distribution of health and illness in human populations. One of the critical insights gained through the use of these analytic methods is that causes of morbidity and mortality are multifactorial. There are indeed few, if any, instances in public health in which there exists a single cause and a simple cure. People who struggle with public policy, e.g., how to prevent and control substance abuse in the population, understand and are often frustrated by the lack of a simple "silver bullet" approach to large-scale intractable problems.

Many models have been proposed to explain the determinants of disease and disability and in turn define appropriate intervention strategies. For example, there is the classic agent–host–environment triangle model (Mausner & Kramer, 1985) in which the determinants of morbidity and mortality are seen as resulting from the confluence of factors associated with the individual (host), exposure to some chemical, biological, or infectious factor (agent), all taking place within an environmental context, e.g., the workplace, home, school (environment). Although an often cited framework, this model is not terribly helpful to the clinician or public health practitioner who may need to consider other aspects of the problem, e.g., what is the potential contribution of the organization and delivery of health services in creating or solving the problem?

In 1974, the Canadian Government published the LaLonde Report, a pivotal document in the evolution of thinking about public health as public policy. Entitled *A New Perspective on the Health of Canadians*, it suggested that there were four categories of factors that had to be considered in developing effective prevention and control strategies (Government of Canada, 1974):

1. Human biological factors. These factors include those that are unalterable, such as age, gender, ethnic background, hereditary factors, and those that can be altered, such as immune status, cholesterol level, blood pressure.
2. Environmental factors. Included are elements of the physical environment such as chemicals, noise, pollution, tobacco smoke. However, the LaLonde Report also speaks more broadly of the political, social, and cultural environment in

which people live and work as a source of concern, such as the tolerance for violence as a means of resolving disputes and attitudes about sexual behavior.

3. Life-style/behavioral factors. One of the conceptual breakthroughs reflected in this report is the inclusion of individual behavior as one of the critical determinants of health. The framework reminds us of something every practicing physician knows, namely, that individual behaviors are as important determinants of health status as pharmacologic and other therapeutic interventions. Choices that people make about diet, exercise, use of licit and illicit substances, seat belts, helmets, and other protective devices are all critical factors in moderating or eliminating the risk of adverse health outcomes.

4. Organization and access to medical care. One of the fundamental insights of the LaLonde model is that it underscores the importance of the organization, financing, and availability of medical care as an instrument for the prevention of disease and the protection of the public. Timely, appropriate, affordable, and accessible care, while the cornerstone of clinical practice, must also be seen as a major axis for crafting population-based intervention strategies.

Implicit in the LaLonde approach is a population-based perspective that is essential for the clinician to keep in mind in crafting an effective management plan to address illnesses or diseases with a known environmental etiology. Using this framework can help the physician craft a management plan that is at once responsive to the needs of the patient, the extended family, and the community. Viewing problems in terms of the four categories of the framework enables the physician to consider how interventions can be identified that will address each of these contributing groups of factors. The inescapable conclusion that one reaches in this process is that preventing and controlling environmentally induced illness requires a multifactorial approach and hence the coordinated action of an interdisciplinary group of professionals.

Maria of Case 9-4, as is often found in dealing with medical problems that have an environmental etiology, potentially represents only the "tip of the iceberg." The physician must consider all of the family members at risk, such as sibling Kenneth, who may already be showing signs of low-level lead exposure, Maria's mother, who is at risk of becoming pregnant again and who may as a consequence place her unborn fetus at risk, and certainly Frank, Maria's father, whose job may indeed be the source of the lead exposure in this instance. At the next level, quite literally, are the families who live in the same building and who may unknowingly also be exposed to high lead levels in the environment and who also may require medical care. Finally, there is the responsibility to protect others within the community.

While we have already addressed the physician's responsibility to act on behalf of others, she cannot possibly hope to manage this complex situation without the active involvement of others. Just as the physician dealing with a child who is suffering from a chronic long-term condition such as asthma requires the assistance of a broad range of helping professionals, so too the physician managing the acute and chronic effects of an environmental exposure must rely on the expertise, advice, and action of other health professionals. This need requires alerting state, local, and sometimes federal officials depending on the nature of the exposure and requires working with health and allied health professionals whose roles and responsibilities are sometimes foreign to those who have worked all of their lives in clinical settings. In the worst case, management of these problems can sometimes lead to a "circus-type" atmosphere in which a huge cast of

Table 9.3
Steps to Take in Addressing Lead Poisoning and Other Environmental Health Problems

1. Screen all children in the nuclear and extended family who may be at risk. (Determine if there are any other children potentially at risk.)
2. Conduct appropriate diagnostic tests and initiate treatment where indicated.
3. Educate parents about ways to reduce exposure levels.
4. Educate children about avoiding exposures, if age and developmental level are appropriate.
5. Alert local public health authorities.
6. Make certain that you, or a designated health professional, coordinate and manage the various aspects of the case.
7. Ensure that all poisoned children are followed up and receive appropriate care.
8. If needed, advocate for changes in policy.

characters swirl around the child and family and everybody's business becomes nobody's responsibility.

In the more usual case, physicians will discover, particularly in dealing with a well-recognized problem such as lead poisoning, that there is a large cadre of helping professionals in both the public and private sectors who are available, who are experienced, and who share concern for the best interests of the family and child. Over time physicians learn which aspects or components of the problem they feel competent to address and which aspects are best left to others. Physicians develop a better understanding and appreciation for contributions and competencies of others while at the same time fulfilling their responsibility to serve as an advocate for both their patients and their community.

Table 9.3 provides a summary of the basic steps physicians should follow in crafting management plans to assist in the clinical management of lead poisoning as well as other environmentally induced illnesses. Following these steps will not only assist in clinical management but will also help the family and protect the larger community of families living in the area.

CASE 9-5

Amanda Stuart has been in practice for just 3 years. She and her husband, who is also a physician, decided to join the same staff model HMO, he with a general primary care practice and she with a subspecialty in pulmonary medicine. As part of her staff role and responsibilities, she works a half day each week in the HMO's employee health service providing both primary care and specialty consultation in pulmonary medicine.

During the course of the last 6 weeks she has seen a total of seven employees each with similar nonspecific complaints related to eyes watering, wheezing, coughing, headache, and nausea. A thorough workup including history, physical examination, and laboratory tests revealed no basic underlying etiology for the complaints. Furthermore, there seemed to be no common work history or work exposure that might provide a plausible explanation for the symptoms.

The clustering of these symptoms bothered her since, though nonspecific, they appeared so striking in their presentation. After thinking about them for several days, she attributed them to coincidence and her lack of experience and went about her routine as before.

THE ROLE OF PHYSICIAN AS SENTINEL REPORTER

Physicians, because of their background and training in science and the scientific method and because of their close contact with individual patients and their families, are in a unique position to provide early warning of the adverse effects of environmental exposures. While surveillance systems exist at both state and federal levels to alert officials of the existence of threats to the public's health, it is physicians in practice who are most likely to be the suppliers of these data. The alert clinician who sees seven cases of upper respiratory discomfort in her practice over a 1-month period (Case 9-5) should consider the possibility that these are not isolated random events. Do these cases have anything common? Do the patients work in the same setting? Are they neighbors? Are they using the same water supply?

The basic principle that underlies the functioning and operation of any of the state or national reporting systems is that taken alone, seven cases do not mean very much. By aggregating data over a broad geographic or temporal expanse, one can begin to look for patterns or common characteristics in the distribution of cases. Once identified, such patterns may well provide clues either to the etiology of the illness or disease or to methods for its prevention. Often, many reported cases are needed before these patterns become apparent. Unless an outbreak is a massive and geographically restricted event, e.g., the Legionnaires' disease outbreak in Philadelphia in 1976, it is quite likely that it may go unrecognized for a long time. Advances in communications technology and the use of computers to aggregate and manage data have shortened the time it takes to identify new manifestations of disease or illness and the patterns that are inherent within them.

There are times when the savvy and observant clinician is in the position to serve as an observer and reporter of patterns and trends in health events. As physicians develop their observational skills as part of clinical practice, they also need to remain highly alert to the possibility of unusual patterns or distributions in the events that they observe. Depending on the type of data and situation, physicians need to be conversant with the different reporting systems that exist at the state health department level. A discussion of a cluster of cases with an epidemiologist or other expert in the field will help determine whether or not a more thorough investigation is warranted.

CASE 9-6

Dr. Frank Fulton had lived and practiced medicine in Jefferson township for over 15 years. His two kids had grown up in the community, gone to elementary, junior high, and high school, and were now sophomores and seniors, respectively, in the high school. Jefferson was an economically struggling community in the southeastern United States having lost its last remaining textile mill to foreign competition 5 years ago. Notwithstanding these realities, Dr. Fulton had a good practice and had achieved a high level of prominence in the community.

Recently, a wave of optimism and euphoria had swept through Jefferson when it was announced that the community had secured a contract with a huge waste management company to build a massive waste management facility at an abandoned mill site a mile and a half from the center of town. Part of the site would be used to construct and operate a high-temperature waste disposal incin-

erator to handle nonradioactive medical and infectious waste from regional hospitals and medical providers. While acknowledging that special care would be
needed to handle infectious waste and contaminants contained in the residual ash
from this facility, the company had convinced city, county, and state officials that
the state-of-the-art facility posed no health risks to the community.

Dr. Fulton was not so sure. He had read about studies in which dioxin and
other potent carcinogens had been identified in the breast milk of women living in
proximity to waste incinerators. He also had concerns about possible contaminants from stack emissions since the regulations for waste incinerators had been
loosened considerably in recent years. He was concerned for his patients, his
family, and his community and he knew that he had sufficient credibility in
Jefferson such that his voice would be heard. What concerned him the most was
what the impact would be on his practice, his family, and the economic well-being
of his community if he raised his voice too high.

——— THE ROLE OF PHYSICIAN AS CITIZEN ———

Implicit in the notion of the physician as sentinel reporter is that of the physician's
responsibility as a citizen of a broader community. Because physicians have background
and training in the basic and clinical sciences, they are often afforded wide-ranging
credibility on a variety of issues that sometimes transcend their training and knowledge. It
is not unusual for community-based physicians to be asked to comment on or interpret
information from diverse technical and scientific sources. While there is always the
danger of falling into the trap of implied expertise, it is equally easy to avoid playing a role
as an interpreter and advocate regarding public health/public policy issues that are highly
charged and value-laden, e.g., the case of a major employer that may be endangering the
health of its employees and the community, as described in Case 9-6.

In addition to being providers of healthcare services in a community, physicians and
their families are also members of that community, a fact that often complicates the
physician's role. Nor are there any easy rules or guidelines to follow in assessing what
courses of action to take when presented with a particularly difficult clinical and/or public
health problem. Threats to one's personal standing and influence, the potential for exposure to civil liability, the fiscal integrity of one's practice, and the effects on one's own
personal life and family have to be weighed against the moral imperative to act to protect
the health both of patients and of the community. The availability of federal, state, and
local agencies, whose responsibilities include protection of all citizens, will not always
make these choices any easier.

CASE 9-7

Cynthia Burdick is a 13-year-old who was diagnosed with asthma at the age of 10
by her family's physician, Dr. Herbert Robinson. Her condition has been generally well managed by her mother, who lives with Cynthia and her brother, Brian
aged 8. Cynthia's mother has struggled to make a living on the farm that she
inherited from her husband when he died in an automobile accident 6 years ago.
Both children attend school 6 miles away. Brian has been actively involved in
school sports, but Cynthia has been unable to compete in athletics, which is her

first love, because of her asthma. Recently, Cynthia has become moody and temperamental and with her mood swings has had two recent asthmatic attacks, one of which required hospitalization in order to stabilize her condition.

Adding to the stress in the household, Mrs. Burdick's brother Edwin, his wife, and their 1-year-old are staying with the family while they look for a place of their own. Edwin and his wife both smoke a pack and a half of cigarettes a day. Although Mrs. Burdick has asked them not to smoke in the house because of Cynthia's asthma, they have not paid very much attention.

ENVIRONMENTAL EXPOSURES: IMPLICATIONS FOR CLINICAL PRACTICE

Estimates are that asthma affects approximately 10 million people in the United States, 2.7 million of whom are children, making it the most common chronic disease of childhood (Schoenborn & Marano, 1988). The incidence of asthma in the United States is gradually increasing; the Centers for Disease Control and Prevention estimates the increase to have been 29% between 1980 and 1987 (DHHS, 1990c, 1995a). Asthma remains the most frequent admitting diagnosis in children's hospitals across the country, while the direct healthcare costs exceed $4 billion annually (Weiss *et al.*, 1992). These figures on economic impact do not include indirect costs, such as the $900 million estimated lost income for parents who missed work to care for their asthmatic children (Weiss *et al.*, 1992).

As is the case with so many chronic diseases, asthmatic death rates for blacks are higher than for whites (DHHS, 1995a). Among Puerto Rican children residing in the United States, the prevalence of asthma is higher than in the non-Hispanic or black communities. Epidemiologic evidence suggests that race/ethnicity may serve as a proxy for socioeconomic status, which is itself another known risk factor for asthma. Additionally, urban dwelling clearly poses its own risks, with dust, pollution, ozone, and other ambient air factors contributing to asthma development. In summary, asthma provides a convenient paradigm for examining the synergistic and potentiating effects of race/ethnicity, poverty, housing, and geography on the natural history of a chronic disease.

Aggressive medical management of the asthmatic child with brochodilators and anti-inflammatory agents along with careful monitoring using peak flow meters are most often the bases for therapy. Of critical importance to the success of this therapeutic approach is the provision of careful instruction and training for both the child and parents so that they will be able to deal quickly and effectively with an asthmatic episode. In fact, several studies have demonstrated that increasing parental knowledge of asthma is effective in decreasing the subsequent use of healthcare services (Brook *et al.*, 1993; Clark *et al.*, 1986).

Strangely, there is little discussion in the clinical literature of the role of in-home management of pollutants and/or the role of pollution prevention in the home environment as a critical component of asthma management practice. For people who spend a significant proportion of their time indoors, as is the case for many urban dwellers, the concentrations of many indoor air pollutants can exceed those found in ambient air. Development or exacerbation of asthmatic episodes has been associated with dust, dander (from cats and dogs), cigarette smoke, mold spores, and vapor and mists from chemicals and cosmetics.

Anyone with children understands how difficult aggressive in-home pollution control measures are to implement. While it may be possible to control the myriad indoor factors likely to participate or exacerbate an asthmatic episode for a short period of time, it takes an extraordinary amount of effort and commitment to engage in such behaviors over long periods of time. If one couples this with the difficulties attendant with various sources of pollution likely to be found in certain other venues, e.g., living on a farm, the scope of the problem becomes enormous.

While anxiety and stress are a part of Mrs. Burdick's life in Case 9-7 and also a factor in the clinical management of Cynthia's asthma, these factors are not often easy to eliminate. Similarly, occupational exposures in a farm environment to dust, pollens and other allergens, and the like cannot be easily eliminated from the family's life without a change of venue. The primary care physician does have a role to play in counseling family members about ways to reduce exposure to these factors through the use of barrier techniques, e.g., a dust mask, or through anticipatory guidance, such as having Cynthia perform chores that are least likely to expose her to environmental factors that will exacerbate her condition.

There are, however, exposures such as environmental tobacco smoke (ETS) that pose a very real threat to the health and well-being of the asthmatic child or adult but that are far more easily preventable or avoidable. The U.S. Environmental Protection Agency (U.S. EPA), in its Scientific Advisory Committee Report on Environmental Tobacco Smoke, stopped short of identifying ETS as a "cause" of asthma but they did conclude that "ETS is a known cause of exacerbation of asthma in persons known to have the disease" (U.S. EPA, 1993).

While it may not be possible for Mrs. Burdick to refuse her brother and his family a place to stay, it is critically important for Cynthia's physician to emphasize the importance of Cynthia's avoiding any unnecessary exposure to ETS. The evidence implicating ETS in the etiology of a range of chronic and acute conditions is mounting rapidly. ETS exposure has been linked to lung cancer, asthma, lower respiratory tract infections, otitis media, and, most recently, SIDS, coronary heart disease, and cervical cancer (U.S. EPA, 1993; Klonoff-Cohen, 1995; Glantz, 1995).

Recognizing the adverse health effects of ETS exposure and fearing potential liability, several well-known restaurant chains that cater to children have banned all smoking in their establishments. Similarly, large businesses and employers are increasingly moving in the direction of restricting or banning smoking altogether, even as the U.S. Occupational Safety and Health Administration (OSHA) considers imposing tighter controls on smoking in the workplace.

While always a potentially volatile subject for discussion, Edwin Burdick's seeming unwillingness to alter his smoking behavior in Case 9-7 to protect his niece and her family from involuntary exposure to ETS requires careful attention. Dr. Robinson may need to explain to Edwin the likely negative effect of his behavior not only on his niece but also on his own child, citing the data on otitis media, lower respiratory tract infections, and SIDS. While Edwin certainly should be encouraged to stop smoking, failing that, a reasonable goal would be to have him agree to only smoke when he is outside and not near to Cynthia and her family. Research shows that even among smokers there is an acknowledgment of the need to keep children from initiating the behavior as well the need to avoid their involuntary exposure to tobacco smoke. Chances are that a little judicious counseling will go a long way to removing this very important modifiable risk factor.

As with lead and other environmental exposures, there is clearly a role here for Dr. Robinson and his colleagues to become involved in efforts to control involuntary exposure to ETS. He should consider joining with local and county public health officials working on the development of ETS regulations and curbing youth access to tobacco. Similarly, large employers and insurers in the area should be approached about reducing involuntary exposure to ETS and other pollutants. Because so many sources of pollution are inaccessible to the average consumer and provider, it is essential to not miss the opportunity to act when it presents itself.

Asthma, along with other diseases having important environmental cofactors, poses many dilemmas for the clinician. While effective pharmacologic agents exist to help in the clinical management of the disease, long-term success requires a three-fold approach:

1. It is essential that the patient receive clear and precise instructions concerning when, where, and how to use the standard medications that you prescribe. To assist in this effort, several excellent materials have been developed to deal with patient education and instruction (NHLBI, 1992).

2. It is essential that the patient and family have access to clinical care when needed to manage any exacerbations that may occur. Since asthmatic attacks can be life-threatening, it is essential that patients and their families have easy access to emergency care when needed.

3. It is essential that families receive assistance evaluating the sources of environmental exposure in their living spaces as well as assistance in taking steps to ameliorate and reduce these factors to the lowest possible threshold levels. Pollution prevention and pollution control are every bit as important in the environmental management of the asthmatic child as they are in the larger environment.

CONCLUSION

In this chapter we have emphasized four points of critical importance to the primary care physician faced with the clinical management of a problem having an environmental etiology:

1. Practicing physicians must be vigilant for situations involving disease and illness that may have an underlying environmental etiology. This implies paying special attention to exposures that may be peculiar to the geographic location of the physician's practice. It also requires special care and attention when obtaining a history to cover areas of possible environmental exposure.

2. Physicians in primary care practice have an important responsibility to serve as sentinel reporters of adverse health events that may be associated with environmental exposures. This requires that physicians be familiar with the various state and local agencies having responsibility for receiving and aggregating reports of environmental disease and illness.

3. Primary care physicians have important roles to play as "risk communicators" sharing information with the communities in which they live, as well as their patients and patient families, about the relative importance of various environmental exposures and methods of avoiding them.

4. The physician faced with environmentally induced illness must look beyond the individual patient and consider the population health consequences of environmental exposures. The effective management of environmentally induced disease forces the physician to assume both roles of medical doctor and public health physician.

The dilemma that physicians in practice often must face is that while these various roles are important, there is little in current traditional medical education that prepares the primary care physician to assume these roles. It is little wonder therefore that many physicians shy away from dealing with problems having a suspected environment etiology. However, attention to the basic principles outlined in this chapter should make that experience both rewarding and meaningful.

———————— CASES FOR DISCUSSION ————————

CASE 1

A young male office worker comes to your clinic with a chief complaint of a rash on his hands and wrists that appeared 5 days ago. The company he works for is the largest employer in your community and is just beginning to recover from a dramatic series of "downsizing" layoffs triggered by cutbacks in the defense industry.

He has just relocated to an older building that has been totally remodeled. Private offices were replaced with cubicles and a large open work environment, new carpeting was laid throughout the work area, and the walls were finished with new wallboard and painted.

Many of his coworkers also have reported a wide range of symptoms from fatigue, lightheadedness, watery eyes, and an assortment of GI symptoms. He reports that to his knowledge he is the only one who has developed a rash, although most other employees attribute their symptoms to the new work environment.

1. *What areas would you want to cover in taking a history?*
2. *What other possible non-work-related exposures might account for these symptoms?*
3. *What obligations do you have to validate the reports of other affected employees?*
4. *To whom would you turn at the state and local level to assist you in unraveling the etiology of this illness episode?*

CASE 2

For years residents of the Fairview neighborhood have been complaining about the foul odors emanating from the abandoned landfill adjacent to the nearby river. The state Department of Environmental Management closed the landfill 5 years ago, installed vents to bleed off methane from beneath the landfill, and instituted a monitoring program to sample groundwater for volatile organic compounds. A nearby elementary school is adjacent to the landfill.

Articles have recently appeared in the local paper suggesting that an "abnormal number of cancer deaths" have occurred in the Fairview neighborhood among long-time residents of the area. The mayor has notified the county health department and has asked you to represent the medical community on an advisory board he is establishing to investigate these allegations.

1. *How would you determine whether or not this reflects a true cluster of cases or is the result of chance?*
2. *How would you define a "case"?*
3. *What type of investigation should be conducted? Who should be interviewed? What about those who have left the area?*
4. *How would you define the exposure? How would you measure it?*
5. *What would you tell your patients who live in the area or whose children attend the elementary school about the risks?*

CASE 3

A mother with two young children calls your office in a near state of hysteria having just seen a report on national television on the association between leukemia and electromagnetic fields. She and her family live two blocks from a major power substation just like one of those implicated in the television documentary. She wonders what she can do to protect her children while she contemplates putting her house on the market. You admit to her that you are not totally familiar with the recent research on electromagnetic fields and human cancer but that you will get back to her once you have done some research and made some inquiries of your own.

1. Where would you look for information about an exposure with which you were unfamiliar? What state and local agencies might you contact for additional information?
2. Does common sense provide any clues as to what steps this mother ought to take?
3. Assuming the data you gathered were equivocal, as they often are, what would you tell this mother about the risks? Should she sell her house?

CASE 4

Over 40 hours, 19 patients have come to your clinic complaining of feverishness, abdominal cramps, and diarrhea. Nine of these patients are women and ten are men. They range in age from 6 to 71.

1. How would you go about determining if this was a foodborne or waterborne outbreak with a common source of infection?
2. When and to whom would you report this outbreak?
3. How would you determine if there were additional cases in your community that might be part of this outbreak?
4. Without yet knowing the cause and the source of this outbreak of illness, how would you advise your patients in order to further minimize spread of this illness?

CASE 5

You have just treated the second case in a month of a child with persistent upper respiratory symptoms. The only unusual aspect to the two cases was that the parents reported that the symptoms appeared after the purchase and use of an ultrasonic humidifier. After seeing the second case, you asked both sets of parents to stop using the humidifier in their children's rooms. In both instances the parents reported that the symptoms abated and disappeared a few days after the discontinuing of use of the room humidifier.

1. Is there a cause-and-effect relationship between humidifier use and the children's symptoms?
2. What subsequent steps, if any, might you take to alert other parents and families?
3. How might an epidemiologic investigation be undertaken to investigate the relationship between humidifier use and symptoms of upper respiratory infections?

———————— RECOMMENDED READINGS ————————

Blumenthal DS, Ruttenber AJ: *Introduction to Environmental Health.* New York, Springer Publishing Co, 1995.

A good basic overview of principles and practice of environmental health. The book contains chapters on epidemiology, environmental health law, occupational health, and an overview of pathways of exposure.

Hennekens CH, Buring JE: *Epidemiology in Medicine*. Boston, Little, Brown & Co, 1987.

One of the best and most widely used texts on epidemiology, this book provides an excellent starting point for obtaining a basic grounding in the theory and practice of epidemiology.

Last JM, Wallace R (eds): *Maxcy–Rosenau–Last Public Health & Preventive Medicine*, ed 13. Norwalk, CT, Appleton & Lange, 1992.

This classic one-volume text of almost 2000 pages covers the principles and practice of public health. The text, which is in its 13th edition, covers epidemiology, environmental health, infectious disease, and the organization and structure of public health in the United States. If one were to purchase only a single book on public health theory and practice, this would be the one to choose.

Levy BS, Wegman DH (eds): *Occupational Health: Recognizing and Preventing Work-related Disease*, ed 3. Boston, Little, Brown & Co, 1995.

This textbook provides a comprehensive introduction to the field of occupational health.

Pope AM, Rall DP (eds): *Environmental Medicine: Integrating a Missing Element into Medical Education*. Washington, DC, National Academy Press, 1995.

An excellent case book and resource guide for developing and implementing environmental health teaching in medical school and residency training settings. The book contains many case studies complete with questions for study, references, and review questions.

Rom WN (ed): *Environmental and Occupational Medicine*, ed 2. Boston, Little, Brown & Co, 1992.

A well-written, comprehensive, and authoritative book on environmental and occupational medicine.

CHAPTER 10

A. Relationships

The Cultural World of the Patient

Howard F. Stein

The patient, a 63-year-old white male being hospitalized for rehabilitation follow-ing a myocardial infarction, suddenly stopped eating, refusing all food and drink. The nurse carefully noted this in the patient's chart and the attending physician, seeking to rule out depression, asked for a liaison psychiatric consult. The psychi-atrist quickly discovered that the refusal to eat occurred on Yom Kippur (the Day of Atonement), a religious day observed with fasting, and that the patient was an Orthodox Jew.

INTRODUCTION

People live in groups, from small, nuclear to large, extended family groups, from face-to-face village-based societies to complex, urban, nation-based societies cemented by electronic communications media. Even in small, bounded societies such as aboriginal hunting-gathering bands, people are never members of only a single group. Even there, they move in and out of several microcultures, although the differences between them are not as dramatic as those in our industrial society. It is in such groups that people become ill, are defined as ill, receive treatment, recover or decline, and eventually die.

Unlike small-scale, face-to-face, closed, kin-based preliterate societies, in our com-plex, secularized, urbanized, and pluralistic society, practitioner and patient often come from different cultural groups. Their values, beliefs, rules, roles, attitudes, expectations, and world views may differ markedly. To further complicate matters, the clinician will have undergone years of socialization in a professional culture that is supposed to super-sede all those earlier ones from childhood that bear the mark of being "lay."

Case 10-1 illustrates problems that can arise if the patient and the physician come from different cultures. Had the team taken a rudimentary social history, been more familiar with the cultural and religious tradition of the patient population, or simply asked the patient why he refused to eat, a psychiatric consultation would have been unnecessary.

This chapter explores the cultural world of the patient and its consequences for sickness and treatment. Following a number of conceptual topics, four types of cultural settings will be discussed: ethnic or nation-of-ancestry, religious, occupational, and popular. The reader should understand, however, that such a classification is at some level heuristic and arbitrary, that all of these overlap, and that culture is a fluid, not a static, process.

As author of this chapter, I wish to serve as the reader's guide on a journey into cultural awareness that did not come easy to me—nor does it now after 25 years of practice. Let me say at the outset that I cannot provide some answers the reader wishes—and that I, too, wish I could provide—even though "answers," "quick answers," "simple answers," and "definitive answers" are what we in the United States are taught to expect of experts. The reader will look in vain for ethnic or denominational formulas that generalize, say, to "all Vietnamese" or "all Southern Baptists." Behind every ethnic or religious label is much diversity, even among seemingly homogeneous tribal groups. Groups change, too, over history, over differing experiences. Twenty years ago, during the Black Power era, I served on the faculty at Meharry Medical College in Nashville, Tennessee. I can still remember the astonishment and disbelief on the faces of medical students who had grown up in New York City as they heard their ethnic brothers and sisters from New Orleans speak of how they left their homes and cars unlocked at night. Ideologically, they thought themselves to be "the same." In experience, they discovered much unwelcomed difference.

No outsider's cultural formulary or "recipe book" can substitute for the physician's painstaking, time-consuming, but rewarding familiarity with the lives of patients and the communities from which they come. This does not make my chapter somehow "too advanced" for medical students—as though a more elementary text should offer ethnic pablum that falsifies the cultural reality the reader will soon see every day in practice. In a real sense, the reader needs to be equipped to be a better clinical anthropologist than I am, because long after the reader has forgotten this chapter, she will have to be making difficult cultural assessments about patients' beliefs, values, attitudes, expectations, feelings, and roles. Behind the myriad of facts and vignettes in this chapter is *a method for learning about culture.*

In my 25 years of medical teaching, many medical students and residents have protested to me during their training that "cultural stuff" is interesting but not "real medicine." "If I had the time, I'd find out about patients' culture, but who has the time?" The trouble is that culture is never mere "background." It is as much foreground as is any tissue or organ system. It may lurk behind the very disease etiology we seek to explain and that we wish to cure. Culture is part of every one of those key words we use everyday in biomedicine: diagnosis, symptom, outcome, satisfaction (the physician's as well as the patient's), compliance, prevention, wellness, and, yes, litigation. Culture is not extrinsic to medicine or on the periphery. The challenge for busy medical practitioners is to be attentive enough to take culture seriously, while attending to everything else as well. And I know that is never easy.

CASE 10-2

The Vietnamese-American parents of a 4-year-old boy brought him to a primary care physician for persistent cough, sore throat, fever, diarrhea, upper respiratory distress, and poor appetite that had lasted a week. On physical exam, the physician found six symmetrical ovoid bruises (ecchymoses) on the boy's back and two on the front of his neck. He immediately suspected child abuse, especially since the child seemed so quiet, docile, and compliant. He wanted immediately to contact child protective services and have a social worker begin an investigation of the boy's home situation.

APPROACHES TO THE CONCEPT OF CULTURE

What is culture? How can physicians look and listen for culture? How can physicians recognize and work clinically with culture—that of their patients, themselves, and their clinical colleagues? Let me offer several perspectives, like a surveyor trying to assess a landscape. A crucial distinction that must be made is between the view of culture offered by a member of that group (insider) and a view of that "same" culture by someone external to that group (outsider), such as a physician. We need to correct the deficiencies and blind spots of each group.

At its most basic—and contrary to a widespread view among social scientists—culture does not consist primarily of trait lists of, say, values, language, attitudes, beliefs, and expectations, all of which somehow add up to influence health beliefs and behavior. Rather, *culture is first and foremost that sense of "us," "we," "our way,"* the contents of which can and do change over time. Central to the concept of culture is that of group boundary and group identity: what is inside and what is outside.

Culture is the social unit, or often one among many units, to which the sense of belonging and loyalty are attached, the unit associated with one's social boundary. It is as if to say: "This is who and what I am; this is who and what we are; this is what we do." Or: "That is not who and what I am; that is what we do not do." Cultural content here serves to define what is "me" and what is "not me." For example, many male members of the "cowboy culture" of the North American Great Plains associate cowboy boots as an intrinsic part of the self and of one's masculinity. Other forms of footwear are viewed as alien, feminine, if not downright wrong. If a cowboy injures his foot, the prospect of not being able to wear cowboy boots is experienced as a threat to the self. Of course, group boundaries are permeable. At any given moment, and over a lifetime, one can have multiple "group" identities and affiliations—all of which affect health beliefs and behavior.

As a "design for living," culture is a normative system, with both prescriptive and proscriptive rules, values, attitudes, roles, expectations, and the like (Parry, 1984; Spiegel, 1971)—much like physicians' *prescriptions* to patients. It is full of "Thou shalt's" and "Thou shalt nots." Understood this way, culture consists of patterned, preferred solutions to common problems, solutions that often lead to standardized, stereotyped responses to these problems. For instance, among many Irish Catholics the lively sense of sin and guilt leads them to believe that if a medicine is truly beneficial, then it must taste bad or hurt when applied to the body: "Good [powerful] medicine tastes bad."

When we describe people's cultures (our own or others'), we often think only in terms of the "object" we are describing rather than also in terms of the "subject" doing the describing. In many ways, physicians and anthropologists are in the same boat, as they try to understand and work with people whose cultures differ from their own. Here, culture is an abstraction constructed by outside observers and interpreters, an abstraction that may be welcomed or condemned by those whom we are describing. Our own cultural lens as healthcare professionals may help us to see better, or distort our vision.

One virtue of an outsider's viewpoint for biomedicine is that an outsider, say, a physician, might detect a pattern that members of the patient's culture or community do not notice or simply take for granted. Further, what people claim about their way of life often differs from what an outsider sees or hears them actually do (Stein & Hill, 1977). A physician can describe a culture statistically, in terms of population characteristics, then interpret it not only to an individual patient, but also to the wider community (from county medical society meetings to newspaper articles). Through careful study of medical records of one-patient-seen-at-a-time, broader community patterns may emerge. At one clinic where I work, for example, "like clockwork" in the middle of March there will be several three- and four-wheeler vehicle [all-terrain vehicle (ATV)] accident victims, mostly teenagers, in the hospital. With the first sign of a break in the winter weather, young people will take their restless energy to daredevil courses on the clay mounds and in the fields.

No culture stands still over time. Cultures change as their ability to fulfill human functions diminishes. People create and change culture in order to meet needs, whether these needs be rational, reality-oriented, or irrational. For instance, once the Spanish and their horses had arrived in North America, Native Americans' hunting and raiding by foot on the Great Plains was succeeded and replaced by equestrian hunting and warfare. But initially this was done only among some groups—others ate the horses as meat. To turn to a medical example: Until the 1950s, entire children's hospitals in North America were filled with iron lung machines for patients with polio. The revolutionary vaccination developed by Jonas Salk was quickly accepted, and by now the massive iron lungs (Drinker respirator) have virtually disappeared. At the same time, the equally revolutionary antiseptic procedure of washing one's hands with chlorinated lime, developed in nineteenth-century Vienna by Ignaz Phillip Semmelweis, was met with fierce and persistent opposition by Western professional culture. As we try to understand the history of Western biomedicine, like the history of all culture, we must realize that, on the one hand, even cultural ideas to which people are committed do change. But on the other hand, the abundance of counterrevolutionary movements over history attests to the fear of change, resistance to change, and the threat of loss of whole ways of life.

Not only do all cultures undergo change over time (often more at the surface than at the core), but all cultures also have some degree of intracultural variation. This internal differentiation is more pronounced and more tolerated in complex, secularized, urban society. In complex society, people move in and out of numerous subcultures, whereas in more primitive, small-scale society, these would tend to merge or at least greatly overlap. The more complex the society, the less homogeneity and the more heterogeneity is found. For instance, in a hunting-gathering band, one's kin group is also one's occupational group and one's religious congregation.

Those of us in healthcare professions need to be able to distinguish between scientific *generalizations* about culture and *stereotypes* we might indulge in about others. It is often difficult to know which form of "discrimination" we are making. (And remember that a good differential list marks the beginning of that crucial form of clinical discrimination called diagnosis!) In theory at least, scientific thinking is open-minded, and theories can therefore be modified, while no amount of new evidence can loosen a stereotype, which people use to defend themselves against thoughts and feelings. However, healthcare practitioners are not the only ones who have stereotypes. All cultures have their stereotypes about themselves and about others (Henry, 1963). That is what ethnocentrism is all about: It says, "*We* are the real human beings; *you* are the dirtballs." Such stereotypes feel and ring true because they perform vital functions of preserving self-esteem and cohesiveness.

But the price of stereotypes is that they distort reality. Groups cannot learn when they feel that they cannot afford to perceive the world differently. For instance, cultural groups that are rife with suspicion and mistrust, and that abound in malevolent supernatural beings who inflict disease and death, will be unlikely candidates for easy acceptance of the more neutral and impersonal biomedical disease model. Similarly, one can only wonder what the effect of the competitive battle among HMOs and their allied physicians for patients will have on physician collegiality in the future culture of U.S. medicine.

To summarize: To say that culture is a *system*, and not a mere collection of elements or traits, is to say that culture is an *organizing principle* of people's lives. This can be taken too far as much as it can be overlooked. Physicians, mental health practitioners, social scientists, and public policymakers frequently use cultural formulations to "pigeonhole" people, to adopt cultural profiles as cookbooks, to turn description, inquiry, and interpretation into stereotypes that oversimplify and distort rather than illuminate. Especially in complex, pluralistic society, statements about a person's ancestral ethnicity, a label about their personal or parental religion, a classification of their job, or a statement that they largely self-medicate based on popular U.S. folk culture should not be construed to be the whole story.

There can be no substitute for the painstaking and time-consuming elicitation of the patient's story, including the patient's family and wider intimate network, a fact that is no less true in the era of corporate medicine and managed care than it was in the prior era of fee-for-service practice (Stein & Apprey, 1987). To know that a person is African-American, Ashkenazic Jewish, Latin Rite Catholic, Great Plains wheat farmer, or avid reader of *Reader's Digest* and *The National Inquirer* as sources for medical advice is rightfully to generate a set of hypotheses that may help to understand and culturally calibrate the *individual* (Hill *et al.*, 1990). On the other hand, uncritical extrapolation from a mere cultural label or stereotype is an indulgence that reveals more the projections of the observer than the cultural worlds inhabited by the one ostensibly under observation.

In Case 10-2, consultation with a behavioral science faculty and subsequent inquiry of the parents revealed a different picture, however. The parents practiced an ethnomedical treatment regimen that they widely shared with coastal Vietnamese peoples. Many diseases are believed to be caused by "bad winds" that enter the body and cause an imbalance. "Winds" are believed to be one among the major elements of the universe. This Vietnamese theory of disease is a local variant on a balance theory widespread throughout the Buddhist/Confucian-influenced Orient. To help their son, the parents resorted to custom to try to help restore the body's natural balance. They took a highly polished coin and rubbed it with an ointment (lubricant) at several places on their son's back and neck until these polaces bruised, thereby creating openings for the "bad winds" to escape from entrapment in the body, thus enabling the boy's body to restore its natural balance. This procedure is called *Cao gio* ("scratch away the wind": *cao* = scratch away, *gio* = wind) (Primosch & Young, 1980).

The boy and his parents alike described the practice as soothing, a little like a massage, and that the warm ointment felt good being rubbed. The boy insisted that "it didn't hurt." The parents became concerned when their efforts did not result in the boy's rapid return to health. With this explanation, the physician was persuaded that he did not need to pursue a child abuse investigation. It turned out that the boy had an especially virulent form of the flu, one that typically lasted around 10 days; the parents likewise felt reassured on hearing this.

CASE 10-3

The scene is a rural North Carolina primary care clinic. During an office visit in which the presenting complaint was a "bad cold," the physician also diagnosed his 35-year-old African-American patient as having hypertension. He gave her some samples from the clinic cabinet of a diuretic medication and recommended a low sodium diet and exercise. As he concluded the interview, he asked her whether she understood what he had explained and whether she had any questions. She averted looking directly into his eyes, and quietly said she had no questions. He asked her to schedule a return visit in 2 weeks; he wanted to monitor her blood pressure. She left the waiting room without rescheduling. When she arrived home, she said with obvious frustration in her voice to her mother with whom she and her husband and children lived: "I don't understand why this doctor gives me these pills for high blood. How's that supposed to thin out my blood? It doesn't make sense to me." Trying to reassure her daughter, her mother said to her: "I'll get you some pickle juice, and tonight when you sleep, sit up a little so the thick blood can drain down easier. That'll be better than these pills—although it was nice that he didn't give you a prescription you'd have to pay for." The patient felt better now that she thought she understood what was going on with her.

PATIENTS' INFORMAL CARE NETWORKS, ROLES, AND TREATMENT CHOICE

Most people's illness are totally treated outside the formal healthcare system (see White *et al.*, 1961). Even when this system becomes involved, it is usually after a number of assessments and interventions by the *patient's own personal network*. Indeed, it is helpful for the physician to see the act of "going to the doctor" as an act of including the physician's world within the patient's expanding cultural world, and to ask, "What is the patient seeking in doing so?" Chrisman (1977) has identified five steps that characterize the health-seeking process: (1) symptom definition, (2) illness-related shifts in role behavior, (3) lay consultation and referral, (4) treatment actions, and (5) adherence.

People consult with and seek treatment from a variety of others in the popular (lay) folk (e.g., root-worker, medicine man) and professional sectors (Foster & Anderson, 1978). This can be sequential or concurrent. For instance, a person might consult an aunt, a local pharmacist, a chiropractor, and a physician for different facets of the same illness episode, as described in Case 10-3. Or the person might seek help from them in some sequence, as a result of the progression or nonresolution of symptoms. Whether a practitioner is defined as "folk" or "professional" also depends on who is doing the defining: Consider only the controversy over chiropractors among biomedical physicians! Johnson and Kleinman (1984) note that

> most illness episodes are dealt with in the context of the family, regardless of ethnic background. This may involve special diets, foods, herbs, massage, exercise, religious treatment, and prescribed or nonprescribed medications. [They] also may consult with

folk practitioners such as *curanderos* among Hispanics, root-workers and spiritualist ministers among blacks, herb doctors and acupuncturists among East Asians, voodoo specialists among Haitians, and medicine men among Native Americans. It is common for patients to engage in lay healing practices and to consult traditional practitioners while simultaneously seeking health care from physicians. (pp. 279–280)

215

PATIENTS'
INFORMAL CARE
NETWORKS,
ROLES, AND
TREATMENT
CHOICE

Almost two decades ago, Kleinman (1978) introduced a useful conceptual distinction between disease and illness, defining "disease" as "malfunctioning and maladaptation of biological and/or psychological processes" (p. 428), and defining "illness" as "the personal and social significance of and life problems created by the experience of perceived disease" (p. 428). Disease is the conceptual domain and chief interest of the medical professional, while illness is the conceptual domain and chief interest of the patient. The degree of congruence between the physician's and patient's cultural models of the illness episode and expectations for treatment deeply affect the clinical relationship and the degree to which a mutually satisfying treatment plan can be developed (Chrisman & Maretzki, 1982; Eisenberg & Kleinman, 1981; Kleinman, 1982). Lack of congruence between physician and patient in this important area often leads to nonadherence, as in Case 10-3.

The following questions are helpful in eliciting the patient's culturally based "explanatory model" of the illness episode (from Johnson and Kleinman, 1984, p. 282; Kleinman *et al.*, 1978; Kleinman, 1980):

1. What do you call your problem?
2. What do you think has caused your problem(s)?
3. Why do you think it started when it did?
4. What does this sickness do to you? How does it work?
5. How serious is this illness? How long will it last?
6. What kind of treatment is best for this illness?
7. What results do you expect from treatment?
8. What are the chief problems your illness has caused you?
9. What worries you most about being sick?

All patients have a rationale for their medical actions. This rationale might not be organized into an Aristotelian explanatory system, nor might it follow the same rules of evidence that biomedical decision-making at least officially strives to follow. While many ethnomedical practices might contain irrational elements or aspects (Boyer, 1983), it is prejudicial automatically to infer that simply because a practice is different from one's own, or from one's official medical model, it is ipso facto inferior, wrong, crazy, or dangerous. On the other hand, it is dangerous to romanticize folk or popular medical practices. It is important to become intimately familiar with patients' various cultures, so that one might know what types of questions to ask the patients.

In the late 1980s I presented Case 10-2 about the Vietnamese-American boy to a group of Family Medicine residents; the topic was patients' and physicians' explanatory models. Their response was far from enthusiastic; one resident said monotonously, "We saw this kind of stuff at the Mecca [teaching hospital]." I then sought to draw a parallel between this "exotic" and "alien" cultural presentation and something perhaps more within their orbit. I said that the Vietnamese model is one among many "balance" theories of sickness, treatment, and health. I continued:

Many of us in this room probably grew up with some degree of humoral folk medicine. Did your mother ever tell you that, when you finish a hot shower or bath, to be sure to run some cold water on yourself to be sure your pores closed? Otherwise, if you went outside or walked on the cold floor, you could catch a draft and get the flu or a cold.

The group brightened, joking about some of the stories they remembered from their childhoods 20 years earlier. Suddenly, the Vietnamese theory of ill winds gained some experiential plausibility. It was not simply silly, prescientific, and foreign. Rather, we all found aspects of our own lives that could be used to identify with those of a different culture.

Questions about explanatory models that a physician might ask can only go so far in data gathering and in building rapport—whether in the medical history or in a social history. Questions that the physician might consider appropriate might be experienced as intrusive, embarrassing, or judgmental to the patient. Careful listening and attentiveness to a patient's changed emotion, tone of voice, eye movements, or gestures can all provide important cues. We Americans ask many direct questions as a standard mode of communication. In many other cultures, indirectness and modesty are greater virtues. Physicians need to gather information; at the same time, they need also to be aware of both the meaning particular questions might have to patients and that questioning itself as a mode of communication may have entirely different meanings to the physician as to the patient.

Sickness and healer *roles*, together with the definition of what qualifies as legitimate illness, are inseparably bound up with shared notions about the self and its boundaries. This collective self-image, together with the range of deviation allowed within the cultural category of "normal," is not only a social fact, but also an important value. In the United States, for instance, disease conceptualization and treatment are embedded in the value system of self-reliance, rugged individualism, independence, pragmatism, empiricism, atomism, privatism, emotional minimalism, and a mechanistic conception of the body and its "repair" (Kluckhohn & Strodtbeck, 1961; Ohnuki-Tierney, 1984). The horror of dependency (the conscious expression of a repudiated wish) is a powerful fuel that influences and confers authority on the biomedical conceptual, diagnostic, and treatment system. Hocking (1987) writes that

> Because the sick are dependent, sickness is seen as deviant behavior, undesirable, and only to be legitimated on certain terms ([Talcott] Parsons sick role concept). Legitimation of sickness has become the prerogative of the medical profession which uses the biomedical concept of disease as its yardstick. (p. 526)

In U.S. culture, the biomedical conceptualization of disease has been welcomed and widely adopted precisely because it fits so well with the image of the self as a physical thing that can be broken but easily repaired.

ILLNESS-RELATED WORDS AND THEIR MEANINGS

Language is a common area of misunderstanding and ill will between physician and patient (Dirckx, 1982). Physicians often discount irrational-*seeming* patient folk expressions. However, some of the worst impasses occur when the words physicians and patients say *seem* to be the same, but carry divergent meanings. Many African-American patients, for example, visualize illness in terms of blood imbalance. Physicians talk about high and low blood *pressure*, whereas many lower-socioeconomic-class blacks talk about high and low *blood* (and parallel terms *thick/thin* and *sweet/bitter blood*) (Snow, 1974, 1983; Hill & Mathews, 1981), as in Case 10-3.

According to this classification, the terms *high* and *low blood* "may refer to either the amount of blood in the body or a shift in its location, that is, 'high blood' may be too *much* blood or it may be that a normal amount of blood is present in the body but has suddenly shot up into the head. Changes in blood volume and shifts in location can result from improper dietary practices or emotional shock or both" (Snow, 1983, p. 824). Foods considered as too rich or red in color are included in the etiology of "high blood": Among these are red meat (especially pork), beets, red wine, carrots, and grape juice. Blackouts, especially in males, are often regarded as a symptom of high blood. Lack of energy, fainting spells, and constipation are common signs of low blood. Diet modification, herbal remedies, and family counseling to deal with interpersonal relations related to stress are among the treatments for these illnesses (Hill & Mathews, 1981, p. 316).

Typical remedies for high, sweet, thick blood are substances believed to help thin down the blood: bitter herbs, epsom salts, vinegar, garlic, peach leaf, horehound, snake root, and pickle juice (Hill & Mathews, 1981, p. 317). Many of these ingredients increase the patient's sodium intake and are thus anathema from a biomedical viewpoint. In lowering "high blood," the goal is to try to sweat the excess out through the pores, to try to eliminate it through the bowels, or, in women, through menstruation (Snow, 1983, p. 824). In part, conditions of "high" and "low" blood are related to gravity. Elderly black patients who diagnose themselves as suffering from "high blood" might drink pickle-brine to *dilute* their blood and might *sleep sitting upright* in bed (propped up with boxes and pillows) so that their thinned blood could run down from their head and redistribute itself in the rest of the body.

Many Americans believe the diagnosis "hypertension" to mean that they are hypertense, anxious, nervous, irritable, high-strung, and that the logical cure is relaxation (Blumhagen, 1982). In such a scheme, drastic diet management, exercise, and medication for life often makes little sense. Also within U.S. popular culture, the heart is a deeply metaphoric subject; one has only to think of its association with Valentine's Day (love, intimacy), sadness and depression (having "a heavy heart"), pride ("a stout heart"), and so on. Americans are attentive to cardiovascular imagery akin to the French and Latin focus on the liver, and the Japanese on the stomach (*hara*). These metaphorical meanings may cause misunderstandings between physician and patient, since physicians are often looking for a mechanical malfunction whereas patients might be referring to a different, personal meaning.

For another example, many Anglo-Americans (narrowly defined, Americans of English ancestry; more broadly, Americans of Protestant, north European ancestry) might feel emotionally "close" to their families and friends, maintaining contact by telephone and travel, yet actually live thousands of miles from them. Mexican Americans (Keefe, 1984) feel deeply close to their families, but such closeness has a markedly different meaning. "Mexican Americans value the physical presence of family members while Anglo-Americans are satisfied with intermittent meetings with kin supplemented by telephone calls and letters" (p. 68). For Mexican Americans, close familism is associated with geographic stability and face-to-face interaction, whereas for Anglos, it is associated with considerable social and geographic mobility.

When patients use familiar-sounding words, it is important to find out from them their own meanings. By doing so, say, with respect to the term *close* family, the physician can assess the extent to which closeness corresponds to his expectation, or is functional or pathological (as, for instance, in "enmeshed" families). Such inquiry can clarify the extent to which the family can realistically function as support system, and which member(s) the physician can rely on or contact during a sickness episode.

Consider, further, the range of cultural meanings of the seemingly self-evident word *togetherness*, and of the clinical misunderstandings between patient (or family) and physician when the physician assumes that her meaning is the same as that of the patient or family. From clinical experience and research, Nguyen Nga, M.D. (1988), a psychiatrist, has discovered that, while many Americans associate "family togetherness" with the notion of spending the weekend together at the lake or going on a picnic, the Vietnamese-American meaning is that of "us versus them," "our family united against other families and against the world." While the mainstream U.S. connotation is inclusive and expansive, the Vietnamese connotation is exclusive and protectively encapsulating. A clinician would miss crucial information if she did not elicit the boundary aspect of Vietnamese family togetherness. For example, in Case 10-2, a physician treating this Vietnamese family should consider the possibility that she would have to expend additional effort at building rapport (the therapeutic alliance), since the medical system was not yet incorporated into the trusted world of "us."

A further distinction lies in the fact that when many Americans speak of togetherness, they mean a collection of distinct selves, each with a personal identity. Traditional Vietnamese, on the other hand, regard themselves more in terms of a shared "family identity" from which each member sees himself as inseparable. This family identity encompasses deceased ancestors for whom the living must perform rites so that their souls do not wander aimlessly forever. Thus, something as seemingly elemental and universal as the definition and the experience of the *self* is influenced by the culture in which one grows up and in which one participates.

In Japan, Korea, and traditional China, the family is also experienced as identical and coextensive with the self. In Confucianism, whose "moral principles . . . supported the legitimacy of [the Japanese] family and state" (De Vos, 1980, p. 121), there is

> no place for individualistic concepts of the person. There are no individuals as such—only family members whose roles change through the life cycle. At no time is the person regarded as separate from his family and social roles, and maturation is a deepening of understanding of one's place in a system, that is, part of a yet larger social unit. One's ultimate duty, as one's ultimate psychological security, is to be found in family or group continuity, not in the continuity of the self.
> . . . Tensions experienced through a conflict of occupational expectations or family role versus disruptive private feelings are most frequently resolved in Japan by directing the individual back toward the family. The goal of attempts to alleviate psychiatric problems are therefore defined in terms of family or occupational integration. (pp. 121–122)

In such families, duty to the family and wider cultural unit predominates over duty to an individual self, a value organization that may make it difficult for the patient from such cultures to "follow doctor's orders" when they conflict with obligations to one's family role. Obligations to one's kinship network often supersede obligations to strangers such as the physician. U.S. individualism and the tightly bounded physician–patient relationship might differ markedly from the value system and expectations of such patients. As Parry (1984) notes,

> seeking help for oneself may be a threat in cultures in which the family or other social networks are more important than the individuals. A set of behaviors that threatens to change a role in a family would be viewed as displaying selfishness, disloyalty, or even hostility. (p. 930).

Thus, for Americans and a number of families of Asian heritage, to speak of birth, adolescence, marriage, and death as "family events" may carry vastly different cultural meanings and burdens.

A behavioral scientist was working with a married, female Family Medicine resident who was irate about a pregnant Chinese-American woman. This patient refused to take the prescribed iron-enriched vitamins and seemed otherwise non-compliant and uninterested in her own pregnancy. The patient had evidently not wanted to become pregnant and wanted to have her baby and be over with it (abortion was out of the question). A consultant was brought in to mediate the conflict. The consultant spoke with the patient in Chinese, and learned that in her culture, pregnant women do not take vitamins because it was felt they would throw the body out of balance. The consultant discovered, however, that within the patient's framework, seaweed figured prominently in her diet. Then the consultant and the resident successfully reached agreement with the patient to increase her intake of seaweed to give her the necessary iron supplement. The resident was relieved that her patient was getting the iron albeit in a culturally acceptable form.

ETHNICITY AND HEALTH BEHAVIOR

Within the United States, the terms *ethnic* and *ethnicity* denote a major *social typology* according to which people are classified by others, and classify themselves, in terms of nation or tribe of origin: Poles, Irish, Slovaks, English, German, Navahos, Hispanics, Iroquois, Jews, and so forth. As has been discussed at length elsewhere, the term *ethnicity* is complex (see Committee on International Relations, 1987; De Vos & Romanucci-Ross, 1975; Glazer & Moynihan, 1975; Stein, 1987d; Stein & Hill, 1977). Jews, for example, are sometimes regarded, and sometimes regard themselves, as a nation, as an ethnic group, as a race, and as a religion.

Until the civil rights and Black Power movements of the 1960s, large numbers of American blacks regarded themselves, and were regarded by the larger society, as a race (and anthropologists were quick to point out that the U.S. folk notions about "race" should not be confused with the concept as is used in scientific biology). Since the mid-1960s, many blacks have renounced the racial classification and have strongly identified themselves as Afro-Americans, that is, in terms of their continent of origin. Not only has the black/white/yellow/red U.S. "racial" classification distorted the deep cultural diversity *within* each ostensibly homogeneous racial category, but "race" has often been used as an "ethnic" category. Moreover, groups that now qualify as whites, e.g., Serbians, Poles, Ukrainians, Italians, Spaniards, and Greeks, were, earlier in the twentieth century, regarded as inferior, darker races, by those "whites" who feared that the north European, Protestant culture of their United States would be defiled.

The important point to keep in mind in all aspects of medical care is that *anything* can have group-shared, symbolic significance that bears consequences for clinical outcome. Consider food, whose symbolic weight is at least as great as its objective, nutritional value. One immigrant Italian-American male in his 60s was recovering postsurgically in the hospital. His physicians and nursing staff were becoming alarmed that he was hardly eating anything from his well-stocked hospital tray. Finally, an Italian-speaking social worker was brought in to find out what was wrong. It turned out that the soft-spoken patient objected to the *way* the food was served: it was so unappetizing that he could not bring himself to eat it. Yet to regain strength from the surgery he had to eat. He protested:

"Couldn't they make the same meat into a nice patty or meatball and put some garlic and spicy tomato sauce on it?"

For another example: In a largely Protestant and Catholic small town lives a retired, Jewish widower in his late 80s, my father. He contacted the local hospital-based "Meals on Wheels" organization to bring his lunch and dinner meals five days a week. Although he was unable to keep a strictly kosher diet (that is, one in complete accord with Orthodox Jewish dietary law), he was able to arrange that the Meals on Wheels kitchen send him sandwiches and hot meals without pork products (the meat of the pig was perhaps the most forbidden). Through this arrangement, Meals on Wheels could provide him with nutritionally high-quality food that at the same time met his sense of religious obligations.

The *form*, rather than the *substance*, of prescribed medication may become a source of conflict, as illustrated in Case 10-4. Many traditional Hispanic Americans prefer to have their medicine in the form of a "shot" (which is more masculine) than in the form of a "pill" (which is more sissifying). A 73-year-old Irish Catholic patient once told me, "Good medicine tastes bad. If it don't hurt going down, it mustn't be very strong." For him and many of his religious/ethnic culture, "taking your medicine" is as much a form of punishment as it is a form of treatment. To soothe the conscience as well as to perform its biomedical function, medicine that is acceptable must inflict some physical pain.

Many traditional Hispanic-American patients (Mexican-American, Puerto Rican) adhere to the Hippocratic, humoral theory-derived "hot–cold" (*caliente–frio*) model of disease (Harwood, 1971, 1981). According to this system, certain diseases are classified as hot, cold, and "cool" (an intermediate category). "Cold-classified illnesses are treated with hot medication and foods, while hot illnesses are treated with cool substances" (Harwood, 1971, pp. 1153–1154). Hispanic women on diuretics might discontinue such physician-prescribed potassium sources as bananas, oranges, or raisins during menstruation (a cold condition, and these foods are likewise regarded as cold or cool). The physician could prescribe potassium in the culturally acceptable form of vitamins (which are "hot"), together with such "hot" foods such as coffee and cocoa, which are rich in potassium (p. 1155). Or, consider pregnancy, a "hot" condition during which "many women will not take hot iron supplements or vitamins. These patients might be encouraged to take these prescriptions with fruit juice or an herb tea [both of which are cool] to 'neutralize' them" (p. 1157).

I continue with another example drawn from Hispanic American culture to illustrate a central issue in physician–patient relationships, namely, attitudes toward authority. Many patients from Central American countries have a tall, hierarchical view of religious and secular authority, ranging from the Roman Catholic priest to the "strong man" leader or *caudillo* who will protect them from marauding outsiders. Like these other authorities, the physician, especially a male physician in this patriarchal culture area, is to be respected, deferred to, and never questioned, at least in face-to-face behavior. Position or place is important in regulating all relationships. The modern-trained physician who cultivates patient autonomy and informed consent is likely to be frustrated by traditionalist Mexican, Guatemalan, or Honduran patients who live more according to an older "paternalistic" model of care wherein the physician is less concerned with seeking thoroughgoing "informed consent" than with directing the patient to follow the proper course of care. Here, a "You decide from a menu of options" collides with "You're my doctor in whom I put my trust; you tell me what I need to do." Moreover, to many Hispanic patients, physician–patient relationships fall into the category of patron–client relationships (as in godparenthood throughout Catholic Europe and Central/South America) in which each person has a personal obligation to the other. An impersonal, professionalized, almost mechanized view of the clinical relationship and of treatment is foreign to such a hierarchical, intimate view and expectation.

In fact, the appearance of respect and conformity with authority's judgment is often far more important than carrying out the "doctor's orders." Hispanic patients, not that unlike, say, many Great Plains whites, African-Americans, or Marshall Islanders from Micronesia, are practical, pragmatic, instrumental in medically related decision-making. They wish to avoid open conflict, confrontation, and ridicule. As a consequence, saying "Yes" in the presence of the physician may well mean a later "No" that could never be said directly. Behind the scenes, privately, or with a different "public," with their own family, neighbors, or coworkers, they will compare the physician's prescription with that of their inner and interpersonal standards, and they may decide to "comply" with family than with physician.

East European Jews tend to be as concerned about the meaning of pains as with their immediate alleviation through analgesics. Although U.S. physicians of various ethnicities perceive both Jews and Italians to be vociferous about their pains, they often fail to perceive that the purpose or function of the complaint differs between the groups. Anglo-American patients, like Jews, tend to be health-conscious, but attach very different significance to the search for health. Jews have been depicted as generally worried that something profoundly terrible might be wrong, whereas Anglo-Americans may be seen as viewing the body in a machinelike utilitarian way: When something seems broken, one is obligated to take care of oneself and bring one's body to the physician to be fixed (Zborowski, 1969). Jews may see in the most minor symptom the harbinger or symbol of tragedy; Italians may primarily want to feel better and place less emphasis on the entire prescribed medical regimen; Irish patients might ignore their symptoms as long as possible, report only a few, and avoid the sense of sin that goes with too much preoccupation with the body; and WASP patients might believe that rationality, hard work, control, and "pulling yourself up by your bootstraps" should suffice, in the treatment of disease as with the rest of life.

Ethnic symbolism often appears in what is to us in biomedicine some of the most unexpected places. For example, in a study of diabetes and diabetes management on the Devil's Lake Sioux Reservation in North Dakota, Gretchen Chesley Lang (1985) found that "food preferences, expense, and lack of time in a large household were the most frequently given reasons for lack of compliance" (p. 252) with the diabetes program. As is true in many other ethnic groups as well, for many contemporary Dakota people bigness and heaviness mean well-being and health. Three widespread Dakota perceptions about diabetes are that (1) diabetes afflicts the Dakota because their way of life is out of balance; (2) diabetes is the most recent among diseases spread by the white man to destroy Indian society; (3) because few medicine men have the power to treat it, diabetes may not necessarily be treated by traditional Dakota means. As among many other peoples, Dakota people highly regard traditional food and medicinal plants, and eating marks social occasions (p. 255). Further, many Dakota believe the presence of diabetes itself signifies the white man's destruction of their society, i.e., that the source of the disease is outside rather than inside their group. Low compliance with medically prescribed diets often serves the purpose of cultural resistance (pp. 255–256). Thus, not only are there cultural and religious aspects to food and diabetes, but *political* ones as well. The presence of a disease, and the way a group responds to that presence, may be used to affirm that group's identity and boundary. Thus, at a very practical level, for one to choose to become more healthy may endanger her inner sense of Dakota-ness and become a source of alienation in others' perceptions as well.

Just as cultural differences between patient and physician can make for misunderstandings and conflict, so—surprisingly, perhaps—can similarities. In a paper on physicians' "cultural blind spots" with regard to patients, Elizabeth Hiok-Boon Lin (1983), a Western-trained Chinese physician, challenges the popular assumption that similarities in cultural background between patient and physician invariably enhance clinical communication and outcomes. A common cultural heritage does not rule out intraethnic variation influenced by age, sex, personality, political orientation, socioeconomic class, rural/urban background, region of origin, dialect spoken, religion, occupation, education, family structure, or extent of acculturation (e.g., Americanization). Especially when the physician identifies herself as belonging to the same ethnic group as the patient, "cultural stereotyping results in superficial generalizations that are often misleading in the case of individual patients" (p. 92). Lin's caution extends beyond ethnicity or nationality of origin to religion, occupation, and common popular cultural participation. The clinical error in all of these is the assumption that "You are the same as I," a psychological merging that prevents the physician from taking notice of potentially important differences between herself and the patient. The reverse is also possible, where the patient tries to persuade the physician that they are the same. Both of these can be seen to be a variation on physician countertransference/patient transference issues. When one wants to see the patient as the same as oneself, the question to ask is: "What am I trying not to see in the patient?" (Devereux, 1980; Stein & Apprey, 1985).

CASE 10-5

During the early 1980s I conducted lengthy counseling with a woman, Carol, who had suffered a spinal cord injury in an auto accident. She had some loss of function in her right hand and leg. [The full description of the case is discussed elsewhere (see Stein, 1987e).] In work with her, I learned of the intimate connection between her sense of self, her Southern Baptist religion (as belief system, as network of community relationships), and expectations she had of herself for full recovery of function. The auto accident and its aftermath stretched her values to the breaking point. These values then exacted from her more than she could physically give.

In Carol's Southern Baptist world of the rural Great Plains small town, self-control was prized. If she had lost it through the auto accident (in which she had been a passenger), she expected to regain it—by herself. It was a test. If she regained complete use of her hand, arm, and leg, it would be proof that she was worthy in the eyes of God. If she failed, it would show to all that she was a failure. She severely reproached herself for not being able to restore herself to perfection (e.g., through exercise or physical therapy) to walk well, to carry even the heaviest casserole, to be a good enough wife, mother, and Christian.

Carol felt very much alone in her attempts at recovery, and in her attempts at differentiating between what were realistic goals and what were magical ones. Her fear of failure and shame dominated much of the therapy. In her personal, family, and religious world, everything was a matter of good or evil. Much of the counseling dealt with her haunting quest of how she could be a good woman and a good Christian if and when she could not make her body return to its condition of health prior to the accident.

Religion is the domain of human life that concerns the belief in, and the experience of, spiritual beings and supernatural forces, as well as the consequences of these beliefs for the conduct of life. In simpler, preliterate societies, and in earlier historical epochs in the West, religious life was inseparably interwoven with "ethnic," "occupational," and "popular" aspects of life. Early German Lutheran, Dutch Reformed, and Hasidic Jewish religion are instances of this fusion. It is only in more secularized, urbanized, industrialized, cosmopolitan settings that the pluralistic separation of religion and nation ("church" and "state") has occurred.

Physicians should keep in mind that patients' and families' religious beliefs, meanings, and practices may well influence any and all aspects of health-related decision-making. Even where patients might accept the naturalistic, mechanistic, diseased entity-oriented biomedical model for certain aspects of their disease and its treatment, they may well harbor more personalistic (Foster, 1976) ideas of why they are sick *now*, why *they* and not another have fallen ill, *what* they might have done in their relations with other people or with God that might have resulted in their "susceptibility" to disease or accident, and what to *do* about it now. Often patients, families, and physicians come to an impasse over how and whether to talk about these issues. Patients and physicians often think that the other only wants to talk about the "strictly medical" matters; or patients may feel afraid to bring up religious beliefs for fear of looking foolish or superstitious in the physician's eyes. On the other hand, patients may compartmentalize their medical care, allocating the corporeal "why" and biomedical treatment to the physician, while allocating the spiritual or psychological "why" and its restoration to their pastor.

In conversations related to Case 10-5, a Southern Baptist family physician colleague who had counseled many ministerial couples and served as their family physician told me of one Baptist minister's wife's symptoms. He had treated her for multiple physical complaints, none of which could be attributed to an organic disease process. When he offered to her the interpretation that the symptoms might be stress-related, she adamantly replied: "I am a Christian. I *can't* have stress," a statement that the physician, I believe accurately, construed as meaning that as she expected herself and her marriage to be perfect, any flaw in that perfection must be denied. In Case 10-5, Carol's self-blame, and its association with evangelical Protestant religious values, was not idiosyncratic or isolated, but characterized the expectations of many born-again Christians and those seeking or awaiting spiritual rebirth.

In keeping with the mind–body dualism that has dominated Western religious and philosophical thought since the late Renaissance, it is acceptable for the body to be sick, though symptoms may have highly symbolic meanings. It is not acceptable, however, for the mind or soul to be sick; nor may the "soul" be permitted to have an influence on the "body." The split must be absolute for moral, religious reasons. Physicians and other healers and therapists who harbor "psychosomatic" or "family-somatic" diagnostic models (i.e., investigating family influences on disease etiology, severity, persistence, and remission) often encounter difficult communication processes when working with such patients for whom the somatic is the only personally and religiously acceptable idiom in which to be ill. Somatization also functions as a complex compromise: for through it one can demand to be cared for, one may be punished for making such demands, one may indirectly punish others through one's symptoms, and one may preserve the personal and family belief or myth that one remains good and Christian.

Four religious groups often misunderstood by U.S. physicians are Christian Scientists, Pentecostals, Seventh-Day Adventists, and Jehovah's Witnesses. The Church of Christ, Scientists (Christian Science), founded in 1879 by Mary Baker Eddy, emphasized the importance of mind-over-body in health, disease, and healing. Disease occurs when that dominion fails. To Christian Scientists (see Eddy, 1886), Jesus is the one and only physician, and God's will determines illness outcomes. Divine Mind is to human mind as Reality is to illusion. Metaphysical doctrine is Truth, while human doctrine, including secular science, is Error. Christian Scientists are instructed to go to their own "practitioners" (as they are called) and to trust in God's will that they will be healed by prayer and proper attitude. Christian Science distinguishes between the Great Mind of God, which produces Truth, Healing, Life, and the mortal mind of humans, which produces error, sin, sickness, and death. The goal of life and of healing is to harmonize the human mind with God's Mind. Through right thinking and prayer, one can avert disease and heal all disease. The expectation of personal control over one's life and health occupies the core of Christian Science belief. If one lives right, one is well; disease is a sign that one has lived wrong, sinfully. The locus of control is inside oneself; one is responsible for one's medical outcomes—an individualism that tends socioeconomically to be more a middle-class than working-class orientation to health. To go to a biomedical physician, then, is not only to show lack of faith, but also to violate the faith. Sickness is equated with and is derived from sin, which a physician cannot treat. Group pressure also supplements individual guilt, shame, and doctrinal belief. For example, fellow Christian Science elders from the church might come to an ill person's home to pray for him, making it even more difficult to violate the church by going to a physician. In summary, Christian Science doctrine distinguishes radically between sacred and secular authority; the two should not be mixed.

The same split and separateness from mainstream U.S. culture (Yinger, 1957) holds for a wide range of U.S. Pentecostal groups (Evangelical Holiness Church, Assembly of God, for instance), except that among these groups the method of healing is not the rationalist, individualistic, somewhat impersonal, "positive thinking" (Norman Vincent Peale, 1948) approach but rather public ritual, reliance on the personal "charismatic" authority of the healer, highly expressive drama, and the experience of miraculous cures. Among Pentecostals there is the belief that only the healer's power, derived directly from God, is capable of affecting a cure—no physician, and nothing one can do or think for oneself. In its powerful expressiveness, this aura and drama of Pentecostal faith healers closely resembles shamanistic healing among North American Native Americans, shamans whose very name means "power man" or "mysterious man" (Hultkrantz, 1992, p. 18).

In contrast with both of these Protestant religious systems, Seventh-Day Adventists (whose Sabbath is the seventh day of the week) use science as an extension of religion rather than its foe or an irrelevant distraction. Meat-eating, tobacco smoking, and alcohol are prohibited. Sickness is not equated with sin, but is instead seen as a more natural, unfortunate process; prayer can be an ally of medicine, just as science can be an ally of God. Within the Adventist system of hospitals, healthcare personnel, not just chaplains, offer to pray with patients as well as minister biomedically to them. Physicians working with patients of the Adventist faith might inquire into details of the patients' diet when questions of nutritional status arise, since an individual's vegetarian diet might not correspond to what the physician expects of a "typical" U.S. patient.

Different Judeo-Christian denominations and sects base their beliefs and practices on different understandings of the Bible. Biomedical practitioners are most familiar with

Jehovah's Witnesses through their prohibition of the medical use of any blood products in the care of any of its adherents (e.g., transfusion). This obviously becomes medically important in such situations as complicated obstetrics, uncontrolled bleeding, surgery, hemophilia, and the like. Four Biblical texts are commonly cited as the basis for prohibiting the use of blood and blood products (*Genesis* 9:14,16, *Leviticus* 17:10–14, *Acts* 15:28–29, and *Acts* 21:25). Blood is simultaneously seen as sacred (belonging only to God), profane (defiling), and something that is eaten by alien peoples. Further, by analogy, if blood is not to be eaten, then it is forbidden to enter the human body by any route. To do so would desecrate, violate, the spiritual body. Many physicians with whom I have worked over the years emphasize to me that as a rule their patients from the Jehovah's Witness faith tend to be quite medically "compliant," and apart from the question of blood and blood products, are not particularly different from other mainstream U.S. patients.

Culturally not far removed from Seventh-Day Adventists and Jehovah's Witnesses are more mainstream Christian and Jewish physicians who maintain a secular practice, but who nonetheless regard medical science as an ally of God and who see themselves and biomedical treatments as God's agents. Even though they might not officially or even consciously espouse religious beliefs in the medical practice, their very practice silently lives it. In the Great Plains where I teach, many devout Christians of mainstream Protestant denominations (e.g., Lutheran, Southern Baptist, Methodist, Disciples of Christ, Presbyterian) believe their physician's hand to be guided by the hand of God, and that their physician's judgment is a tool of God. God's will is manifested through the physician. Physicians, for their part, utilize or accept their patients' belief as an additional tool of the therapeutic alliance, either as "placebo" effect or as a sign that their own healing derived from a power beyond their own abilities. Here, the "faith healing" is often an implicit "transference" rather than an explicit drama as in, say, Pentecostal healing rites. Faith in God supplements the widespread popular "faith in science."

Before ending, I offer the caveats that (1) the official, doctrinal, formal side of any religion must be distinguished from the actual experiential, practical, or folk side of that religion (Spiro, 1982); (2) health-related beliefs, values, customs, practices, and remedies are mediated by family and unconscious forces that, in a sense, "use" religion in their own service; and (3) religious affiliation, intensity, and type of belief often shift during the course of a person's lifetime and over family generations. Thus, in religion as with ethnicity in complex Western society such as ours, one cannot take for granted the monolithic "sameness" that we often (mistakenly) ascribe to preliterate, tribal, societies. In religion as in all culture, patients come one person at a time.

In summary, each religious denomination has a view of *authority*, and of the relationship between *sacred* and *secular* (even *profane*), as these affect the healing of disease and the identification of who is responsible for that healing. Knowledge of these helps the physician to inquire what a patient will expect or even allow.

CASE 10-6

"Tinker syndrome": For six years (1979–1985) I coordinated behavioral science teaching at the Family Medicine residency program in Shawnee, Oklahoma, a clinic in which many workers from Tinker Air Force Base sought their primary care. Over the years, several residents came to formulate what they wryly referred to as the "Tinker syndrome." The syndrome was characterized by feelings of job dissatisfaction, low productivity, punching the clock, and collecting a paycheck.

Many workers came to the clinic intermittently through the year, acknowledging depression or with multiple organic complaints. Toward early spring (March, April), the Family Medicine residents noticed that many of these workers would come into the clinic with symptoms they would relate to stress (anxiety, can't sleep, nervousness).

Early spring was the time of an annual site visit and major review of the air force base, when supervisors were expected to show efficiency and productivity, and units were evaluated for their performance. Suddenly, the base became self-consciously more active and busy. The physicians surmised that many of their patients were situationally anxious or suffering from vague guilt and fear of being judged and found inadequate, which they expressed in a wide spectrum of physical symptoms. During this "Tinker syndrome" influx, there were biomedically bona fide physical complaints as well. Some workers would literally strain themselves by trying to cram 12 months of physical labor into 2 to 3 weeks prior to the annual site visit. Unaccustomed to regular strenuous physical labor, some workers injured themselves when they attempted to perform intensive physical labor on their jobs.

Apart from this latter group, a visit to the physician usually resulted in reassurance that no severe disease process was taking place. The workers were able to ventilate about their variously frustrating and bureaucratic governmental jobs and confess some anxiety, guilt, and shame for their lack of enthusiasm at an unrewarding job. Through their symptoms they received some degree of punishment for their lackluster attitude toward work and received assurance that neither their body nor their spirit was in that terrible a shape, only to return to the base to commence the cycle anew. It required rather sophisticated cultural thinking on the part of these residents (1) to recognize an epidemiological pattern rather than think exclusively of patients on a one-by-one basis and (2) to interpret a plethora of physical complaints as a metaphor for a disorder related to the culture of the workplace. (Gratitude is expressed to James Michael Pontious, M.D., for his collaboration on this case.)

OCCUPATIONAL CULTURE AND HEALTH BEHAVIOR

The culture of the workplace is yet another source of health behavior-related norms. These are often learned not via intergenerational socialization of the young (as is more characteristic of long-term ethnic and religious cultures) but through learning as a participant in one's work culture (an exception, discussed later in this section, is the culture of family farming). One is subject to similar external stresses and expectations. One negotiates common meanings and interpretations of events from day-to-day interaction with superiors, coworkers, and subordinates.

Although the family farm, the family grocery store, the hospital, and the corporation, for instance, can all be labeled "occupational cultures," one must keep in mind that they differ markedly in the process of recruitment. Family farms and family businesses recruit from within, through procreation and socialization of the next, succeeding generation. However, "Organizations [such as hospitals and corporations] are not self-renewing but must replace their memberships from the outside society" (Grieco, 1988, p. 85). Those recruited from without are already culture-bearers, albeit those whose values are congruent with those of the organization and who are most easily socialized.

As the Tinker syndrome illustrates in Case 10-6, a major element in the healthcare process is *timing*: When does the patient (in league with relatives, coworkers, drinking partners, and others) decide to come in for medical care? Physician and patient often become embroiled in conflict from the start, because the physician's sense of timing does not correspond to that of the patient. Consider this issue from the viewpoint of the culture of Great Plains wheat farming families, a regional cultural group congealed over the generations from immigrants and their descendants from western and central Europe, Great Britain, and Ireland. A typical farmer's presenting complaint at the emergency room or in the clinic is frequently a variation of the following:

> My wife made me come. She's been on my back for 2 weeks now. I've had just a little
> pain in my chest, nothing that working out in the yard or on the tractor won't cure in
> time. But the only way I could get her off my back is to come in and prove it's nothin'.

Moreover, it is often difficult if not impossible to elicit a "complete history" from the taciturn, terse farmer (who keeps words to a minimum, wants to avoid stirring a fuss over nothing, and serves up plenty of *Yup*'s and *Nope*'s); therefore, it becomes the role of the wife to provide the history of the symptoms. She is the person from whom the explanatory model can often be elicited. As described elsewhere in detail (Stein, 1987a,b), the preharvest months and harvest proper are times when only a seriously ill infant or child will be brought to the physician; similarly, during holiday times of family togetherness (Thanksgiving, Christmas) trips to the physician will be postponed (Stein, 1987a,b).

CASE 10-7

Many rural "white" farming families, like countless of their urban counterparts in the mainstream United States, routinely take sodium bicarbonate (baking soda) frequently for a wide variety of gastric discomforts. Baking soda thus occupies the same place in popular culture as, say, Vicks once did. Also, these farming families usually do not consider baking soda to be a "medicine" or "drug." Thus, when a physician inquires, "What medications are your currently taking?," baking soda (like birth control pills, aspirin, and vitamins) is likely to be omitted from the list. The frequent use of sodium bicarbonate could complicate, or at least compromise, the course and medical treatment of hypertension and related cardiovascular diseases, since it increases rather than decreases the sodium in the body.

—— POPULAR CULTURE AND HEALTH BEHAVIOR ——

In many ways, of the four cultural regions covered in this chapter, this section may be the most difficult for the reader to "stomach" precisely because it comes closest to home. It may feel too personal. For many readers it may be more tolerable to read about ethnic groups, religious groups, and occupational groups that seem sufficiently alien to be safely distant from one's own. But when we examine popular U.S. culture and its link to health beliefs and health behavior, the reader is likely to rear up, as it were, and say: "Wait a minute, buddy, you're talking about *me*!"

There is safety in scrutinizing, even compassionately criticizing, something or some-one who seems "foreign," but we are quick to muster our defenses to protect our bound-aries when we feel scrutinized ourselves. Yet unfair scrutiny is not my intention; nor do I wish to make any group more foreign-seeming than another. If anything, my goal all along in this chapter is to help make the familiar a little more unfamiliar, to make it a little more remote, and to make the more unfamiliar feel closer to ourselves. I raise the question: How do we in biomedicine think compassionately yet critically about the many links between our own professional culture and national culture? Can we be at once loyal while some-times critical? If in describing popular U.S. culture, I come uncomfortably close to the home of the reader, I am likewise looking at my own cultural household!

The culture most difficult to gain distance from, and then to be carefully critical of, is one's own. It is much easier to be leery of "their" health practices than of "ours." Don't we all assume that "our" practices (of any kind—food, clothing, gesture, speech—not only medical) are human, natural, while "their" practices are "cultural" if not suspect? When we think of language, do we ever imagine *ourselves* to have an "accent"? Certainly not. Only those who "talk differently" from us have "accents"—but then to them, we have an accent, too! For the sake of patient care, we deserve to increase our own tolerance of anxiety about "difference" and place our own popular culture health beliefs and practices under the same microscope and "macroscope" we do to understand the foundations of others' health values and behaviors.

Powerful folk medical currents exist within mainstream U.S. popular culture (and not only isolated religious sects and newly arrived ethnic groups), currents that flow into official professional culture as well. In recent years popular interest has grown in what has come to be called "alternative medicine" (Murray & Rubel, 1992; Fuller, 1992) (e.g., herbal teas, crystals, chiropractic, therapeutic touch, meditation, acupuncture). As the reader has no doubt already discovered throughout this chapter, the designation of cultures and their health-related practices as "professional," "popular," "ethnic," "occupational," "alternative" is ultimately contextual if not arbitrary. A healthy sense of medical history is required to realize that what in one decade is marginal, if not anathema, might in another decade be incorporated into the biomedical "armamentarium" (biofeedback, acupuncture, family therapy)—and vice versa (psychoanalytic theory and therapy in psychiatry, now almost entirely supplemented by psychopharmacology).

In one Family Medicine residency setting I have known intimately for nearly two decades, allopathic and osteopathic physicians (M.D.s and D.O.s) train together. Busy M.D.s with neck and back strains often quietly ask their D.O. colleagues to take them into a nearby exam room and "manipulate" them back into shape so that they will be without pain and able immediately to resume allopathic patient care! Still, the anxious "D.O. jokes" persist. Years ago, an especially perceptive allopathic physician-colleague said to me: "Isn't it strange that we are so hard on chiropractors, but then we turn around and send patients to physical therapists in the hospital?"

We take for granted elements of U.S. popular medical culture, although they become evident as soon as they are pointed out. Over-the-counter, patent medicines available at pharmacies and supermarkets are part of this popular, folk-American culture. The wide-swinging deification and vilification of physicians (who can do nothing wrong and who can do nothing right) is intrinsic to popular culture. The common preference for medica-tion in pill (oral) form, together with the search for a pill-for-every-ailment, "magic bullets," are popular ethnomedicine. Similarly, much of the impetus for high-technology solutions to human suffering come from this cultural "grass roots." Television commer-cials (from prime time to soap operas), newspaper and magazine ads, and articles in the popular press are rich treasure troves of fantasies and ideologies and practices within U.S. popular medicine.

Consider the term *germs*. The word blurs fantasy and reality. As science, they refer to viral and bacterial entities and their adaptation to human hosts; as a folk category they have (like cancer) assumed mythic, malevolent proportions. They are akin to the nuclear mutagenic aliens who threatened to overtake us in films from the 1950s. Every housewife (and now, house husband) is taught by TV commercials to dread the presence of even a single "germ" in the kitchen or bathroom—or on the floor anywhere. With the threat of AIDS and hepatitis B, the return of the nearly banished tuberculosis, and the emergence of drug-resistant streptococcus, *Time* magazine even featured a cover story in 1994 entitled "Revenge of the Killer Microbes: Are we losing the war against infectious diseases?" The listing in the table of contents continues the imagery of assault: "The Microbes Strike Back"; and later, "Counterattack" (p. 3; note of course the widespread military metaphor in biomedicine).

A strong theme within U.S. popular culture is that of *germ phobia*, a long-term preoccupation of Americans, into which the growing list of sexually transmitted diseases and tuberculosis now fits grimly well. In popular culture, much of the painstaking, scientific method that officially characterizes the ideal self-image of biomedicine is replaced by abundant magical thinking, of which supernaturalized, menacing "germs" are the result. The popular medical cult of cleanliness is obsessed with the ritual purification of the body, both inside and outside. We cleanse and purge ourselves with folk remedies ranging from laxatives through laundry detergents (as in the Ivory Snow commercial's slogan, "99 and 44/100% pure"). The popular image of the physician, conqueror, warrior, doer, teacher, wise caretaker, and master of high technology holds that the physician is the one in whom the hope rests for the secularized purification of the body for life here on earth.

The deep embeddedness of biomedicine in the national imagination can be immediately attested to by the consistent popularity of medical programs on television: e.g., *Marcus Welby, M.D., Ben Casey, Medical Center, MASH, After-MASH, Trapper John, M.D.*, and most recently, *ER* and *Chicago Hope*; the daytime soap operas, such as *General Hospital*; and countless local call-in physician talk shows. Moreover, medical "miracles" and "breakthroughs" are featured on local and national "news" on radio and television, in the newspaper, and in national magazines. To be so worthy of prominence in the genres of "news" and "entertainment," medicine must tap deeply into the dominant meanings and fantasies of our time.

Professional culture is never far removed from popular U.S. culture. An example is the prevalence of "management" imagery, language, and organization within biomedicine. In the 1910s, the movement led by Frederick Winslow Taylor (1911) introduced principles of "scientific management" into industry and organizational settings. Three decades later, Peter Drucker's (1954) rationalist approach called "management by objective" became widely accepted throughout U.S. business culture. Work was conceived to be a strictly and narrowly linear, impersonal enterprise, having expected outcomes and precise ways of reaching them and measuring productivity along the path toward that outcome. One might say that this managerial worldview was a decontextualized one or, rather, one in which the only contexts to be considered were those regarded by the managers as important (e.g., specifically, variables that were supposed to be incentives for greater worker productivity).

This management ethos rapidly diffused throughout various cultural institutions, medicine among them. Common expressions are "medical management," "case management," "management conference," "It is a clinical management problem," and so forth. Not only the language, but the way of imaging or conceptualizing medical problems, the way of treating them, and the way of relating to other medical colleagues in the treatment process—these are all consequences of the popular culturally managerial style of thinking. Clinically and elsewhere in life, people act toward themselves and toward others in terms of how and what they think of themselves. In medicine as in life, metaphors often become destinies.

In a powerful interpretive passage, Scheper-Hughes and Lock (1987) show how professional and medical cultures collude in the production of the obsession with anorexic fitness and ascetic wellness. In a sinister way, hypochondriasis is transformed from disease into cure!

> In our own increasingly "healthist" and body-conscious culture, the politically correct body for both sexes is the lean, strong, androgynous, and physically "fit" form through which the core cultural values of autonomy, toughness, competitiveness, youth, and self-control are readily manifest (Pollitt 1982). Health is increasingly viewed in the United States as an achieved rather than an ascribed status, and each individual is expected to "work hard" at being strong, fit, and healthy. Conversely, ill health is no longer viewed as accidental, a mere quirk of nature, but rather is attributed to the individual's failure to live right, to eat well, to exercise, etc. We might ask what it is our society "wants" from this kind of body. DeMause (1984) has speculated that the fitness/toughness craze is a reflection of an international preparation for war. A hardening and toughening of the national fiber corresponds to a toughening of individual bodies. In attitude and ideology the self-help and fitness movements articulate both a militarist and a Social Darwinist ethos: the fast and fit win; the fat and flabby lose and drop out of the human race (Scheper-Hughes and Stein 1987). Crawford (1980, 1985), however, has suggested that the fitness movement may reflect, instead, a pathetic and individualized (also wholly inadequate) defense against the threat of nuclear holocaust. . . . Crawford (1985) has interpreted the eating disorders and distortions in body image expressed in obsessional jogging, anorexia, and bulimia as a symbolic mediation of the contradictory demands of postindustrial American society. The double-binding injunction to be self-controlled, fit, and productive workers, and to be at the same time self-indulgent, pleasure-seeking consumers is especially destructive to the self-image of the "modern," "liberated" American woman. Expected to be fun-loving and sensual, she must also remain thin, lovely, and self-disciplined. Since one cannot be hedonistic and controlled simultaneously, one can alternate phases of binge eating, drinking, and drugging with phases of jogging, purging, and vomiting. Out of this cyclical resolution of the injunction to consume and to conserve is born, according to Crawford, the current epidemic of eating disorders (especially bulimia) among young women, some of whom literally eat and diet to death. (1987, pp. 25–26)

At individual, family, workplace, and larger cultural levels, these U.S. eating disorders condense the dread of death, the quest for immortality, preoccupation with and intense ambivalence about sexuality, an obsession with elusive perfection and control, and the unreliability of people in the face of plentiful food.

Family Medicine and Sports Medicine physician and faculty colleague James R. Barrett (1994) recently described a syndrome of "exercise addiction," complete with the triad of dependence, tolerance, and withdrawal symptoms. As often happens in all human culture's attempt to solve life's problems by vicious cycles of anxiety and defense, one day's solutions often become the next day's burdens. Alas, the recent history of medicine's linkage of "wellness" and "fitness" with preventive medicine may be one such triumph and casualty. At its extremes, "wellness" could be considered a culturally acceptable expression of hypochondriasis.

A powerful link between professional biomedical and popular U.S. culture is "illness somatization [that] has become a dominant metaphor for expressing individual and social complaint" (Scheper-Hughes & Lock, 1987, p. 27). Physician, healthcare system, third-party payers, patients, families, and society jointly collude in the diversion of attention from affect (emotion), conscious and unconscious meaning, and the experience of social injustice. Paradoxically, by defining virtually all problems and issues somatically, patients and families inadvertently surrender to physician control much of the autonomy and self-responsibility for which the medical consumerist movement of the 1970s fought so strenuously. Scheper-Hughes and Lock point ironically to "the usefulness to the body politic of filtering more and more human unrest, dissatisfaction, longing, and protest into the idiom of sickness, which can then be safely managed by doctor-agents" (p. 27). In a now-classic article on premenstrual syndrome (PMS) as a Western culture-specific disorder, Johnson (1987) underscores this very point.

Yet another link between health beliefs in professional biomedical and popular U.S. cultures is an alternate model of alcoholism that diverges from the official disease model endorsed by many physicians and by Alcoholics Anonymous, to whom physicians often refer patients. Its essence is captured by patients, spouses of patients, friends, and co-workers of patients who often say, for instance:

- "I'm just a different person when I drink."
- "I'm not myself when I drink."
- "She's not herself when she drinks."
- "I just don't know what gets into him when he's drinking."
- "It's not him talking, it's the liquor."
- "I don't know what overcame me to get into that fight last night—I'm really a quiet person; it must have been all those beers I had at the [football] game."

Within what explanatory frame(s) of reference do statements like these make sense? We Americans have long prided ourselves on our hard-bitten realism, our practicality (pragmatism), our rationality, our goal of objectivity. One could even claim that "medical science" is one of our chief contemporary religions, at least with respect to the salvation and preservation of the youthfulness of the body.

Yet, from research I have conducted over the course of medical teaching (Stein, 1982, 1985a, 1987c, 1993), a widespread model of alcoholism departs markedly from how we prefer to view ourselves. Alcohol is not only *substance* but also *symbol* (Stein, 1993). This symbol serves as a collective excuse for individuals, family members, coworkers, friends, to do and condone for others to do what we secretly wish to do, but which also violates our conscious values, feelings, and roles. Our model of alcohol and alcoholism is the compromise. Foreign as it may seem to the reader, I have come to the conclusion that an implicit popular cultural theory of "possession" underlies the official, professional pharmacological biomedical theory of alcoholism and drug abuse in United States (Stein, 1982, 1985a, 1987c, 1993).

In this folk model, alcoholism and chemical dependency constitute a form of what I have called *secular possession*. In arguing so, I am quite aware that I am suggesting that we, too, even though we have gone to the moon and returned, are also "primitive" in many ways! In imbibing the spirits, one incorporates the impersonal anima or "spirit" that has been bottled or canned, and is soon possessed by it. Just as religious knowledge is said to come from the outside in, by divine "inspiration" or "revelation," likewise does drunkenness or drug-induced highs. All one need do to confirm this is to consult our cultural semantics, vividly illustrated by the earlier clinical example.

Everyday language offers clues about the meaning alcohol has for us. We say one becomes "in-toxicated" or "in-ebriated" after consuming alcoholic beverages. We speak of someone being "under the influence" of alcohol or "driving under the influence" (or "while intoxicated"). The term has even made it into the legal vocabulary ("DUI" or "DWI"). Alcohol is associated with being "influenced by" the profane, with badness, with poison that enters the body and does its evil work (e.g., demon rum). Not unexpectedly, the initial part of our cultural ritual cure for alcoholics is a form of exorcism: *detoxification* to expunge the poisons (toxins) from the body, often performed in special inpatient hospital wards or mental health units. Since possession by the debasing, alien agent of ethanol caused the intoxication in the first place, detoxification will expel the noxious substance from the body. But expulsion is never complete ("Once an alcoholic, always an alcoholic," we Americans also often say). Alcoholics, even after the exorcism (similar to drug abusers following chemical detoxification), remain vulnerable to being possessed once again by the vile, but fascinating, substance.

We realist Americans scorn as mere superstition the notion of spirit possession. Yet we also practice what we claim not to believe. Scientific theory can serve as a scarcely veiled supernatural, animistic possession in an acceptable cultural form ("It's the booze talking, not him!"). Two cultural models of alcoholism, one official (scientific, disease, naturalistic) and the other unofficial (folk, possession), can coexist alongside each other in the same people's minds. One or both can be used to divert the attention of patient, family, physician, healthcare institution, and the wider culture away from the system of meanings, conscious and unconscious, of which alcoholism or drug abuse are only "the tip of the iceberg."

Sadly, much of human culture—not only U.S. popular health culture—serves precisely the function of allaying anxiety, guilt, shame, and other dysphoric feelings by directing our attention only to the tip of that iceberg. Unfortunately, culture can have both adaptive and maladaptive sides.

CONCLUSIONS

This chapter has introduced the reader to the cultural world of the patient, and perhaps has *re*introduced the reader to the cultural worlds he inhabits. In all clinical communication, the practitioner gains access to realms of the patient's experience, values, beliefs, expectations, explanations, feelings, meanings, and conflicts by having free access to those realms within oneself. The self of the clinician remains one of the finest instruments of observation, assessment, and treatment available. Physicians, no less than patients, are creators and bearers of culture and suffer the consequences from unexamined assumptions about others' cultures.

All of us in U.S. medicine wish to make the work of medical practice more simple. Physicians conduct thorough physical exams, "take" thorough histories, order numerous tests, all in an attempt to obtain a definitive diagnosis and proceed with a decisive treatment plan in order that they succeed rather than fail (two culturally loaded words in biomedical culture). But often the more we know biomedically, the more complicated knowledge and decision making become. It is no different with the culture of the patient: Despite our wish for simple cultural answers, the more we know of a patient's, a family's, a physician's culture(s), the more complicated the clinical picture becomes (that is to say, the more real). Just as I wish it were different on the organic side of medicine, so I also wish it were different from the cultural side. But it is not.

Interest in the patient's culture, however, can lead to some surprising turns in the physician–patient–family relationship, and to wisdom about people outside the ethnic group or tribe one is currently thinking about. Consider, for example, the widespread practice among Jews of circumcising newborn males on the eighth day, or the widespread practice among Muslims of female circumcision—or, for that matter, the belief among many U.S. physicians that male babies should be routinely circumcised at birth, and further that such procedures do not require pain control, or much pain control, because infants supposedly do not feel pain or presumably will not remember it in later life anyway. Or consider the question of whether Muslim women should be routinely assigned a female physician to conduct the physical exam. For one thing, there is considerable intragroup variation, which is often to say controversy, among Jews, Muslims, and physicians as to what is culturally acceptable.

Any group's health-related practices (including our own as Americans, as physicians) should be open to further inquiry as to their personal and family meaning. To say simply: "Custom A is practiced in Group B means we should uncritically and automatically abide by it" is to suspend the very judgment we regard as critical in areas we call "clinical." On the other hand, sensitivity to cultural *questions* (e.g., physical exams, pelvic exams with female Muslim patients) can be a cue for physicians to ask key questions about gender, modesty, sexuality, exposure of the body, expectation, and the like, of *any* female patient: for instance, "Are you comfortable having a male physician examine you? Doing a pelvic? Would you like anyone else in the room with you during the exam?" Often, too, a physician must infer a patient's comfort from nonverbal messages such as facial expression, because many patients would feel it to be disrespectful to ask something, let alone to tell a physician not to do something. Just as physicians often fear retaliation from patients (e.g., lawsuits), patients, especially those from newly immigrant families and countries, often fear rejection if not retaliation from their physicians if they are too outspoken or demanding. Cultural issues, alas, far from being mere "background" or "academic" in the medical encounter, may turn out to be among the most intellectually, emotionally, and ethically demanding facets of medicine.

In this chapter, after several approaches to the concept of culture were discussed, two aspects of culture were considered: (1) patients' informal care networks and (2) illness-related words and concepts, together with their meanings. Four cultural domains that affect patients' health behavior were then explored: (1) ethnicity, (2) religion, (3) occupation, and (4) popular U.S. culture. It is tempting for the practitioner to memorize lists of cultural traits, just as in medical school the student must memorize thousands of anatomical parts, biochemical terms, physiological processes, and pharmacological actions. The result, however, would be less an intimate understanding of a real other person and family than the imposition of a stereotype and the mistaking of that stereotype for the patient's reality. It is admittedly more difficult, yet at the same time more rewarding, for the physician (or other healthcare provider) to take an interest in the patient as a person, an interest that will quite naturally lead to inquiry into the universes of meaning the patient inhabits, and in turn to a more satisfactory, productive, clinical relationship.

——————— CASES FOR DISCUSSION ———————

CASE 1

The following case is based on Macquire (1978) and Hocking (1987, p. 527). It highlights the fact that (1) pathology occurs in workplace culture and (2) work culture pathologies occur not only in individuals one at a time but also in groups where persons identify with one another as members of groups. In many U.S. communities, family physicians and general internists have long served as the "company doc" for oil refineries and factories. More recently, in large industries and corporations, occupational medicine physicians, PAs, nurses, and industrial hygienists, among others, serve in this capacity. Although the case below occurred in England, it easily could have occurred in the United States:

> *An outbreak of skin disorders took place in a ceramics factory. Those affected consisted of eight female employees who worked in one room, and two male porters. Subsequently one woman was diagnosed with angioneurotic edema with cholinergic urticaria with impetigo complicating self-inflicted excoriation. The other seven women described that after seeing this woman, they themselves developed transient rashes on exposed surfaces. The two porters had winter eczema. Following an extensive investigation the plant was temporarily closed, the employees were given clear assurance, and the rashes disappeared. Only the first employee had sought medical help. There was consensus among employees that factory management was responsible for the illnesses and that management was likewise responsible for the cure. Employees believed they had lost their sense of individuality and that the factory now consisted only of a system of variously sized, impersonal work-groups. Somatization was the only acceptable way the grievance and protest could take place. The rash was a way to express powerlessness, to exert a small degree of power, and to help the group of employees to redefine themselves as a group. (Hocking, 1987, p. 527)*

When practitioners and educators in biomedicine speak of "infectious disease," we usually refer to viral and bacterial infection. In this case, one might think of a kind of metaphoric infection based on identification. What is symbolically "infectious" here is discontent based on a sense of group isolation and mistreatment. The organizational culture had changed, making it a far more emotionally sterile place to work. The astute clinician of any specialty needs to inquire into the kind of "infection" that is affecting an organization and its timing (why now?) as well. A number of questions emerge from this case:

1. *As a physician in a community or corporate group, how do you learn to think in terms of epidemiological or cultural patterns in addition to thinking clinically, biomedically, one patient at a time?*
2. *As the physician for a corporation or plant, for whom do you work (that is, individual employee, the employee's supervisor, the management, the union)? What role conflicts might you expect in the setting of an industrial or corporate culture?*
3. *Discuss this case in terms of Kleinman's distinction between "disease" and "illness."*
4. *If somatizing responses are corporately and culturally safe, how would you help employees to discuss feelings and grievances if these could be construed by management as threat or rebellion?*
5. *How would you clinically or administratively deal with the issues of female employees' low pay and relative powerlessness—factors over which you as a physician have no control and which management would likely tell you are "off limits" as a medical issue?*

CASE 2

Mary Tinsley, a woman in her mid-60s, presents at the office of her family physician with a complaint of mid- and low-back pain. It is late September, and her annual visit(s) are like clockwork. Her ritual has been going on for some 30 years. She alleges that years ago she had some back injury but no vertebral fractures or compressions can be detected. Recent workups confirm the present physician's conviction that the problem is psychosomatic. The present physician is one in a distinguished line of family physicians, general practitioners, and orthopedic surgeons, all of whom were able to "find nothing."

Every year during the September planting season, John Tinsley, her husband, a man in his late 60s, spends nearly 2 weeks away from the house, working in the field. Mary feels isolated, abandoned. She felt this way even when their children were young and lived with them in a house on the farm. She feels the same, now that she and her husband have moved from the farm to a nearby town. Thirty years ago, her back pain was so bad that she had to move about in a wheelchair, and her irate husband and children had to take care of her. Over the years, she has admirably run the household, reared the children. During the rest of the year, she is not sick a day. But come September and planting, her low-back pain is as predictable as is the change of season. The annual onset of symptoms coincides with John's departure. By the time plowing is finished, she has become veritably incapacitated (while continuing to perform domestic duties to a fault), and seeks medical relief. The physician prescribes meperidine HCl (a narcotic pain medicine) or flurazepam HCl (a tranquilizer) to alleviate the pain.

Mary reports that her husband berates her as "excess baggage," accusing her of not holding her own in her responsibilities around the house. As both have grown older, Mary has apparently "aged" more than John—who even now cannot seem to work enough. John wants the freedom to work his farm, to come and go as he pleases, to be accountable to no one, and to not be tied to home or wife. Over time John's expectations have not at all diminished, while Mary resents being saddled with these expectations, feeling unappreciated for her role and abandoned and ridiculed as "excess baggage." (Adapted from Stein, 1987a, pp. 170–171)

1. *Explain the timing of the wife's symptoms.*
2. *Speculate on the role of her symptoms in her marriage.*
3. *How would you as a physician go about inquiring into the meaning and function of her physical symptoms?*
4. *How would you avoid the temptation to do a "million-dollar workup" on a patient of this kind—who is "presenting" somatically?*
5. *How would you introduce "psychosocial" issues to a patient whose familial–cultural–religious beliefs militate against such an interpretation?*

CASE 3

A farmer in his early 50s was scheduled for gallbladder surgery. Hospitalized, he was being prepped for surgery, his family gathering in the waiting area. As the anesthesiologist approached the patient, he developed supraventricular tachycardia, whereupon she stepped back and waited for him to calm down. She tried this unsuccessfully several times. Finally, she decided to postpone the surgery until a later time—when the patient would presumably be less nervous.

In the waiting area, the family wondered why it took so long for him to be readied for surgery. First, the anesthesiologist attempted to explain the problem by saying that the patient had developed supraventricular tachycardia; she explained anatomically all that was involved; she even drew an elementary diagram. The family didn't understand, standing around puzzled, wondering whether something undiscovered was wrong. The surgeon then attempted to redeem the situation, going basically through the same explanation as had the anesthesiologist—with similar results.

Down the hall walked a family physician who overheard the vain attempts to explain to the family through recourse to anatomy and physiology. He put his arm around the shoulder of one of the members of the family, and said: "Your father's heart is shimmying like the front end of an old Chevy." The family said, with one voice, "Oh!"—finally feeling that they understood what was wrong. Satisfied, they were ready to leave until the next attempt could be made. (From Stein, 1985b, pp. 87–88)

1. How would you have tried to explain the patient's cardiac reaction to the patient and family?
2. How do you think you would have responded (feeling, behavior) to the patient's and family's incomprehension of an accurate, elegant biomedical explanation you had just offered to them?
3. What cues would "tell" you that you need to talk with them in a different language?
4. Why do you think that the family practitioner's explanation succeeded, since a heart is not the same as the front end of a pickup truck?
5. Had this been an emergency situation, how would you have proceeded medically?

CASE 4

Internist and family physician Robert E. Pieroni, M.D. (1981), reported the following case of hypokalemia, here paraphrased: He was asked to evaluate a 42-year-old black female with a dangerously low serum potassium level. She was 8 months pregnant and had been admitted to the hospital because of weakness and marked hypertension. She reported no significant vomiting, diarrhea, or use of drugs that could have contributed to her considerable loss of potassium. He then questioned her about pica (an abnormal craving), which was frequently found in their region (the deep South). She reported that she had not eaten starch, dirt, or clay, but when directly questioned she did state that she had used chewing tobacco to ease her morning sickness. Such a practice is not uncommon in the deep South and has probably been handed down from generation to generation. Many brands of chewing tobacco, including the brand his patient was using, contained licorice, which not only can deplete the body of potassium but can also cause marked hypertension, weakness, and swelling. Fortunately, her potassium was corrected before further harm was done, and she went on to deliver a healthy baby. She now spreads the word that chewing tobacco is not a panacea for morning sickness (1981, p. 7).

1. Describe the two cultural explanatory models (professional and ethnic or folk) that were in conflict.
2. How do you decide whether to try to work within a patient's cultural framework or to persuade a patient to change it?
3. When you as a physician are unfamiliar with a patient's cultural practices, how would you go about inquiring into them so as to lead—for example—to thinking about licorice?

CASE 5

In U.S. religion, as in ethnicity, there is considerable intermarriage and culture change over the generations. If for some people religion is a dominant, organizing force in their lives, for others it is situational; that is, it ranges from worship services on Sunday or Wednesday night to serving as a source of comfort or guilt during stressful times of life. This perspective complicates any simple view that religious sect, denomination, or national culture remains static over time. It likewise complicates assessment of cultural implications for health behavior and healthcare. Consider the following vignette:

A family physician in Chicago has taken care of the health needs of an English-American Presbyterian couple in their 30s, and their three children, for nearly a decade. The family physician receives an anxious phone call from the wife, Sarah Jones, who says that her New England in-laws, now in their 70s, will soon be coming to live with them in their home, that they have just become unable to live independently any longer. She wants to be a good daughter (she says, not daughter-in-law) to her husband's parents; and her husband, Ralph Jones, wants to give his parents some good years.

Her mother-in-law, Sally Jones, has had chronic, worsening asthma. Philip Jones, Sally's husband of 40 years, has gradually developed increased shortness of breath and fatigue with exertion of effort. He has helped the Boston couple to get by with shopping and other errands since his retirement from a career in railroad maintenance. However, with the development of these (cardiovascular?) symptoms, he is just unable to compensate for Sally's increased inability (disability?) to take care of chores and other family roles that were hers. He has lately been trying to do the work of both of them.

Sarah explains that her husband's parents have been practicing Christian Scientists all of their lives, and that both their families "go way back" in the Church. Now and then they will go to a Christian Science practitioner. They pray a lot. Much of their reading consists of the Bible and of books written by Dr. Norman Vincent Peale. They are a very private couple, she says, and prefer to take care of their own problems, "real New England types," Sarah calls them. Sarah and Ralph have for years in long-distance phone calls and in annual visits with their children, tried to urge her husband's parents to seek medical care from a family physician, an internist, a pulmonologist, anyone in biomedicine who could investigate what might be going on physically inside their bodies. Sally and Philip keep insisting that there is nothing "physically" going on that right living and prayer would not correct.

During his own adolescence, Ralph had rejected the religion of his upbringing, and with it, the health practices and beliefs of his parents. When he married Sarah 15 years ago, he joined her Presbyterian Church, in which they are nominally raising their own children. Ralph did not have the heart to make the phone call to their family physician himself, so Sarah called on behalf of both of them. What, she asked, were they supposed to do with the family who would soon join them? "Just watch them go downhill? Do nothing?"

She wondered whether her family physician had any advice for her. She, a Presbyterian whose family of origin prided themselves in Sunday church attendance, prayer before meals, medical science, and "common sense," said that she expected to be the primary "health" provider at home. But, she asked, "How do you provide even minimal healthcare to people who don't believe in healthcare? We all talk English, but talking to them is like speaking in a foreign language!" If she could not prevail on them to seek medical care, was there any way, she wondered aloud to her physician, he could "coach" her over the phone.

1. Describe the interplay of religious and family functions in this case of asthma.
2. Describe some of the conflicts the physician would have in this case—for example, who is (are) the patient(s)?
3. Describe some of the key Christian Science beliefs and practices in this case.
4. In what sense is everyone who is involved in this complex cultural case "out of control"?
5. If you (the reader) had been the physician telephoned, what would you have done? What is your rationale?

RECOMMENDED READINGS

Abel TM, Metraux R, Roll S: *Psychotherapy and Culture*. Albuquerque, NM, University of New Mexico Press, 1987.

> Abel, Metraux, and Roll offer a view of the therapeutic process based on a psychodynamic model of human relationships and meanings.

Chrisman NJ, Maretzki TW (eds): *Clinically Applied Anthropology*. Dordrecht, The Netherlands, Reidel, 1982.

> This edited volume describes the clinical contributions of applied anthropologists who conduct research and teach in health science settings.

Harwood A (ed): *Ethnicity and Medical Care*. Cambridge, MA, Harvard University Press, 1981.

> This edited volume offers rich accounts of the role of cultural values, attitudes, expectations, language, and beliefs in a wide array of ethnic groups' members' health behaviors.

Henry J: *Culture Against Man*. New York, Random House, 1963.

> Henry critically examines family, education, values, political ideologies, attitudes toward aging, and much more in this classic work on U.S. culture.

Johnson T, Sargent C (eds): *Medical Anthropology*, ed 2. Westport, CT, Greenwood Press, 1995.

> This encyclopedic volume represents a state-of-the-art review of the conceptual, methodological, and clinical issues in culture and medicine, including a focus on gender and health and HIV disease.

Stein HF, Apprey M: *From Metaphor to Meaning: Papers in Psychoanalytic Anthropology*. Charlottesville, VA, University Press of Virginia, 1987.

> Stein and Apprey offer interpretations of the intrapsychic story that is simultaneously represented and veiled by culture. They demonstrate how deceptively simple personal, familial, clinical, and larger cultural symbols condense complex ideas and feelings.

Stein HF: *American Medicine as Culture*. Boulder, CO, Westview Press, 1993.

> Stein presents a description and interpretation of U.S. biomedicine as an occupational culture. Topics include values, metaphors, control, group dynamics in clinical decision-making, money and medicine, the process of becoming a physician, and the self of the physician.

CHAPTER 11

A. Relationships

The Healthcare System

James W. Mold*

Dr. S. had become increasingly active on the staff of a rehabilitation hospital. He was particularly interested in geriatric rehabilitation, the most frequent admitter of older patients to the facility. With the encouragement of the chief of staff and administrator of the hospital he began having meetings with the staff to discuss ways to improve the care of older rehabilitation patients. One of the ideas he presented to the group made up of physicians, nurses, speech–language pathologists, occupational therapists, physical therapists, recreational therapists, social workers, case managers, and dietitians was to have each member of the team document her portion of the initial assessment in a single unified section of the chart and to put all progress notes within another unified section using a goal-oriented, rather than a problem-oriented, format.

Dr. S. was surprised at the resistance to his ideas. The physicians did not want other providers writing in the (physicians') progress notes section of the chart and they felt that a problem-oriented format was more appropriate than a goal-oriented system. The nursing staff was using a separate chart altogether, had put a great deal of effort into developing it, and saw no reason to change their system. Many of the therapists were enthusiastic about the idea, but were concerned about who would be involved in constructing the goals list, specifically wondering whether the physicians would control the process.

*With the assistance of Barbara Barrett, D.P.M.; F. Tohgi, D.C., L.Ac., Ph.D.; Dan Gentry, P.T.; Andre F. Fountain, R.N.; Kevin T. Avery, D.M.D.; Julia Eyer, Ph.D., CCC-SP; Martha J. Ferretti, M.P.H., P.T.; Marjorie Greer, LPT; Don Lanquist, RRT; Carol McCoy, Ph.D., MT (ASCP), CLS; Earl Schmitt, O.D., Ed.D.; Roberta Warner, R.D./L.D.; Terry Pace, Ph.D.; Linda E. Reed, P.A., M.Ed.; Bob Shahan, R.T.; Carole A. Sullivan, M.Ed., R.T.(R)T, FASRT; Sheila Tiarks, M.S.W.; Shirley Wunder, R.N.

INTRODUCTION

Although typically considered to be the principal providers of healthcare, physicians represent only one of a large number of disciplines that make up the healthcare system. Many of the other disciplines are comparatively new, reflecting the increasing complexity of modern healthcare. Table 11.1 is a partial list of "traditional" healthcare providers. In addition to these mainstream healthcare disciplines, a variety of "alternative" healthcare practices have gained prominence in recent years (Table 11.2).

For such a large and complex system to be effective and efficient, a certain amount of teamwork is required. Unfortunately, the training received by the practitioners in each discipline is usually discipline specific, with surprisingly little integration with the training programs of the other disciplines. As a result, conceptual approaches to healthcare and even the terminologies used by providers from the various disciplines often differ considerably. In addition, because of differences in responsibilities and rewards as well as some overlap of competencies, there is a natural tendency for the various groups to be sus-

TABLE 11.1

Characteristics of "Traditional" Healthcare Professionals

Discipline	Year and number of practitioners in U.S.		Length of training	Degree
Physicians				
Allopathic[a]	1993	670,336	5–11 years	M.D.
Osteopathic[b]	1993	33,514	5–11 years	D.O.
Podiatric[d]	1991	12,600	6–7 years	D.P.M.
Psychologists[d]	1990	22,888	5–8 years	Ph.D.
Social workers[d]	1990	53,487	4–8 years	B.A., M.S.W., Ph.D.
Speech pathologists/audiologists[d]	1988	52,600	4–6 years	CCC-SP; CCC-A; CCC-SP/A
Pharmacists[d]	1991	163,600	5–6 years	Pharm.D.
Physician associates[c]	1994	26,000	2–4 years	P.A.
Dental practitioners[b]	1992	155,058	4 years	D.D.S.
Nurses				
Registered nurses[b]	1991	1,758,000	2–4 years	R.N.
Licensed practical nurses[e]	1993	886,597	1 year	L.P.N.
Optometrists[d]	1991	26,500	4 years	O.D.
Dietitians[d]	1991	35,294	4–5 years	R.D./L.D.
Medical technologists[d]	1991	161,087	3–5 years	
Occupational therapists[d]	1991	33,000	4–8 years	O.T.R.
Recreational therapists	1995	13,260	4 years	
Physical therapists[d]	1991	70,000	4–5 years	P.T.
Respiratory therapists[d]	1989	82,400	2–5 years	RRT/CRTT
Radiology technologists	1994	235,763	2–4 years	RTR/RT(N)/RRT RT(US)/RT(CT)

[a]American Medical Association, *Physician Characteristics and Distribution in the U.S.*, 1994 edition.

[b]Health Care State Rankings, *Health Care in the 50 United States*, O'Leary K, Morgan S, Quitno N (eds) Lawrence, Kans, Morgan Quitno Corp, 1994.

[c]*1994 Physician Assistant Programs Directory*, Alexandria, VA.

[d]*Health United States 1993*, U.S. Department of Health and Human Services, Hyattsville, MD, 1994.

[e]National Foundation of Certified Nurses, Research Division, Chicago.

Table 11.2
Partial List of Alternative Healthcare Disciplines
and Practices

Acupuncture	Iridology
Ayurveda	Macrobiotics
Chelation therapy	Massage
Chiropractic	Meditation
Herbal medicine	Naturopathy
Homeopathy	Reflexology
Hypnosis	Rolfing
Imagery	Spiritual healing

picious and sometimes envious of each other, a tendency that, at its worst, leads to what is commonly called protecting one's turf (territory), as illustrated in Case 11-1.

When the healthcare system can overcome the barriers between disciplines, it can function in a truly interdisciplinary way. Cooperation such as this results in improved coordination of healthcare with less duplication of efforts. More overall energy can be applied to patient care.

The goals of this chapter are to introduce the major healthcare providers, both traditional and alternative, including information about roles, practice settings, training, and certification. The consultation and referral process is described. The concept of interdisciplinary teamwork is introduced and described. Some of the obstacles to implementation of a team approach are discussed, and suggestions are made regarding ways to overcome those obstacles.

CASE 11-2

Mrs. B. F. was a 68-year-old woman who had coronary artery bypass surgery 6 years earlier and now was experiencing recurrent symptoms related to her severe coronary artery disease, uncontrolled by medications. Her physician, Dr. J., requested a cardiologist's opinion regarding the risks and benefits to Mrs. F. of another coronary artery bypass operation. The cardiologist, after evaluating Mrs. F., agreed that surgery was a possible option and requested the additional input of a cardiothoracic surgeon. The surgeon, after reviewing the cardiac catheterization results, recommended against surgery because of the high operative risk for this particular patient.

However, Dr. J. felt that his questions had not been properly answered. He already knew that the risk associated with a second cardiac surgery would be high, but he believed his patient might be willing to take a substantial risk because of the persistence of her chest pain after trying all other available treatments. What Dr. J. really needed to know were the probabilities of benefit and of the various possible adverse outcomes associated with surgery for his patient so that he could intelligently help Mrs. F. to make the best possible decision taking into account her own values and preferences.

PHYSICIANS

Practitioners of several different disciplines use the title "physician" and/or "doctor." These include allopathic physicians, osteopathic physicians, doctors of podiatric medicine, doctors of optomety, chiropractic physicians, and homeopathic and naturopathic physicians. At present, allopathic and osteopathic physicians are most similar in terms of training, credentialing, practice activities, and stature. For this reason, after a brief review of their different philosophical origins, they will be discussed together, while the other groups will be discussed individually later in the chapter.

The terms *allopathy* and *allopathic medicine* were coined by Hahnemann around 1849 to distinguish "ordinary" medical practice from the emerging field of homeopathy. They imply an active approach to the treatment of disease using medications and surgery to do what the body is unable to do itself. Allopathic physicians are currently the predominant type of physician in the United States. Their education involves an undergraduate college degree including a variety of prerequisite—mainly science—courses, 4 years of undergraduate medical education leading to the M.D., medical doctor, degree, and from 1 to 7 years of residency training.

OSTEOPATHIC PHYSICIANS

Osteopathy was founded by Andrew Still on the following principles, which he felt to be sufficiently distinct from those of allopathic physicians at that time (Jones, 1978):

1. The body is an integral unit, a whole. The structure of the body and its functions work together, interdependently.
2. The body systems have built-in repair processes, which are self-regulating and self-healing in the face of disease.
3. The circulatory system or distributing channels of the body, along with the nervous system, provide the integrating functions for the rest of the body.
4. The contribution of the musculoskeletal system to a person's health is much more than providing framework and support.
5. While disease may be manifested in specific parts of the body, other body parts may contribute to a restoration or correction of the disease.

Dr. Still had become fascinated with the musculoskeletal system, spending large amounts of time studying it in great detail. At the same time he opposed many of the medicinal remedies that were in vogue at the time, and was therefore interested in non-pharmacological treatments for disease that could enhance the body's natural repair mechanisms. He become convinced that manipulation of the musculoskeletal system could affect beneficial changes in all other systems, particularly the circulatory and nervous systems, which he felt were critical to the body's natural reparative mechanisms.

Although musculoskeletal manipulation is now a relatively small part of the practice of osteopathic physicians, it has been emphasized during the historically aggressive and persistent, though now weakening, campaign by allopaths to discredit and ostracize osteopaths. It has only been within the last two decades that osteopaths have been allowed to be members of the medical staffs at predominantly allopathic hospitals. It is still more difficult for osteopaths to obtain malpractice insurance in many areas.

Currently osteopathic physicians receive essentially the same quantity and quality of training as allopathic physicians, with only minor differences in philosophy and emphasis.

Their terminal degree is the D.O., doctor of osteopathy, degree. Although barriers and philosophical distinctions between the two physician groups are diminishing, there are no obvious signs that they intend to unite in the near future. For a variety of reasons, including the basic principles of the discipline, osteopaths have always been trained as generalists first and foremost, and although specialty training is available in all of the traditional areas, a larger percentage of osteopaths end up in general practice compared with allopathic physicians. Osteopathic physicians have also been more likely to practice in rural settings than their allopathic counterparts, a fact that has not gone unnoticed by state legislatures, resulting in substantial political power for osteopaths. Many osteopaths do osteopathic or allopathic residency programs in a primary care or subspecialty after medical school.

Physicians have tended to occupy the highest leadership roles in the healthcare delivery system, reflecting their extensive training and a highly revered position in society. They often chair hospital committees and are frequently the directors of peer review organizations (PROs). They often hold important positions within health insurance companies and managed care systems as well. State and national physician organizations, such as state medical societies and the American Medical Association, exert a powerful influence on legislators. Although administrators are now taking away some of the authority and responsibility that has traditionally belonged to physicians, among healthcare providers it is still physicians who most frequently give the orders that other providers are expected to follow. And it is physicians who bear the greatest liability when something goes wrong. Many physicians believe strongly that other healthcare professionals are, or should be, under their direct control and should only be involved in patient care by direct order of a physician.

Because of the current dominance of the biomedical model of health, physicians, as the most highly trained biomedical applied scientists, are the most powerful members of the healthcare team. Other health professionals are often forced, then, to function in supporting roles. There is some reason to believe, however, that the current biomedical model may soon undergo a transformation that may alter the traditional hierarchy to some degree. The pressure for such a paradigm shift comes from consumers who have become increasingly dissatisfied with the current biotechnical, physician-dominated approach, which they view as too impersonal, mechanistic, and expensive (Freymann, 1989).

While in the past physicians have traditionally been male and other healthcare disciplines predominantly female, since 1967, the percentage of female physicians has increased substantially. Differentials in average income undoubtedly reflect differences in training and responsibility and perhaps also a measure of sexism. As more women choose to become physicians and more men become nurses and allied health professionals, these differences may become less significant.

INTERACTIONS AMONG PHYSICIANS

As the field of medicine has become more complex, physicians have become increasingly subspecialized. Table 11.3 lists the major medical and surgical subspecialties. Many of the same kinds of turf issues that occur between healthcare disciplines also occur between subspecialties of medicine for similar reasons. Subspecialized physicians tend to have greater status and higher incomes than generalists. This is in contrast to most modern corporations in which individuals with the most specialized training head divisions, whereas corporate leaders are, of necessity, generalists. Part of the income differential between subspecialists and generalists is the result of third-party reimbursement practices.

Table 11.3
Major Medical and Surgical Specialties

Allergy and immunology	Otolaryngology
Anesthesiology	Pathology
Colon and rectal surgery	Pediatrics
Dermatology	Physical medicine and rehabilitation
Emergency medicine	Plastic surgery
Family practice	Preventive medicine
Internal medicine	Psychiatry and neurology
Neurology	Radiology
Nuclear medicine	Surgery
Obstetrics and gynecology	Thoracic surgery
Ophthalmology	Urology
Orthopedic surgery	

Despite their higher incomes and status, subspecialists are dependent on generalists for consultations and referral of patients. Thus, there is some pressure on subspecialists to be gracious and to return patients to the referring physicians as promptly as possible. These courtesies often break down within medical centers and other larger organizations in which, for one reason or another, subspecialists are less dependent on, or are less aware of their dependency on, primary care physician referrals, as in Case 11-2.

Patients interested in obtaining the best possible medical care are faced with the choice either of seeing the appropriate subspecialists for each of their health problems or of seeing a generalist (family physician, internist, or pediatrician), whom they must trust to refer them to subspecialists when appropriate. Studies indicate that family physicians manage 85 to 95% of the healthcare problems that their patients present to them without consultation or referral (AAFP, 1991). Because of their familiarity with specialist colleagues and with the local healthcare system, generalist physicians are often in a good position to advise their patients when consultation with other providers is necessary and which subspecialists would provide the best service in specific situations.

However, generalists are less likely to recognize and diagnose unusual problems as quickly and accurately as subspecialists. They are therefore susceptible to *errors of omission*. Subspecialists, on the other hand, often have less familiarity with the patient, are less able to view health problems in context, are expected not to make errors of omission, and have more technology at their fingertips, making them more susceptible to *errors of commission*, doing too much. Errors of omission are more obvious than errors of commission, but they are not necessarily more harmful. Increasingly aggressive attempts, through testing and other interventions, to reduce uncertainty and the anxiety that accompanies it at times may result in an avalanche of unwanted consequences. This phenomenon has been called the "cascade effect" (Mold & Stein, 1986). Clinical cascades may be catastrophic and obvious but are more often inapparent and unrecognized.

Increasingly, insurance companies are dictating the choices that patients can make regarding the level of care appropriate for particular problems. The system is moving toward a greater reliance on primary care with somewhat fewer subspecialists for reasons of cost effectiveness. With the advent of managed care as the dominant healthcare delivery model, primary care physicians will assume a much more prominent and influential role.

Integral to the professional relationship between physicians is the consultative process. Classically, a physician asks a consultant on behalf of his patient for advice regarding the diagnosis or treatment of a particular health problem. The request may be communicated by phone, letter, or by the patient. The more effectively the request is communicated, the more likely the consultant is to be helpful by providing the answers to the referring physician's questions. Once the consultant has reached an opinion, he communicates it to the patient and primary physician and returns the patient to the care of the primary physician unless requested to do otherwise (McWhinney, 1989c). Obviously, good communication between physicians is essential to the consultative process, but for several reasons, including time constraints, fear of disclosing incompetence, and lack of training in the consultative process, it doesn't always occur.

A proper request for consultation should include the specific questions that are being asked of the consultant and specific directives as to the extent of involvement requested of the consultant in the evaluation and management of the patient. The physician requesting the consultation may, for example, request that the consultant render an opinion regarding diagnosis or treatment but not assume responsibility for implementation of the recommended treatment or for ongoing care. At times it is necessary and appropriate for one physician to refer a patient to another physician for ongoing management of one or more problems. This process, which is called *referral*, requires the same careful communication as described for the consultative process.

Although the opinion of the consultant should obviously be given a great deal of consideration, it is in no way binding. Neither the physician requesting the consultation nor the patient is under any ethical or legal obligation to follow the advice of the consultant. It should be remembered that although the consultant brings specialized knowledge and skills to bear on the problem in question, the referring physician and patient have equally important information that must be considered before a final decision can be made. Under no circumstances should a consultant send the patient to a second consultant without the authorization and approval of the primary physician, as was done in Case 11-2. Unfortunately, even when the request for a consultation is communicated effectively, the consultation does not always prove helpful. In such a situation, the physician involved may need to communicate the request again directly, or it may be necessary for the primary physician to consult a different subspecialist.

PHYSICIAN ASSOCIATES/ASSISTANTS

Once called "physician extenders," physician associates (PA) are healthcare professionals who provide services to patients under the supervision of physicians. PAs take medical histories, perform physical examinations, and order laboratory tests. Under the direct or indirect supervision of either an allopathic or osteopathic physician, they make diagnoses and initiate treatment plans. PAs also perform patient education and counseling. They practice in private practices, health maintenance organizations, nursing homes, student health services, urban and rural clinics, correctional institutions, and industry. In addition, some PAs have become involved in medical education, health administration, or research.

PAs are trained in programs accredited by the Committee on Allied Health Education and Accreditation (CAHEA). The first phase of the 2-year curriculum includes classroom and laboratory instruction in the basic medical sciences. The second phase consists of structured clinical rotations providing the students with direct patient contact. These rotations are intensive hands-on learning experiences in private and institutional medical settings that emphasize training in primary care (family practice, internal medicine, and pediatrics) but also include experience in obstetrics and gynecology, surgery, and emergency medicine.

Degrees awarded on completion of a program vary, depending on the institution offering the program and the educational background of the student. Most programs offer a baccalaureate degree on graduation. A few masters-level and residency programs are available either within the core PA curricula or for postgraduate specialization in such areas as occupational medicine, surgery, and pediatrics.

PAs, working with other members of the healthcare team, improve the overall distribution of healthcare services and access to care in rural areas and underserved communities. They also increase the efficiency of ambulatory care practices, reduce patient waiting time, and allow physicians more time for difficult cases. By stressing preventive health maintenance and periodic screening, they may help to reduce excess morbidity and mortality (Jones & Cawley, 1994).

CASE 11-3

A 40-year-old insulin-dependent diabetic, E. W., who had previously achieved excellent diabetic control, had recently begun to have blood glucose levels in the 200 to 300 mg/dl (normal ≤ 100 mg/dl) range for reasons that were unclear to him. His physician seemed equally puzzled. Because of some gum swelling and irritation, he saw his dentist. The dentist discovered an abscess under one of E. W.'s teeth, which he treated with antibiotics and surgical drainage. One week later, E. W.'s diabetes again came under good control. No communication occurred between the two health professionals involved.

DENTISTS

Approximately 85% of dental practitioners in the United States are generalists. Only one state (Delaware) requires a year of residency training following the 4 year dental school curriculum. Most states require National Board examinations, and practical clinical examinations are also conducted in most jurisdictions. In some areas, regional clinical board examinations have been organized. The American Dental Association (ADA) recognizes eight dental subspecialties: orthodontics, oral surgery, oral pathology, endodontics, pediatric dentistry, dental public health, periodontics, and prosthodontics, all of which require several years of additional training beyond dental school.

Dentists provide a wide variety of services: prevention, diagnosis, and treatment of dental caries; gingival and periodontal disease; malocclusion; temporomandibular joint dysharmony; soft tissue pathology; and various cosmetic problems. The dental caries rate in the U.S. population has been substantially reduced as a result of water fluoridation. As a result, the rate of edentualism is much lower, and many more people are at risk for periodontal disease. The profile of services that dentists provide has therefore shifted to include fewer fillings and extractions and more endodontics, periodontics, and cosmetic restorations (Ring, 1985). Part of this shift is also related to new technology and to patient expectations. People now expect to keep their natural teeth over a lifetime and are demanding treatment in order to do so. In 1988 the U.S. population spent more than $37 billion on dental care. Half of that amount came directly from patients, almost half from third parties, and very little from the government.

Physicians and dentists working together could better educate their patients, identify problems early, and make appropriate referrals in contrast to what often happens, as illustrated in Case 11-3. Most dental diseases are either preventable or much easier and less costly to treat in the incipient stages. Particularly critical to oral health are episodes of severe physical illness when resistance is compromised and oral hygiene is likely to be less adequate. Physicians must be particularly alert to the potential need for dental evaluation and treatment during or following such episodes.

CASE 11-4

Mrs. R., a 60-year-old debilitated white female, was admitted for pneumonia and dehydration. Her regular physician, Dr. P., was on vacation. His associate did not know Mrs. R., nor did he have access to her chart in the emergency room. The physician's orders at admission included a regular diet, an intravenous infusion of 5% dextrose and normal saline, and penicillin to be given intravenously.

During the admission assessment by a registered nurse, Mrs. R.'s daughter arrived. Prior to instituting the physician's orders, the nurse interviewed the daughter and discovered that Mrs. R. had insulin-dependent diabetes mellitus and had not eaten or taken her insulin in the last 24 hours. She also discovered that Mrs. R. was allergic to penicillin. The nurse placed a call to the physician and, while waiting for his return call, started the intravenous infusion with normal saline, withholding dextrose until appropriate insulin and diet orders could be given. The nurse then called the pharmacy and put a hold on the penicillin order and clearly marked the chart so that the penicillin would not be given inadvertently by another nurse.

NURSES

Florence Nightingale described a nurse's role as "putting the patient in the best condition for nature to act upon him." In 1980, the American Nurses' Association redefined nursing as "the diagnosis and treatment of human responses to actual or potential health problems," reflecting a somewhat more expansive concept of the involvement of nurses in patient care (Friedman, 1990). In most clinical settings, nurses spend a greater amount of time working directly with patients than any other healthcare professionals. Their impact on outcomes is often underestimated. For example, studies of postoperative mortality rates between hospitals have consistently pointed to the experience and qualifications of the nursing staff as one of the major variables determining outcome. Case 11-4 is another example of good nursing care that could easily go unrecognized and unrewarded by other members of the healthcare team.

Collaboration between physicians and nurses, though vitally important for optimal patient care, is too often suboptimal (Stein *et al.*, 1990; Friedman, 1990; Fagin, 1992). Physicians frequently regard nurses as subordinates whose major responsibility is to carry out their orders. Nurses, on the other hand, consider themselves as healthcare professionals in roles as equally important and distinct as physicians. Although nurse practice acts vary from state to state, several legal opinions have held nurses responsible for failing to take timely and responsive action, such as failing to communicate patient condition changes to the physician and failure to discover conditions not found by the physician.

Mechanic (1983) described the tension between nurses and physicians regarding clinical decision-making responsibilities as follows:

> Clinical decision making is the major source of continuing tension between nurses and physicians in the hospital context. Nurses have been cast in roles where they frequently must make clinical decisions, some of critical life-and-death significance, but they work under institutional rules that recognize only physicians as having authority to make independent professional decisions about patients. . . . Much of the continuing conflict between nurses and physicians could be reduced if better agreements regarding decision making could be achieved which appropriately recognized nurses' levels of expertise and their particular responsibilities for seriously ill patients.

Like medicine, nursing has begun to develop a subspecialty structure, allowing nurses to develop greater expertise in more limited areas. This should result in increased status, income, and decision-making responsibility. Nursing clinical specialties have for the most part been organized around medical subspecialties, but with a clearer differentiation between ambulatory and hospital-based practice. Subspecialty-trained, master's degree nurses in hospital practice are called clinical nurse specialists, whereas those in ambulatory settings are more often educationally prepared as nurse practitioners or as nurse midwives (Kassirer, 1994; Maule, 1994). Their training differs, reflecting different roles and responsibilities.

CASE 11-5

O. L. was a 79-year-old man admitted to the hospital because of intractable pain and disability resulting from a vertebral compression fracture. His physician pursued a diagnostic evaluation and ordered narcotics for the pain. He consulted a physical therapist for advice regarding pain management and mobilization. The physical therapist with the assistance of orthotist fitted O. L. with a thoracolumbar extension brace and taught him to use a transcutaneous nerve stimulation unit. She taught him bed exercises and provided him with a walker for trips to the bathroom.

In several days, although he was much more comfortable, O. L. felt that he would benefit by a short nursing-home stay before returning to his home to care for himself. The hospital social worker helped him make the necessary arrangements and discussed home care options in case he should need them once he returned home. He also mentioned to O. L. that an occupational therapist might be able to suggest some home modifications and adaptive equipment that might allow O. L. to return home more quickly.

——————— ALLIED HEALTH PROFESSIONALS ———————

The major allied health professions are listed in Table 11.4. During this century, the rise of the allied health disciplines has been one of the most dramatic developments in the healthcare delivery system, reflecting both the increasing complexity of patient care and the increasing use of technology for diagnosis and treatment.

The relationships among the various allied health professional associations, the American Medical Association, and the certifying and licensing bodies governing each

Table 11.4
Allied Health Professionals

Audiologists
Dietitians
Laboratory professionals
Medical technologists
Medical laboratory technicians
Cytotechnologists
Histological technicians
Occupational therapists and OT assistants
Physical therapists
Radiologic technologists
Nuclear medicine technologists
Radiation therapists
Ultrasonographers
CT/MRI technologists
Mammographers
Recreational therapists
Respiratory therapists
Social workers
Speech pathologists and audiologists

discipline are somewhat complicated, at times strained, and subject to fairly frequent modifications. An additional complicating factor in recent years has been the tension between the federal government (Medicare, Medicaid), state governments (Medicaid), and the private sector created by efforts to contain costs while assuring quality.

CLINICAL DIETITIANS

Nutritional status is obviously a very important component of health. The evaluation of current nutritional status, calculation of adjustments needed to achieve nutritional well-being, development and implementation of a plan to meet those goals, and education of the patient and other caregivers are all important and expected responsibilities of clinical dietitians.

Most accredited hospitals and rehabilitation facilities require that nutrition support be provided by a *registered* or *licensed* dietitian. These titles denote a level of expertise acquired through an American Dietetics Association (ADA)-regulated combination of didactic and clinical learning. Many facilities require ADA registration, which documents passage of a professional examination and monitored maintenance of continuing education hours in compliance with ADA regulations. Some states have also implemented a licensing procedure through state medical licensure boards, which protects the consumer from persons practicing under false credentials and guards against inappropriate practice behavior of its members. The initials R.D. or L.D. will appear with the person's signature if these higher levels of certification have been achieved. The term *nutritionist* has been used by many to imply professional expertise in the area of human nutrition. However, this title is not protected from misuse by persons with questionable educational background and sometimes inaccurate or unethical presentation of information to the consumer.

A. R. was an 8-year-old girl brought to the emergency room by her parents for evaluation of recurrent leg pains occurring at night, preventing her from sleeping. The episodes had been occurring occasionally for 4 months but had been getting more frequent and severe for the past 2 weeks.

Dr. Y. was working in the emergency room on the night that A. R. came in. Results of his examination of her were completely unremarkable. However, he ordered a complete blood count (CBC) with a differential count and an erythrocyte sedimentation rate (ESR) as a precaution. The machine-run CBC results showed normal parameters. Review of the differential white blood cell count by the medical technologist revealed the presence of immature white blood cells. To further investigate the possibility of acute leukemia, a bone marrow biopsy was performed. With the results of the special stains performed by the medical technologist and review of the bone marrow aspirate by the pathologist, the diagnosis was confirmed. A. R. was expected to have a good prognosis because her disease was diagnosed at such an early stage.

MEDICAL TECHNOLOGISTS/CYTOTECHNOLOGISTS

Laboratory professionals represent the single largest group of allied health professionals. This reflects the heavy reliance of modern patient care on analytical laboratory testing and procedures for the diagnosis, treatment, and monitoring of patient care. There are several categories of laboratory professionals. Educational requirements differ based on scope of practice.

Medical technologists represent the largest group. Both hospital-based and university-based programs utilize the clinical setting in hospital laboratories for this part of the educational experience. All programs integrate theory with analytical testing performed in the clinical laboratory.

The medical technologist performs analytical testing, evaluates the validity of the results, and reports the results to the physician who requested the test, as illustrated in Case 11-6. If there is a question regarding the clinical correlation of the results and the patient's condition, a clinical pathologist provides the consultation.

Medical technologists are able to work in any of the clinical laboratory specialties, i.e., blood bank, chemistry, toxicology, microbiology, and hematology. They are employed in hospital and independent laboratories as well as medical and industrial research laboratories. Some obtain specialty certifications after the medical technology certification. Many supervisors and managers hold master's degrees.

A *cytotechnologist* screens slides for the presence of cancer and other disease states. Any diagnosis of malignancy is confirmed by an anatomic pathologist. The largest portion of the work performed by a cytotechnologist is in the screening of Pap smears. Cytotechnologists also screen many nongynecological specimens such as bronchial washing and fine-needle aspirations of masses for the presence of cancer cells. Some take additional training and are employed in cytogenetics laboratories.

Histological technicians prepare tissue specimens for viewing by a pathologist. The histology laboratory has recently expanded its diagnostic capabilities via special types of stains, e.g., immunochemistry.

Physical therapists are mobility experts. Through neuromusculoskeletal evaluation   **ALLIED HEALTH**
and the use of a variety of treatment modalities they help patients to maintain or improve   **PROFESSIONALS**
their ability to move about. Physical therapists practice in a variety of settings, providing
inpatient, outpatient, and community-based services. Unique settings include community
health centers, public schools, private practices, athletic centers, and specialty medical
clinics as well as hospitals and rehabilitation centers.

Opportunities for specialization following entry-level education are increasing. The
American Physical Therapy Association (APTA)-sponsored American Board of Physical
Therapy Specialties presently offers board certification in six specialty areas: pediatric
physical therapy, orthopedic physical therapy, sports physical therapy, clinical electro-
physiology physical therapy, cardiopulmonary physical therapy, and neurological physical
therapy.

A physical therapy assessment may include determination of motion, strength, and
endurance abilities of the patient; evaluation of balance, coordination, and postural (static
and dynamic) abilities; establishment of quantitative and qualitative profiles of movement
abilities; development of a profile of the cardiopulmonary abilities of the patient; and
definition of electrophysiological responses to various electrical modalities. Therapeutic
regimens consist of a wide range of interventions, from the application of specific modalities, heat, ice, ultrasound, diathermy, and so forth, to exercise, musculoskeletal rehabilitation, and the reeducation of various functions. In addition to treatment of physical impairments, physical therapists provide a wide range of consulting services in areas such as
health promotion and fitness, prevention of athletic injuries, and the prevention of work-
related injuries and trauma.

OCCUPATIONAL THERAPISTS

Occupational therapists use selected educational, vocational, and rehabilitative activities to help individuals reach the highest functional levels possible, become self-reliant,
and build a balanced life-style of work and leisure. In partnership with their clients, they
frequently work with other members of a healthcare team and with community agencies
not only to treat patients with disabilities but also to attempt to prevent disabilities from
occurring. Whereas physical therapists focus on mobility, strength, and endurance, occupational therapists more frequently deal with activities of daily living such as bathing,
dressing, cooking, and driving (see Case 11-5).

Occupational therapists work in hospitals, clinics, schools, rehabilitation centers,
home care programs, private practice, community health centers, nursing homes, day-care
centers, and psychiatric facilities. A registered occupational therapist (OTR) carries professional and administrative responsibilities for occupational therapy programs and services and is responsible for evaluating clients, deciding on program goals, working with
clients to implement those goals, and evaluating progress. In addition, OTRs educate
students entering the field and may be involved in research.

Certified occupational therapy assistants (COTAs) work under the supervision of an
OTR. They are high school graduates or the equivalent who complete an associate degree
program in an accredited university or community college or a 1-year certificate program
in an accredited educational institution. A minimum of 2 months of supervised fieldwork

is also included. Graduates are eligible for certification as a COTA on passage of a national certification examination.

RADIOLOGIC TECHNOLOGISTS

Radiologic technologists can be subdivided into four major groups: radiographers, nuclear medicine technologists, radiation therapists, and diagnostic medical sonographers. Members of the first three groups, who are involved in the use of radiation of various types for either diagnostic or therapeutic purposes, are different in several other ways from diagnostic medical ultrasonographers, who are involved in the use of high-frequency sound waves. Diagnostic medical sonographers are credentialed by the American Registry of Medical Sonographers, whereas the others receive their credentialing through the American Registry of Radiologic Technologists.

Radiographers [R.T.(R)s] are responsible for obtaining radiographs (X rays) as requested by a physician to be interpreted by a radiologist. This involves working closely with patients and with a variety of sophisticated equipment. They must know how to properly position the patient, set the proper radiation exposure levels, protect the patient from unnecessary radiation exposure, and determine whether adequate images have been obtained. With the development of computed tomography, magnetic resonance imaging, and mammography, special training and certification are now required to operate these instruments.

Nuclear medical technologists [R.T.(N)s] administer radiopharmaceuticals to patients and operate a variety of scanning instruments that produce radiographic images of various parts of the body for diagnostic purposes. Brain, bone, liver, and thyroid scans as well as dynamic cardiac and pulmonary scans are examples of the tests they routinely perform.

Radiation therapists are involved in the administration of ionizing radiation primarily to cancer patients for therapeutic purposes. Because of the nature of cancer, and since treatments are generally given repetitively over a period of time, radiation therapy technologists often develop close relationships with patients and their families and are therefore called on to function as members of interdisciplinary teams.

Although most radiologic technologists frequently work in hospital settings or in large clinics, *diagnostic medical ultrasonographers* work in a variety of settings. Cardiologists, obstetricians and gynecologists, and occasionally general surgeons and primary care physicians may employ ultrasonographers to assist them in the evaluation of common problems such as valvular heart disease and congestive heart failure, pelvic masses, pregnancy dating, gallstones, and peripheral vascular diseases.

RECREATIONAL THERAPISTS

Recreational therapists constitute a diverse group of professionals. Some areas of interest and expertise of recreational therapists are (1) self-esteem/confidence building, (2) independent living/self-reliance building, (3) self-expression/enrichment of life, (4) group acceptance/development of interpersonal skills, (5) hospital and play therapy/fear reduction, (6) art and music therapy/self-expression and fulfillment, and (7) physical activities/physical condition and stress reduction. They are employed in a variety of settings, including hospitals, rehabilitation centers, nursing homes, mental health centers, community parks and recreation departments, schools, sheltered workshops, and correctional centers.

Recreational therapists must complete an approved associate's degree program. Certification is awarded by The National Council for Therapeutic Recreational Certification after satisfactory completion of a certifying examination. Licensure or registration is also required in many states, often through the state's Board of Medical Examiners.

RESPIRATORY THERAPISTS

On successful completion of the registry examination of the National Board for Respiratory Therapy, respiratory therapists become registered respiratory therapists (RRT). Under the direction of a physician, respiratory therapists are responsible for the administration of therapeutic gases, oxygen, carbon dioxide–oxygen mixtures, aerosols and humidity, bronchodilators, corticosteroids, aerosolized water, assisted ventilation, respirators, positive airway pressure, chest physical therapy to mobilize secretions and stimulate cough, breathing exercises, and more. They perform blood gas sampling and pulmonary function testing, and they provide individualized patient education and follow-up.

SOCIAL WORKERS

Social work practice focuses on the relationship between individuals and their environment and is directed toward defining and resolving problems that develop in this relationship. Social workers are therefore trained to evaluate the psychosocial aspects of an individual's situation. They are often able to provide supportive counseling to individuals and families and act as their advocates in situations where environmental changes would be helpful, as in Case 11-5. They are especially well trained to locate community resources that may enhance the quality of life of an individual or family.

A majority of practicing social workers have a master's degree (M.S.W.). Social workers who have received special training in mental health services such as individual or family therapy are called *psychiatric social workers*.

The specific activities of a social worker depend somewhat on the occupational setting in which the social worker practices and the amount and type of training he has received. Common practice settings include medical and psychiatric hospitals and clinics, schools, nursing homes, special shelters, government agencies, the workplace, family service agencies, churches, and private practice. Social workers often function as case managers in settings in which interdisciplinary teamwork is practiced.

SPEECH–LANGUAGE PATHOLOGISTS AND AUDIOLOGISTS

Speech–language pathologists and audiologists are health professionals who deal with the normal and developmental aspects of human communication, communication disorders, and clinical techniques for evaluation and management of these disorders. Their training involves a minimum of 300 hours of supervised clinical experience and 9 months of full-time professional experience, termed a *clinical fellowship* (American Speech–Language–Hearing Association, 1989), in a variety of settings, including hospitals, rehabilitation facilities, and public and private outpatient settings. They often work closely with otorhinolaryngologists, neurologists, psychiatrists, dentists, and plastic surgeons. Much of their work involves children with congenital and development disorders and the elderly who have acquired disabilities such as deafness and aphasia.

Audiologists are concerned with diagnosis and remediation of hearing loss. Responsibilities include prescription and fitting of amplification. They are accountable for provision of auditory, speech, and reading training. Speech and language pathologists diagnose and remediate speech disorders (e.g., problems of fluency, voice, and articulation) and language disorders (e.g., aphasia, reading disorders, and delayed language development). Many are also involved in the evaluation and treatment of eating and swallowing problems, augmentative communication devices, and alternate forms of communication such as sign language and esophageal speech.

PHARMACISTS

Pharmacy is the third largest health profession after registered nurses and physicians. Over 1.5 billion prescription orders are dispensed annually from community and hospital pharmacies in the United States (Smith & Knapp, 1987). Pharmacists are involved in the dispensing of nonprescription, over-the-counter (OTC) medications as well.

Almost 90% of active pharmacists are practicing in clinical settings. Another 10% are involved in the development, production, or distribution of drugs, teaching, research, legal and regulatory activities regarding pharmaceutical practice, public health activities, association work, and journalism. The clinical work of pharmacists includes community pharmacy, hospital pharmacy, drug information centers, poison control centers, and supervision of dispensing practices in long-term care facilities such as nursing homes. An increasing number of residencies and fellowships are available for academic and clinical pharmacists in specialized areas such as psychiatry, geriatrics, internal medicine, pediatrics, pharmacokinetics, family medicine, and others.

Pharmacists are involved in many clinical activities: verification of prescriptions for accuracy, legality, and physical and chemical compatibility; advice to patients and other healthcare providers regarding proper administration, potential side effects, and potential drug–drug and drug–nutrient interactions of prescription drugs; advice to patients and other healthcare providers regarding proper use and choice of OTC medications; advice to patients regarding personal health habits, smoking, drug abuse, etc.; referral of patients to other health professionals; instruction of patients and other healthcare providers regarding proper use of medical or surgical appliances, inhalers, colostomy bags, splints, and bandages; participation in mass screening programs, stool occult blood testing, hypertension screening, etc.; and participation in utilization review, medical audits, and other medical care evaluations in hospitals, nursing homes, etc. Other services of a more innovative and advanced nature include pharmacokinetic and nutrition consultations and primary care of patients, with special emphasis on hypertension, diabetes mellitus, hyperlipidemia, etc. Advanced trained pharmacists are also now able to conduct drug research with human subjects provided that a physician is part of the study team (Schulz & Brushwood, 1991).

Pharmacists may be the nation's most accessible healthcare professionals. However, in retail community pharmacy practice, an important factor that limits the ability of pharmacists to provide good care is their lack of access to complete patient-related information. Pharmacists, more than any other healthcare professionals, are often relatively isolated from other professionals. Patients would benefit greatly from improved communication between physicians and pharmacists particularly.

OPTOMETRISTS

Optometrists evaluate, diagnose, and manage a variety of ocular pathological conditions. Binocular and refractive conditions, along with accommodative and convergence relationships that can influence reading, learning, and other visual tasks, are major professional concerns. As is the case with other primary healthcare professions, the scope of optometric practice is governed by individual state laws. Optometrists may prescribe topical diagnostic pharmaceuticals throughout the nation and may administer a wider selection of therapeutic agents in half of the states.

Optometric training leading to the O.D., doctor of optometry, degree requires 4 years in an accredited school or college of optometry. Preadmission and undergraduate optometric requirements are parallel to those of other major health professions and include basic science courses such as biology, physics, advanced mathematics, organic chemistry, and microbiology. Postdoctoral residency programs are widely available. In order to obtain licensure, the optometric graduate must pass a board examination administered by the state in which he would practice.

Demarcations are sometimes indistinct between the professional roles of optometry and ophthalmology. Matters of serious ocular pathology and surgical intervention clearly require the expertise of an ophthalmologist, as well as systemic therapy, as might be suitable to remedy ocular pathologies and related disorders at a secondary or tertiary level of referral. Otherwise, in primary ophthalmic healthcare, the clinical activities of the two professions are very similar. Optometrists are employed as members of HMOs, in group practices, as industrial and sports vision consultants, in research capacities by ophthalmic companies, and in academic institutions.

PODIATRISTS

Podiatrists are clinicians trained to manage health-related conditions of the feet and ankles. Their 4-year training program, often supplemented with 2 to 3 or more years of residency, prepares them to utilize all of the same diagnostic and treatment approaches employed by allopathic and osteopathic physicians, including prescription of medications and various kinds of adaptive equipment (e.g., special footwear, orthotic devices, casts and splints) and performance of surgery. Many have hospital and operating room privileges. Most work out of private offices while others are employed by various healthcare facilities. Certification as a doctor of podiatric medicine (D.P.M.) requires a case study preparation and final examination by the American Board of Foot Surgery and successful completion of the National Board Examination. All states require state licensure as well.

MENTAL HEALTH PROFESSIONS

As in other healthcare professions, the decades since World War II have seen dramatic developments within the mental health and clinical behavioral science professions. These developments have been spurred by the maturing and professionalization of these relatively young disciplines. The emergence of new theoretical perspectives on mental health, an accumulating empirical data base, demonstrations of effective and generalizable clinical procedures and programs, and broader social acceptance of mental health concerns have all contributed to the growth of the mental health professions (Richardson, 1988). The development of the biopsychosocial (Engel, 1977) and multisystem (Tapp & Warner, 1985) theories of health and illness along with theories of stress and coping (Lazarus, 1966; Selye, 1976) have blurred the distinctions between physical and mental health and resulted in the development of the fields of behavioral medicine (Schwartz & Weiss, 1978) and health psychology (Millon *et al.*, 1982). Mental health professionals have been increasingly integrated into medical settings.

These developments have resulted in a diverse array of distinct yet overlapping clinical mental health professions. The primary mental health professions include psychiatry, psychology, counseling, marital and family therapy, social work, and psychiatric nursing.

Psychiatrists are physicians who specialize by completing a 3-year psychiatric residency during which they receive training and experience in the diagnosis and treatment of major mental illness. They may further subspecialize in order to work primarily with adults, children, or other identified groups.

There are two major schools of philosophy and training regarding U.S. psychiatry (Richardson, 1988). The traditional approach emphasizes the biological aspects of psychiatric illness. A second approach is primarily social and emphasizes environmental aspects of psychiatric illness. Most contemporary U.S. psychiatrists have a strong biological orientation and are highly trained in the diagnosis and pharmacological treatment of major mental illness. Depending on training and interest, psychiatrists may also be skilled in psychotherapy and other forms of psychosocial treatment. As physicians, psychiatrists are licensed to practice medicine by each state and, after completion of an approved residency and comprehensive examination, are certified by the American Board of Psychiatry.

Psychologists are nonphysician, doctoral-level behavioral scientists, typically holding doctor of philosophy (Ph.D.), doctor of psychology (Psy.D.), or doctor of education (Ed.D.) degrees. The American Psychological Association recognizes four professional specialties within psychology: clinical psychology, counseling psychology, school psychology, and industrial–organizational psychology (American Psychological Association, 1981). Three additional professional specialty areas are emerging: neuropsychology, health psychology, and forensic psychology. Diplomate status granted by the American Board of Professional Psychology requires at least 4 years of postdoctoral experience in the specialty area, a written examination, and direct peer review of clinical skills. Professional psychologists are licensed for independent practice by all states.

Clinical and *counseling psychology* have evolved out of different historical contexts (Tipton, 1983; Whitley, 1984). Clinical psychology has traditionally had a greater emphasis on the diagnosis and treatment of children, severe psychopathology in all ages, and services delivered in inpatient mental health settings, whereas counseling psychology has had a greater focus on assessment and treatment in rehabilitation settings, vocational, educational, and family counseling agencies, and with persons experiencing adjustment problems and other less severe forms of psychopathology. Despite these differences, it has been estimated that these two specialties have 80 to 90% overlap in training skills, work settings, and professional roles (Watkins *et al.*, 1986). Clinical and counseling psychologists are employed in many settings, including private practice, medical schools, hospitals, universities, mental health centers, other human service agencies, and research foundations. Their training includes basic and clinical coursework, a doctoral dissertation, and a 1-year clinical internship.

School psychologists specialize in the learning and mental health needs of children in educational settings. School psychologists are usually employed in school systems or academic research institutions. *Industrial–organizational psychologists* specialize in the study and design of organizational settings with regard to human performance and interpersonal relationships and are usually employed by large corporations and public institutions or in academic research settings. *Neuropsychologists* are typically clinical or counseling psychologists who complete special pre- and postdoctoral training in neuropsychology. Neuropsychologists conduct neuropsychological evaluations and contribute to diagnosis and treatment planning of patients with a variety of neurological injuries and rehabilitation concerns. They are typically employed in medical and rehabilitation settings but may also work with school systems and in academic research capacities. *Health psychologists* are also trained as clinical or counseling psychologists but specialize through pre- and post-doctoral work in preventive health and the psychological needs of general medical and surgical patients. Health psychologists work in a variety of hospital and medical settings. *Forensic psychologists* are clinical or counseling psychologists who further specialize in forensic issues and typically work in penal, law enforcement, or psychiatric hospital settings. Individuals trained at the master's level in psychology may be identified as psychological assistants or associates and are licensed by many states to provide limited psychological services under the supervision of a licensed doctoral-level psychologist.

Counselors and *family therapists* are important mental health professionals. The titles counselor, therapist, and family therapist are generic terms and have only recently begun to be defined and licensed by states. Typically, a counselor or family therapist has a master's degree in counseling or family therapy from an accredited college or university and has received a minimum of 6 months to 1 year of supervised clinical experience on at least a half-time basis. A limited number of practicing counselors and family therapists hold doctoral degrees. There are two major organizations that credential and monitor the training of these professions: the American Association of Counseling and Development and the American Association of Marriage and Family Therapy.

Counselors are usually affiliated with the American Association of Counseling and Development. They may specialize through graduate study and work experience in a variety of areas, such as mental health counseling, counseling of children, marriage and family counseling, school counseling, or rehabilitation counseling. Counselors who work with persons experiencing mental health problems should be further certified by the National Academy of Certified Clinical Mental Health Counselors. Certified clinical mental health counselors are licensed for independent practice in 28 states (Weikel & Palmo, 1989).

Family therapists are usually affiliated with and should be certified by the American Association of Marriage and Family Therapy (Nichols, 1984). Often counselors and family therapists belong to both organizations but may prefer to refer to their work as either counseling or family therapy. Counselors and family therapists are employed in a variety of settings, including mental health centers, guidance and counseling agencies, schools, and increasingly in private practice.

As previously discussed, social workers are also major providers of mental health services. Social workers often have unique skills and training qualifying them for roles as case managers within mental health organizations (Richardson, 1988). They may also be trained as psychotherapists or counselors. Psychiatric nurses are also important providers of mental health services. Nursing training is heterogeneous, and as a result there are multiple levels of training that may qualify a nurse to provide psychiatric services. The term *psychiatric clinical nurse specialist* has been suggested as designating an R.N. with a master's degree in psychiatric services. Such qualified nursing personnel may play an increasing role in the delivery and coordination of mental health services, especially in hospital settings (Richardson, 1988).

PASTORAL CARE

Ministers with additional training in either pastoral counseling or pastoral care also provide counseling services. Pastoral counselors are individuals who usually have an M.Div. (master of divinity) degree and have completed an additional 3 to 5 years of residency training in pastoral counseling. Some go on to obtain a D.Min. (doctor of ministry) degree as well. They typically work in outpatient counseling centers, clinics, and through churches and provide both psychological and spiritual counseling services. They are credentialed by the American Association of Pastoral Counselors.

Hospital chaplains who provide pastoral care receive from 1 to 2 years of residency training after their 3-year M.Div. degree program. They are trained to provide pastoral care to people in crisis, and work primarily in institutional settings such as hospitals, mental health facilities, and hospices. The training is provided by the Association for Clinical Pastoral Education (ACPE), The College of Pastoral Supervision and Psychotherapy (CPSP), and/or The National Association of Catholic Chaplains (NACC). Certification for chaplaincy is by The College of Chaplains or the NACC. Many chaplains go on to obtain their D.Min. degree.

CASE 11-7

Francis Tuttle was a 57-year-old stenographer who had for the last year been experiencing migratory muscle and joint pains. She had seen several allopathic physicians who had diagnosed a nonspecific inflammatory condition and prescribed various types of nonsteroidal anti-inflammatory medications, all of which upset her stomach and caused her blood pressure to go up and her ankles to swell. On the advice of a church friend, she decided to see a naturopath. She was pleased that he did not prescribe any medications other than some vitamins and herbs, and after his treatments she actually began to feel a great deal better.

NONTRADITIONAL HEALTHCARE PRACTICES

In addition to the methods employed by the traditional healthcare disciplines, a variety of alternative approaches exist, some of which are listed in Table 11.2. These alternatives to traditional healthcare are becoming increasingly popular in the United States, particularly in the last decade (Eisenberg *et al.*, 1993). Many of these practices are based on entirely different conceptual models of health and illness, and most have not been subjected to the same level of scientific scrutiny as the conventional methods. It should be acknowledged, however, that the efficacy of many conventional practices has never been studied well either. While these approaches are still considered to be "nontraditional, alternative, or unconventional" in the United States, it should be pointed out that up to 70% of the world's population rely on nonallopathic systems of healing (Krippner, 1995).

Interest in alternative forms of healthcare has been growing rapidly in the United States primarily among upper-middle-class, well-educated people. In a recent population survey reported by Eisenberg *et al.* (1993), one in three respondents reported using at least one unconventional therapy in the past year, and a third of these saw healthcare providers for unconventional therapy. The vast majority also sought help for the same condition from a medical doctor. However, three-quarters of them did not inform their medical doctors that they had done so. This may be because physicians in particular have been critical of many of these practices. Other studies suggest that from 10 to 50% of cancer patients use some form of alternative therapy (McGinnis, 1991). Interestingly, the American Medical Association revised its Code of Ethics in 1980, giving physicians permission to consult with, take referrals from, and make referrals to practitioners "without orthodox medical training" (Krippner, 1995). Recently an Office of Alternative Medicine has been established at the National Institutes of Health to direct research involving nontraditional therapies.

TRADITIONAL CHINESE MEDICINE

Chinese traditional medicine has probably been practiced for more than 23 centuries in the Orient. It is a comprehensive form of healthcare based on the view of the human body as an ecosystem, with a language based on metaphors from nature. Health is considered "the ability of the organism to respond appropriately to a wide variety of challenges while maintaining equilibrium, integrity, and coherence" (Beinfield & Korngold, 1995). The human body is believed to be the result of the fusion of shen (psyche), essence (soma), and to be made up of qi (*chee*, energy), moisture (body fluids), and blood (tissue). Disease is thought to result when there has been depletion or congestion of these substances. Qi is believed to flow along distinct paths called *meridians*, which can be evaluated and manipulated. Therapeutic modalities include acupuncture, herbal medicine, exercise, and massage (including energy techniques).

CASE 11-8

Olive Andrews, a 38-year-old woman with chronic shoulder pain resistant to oral medications, physical therapy, and local corticosteroid injections, decided to try acupuncture therapy. The practitioner, a physician trained in traditional Oriental medicine and acupuncture in Japan and subsequently chiropractic in this country, used physical clues (palpation of wrist pulses) and electronic equipment designed to detect energy generation from the skin to determine where to place eight acupuncture needles that he then attached to a source of electrical current. Mrs. Andrews received three 30-minute treatments per week for 5 weeks. Following the course of treatment she reported nearly complete resolution of her shoulder pain and full mobility.

ACUPUNCTURE

Acupuncture is a form of treatment that has been practiced in the Orient for at least 4000 years. It is an attempt to affect the quality and mobility of the life force, *Qi Chee*, which, it is believed, flows in channels or meridians within each of us and is the primary determinant of health and illness. Very fine needles, usually eight to ten, are inserted just beneath the surface of the skin in specific locations dictated by the specific problem being treated. These needles are then manipulated manually or attached to a source of electrical current. Occasionally the needles are heated with a burning herb stick or cone called *moxa*.

Virtually all health problems are believed to be amenable to acupuncture therapy, although in this country its use in chronic pain syndromes and for smoking cessation and weight loss have been emphasized. In China it is often used for anesthesia during both minor and major operations. For treatment of chronic conditions, a minimum of ten treatments is usually required, as in Case 11-8. Acupuncture is also used for prevention of disease. Acupuncture is but one of a number of treatment approaches used by traditional Oriental physicians.

Practitioners of acupuncture can receive their training in an Oriental medical school or in one of more than two dozen 3- to 4-year training programs that have been started in the United States and in other parts of the world since 1970, when James Restin, a *New York Times* columnist on assignment in China, underwent an appendectomy with acupuncture needles as the only anesthetic and focused attention on this form of treatment. In the United States, practitioners of acupuncture are often chiropractic, osteopathic, or allopathic physicians or veterinarians who have received additional training in this method. Length of study varies considerably. Licensure is also quite variable between states, but frequently involves passing both written and skills tests.

HERBAL MEDICINE

The various parts of plants have been used for medicinal purposes for centuries. At least 25% of modern prescription medicines today are derived from higher plants. As the pharmaceutical industry has become more successful in designing more effective and less toxic medicines, many of the herbal remedies of the past have gone by the wayside. However, in the midst of the most recent trend toward "natural" healing methods, more and more people have once again become enamored with herbal remedies. The variety of herbal products sold in health-food stores and increasingly in pharmacies is large and regulations governing product labeling are loose enough that manufacturers are able to make claims about these products that are often misleading or completely baseless.

There is no question that some herbal products have physiologic effects. In fact, the pharmaceutical industry is actively studying a variety of traditional herbal remedies in hopes of discovering new pharmaceuticals. However, the magnitude of the effects, the doses required to achieve them, their potential toxicity, and potential interactions with other medicines or food products have often not been well studied. Fortunately, the quantities of biologically active ingredients in many, if not most, of the OTC preparations available in the United States are insufficient to cause either benefit (beyond the placebo effect) or harm. Nevertheless, sales of these products are now at roughly $1.5 billion per year and growing at a rate of 15 to 20% per year (Consumer Reports on Health, 1995), and a number of healthcare practitioners, both traditional and alternative, are reaping substantial profits from their promotion and sale.

THERAPEUTIC MASSAGE

Massage as a therapeutic modality is practiced by a wide variety of health professionals, both traditional and nontraditional. There are four basic types of therapeutic massage with many variations within types: oriental, athletic, energy, and psychotherapeutic. The major differences between modalities are the intent of the therapist and the amount of pressure and speed of application. All types are noninvasive, nonpainful, and palliative, not curative. The mechanisms of action may include relaxation, stress reduction, mobilization of extracellular fluid, and muscle relaxation. In addition, there is some evidence that therapeutic touch or even possibly no touch, energy, massage may stimulate a variety of systemic responses including, for example, increased red blood cell production.

Certification as a massage therapist can require anywhere from 20 to 3000 hours, usually 500 hours of training. There is no national standard. Currently 17 states have licensure requirements and many cities have ordinances to control prostitution, which has been associated with so-called "massage parlors."

Imagery is a technique in which the patient is asked to create a mental image of a pleasurable event or setting or a desired outcome. This technique can be used to achieve a state of relaxation or to attempt to influence the body's natural defenses. For example, a cancer patient might create a mental image of the cancer melting away or of white blood cells rushing to attack the cancer. The hope is that the mind can encourage and direct the immune system to accomplish the desired task. Because it is relatively easy to do and teach, and has few, if any, side effects, and because of some data to suggest that it may sometimes make a difference (Burish *et al.*, 1991; Post-White, 1993), imagery has become popular in the treatment of a variety of health conditions. It is prescribed by physicians, nurses, mental health professionals, and many others, but is still considered by most nontraditional therapy.

CASE 11-9

Andy Raddisan was a 63-year-old businessman who, when not at work, enjoyed a variety of outdoor activities, including jogging and cross-country skiing. However, over a 3- to 5-year period, he developed discomfort and stiffness in his right hip such that it became increasingly difficult to raise his leg to put on his pants. He also had to change his jogging stride to accommodate the impairment, and his ability to ski became more and more limited because of pain. He saw his family physician, who prescribed a nonsteroidal anti-inflammatory medication for suspected osteoarthritis. He also referred him to a physical therapist who taught him to follow exercise with appropriate periods of rest, and prescribed joint protection strategies and mobilization exercises. He followed this advice but did not see much improvement. A business associate suggested that he see his rolfer.

ROLFING

Rolfing is a system for maximizing human physical structure and function using connective tissue manipulations. The method, developed by Dr. Ida Rolf during the first half of this century, involves the use of the practitioner's hands, knuckles, and elbows to stretch the connective tissues surrounding muscles and joints in an attempt to improve alignment and mobility. Unlike massage, the manipulations involve static pressure applied to specific structures for periods of time. There tends to be some discomfort involved. Rolfers believe that stress-related chemicals may become trapped within contracted segments of muscle, and that when they are released through rolfing these chemicals enter the circulatory system, sometimes triggering emotional reactions including memories of past traumas. Therefore, rolfers must be prepared to provide supportive counseling.

A fundamental assumption of rolfing is that connective tissue disturbances in one part of the body cause compensatory disturbances in other areas. Therefore, a whole-body approach to treatment is necessary. A whole-body realignment is called the "ten series" because it generally requires ten 1-hour sessions to complete. However, depending on the client's needs, a rolfer may choose to use a more focused approach.

There are at least four rolfing institutes in the world that have trained about 800 rolfers. To qualify for admission to one of these institutes one must complete prerequisite courses in anatomy, physiology, kinesiology, and psychology, write a prescribed research paper, and undergo a series of rolfing treatments. Once admitted to an institute, one must complete required course and clinical work, which can take from $1\frac{1}{2}$ to 5 years. On graduation, certification is awarded. There are no licensure requirements at this time. A high percentage of rolfers have advanced degrees in another health science, e.g., M.D., R.N., M.S.W.

CASE 11-9 (*continued*)

Mr. Raddisan saw a rolfer who learned that he had had a complicated appendectomy many years earlier with perforation and subsequent intra-abdominal adhesion formation. He underwent 20 weekly 1-hour treatments involving the ten series plus efforts focused at stretching and mobilizing contracted and adhesed connective tissue in and about the abdomen and right hip. By the end of this series of treatments he had 95% normal painless range of motion in the right hip, was able to jog normally, and had gone cross-country skiing with minimal discomfort. He agreed to monthly maintenance treatments for 6 months followed by less frequent treatments for an undetermined period of time. Mr. Raddisan's health insurance company did not reimburse him for the cost of the sessions.

CHIROPRACTORS

Doctors of chiropractic (DCs) could be considered either traditional or nontraditional healthcare providers depending on the definitions one chooses. Licensed in all 50 states, they are approved for reimbursement under Medicare, Medicaid, and the vocational rehabilitation program. They are authorized providers under worker's compensation statutes. The U.S. Public Health Services classifies doctors of chiropractic among "medical specialists and practitioners," includes them in its *Health Manpower Sourcebook*, and includes a chapter on chiropractics in its *Health Resources Statistics*. However, though it certainly does occur, it is still relatively uncommon for chiropractors to work collaboratively with the other traditional healthcare professionals, and while chiropractic physicians regard themselves as primary healthcare providers, they are rarely mentioned in federal and state policymaking discussions regarding primary care manpower shortages. And while the fundamental principles on which chiropractic are based are compatible with the traditional Western biomedical paradigm, the theories derived from those principles and their application have not been well accepted by physicians particularly.

Chiropractic, from the Greek *chir* and *praktikos* meaning "done by hand," is based on the beliefs that disease processes may be caused or exacerbated by disturbances of the nervous system and that disturbances of the nervous system are often the result of derangements of the musculoskeletal system, e.g., subluxations of vertebrae in the back or neck may impinge on nerve roots resulting in alterations of function in the tissues innervated by those nerves. After a diagnostic evaluation that commonly includes a history, physical examination, and X rays, chiropractors utilize spinal and appendicular adjustment and manipulation, physical modalities, traction, diathermy, ultrasound, massage, heat, cold, nutritional counseling and prescription, and adaptive and supportive equipment to maintain or restore the structural and biomechanical integrity in order to prevent or ameliorate a variety of health problems. While the vast majority of patient encounters involve treatment of "neuromusculoskeletal conditions," nearly 15% of encounters concern the treatment of conditions involving other organ systems thought to have been caused or exacerbated by neuromusculoskeletal imbalances (*Chiropractic: State of the*

Art, 1994–1995). It is their treatment of these latter conditions that most disturbs allopathic and osteopathic physicians. Concerns have also been expressed regarding whether chiropractors are qualified to obtain and interpret radiographs and to provide nutritional and psychological counseling.

To obtain a doctor of chiropractic degree, one must have a minimum of 2 years of college including certain prerequisite science courses, and then complete 4 years at a chiropractic college. The chiropractic curriculum includes many of the same basic science courses taken by medical students, e.g., human anatomy, biochemistry, physiology, human behavior, etc., as well as a variety of clinical rotations. State chiropractic examining boards generally require graduation from an accredited chiropractic college and successful completion of a certifying examination.

CHELATION

Chelation involves the intravenous injection of chelating substances like sodium EDTA in order to bind and ultimately remove from the body substances thought to be responsible for various health problems. It is commonly used, for example, to treat atherosclerosis on the premise that calcium can be removed from the plaques that line the obstructed blood vessels. Other purported benefits include improved lipid profiles, increased effectiveness of hydroxyl-radical scavengers, inhibition of platelet aggregation, and restoration of electromagnetic potential across cell membranes (Chappel, 1995; Margolis, 1995). Diagnostic blood and tissue tests are done to determine the levels of various toxic substances in the body as well as the quantities of various essential vitamins and minerals. Based on the results of these tests and the nature of the presenting problem, a chelating solution is prepared that may include the chelating agent plus supplemental vitamins. Chelation is generally performed by physicians. Training usually consists of attendance at workshops and short courses.

CASE 11-10

Francis Gordon was 28 years old and pregnant with her second child. She had had tremendous problems with nausea and vomiting with her first pregnancy and now at 12 weeks gestation was beginning to experience similar problems with her second pregnancy. Remembering the fear that she experienced when taking physician prescribed medications during her first pregnancy, she decided to consult a homeopath for advice. She was given instructions to take homeopathic doses of ipecac which she was assured would not harm the baby. She found that, in fact, the treatment seemed to help.

HOMEOPATHY

Homeopathy is a healthcare practice based on the principle that "like treats like." Its practitioners and advocates believe that symptoms are the body's attempt to heal itself, and that they therefore should not be suppressed, but rather promoted. To accomplish this, homeopathic physicians prescribe extremely dilute solutions of substances that in larger amounts would cause the same symptoms as the problem being treated. Their prescription is based on both the type of problem and the patient's reaction to it, that is, the patient's personality style.

In Case 11-10, for example, ipecac when given in pharmacologic doses *causes* nausea and vomiting, but in minute doses it is used by homeopaths to relieve it. Ipecac was chosen for Ms. Gordon because of the pattern, severity of the nausea, and certain characteristics of her personality (Ullman, 1988). Most homeopathic remedies can be purchased without prescription in health-food stores or in a rapidly increasing number of pharmacies. Self-care has been facilitated by the availability of homeopathic mixtures containing several of the substances commonly prescribed for particular problems (Debrovner, 1993).

The principles of homeopathy were developed by the German physician and pharmacist Samuel Hahnemann, in the early 1800s. By 1900 there were 22 homeopathic medical schools in the United States alone. However, with the discovery of antibiotics and other advances in allopathic medicine, the practice fell out of favor in the 1940s (National Center for Homeopathy, 1995). In the last 5 to 10 years, homeopathy seems once again to be gaining in popularity. The number of pharmacies selling homeopathic products in the United States has increased tenfold in the last 5 years, and the popularity of homeopathy has far outgrown the number of homeopathic practitioners. Patients must largely depend on their own knowledge or the advice of pharmacists and health-food store owners. Many homeopathy "study groups" have been formed, and the National Center for Homeopathy offers short courses for laypeople.

Individual states regulate the practice of homeopathy. Usually it can be practiced legally by licensed medical practitioners including allopathic physicians, osteopathic physicians, dentists, and veterinarians. In some states, chiropractors and naturopaths may be licensed to prescribe homeopathic remedies. The National Center for Homeopathy lists approximately 800 practitioners throughout the United States whose practices include homeopathy. A majority of these have become educated through participation in multiple short courses and workshops and through self-directed reading. There is no certification examination.

NATUROPATHIC MEDICINE

Naturopathy as a distinct healthcare profession began in the United States about 100 years ago. Its founders, Dr. Benedict Lust and Robert Foster, were concerned that conventional medical practice had become reductionistic and overly reliant on drugs and surgery. They advocated the use of "natural healing methods" designed to assist the body's own healing processes. Modern naturopathy is based on six fundamental principles: the healing power of nature; identify and treat the cause of the problem not just its symptoms; first, do no harm; treat the whole person; the physician as teacher; and prevention. Naturopaths are primary healthcare practitioners whose therapeutic armamentarium includes clinical nutrition, physical modalities, homeopathic strategies, botanical medicine, natural childbirth, traditional Oriental medicine techniques, counseling, and minor surgery.

Naturopathy enjoyed great success during the first quarter of this century but experienced a decline in the 1940s and 1950s. There is now only one college of naturopathic medicine in the United States. Located in Portland, Oregon, its curriculum includes courses in the traditional basic and clinical sciences as well as the areas mentioned above. A 4-year course of study leads to the doctor of naturopathic medicine (N.D.) degree. Licensure is currently required in six states. Scope of practice is specifically defined in the practice acts in the various states that license or regulate naturopathic medicine.

Mrs. G. M. was a 78-year-old widow who lived alone. Because of frequent falls and increasing forgetfulness, she had become essentially homebound by choice. She came to the attention of Dr. S., a general internist, on referral from a social worker from Adult Protective Services (APS) who requested a medical evaluation of her falls, forgetfulness, and the recent onset of a blood discharge from one of her breasts. The APS became involved because of the neighbors' concerns that Mrs. M. was in need of assistance.

Dr. S., after careful evaluation, concluded that there was a possibility of significant heart disease as well as a breast nodule, bilateral cataracts, and mild dementia. He referred her to a general surgeon for breast biopsy, an ophthalmologist for evaluation of the cataracts, and arranged for her to have some cardiac studies, an echocardiogram, and a 24-hour Holter monitor.

The breast nodule was biopsied and proved to be malignant. The consulting surgeon suggested a modified radical mastectomy. The ophthalmologist confirmed the presence of cataracts but was not convinced that removing them would prevent further falls. Results of cardiac studies were normal.

Mrs. M. was admitted to the hospital for breast surgery. Dr. S. visited her in the hospital and met with nurses to develop a plan of care that would prevent falls and minimize the confusion that he anticipated might result from the unfamiliar hospital environment. He asked that the surgeon request a physical therapy consult to help with the evaluation of the falls and to assure that Mrs. M. remained as active as possible during the hospitalization. The surgery was a success, no complications occurred, and Mrs. M. was discharged to her home. Dr. S. then scheduled a house call and invited the social worker from APS to be present for a discussion of further healthcare needs.

INTERDISCIPLINARY TEAMWORK

Patients like Mrs. M. in Case 11-11 require the services of a variety of health professionals simultaneously. How should these services by coordinated? In the above case, Dr. S. took it on himself to coordinate Mrs. M.'s care. However, even though his efforts appeared to have been successful, at no time were more than two professionals able to engage in a discussion of Mrs. M.'s situation at the same time, and there were professionals who were excluded from even those discussions, e.g., the hospital pharmacist, the hospital social worker, the cardiologist who read the cardiac studies, and the anesthesiologist.

As modern healthcare has become more complex because of broader definitions of health, increased medical knowledge, technological advances, and changes in the spectrum of illnesses, so too has the healthcare system become increasingly complex. One aspect of this complexity is the dramatic increase over the last half century in the number of different healthcare disciplines and in the degree of specialization within the more traditional disciplines, particularly medicine, nursing, and dentistry. For such a complicated system to function effectively and efficiently to the benefit of individual patients, teamwork is required.

Interdisciplinary teamwork in healthcare as a concept has been described and advocated for at least 30 years. Enthusiasm was particularly high in the 1960s, when several large demonstration projects were funded. Unfortunately, because of the difficulties involved in implementation and a relative shortage of convincing data proving increased efficacy, the movement lost momentum. However, as health professionals find that they are caring for increasing numbers of chronically ill and disabled patients, there has been a resurgence of interest in interdisciplinary approaches to healthcare. Interdisciplinary teams are now the rule in rehabilitation (Rothberg, 1981), home healthcare, and geriatrics (Rubenstein, 1983), where there is now some reasonably good evidence that interdisciplinary team care is superior to traditional multidisciplinary care (Williams & Williams, 1986).

Of course, any setting in which professionals from more than one discipline work side by side could be considered interdisciplinary teamwork, and that is probably true to a degree. Outpatient clinics, operating rooms, and hospital wards all require interdisciplinary collaboration. However, teamwork in these settings generally means that physicians give orders to the other professionals on the team, who dutifully carry them out. There is very little collaborative decision-making.

What are the barriers to true interdisciplinary teamwork? Several have already been mentioned. Professionals from the different disciplines are trained separately in their own specialized fields with little chance to learn about or even interact with professionals from other disciplines until after they graduate. By that time, "turf" boundaries are well established. Specialization tends to emphasize differences more than similarities between professionals (French, 1979). Issues of power, prestige, financial compensation, sexism, and racism also contribute to defensive and distancing behaviors. Attitudes that develop within a group become firmly entrenched through social support and affiliation (French, 1979).

Physicians in particular are trained to be action-oriented, self-contained, autonomous decision-makers. Thus, they are systemically educated to be poor team players (Goldstein, 1989). If being a member of an interdisciplinary team means being responsible to other team members, then physicians, whether by selection or training, are often unwilling and ill prepared to do so (Charns, 1976). In addition, teamwork results in significant loss of power and control, items valued highly by many physicians, particularly in today's liability-conscious society.

Effective interdisciplinary teamwork requires that professionals from the various healthcare disciplines understand and respect each other, that there be a common language and method of communication between them, and that the goals of treatment and the roles played by each team member can be agreed on by all. To become an effective team member, a healthcare professional must learn her own discipline well and feel comfortable within its boundaries. In addition, she must learn enough about each of the other disciplines to allow colleague-to-colleague communication, consultation, and referral. The consultative process must be mastered. In situations requiring particularly close and frequent interdisciplinary collaboration, such as geriatrics and rehabilitation, group process skills must also be learned.

Perhaps the most important obstacle to a team approach is the traditional departmental organizational structure that exists in nearly all healthcare institutions. Hospitals, for instance, usually have separate departments of nursing, social work, occupational therapy, physical therapy, radiology, laboratory, and pathology. Garner states that the "departmental model places the clients in the middle, where they become pawns in territorial battles for power, control, status, and financial resources." As a result, Garner says, staff members who serve the same clients are not obliged to know each other, to communicate, to plan together, or to support one another" (Garner, 1988). He describes teams and departments as being like oil and water.

The basic requirements for interdisciplinary teamwork are mutual respect and an understanding of the potential contributions of team members from other disciplines, communication through use of a commonly understood language, and an interdisciplinary decision-making process that facilitates the formation of mutually agreed-on goals and strategies. Teamwork also requires training and practice; it does not occur automatically. For interdisciplinary healthcare to become a universal reality, a great deal more interaction must occur between disciplines at every stage of training, and administrators must recognize the need to reorganize healthcare systems into interdisciplinary teams rather than discipline-specific departments. The time required for team meetings must be reimbursed by third-party payers. Liability issues must be explored and addressed. If physicians are to function as leaders of interdisciplinary healthcare teams, strategies will need to be developed at both the selection and training stages that will foster appropriate attitudes and skills.

CONCLUSIONS

Our modern healthcare system is complex. The number and variety of healthcare practitioners, both traditional and nontraditional, provide people a great many options. It also presents a formidable challenge. Despite the explosion of health information available to the public, most people still know very little about the knowledge, skills, and attitudes that characterize each of the various healthcare disciplines. In fact, healthcare professionals often know surprisingly little about other professionals outside their own discipline. It is hoped that this chapter has taken a small step toward rectifying this.

Important changes are occurring in the healthcare system. Driven largely by rising costs, a predominantly medical subspecialty-oriented system is evolving into one in which generalists occupy a more important role. Administrators are becoming more powerful, as are the other health professions such as nursing. As people in our society have become healthier, the healthiest we have ever been in the history of mankind, and better informed, we nevertheless have become increasingly dissatisfied with our health, and particularly with our healthcare system. Interest in nontraditional healthcare methods has grown exponentially in the past two decades. Healthcare reform remains near the top of the political agenda.

Regardless of the changes that occur, there is no question that such a complex system can only run effectively and efficiently when the various providers of care can coordinate their efforts toward the best interests of patients. This requires teamwork, and true interdisciplinary teamwork requires more than good intentions. A critical ingredient is understanding and respect for the skills of others. The consultation and referral process is also essential, but even better methods of communication and coordination are required. Administrative structures may need to be changed, liability issues explored, and record systems revamped. Most importantly, health professionals must be trained to function as members of teams.

CASES FOR DISCUSSION

CASE 1

K. S., a 42-year-old man who had no regular physician, saw a plastic surgeon to have a large lipoma removed from his back. Because of the size of the lesion, which would have required a fairly large dose of local anesthetic, the surgeon ordered an ECG to reassure himself that no heart disease was present. The ECG report was equivocal, showing some minor ST-T wave changes possibly caused by ischemia. He recommended and made arrangements for a consultation with a cardiologist.

The cardiologist took a more complete cardiac history and learned that the patient had had a long history of occasional episodes of palpitations never severe enough to require treatment. In fact, he had never before mentioned them to a physician. The cardiologist ordered some blood tests and recommended an exercise tolerance test and a 24-hour Holter monitor study. Results of the blood work were normal except for a fasting serum cholesterol value of 250 mg/dl. Results of the exercise test were equivocal with 1.5-mm ST depressions at maximal exercise. He recommended that K.S. begin a low-cholesterol and low-saturated-fat diet.

Before the Holter tracing could be done, K. S. had to be seen in the emergency room with the worst episode of palpitations that he had ever had. A rhythm strip showed paroxysmal supraventricular tachycardia. He was converted using digoxin and carotid massage and was sent home only to return several days later with another episode, which was converted similarly. He was then told to continue to take digoxin indefinitely. The Holter monitor was canceled.

The cardiologist then requested an echocardiogram to look for valvular disease and chamber enlargement and an exercise nuclear ventriculogram to further evaluate the possibility of ischemia. These studies demonstrated no chamber enlargement, normal valves, but a borderline low left ventricular ejection fraction of 50% (normal 60% or greater) and no real evidence for ischemia. However, because of the low ejection fraction and atrial arrhythmia as well as the elevated serum cholesterol, the cardiologist suggested going ahead with a cardiac catheterization, which demonstrated clean coronary arteries and again a borderline low ejection fraction.

One year later, K. S. now follows a low-cholesterol, low-saturated-fat diet to which his wife compulsively forces him to adhere, niacin three times daily to further lower his cholesterol, which remained elevated despite the diet, once-daily digoxin, and once-daily baby aspirin. He has had two more episodes of palpitations requiring emergency room conversions, and he anxiously awaits the results of his follow-up nuclear ventriculogram to see if his "idiopathic cardiomyopathy" has worsened. His lipoma remains intact.

1. *What happened? In what ways is K. S. better off for having had the cardiac evaluation? In what ways is he worse off? What do you suspect the impact has been on his family?*
2. *At what points in this clinical cascade could it have been stopped? Who could have stopped it most effectively?*
3. *Can too much information ever be harmful? If so, how can we decide how much is enough?*
4. *What do you suspect would happen if K. S. now developed postprandial epigastric pain?*

CASE 2

Dr. F. L. was fit to be tied when he learned while examining his long-time patient T. Y. that the consultation he had requested 9 months earlier from an endocrinologist—T. Y.'s blood pressure had been difficult to control, and his serum calcium level was borderline high—had led to a pulmonary consultation for a chronic cough, which Dr. L. knew to be allergic in nature and of long standing, and an orthopedic consultation for evaluation of low back pain, which Dr. L. had previously evaluated and found to be associated with marital and job-related stress. Neither of the secondary consultants had known to send the results of their evaluations to Dr. L., since they were unaware that he was the primary physician. Furthermore, the endocrinologist who had handled the blood pressure and calcium questions with the patient had not communicated with Dr. L.

1. *Why did the endocrinologist probably act in this way? What kind of trouble did it cause?*
2. *What do you think Dr. L. should do about it?*
3. *Why didn't T. Y. keep it from happening?*

CASE 3

When Dr. D. W. decided to admit R. P. to the intensive care unit of the county hospital to rule out an acute myocardial infarction, he was told that he would have to speak with the charge nurse in the ICU. When he was informed by the charge nurse that although there was one open bed, there were not enough nurses available to properly care for any additional patients, and she therefore could not authorize the admission, he was livid. How dare a nurse tell him whether or not he could admit a patient to the ICU? He called the intensivist in charge of the ICU but to his surprise was informed that the nurse's decision was correct and would be upheld.

1. *Should nurses be making this kind of decision? Was the nurse's decision in this case an appropriate one?*
2. *Why was Dr. W. so angry?*

CASE 4

A 46-year-old woman suffered a left hemispheric stroke. After a brief hospitalization, she was referred to an inpatient rehabilitation facility. There she was found to have a right hemiparesis, a moderately elevated blood pressure and blood glucose.

1. *Which healthcare professionals should be involved in this patient's care? What would each be expected to contribute to her management?*
2. *Who should be the coordinator of the rehabilitation team? Suggest a method of care that would allow interdisciplinary teamwork.*

CASE 5

S. R., a pharmacist, called Dr. W. G. to clarify a prescription that Dr. G. had written for D. D. for a potassium-sparing diuretic. He wanted to make Dr. G. aware of the fact that Mr. D. was also taking a potassium supplement and an ACE inhibitor and had just bought a box of Lite Salt, all of which, in combination with the diuretic, might be expected to increase D. D.'s risk of hyperkalemia. He was not terribly surprised when Dr. G. seemed somewhat annoyed and told him in essence to quit practicing medicine. Dr. G. added that he had told Mr. D. not to take any more of the potassium supplement. However, when S. R. had asked D. D. earlier, he had not remembered that advice.

1. *What should the pharmacist's role be on the healthcare team? What, if anything, should the pharmacist have done differently in this case?*
2. *What obstacles, if any, exist that prevent pharmacists from taking a more active role in patient care?*

CASE 6

G. C. was 71 years old when he came to see Dr. H. for a checkup at the insistence of his daughter. G. C. had had a heart attack 2 years earlier. Now he was having some mild stable angina, but wasn't taking any medication for it, and had had one episode of sudden vision loss in his right eye which lasted about 5 minutes. After recommending several tests and a medication, G. C.'s daughter revealed that her father had been receiving chelation therapy weekly for the last 6 months.

1. *Could the chelation therapy be contributing to G. C.'s symptoms?*
2. *What would you say to G. C. and his daughter about chelation therapy?*
3. *What kind of practitioners generally perform chelation therapy? What is involved in this kind of treatment?*
4. *What are its purported benefits?*

CASE 7

D. T., on discharge from the hospital after the birth of her second child, when asked to bring the child in for a 2-week checkup, disclosed to you that she would be taking the child to the same chiropractor who had been providing well-child care to her other child for the past 2 years. She said that she was well pleased with his care which included regular spinal manipulations and dietary advice, but apparently no immunizations.

1. *What are your feelings about chiropractors providing well-child care?*
2. *What besides immunizations might the child not be getting that would ordinarily be part of traditional well-child care?*
3. *What advice, if any, would you give to this mother?*

RECOMMENDED READINGS

Lecca PJ, McNiel JD (eds): *Interdisciplinary Team Practice: Issues and Trends.* New York, Praeger, 1985.

> This text is a state-of-the-art review of interdisciplinary team practice, including rationale for development of such an approach, models, and projections for the future. Specific chapters describe various types of team care, including rehabilitation, mental health, and hospice care.

Mechanic D (ed): *Handbook of Health, Health Care, and the Health Professions.* New York, The Free Press, 1983.

> This text is a broad-based book on the determinants of health and illness and the organization and provision of healthcare in this country. Two sections on healthcare delivery and management and health occupations are especially pertinent to this chapter.

Williams SJ, Torrens RR (eds): *Introduction to Health Services,* ed 3. New York, John Wiley & Sons, 1988.

> This text describes the major features of the U.S. healthcare system from a macro level and thus serves as a nice complement to this chapter's microview. It also addresses several economic issues, such as health manpower and the evaluation and regulation of healthcare programs, and concludes with a discussion on health policy.

Wynne LC, McDaniel SH, Web TT (eds): *Systems Consultation: A New Perspective for Family Therapy.* New York, Guilford Press, 1986.

> This text views organizations, using healthcare organizations in the majority of its chapters, from a systemic viewpoint. It describes a method for consultation when such systems are dysfunctional that derives from family therapy. Case examples show that this approach can be remarkably fruitful when other approaches have failed.

CHAPTER 12

B. Values

Medical Ethics

Warren L. Holleman

T. Z. is a fourth-year medical student doing an oncology elective. At team meeting the first day, T. Z. learns about Ms. Ballard, a patient with apparent breast cancer who is scheduled for surgery the next day. The surgeons plan to obtain a frozen biopsy and, depending on the extensiveness of the cancer, to go ahead and perform a lumpectomy or mastectomy. Later that morning T. Z. visits Ms. Ballard and discovers she has serious misperceptions about the nature of her illness and the surgery to be performed. She has no inkling that she has breast cancer, that her disease is life-threatening, or that the surgery might significantly disfigure her. She believes she merely has "a cyst."

T. Z. wanted to believe that too, and wondered momentarily if she misunderstood the discussion earlier that morning. After reflecting, reviewing her notes, and checking with another member of the team, T. Z. confirmed that the oncologist is certain the patient has breast cancer.

T. Z. then wondered if Ms. Ballard might be in a state of denial. Perhaps she knows intellectually the nature of her illness and of tomorrow's surgery, but she is hoping against hope that the physicians have made an error in judgment. So T. Z. spends a little extra time with Ms. Ballard to evaluate her competence, her level of anxiety, and her level of denial. T. Z. finds her to be lucid and, although she is not as curious about her condition as others might be, it is clear to T. Z. that the team has not informed her truthfully about her illness and the surgery.

Now T. Z. is in a difficult position. T. Z. is the lone medical student on a team of experienced faculty, fellows, and residents. It is her first day on the service. One of her patients—well, not exactly T. Z.'s patient, she's just a medical student—is about to be wheeled into surgery, apparently unaware of the disease that threatens her life or that, on awakening, some or all of her breast may be missing.

T. Z. asks the intern whether the patient knows what's going on. "She might. Patients often know more about their condition than we do." "Has anyone told her?" Intern: "Probably not." "Well," T. Z. asks, "don't you think someone ought to tell her?" The intern seems distracted and avoids her question: "You need to check the prostate in 614. He's had catheter problems. Maybe you could be useful there." T. Z. wanted to be useful here, but she doesn't want to be too pushy. "I'll check on Mr. Honda in 614 but first I'm going to talk to Ms. Ballard." Intern: "Don't do that." "Why not?" T. Z. asks. Intern: "Because I said so. She's an old lady. Trust me, I'm a doctor." He walks away as he says this. Then, halfway down the hallway, he stops, turns, and flashes a knowing grin. The grin could be interpreted any number of ways: a clumsy attempt at understanding, a seductive overture, or a conceited way of saying "I'm in charge here." T. Z. thinks it's probably a little of each.

In any other context his smile would have won T. Z. over, but here she finds herself confused, angry, and scared. The patient is 65 years old, the same age as T. Z.'s mother. T. Z. reflects: "My mother doesn't seem that old, and I know she wouldn't want to be treated like this."

T. Z. then took care of the gentleman with the catheter problem and someone else's pain problem but T. Z. couldn't get Ms. Ballard off her mind. In the politest voice she could muster T. Z. asked the fellow to "help" her with her problem. The problem, of course, is that T. Z. doesn't understand why Ms. Ballard hasn't been told the truth, why she's being wheeled off to surgery without giving an informed consent, and why supposedly confidential information about her medical condition is being discussed with her daughter apparently without her knowledge. The fellow begins with a familiar response: "She's an old lady, and we don't want to upset her." Still trying to maintain a courteous pose, T. Z. acknowledges his concern but wonders whether Ms. Ballard might also be upset at being lied to or at waking up and discovering her breasts mutilated. The fellow says that since she's an old lady, and since this is the best treatment for her, she probably won't be too upset. Trying not to become too upset herself, T. Z. asks, "How do you know that this is how she'd want it handled?" The fellow's response: "We're working closely with her daughter, and that's what her daughter says. Her daughter is a nurse herself. We're trusting her judgment."

The fellow gives T. Z. a friendly discourse on how things are done in his home country, where the oldest child routinely handles all medical decision-making. Cancer, prognosis, and death are never discussed with patients: "It's taboo." Attempting to avoid sounding culturally insensitive, T. Z. points out that, until recently, such behavior was considered taboo in many parts of the United States as well. Then T. Z. realized that maybe it still is.

T. Z. had signed up for this elective because of the outstanding reputation of the oncologist and this cancer treatment center. Now, just a few hours into the rotation, she is disillusioned with both.

INTRODUCTION

Case 12-1 is troubling for a number of reasons, not the least of which is that it is true. It happened recently, and at one of the leading cancer treatment facilities in the United States.

Fortunately, this story has a happy ending. T. Z. confronted the oncologist, who responded by admitting his fault, apologizing to the patient, and disclosing truthfully to the patient. The oncologist even thanked the student for her courage and concern. He explained that he generally was very conscientious regarding ethical standards of treatment but that in this case his judgment had been impaired by the fact that the patient's daughter was a nurse, not just any nurse but an oncology nurse, and not just any oncology nurse but *his* nurse! Once the charade ended he breathed a sigh of relief, saying that it was much harder to cover secrets, tell lies, and bend rules than simply to do the right thing, even though in this case that meant telling a patient bad news.

The medical ethics movement of the past quarter-century has made much progress in establishing standards of treatment requiring truthfulness, informed consent, and confidentiality within the physician–patient relationship. Incidents such as the one described in Case 12-1 are becoming less common in the United States. As the foregoing case illustrates, however, deception does happen and for a variety of reasons, including paternalism toward patients, cynicism regarding morality, denial of death, medical hubris, and clumsiness in balancing conflicts of interest.

FACTORS AFFECTING PHYSICIAN COMPLIANCE WITH ETHICAL STANDARDS OF CARE

Paternalism is often fueled by a desire to protect the patient, but without a fundamental respect for the patient the "helpful" physician becomes coercive, dishonest, and untrustworthy. The attending physician in Case 12-1 may have honestly believed he was doing what was best for his patient but his judgment had been clouded by his relationship with her daughter. The patient would soon go home, but the physician would continue to work side by side with the daughter. The physician became confused regarding the primacy of the conflicting loyalties and blurred the boundaries between personal, collegial, and professional responsibilities. In so doing he forgot to show a fundamental respect for the autonomy and integrity of the patient.

Cynicism is common in academic medical centers, often fostered by fatigue, stress, peer pressure, and poor mentoring. While psychological, sociological, and institutional factors influence attitudes and behavior, they do not justify them. Those who feel cynical about the moral enterprise should search their souls to consider basic motivations for pursuing a medical vocation. They should also recognize that many standards of medical ethics have been codified into law. Violators have more than a guilty conscience to deal with: They may face fines, imprisonment, malpractice suits, and probation or loss of their medical license.

Those who have difficulty discussing death, disability, and disease with their patients should recognize that this feeling is normal. It is usually rooted in fear and insecurity regarding one's own mortality or in feeling impotent to do something to change a bad situation. For some students it takes considerable willpower to resist the temptation to flee the bedside of the dying, disabled, or disfigured patient. One rule of thumb I try to follow is: *If I feel the urge to leave, stay. If I find myself staying away from a difficult situation, that's the very place I need to go—right now.* When I get there and feel the urge to leave, I imagine myself on a rambunctious horse and I tell myself to stay in the saddle—that's the only way to learn to ride the tough ones. Similarly, when I feel the urge to leaf through the chart or to carry on small talk with the family, I have another rule: *Don't just do something, stand there.* Or better: sit there. Let the patient comfort you. Then you can begin to care for the patient.

Medical hubris is an occupational disease found among those medical students and physicians who believe that modern medicine can cure every ailment. I have found chronically ill and disabled patients the best teachers in helping rid one of this misconception.

With so many competing interests these days—patients, families, third-party payers, employers, hospital administrations, pharmaceutical companies—it is little wonder that physicians have difficulty weighing the legitimate interests of each party (Morreim, 1991). A thoughtful consideration of ethical foundations and ethical standards of care can go a long way, however, in helping one avoid the most common pitfalls and in learning to juggle multiple competing interests more adroitly.

CHAPTER OVERVIEW

Although the chapter will touch on controversial areas such as euthanasia, abortion, and access to care, the main focus will be the areas in which some consensus has been reached in hopes that this basic knowledge will enable the student to be more competent and confident on clinical rotations. Case 12-1 illustrates many of the areas covered by the chapter.

First, confidentiality vis-à-vis the patient's family and other third parties: Under what circumstances should the physician discuss diagnosis, prognosis, and treatment options with family members or with other individuals not involved in the patient's care? Second, truth telling: Does the fiduciary nature of the physician–patient relationship require that physicians and patients be honest with one another, and are there any circumstances in which the physician or patient might legitimately withhold information from each other or deceive one another? Third, informed consent: What constitutes a free, informed consent, what types of information should the physician provide the patient, and under what circumstances should a physician seek the consent of a proxy decision-maker rather than the patient?

To appreciate the significance of respect for confidentiality, truth telling, and informed consent to treatment, it is important first to understand the foundations on which these ethical standards are based. The next section will examine these foundations.

CASE 12-2

Miguel, a 24-year-old police officer, presented to his primary care physician with a broken nose, an injury sustained 3 months previously while playing soccer. The examination revealed a deviated septum that partially closed the air pathway. Miguel reported mild to moderate difficulty in breathing and sinus allergies and discomforts. The physician, who himself had had a deviated septum for many years and who received a salary bonus at the end of the year for keeping tests, procedures, referrals, and hospitalizations under a certain limit, suggested doing nothing: "No one ever died of a deviated septum, but the other options carry risks." When Miguel asked about those options the physician responded by saying, "There are medicines you could take but they'd probably make you feel worse than you do now. Mother nature is the best healer. If I were you I wouldn't worry."

Soon thereafter Miguel's employer switched to a new health plan and Miguel visited a new physician, who referred Miguel immediately to a head and neck surgeon. After a brief examination the specialist told Miguel he ought to have surgery to repair the deviated septum: "Not only will it open the pathway and improve your breathing, but also the girls will like your new nose." After calculating the cost of meeting his deductible and the 20% copayment, Miguel decided he could not afford the surgical procedure at this time. Six months later Miguel presented once again to the primary care physician with sinus headaches and sinusitis. The physician scolded him for not having the surgery and prescribed antibiotics. The problem resolved temporarily but when it recurred Miguel— feeling shamed by the physician's comments—delayed returning to the physician until the headaches became unbearable. This pattern repeated itself several times over the next year, with the physician prescribing an antibiotic but making Miguel feel the blame for his illness.

Then Miguel's employer switched healthcare plans once again. The new primary care physician, concerned about the frequency of the recurrences and of Miguel's absences from work, took a complete history, reviewed with Miguel the pros and cons of nontreatment and surgery, and suggested a third option, nasal decongestants, to open the nasal pathway. Miguel agreed to try the medication. When he returned 6 months later for a follow-up examination, Miguel said he felt like his old self again. He reported only occasional mild headaches and no bothersome side effects of the medication.

ETHICAL FOUNDATIONS

In every patient encounter, physicians ought to ask themselves four basic ethical questions (Beauchamp & Childress, 1989; Pellegrino & Thomasma, 1993; McCullough & Ashton, 1994). These questions apply whether the patient has a deviated septum or a deviated spine, a cold or cancer. These questions concern whether the patient will be benefited by the treatment (*beneficence*), whether the patient might be harmed by the treatment or the risks, discomforts, and side effects might outweigh the benefits (*nonmaleficence*), whether the patient participates in the decision process (*autonomy*), whether the physician considers the impact of the treatment on other patients, on the patient's family, on caregivers, and on the rest of society (*justice*), and whether the physician's motives reflect personal and professional values and ideals (*virtue*).

The first question to ask is, *What medical benefits can I offer this patient, and what harms are also possible?* In Case 12-2, the medical benefits that can be offered to Miguel are to open his nasal pathway, improve his breathing, reduce his discomfort, and reduce his sinus allergies. These benefits can be achieved by one of two means: surgery and medication. The surgery would permanently correct the problem but would involve considerable expense, 1 week of missed work and postoperative pain and discomfort, and the remote possibility of disfigurement as a result of infection or death as a reaction to the anesthesia. Nasal decongestants usually result in moderate improvement with little risk or cost in the short run. Long-run costs will be much higher, however, and some patients will experience mild to moderate discomfort as a result of feeling "wired" and insomnia. Additional factors to consider when comparing the cost of surgery vis-à-vis medication include the patient's life expectancy and which treatments are covered by the patient's health insurance plan. From a medical and societal perspective, the decision becomes even more complicated when the patient's health insurance reimburses the less desirable or more expensive option.

One reason Miguel received suboptimal care is that the first three physicians failed to spell out the entire array of legitimate treatment options. Each was comfortable with one particular option and tried to force Miguel to accept it, without exploring alternatives and without exploring benefits, harms, and costs. As a result, Miguel was sick much longer than he had to be. When the fourth physician took the time to review each treatment option, physician and patient quickly found a mutually satisfactory solution.

Because each patient will weigh benefits and harms differently, it is important to ask a second question: *What are the patient's values and preferences?* For some patients, such as Miguel, the cost of surgery will be prohibitive. Even those patients who could afford the procedure may prefer to spend the money on some other good, such as a downpayment on a car. If the nasal blockage is minor, the patient will probably prefer conservative treatment or no treatment at all, as in the case of the first physician. What that physician failed to recognize, however, is that the severity of the problem and the tolerance for discomfort vary from patient to patient; he should have assessed Miguel's severity and discomfort more carefully.

For patients whose threshold for risk is low, the risk of anesthesia will seem excessive for an elective procedure. One can imagine, for example, parents of young children deferring the procedure until the children are older. If the discomfort of the nasal blockage and the side effects of decongestants are having a significant impact on one's life-style, work, or parenting abilities, then the risk of anesthesia may seem reasonable. Because values, preferences, and thresholds for risk vary from person to person, it is important for the physician to inform the patient of the risks, benefits, side effects, and costs of the various legitimate treatments—and of nontreatment—so that the patient can make an informed and individually appropriate decision.

Respect for the patient's autonomy includes respect for the patient's right to choose among each of the legitimate treatment options, or to refuse treatment completely. Patients have the right to refuse treatment regardless of whether the treatment is an elective procedure, such as rhinoplasty, or a lifesaving procedure or medication, such as cardiac bypass surgery or chemotherapy. It is quite common, for example, for patients dying of cancer or AIDS to refuse antibiotics for opportunistic infections, even though the antibiotic could prolong the patient's life.

Respect for the patient's autonomy does not mean that physicians are obligated to provide *whatever* treatment the patient requests. If the patient requests a treatment that is outside the standard of care, such as sleeping pills for chronic insomnia, the physician is not obligated to comply. In fact, the principle of nonmaleficence would suggest that the physician is obligated *not* to comply.

More controversial is the patient's request for assistance in suicide or abortion. For many physicians these medical procedures violate personal and professional values. For these physicians there is no legal or professional obligation to comply with the patient's request, even though abortions or medically assisted suicides may be legal or at least permissible in their jurisdictions. Physicians who refuse to do procedures they consider unethical are protected in most states by conscience clauses. Conscience clauses do not apply to emergency abortions in which the mother's life is in danger and do not exempt physicians from the obligation to provide their patients with appropriate referrals.

The third question to consider is, *What is fair in this situation?* Medical decisions have an impact not only on the patient but also on family, caregivers, other patients, and the rest of society. A concern for justice demands that physicians and patients bear this in mind when making decisions about which tests to order and which treatments to pursue.

For example, if the deviation of a patient's septum is minor and the benefits of surgery are marginal, the physician should not recommend surgery even if the procedure is covered by insurance. Wasting scarce resources on marginally beneficial treatments is unfair to others in the insurance plan and, in the case of Medicare, to taxpayers in general. In the case of patients who are dying and for whom curative treatments are deemed futile, the physician should not only ask whether the patient wants the treatment and has the ability to pay, but should consider the cost to other patients in terms of allocation of beds, equipment, and supplies. The physician should also consider the financial, emotional, and physical cost to family and caregivers in providing round-the-clock care: Many spouses become so exhausted in caring for their loved ones that the health of the caregiver becomes a more pressing concern than that of the identified patient.

A concern for justice also demands that nations make primary medical care available to all citizens regardless of ability to pay. Physicians ought to be leading this effort. Unfortunately, too many U.S. physicians are preoccupied with maximizing their incomes or the power and prestige of their specialty.

In light of the tendency to place self-interest above professional service and social responsibility, it is important always to bear in mind a fourth question: *Am I remaining faithful to my values and ideals, and to those of my profession?* One such value is honesty: being truthful with patients, colleagues, and administrators, and on medical records and insurance forms. On some occasions third parties may demand information to which the physician believes they have no right. In some cases other concerns, such as protection of patient confidentiality, must be weighed with the moral demand to be truthful.

Another value is compassion, which means "to suffer with" or "to experience with." Fundamental to compassion is empathy, the ability to understand the thoughts and share the feelings of another, without being overwhelmed by those feelings (Reich, 1989). Compassion and empathy improve the competence of the clinician, enabling her to better assess the needs, values, and preferences of the patient. Compassion and empathy are themselves means of healing. Patients who feel known, understood, and cared for can focus on the healing process rather than worrying whether the physician knows what she's doing or being angry that nobody cares. The physician who fails to feel the pain of her patients not only deprives herself of a powerful diagnostic and therapeutic tool, but also denies her own humanity and runs a higher risk of burnout and job dissatisfaction.

Two other values are courage and humility. Courage enables a physician to face a scary situation, make sound judgments, and perform adroit procedures. Humility enables a physician to recognize when she has reached the limitations of her expertise and needs to ask for help. Humility also enables a physician to recognize the limitations of medical science and medical technology so as to avoid hubris. In Miguel's case, the first physician, who had too high an opinion of his ability to take care of Miguel, lacked humility. The second physician, who referred too quickly, lacked courage.

Finally, integrity is the virtue that encompasses all of the other virtues. Integrity is what Polonius had in mind when he advised his son Laertes, "This above all, to thine own self be true" (*Hamlet* I,3). For the physician, integrity requires being faithful to one's own values and to the values of the profession. In addition to the moral values of honesty, compassion, humility, and courage, there are essential medical values to which every physician must ascribe: enhancing health, preventing illness and disability, preserving life, preserving quality of life, and palliating pain and discomfort. These medical values will sometimes conflict and physicians will differ as to the priority given each of them, but professional integrity requires a conscientious effort to be faithful to each of these values.

The physician who, for financial gain, told Miguel not to treat his problem was not acting with integrity. He should have disclosed his financial conflict of interest and he should have given Miguel sound medical advice and excellent care.

CASE 12-3

Shilpa Chandran presented to Dr. Estrilino Lumicao with fever, chills, and congestion of the lungs. Dr. Lumicao treated her appropriately and, at her request, wrote a note to her employer to indicate that her absence from work was medically justified. The note read as follows: "Shilpa Chandran was seen in my office today. She was unable to work today because of pneumonia."

CONFIDENTIALITY

Most discussions of confidentiality begin with a more dramatic case involving AIDS, alcoholism, a teenager who doesn't want her parents to know that she smokes marijuana or sleeps with her boyfriend, a schoolteacher who is secretly homosexual, a student who is depressed and suicidal, or a husband who goes to a convention, cheats on his wife, and discovers he has a sexually transmitted disease (STD) *after* he has infected his wife. I have intentionally begun this section with a more routine case to make a point: Confidentiality is important in every facet of the practice of medicine, not just the sexy, scary, or scandalous areas.

At first glance, it appears that the physician in Case 12-3 has provided excellent medical care. He did a careful history and physical, ordered the appropriate diagnostic tests, prescribed the right medications, and advised the patient properly regarding rest, diet, and not exposing others to the illness. He judged properly that she was not able to work and was correct in agreeing to write a sickness excuse for her. But he made a serious error in revealing to her employer the nature of her illness.

THE PATIENT'S EMPLOYER

Employers have a right to know whether their employees' absences are legitimate. Thus, the physician could have written, "She was unable to work today because of illness." But the precise nature of the illness is a private matter. The reasons for this are obvious in cases of "embarrassing" or taboo illnesses, such as schizophrenia, AIDS, and STDs. Many careers and reputations have been destroyed by the illegitimate release of such information. The movie *Philadelphia Story* documents one such incident in which a man lost his position with a law firm after it was revealed that he was a homosexual and that he had the AIDS virus. A similar scenario played out in Houston: After discovering that an employee had been infected by the human immunodeficiency virus (HIV), a music company changed its health insurance policy to reduce coverage for HIV from $1 million to $5000 (Holleman *et al.*, 1994). AIDS is not the only taboo: In 1972 Thomas Eagleton was forced off the Democratic presidential ticket after it was revealed that many years previously he had seen a psychiatrist for depression.

At this point the reader may be thinking, "This is all well and good, but certainly none of these disasters could befall Ms. Chandran since, after all, her illness is neither expensive nor socially stigmatic. In fact, by being informed of the precise nature of her illness, and because of the fact that her symptoms are not vague but rather are verifiable, the employer will be assured that she is truly sick and is not malingering. So it is in Ms. Chandran's interest that the physician reveal this information to her employer." This reasoning is specious for several reasons. One is that the employer will become accustomed to being informed of the nature of the illness and when that information is absent will suspect that the employee has an expensive or embarrassing illness (Holleman & Holleman, 1988). Another is that, since pneumonia is a common complication of HIV, even pneumonia could be viewed by a xenophobic employer as a justification for firing or discriminating against an employee.

THE PATIENT'S FAMILY

Another area in which confidentiality must be guarded delicately is in relation to families of patients. Sometimes they want to know what's going on but don't want the patient to know what's going on. Sometimes they don't want the patient to know that they know. If the physician isn't careful to protect boundaries, the diffusion of information can get out-of-hand, more like a soap opera than a textbook case.

In the case of severely ill patients, physicians often prefer to talk with family members: The families may be more lucid and the physician doesn't have to face the angst of the patient. While such an approach may be expedient in terms of time and emotional energy, it is inappropriate as long as the patient is able to communicate with the physician. In some cases, often as a result of cultural traditions, the patient may request that the physician deal directly with a particular family member. Such an approach should not be encouraged and, if adopted, every effort should be made to ensure that the patient was not coerced. The patient's waiver of confidentiality should be expressed in writing and included in the chart.

Patients presenting with STDs often request that their spouses or partners not be informed of the nature of their illnesses. Adolescents seeking treatment related to pregnancy, abortion, STDs, and drugs often make similar requests regarding their parents. The first situation is problematic because the partners are often at risk and the second because the child is still dependent on the parents and the parents are usually footing the bill. Judgments in these cases are often based on the seriousness of the disease, the risk of transmission, the legal reporting requirements, the attitude of the patients, and the degree of trust between physician and patient. Usually the physician will encourage the patient to discuss the matter with the third party, but when persuasive efforts and goodwill fail, the physician is faced with a difficult decision.

THE ADOLESCENT PATIENT

Many of these problems can be alleviated by conscientious attention to "preventive ethics" (McCullough & Ashton, 1994). With regard to adolescents, for example, physicians ought to establish policies of meeting alone with the patient at each visit, as well as meeting with the parent and child together. By following this process in all cases, the parent does not become suspicious when the physician unexpectedly asks the parent to leave the room. Physicians and parents also ought to establish an agreement for treating adolescents whereby the parents agree to let the adolescent see the physician privately without requiring patient or physician to report to them. It has become a custom for physicians to treat adolescents for sexual and substance-related problems without insisting on notification of the parents, but an up-front agreement could help prevent many problems caused by secrecy, cover-ups, and the threat of disclosure.

Privacy is particularly important for teenagers. Many will not seek treatment if confidentiality cannot be guaranteed. Many are too embarrassed to reveal their life-styles to their parents. In many cases embarrassment is but the tip of the iceberg. Many fear physical violence in retaliation for breaking their parents' rules.

For many pregnant teenagers, the father of the child is, well, the father of the child. Or, the stepfather, uncle, a friend of the father's, or some other adult man. A colleague once told me of a case in which a young physician refused to prescribe birth control for a 12-year-old patient, insisting that the girl was too young for sex. Soon thereafter she became pregnant and asked for an abortion. The physician refused to discuss abortion with her and advised her once again to practice abstinence. After the girl delivered the baby she asked once again for birth control. The physician refused and, as before, did not offer a referral. The next time the girl presented to the clinic the physician, a family practice resident, was on another rotation and the girl was assigned a different resident physician. Instead of refusing to discuss sex with the girl outside the presence of her parents, the physician listened and discovered the girl's father to be the father of the baby. As a result of this discovery, the girl's primary physician was placed on probation.

As this tragic case illustrates, one purpose of confidentiality is to create a space in which patients feel safe, comfortable, able to be vulnerable, and able to trust their physicians. Only in such an atmosphere will patients reveal embarrassing symptoms, family problems, life-style preferences, and other information essential to good medical care.

CONFIDENTIALITY AS A CORNERSTONE OF THE PHYSICIAN–PATIENT RELATIONSHIP

Respect for the patient's privacy is among the oldest and most time-honored traditions in the practice of medicine. The Hippocratic oath regarded medical information as "holy secrets" (Reiser, 1977). More recently, the American Medical Association's Code of Ethics has forbidden the physician from revealing "the confidences entrusted to him in the course of medical attendance, or the deficiencies he may observe in the character of patients, unless he is required to do so by law or unless it becomes necessary in order to protect the welfare of the individual or of the community" (American Medical Association, 1957). As these documents indicate, confidentiality is not simply a "good idea" or "a nice thing we do for our patients." Confidentiality is the cornerstone of the physician–patient relationship. Without it, often there would be no meaningful exchange of information and no effective therapeutic relationship.

EXCEPTIONS

Even so, there may be times when the responsibility to protect the patient's confidentiality must be weighed against other responsibilities. I have already discussed the responsibility of the physician to protect the public's health, as in the case of certain infectious diseases. There may be an ethical obligation, for example, for physicians to notify persons exposed to TB, syphilis, and HIV (Brennan, 1989; Dickens, 1988). The physician's minimum legal obligation is to report the information to the local health department, which in turn notifies endangered parties. The parties are not told the source of their exposure although they often are able to deduce the source.

The famous *Tarasoff* decision (*Tarasoff v. Regents of the University of California*, 1976) dealt with another type of exception, that of a patient who threatens to murder a particular individual. In this case a distraught young man killed his ex-girlfriend after disclosing to his psychiatrist his intention to do so. The psychiatrist had contacted the police but not the young woman. The courts ruled that the psychiatrist had a duty to warn the woman directly. Not every state has made such a strong ruling, and the legal requirements outside California are not yet clear. There does seem to be a consensus among ethicists, however, that in cases where the patient's homicidal threat is specific and there is a reasonable likelihood that the patient will follow through, the physician's ethical obligation to respect the patient's confidentiality is superseded by an ethical obligation to protect the lives of endangered human beings (Cooper, 1982). Thus, notifying both the police and the endangered individual or individuals is in order in such cases.

One problem with notifying potential victims, of course, is that they may initiate a preemptive strike and commit a crime themselves. States vary as to the reporting requirements of physicians in this situation, so for legal guidance the medical student is advised to examine his state's laws. For ethical guidance, physicians must rely on their knowledge of the persons involved and on the counsel of colleagues and law enforcement officials. My own experience is that lawyers will advise you to do the minimum legal obligation in order to avoid litigation, but will not advise you regarding the ethically responsible action.

One other area in which traditional views of confidentiality need rethinking is in the large medical center, where the "dyadic" physician–patient relationship is replaced by the patient being cared for by a team of physicians, nurses, and other medical personnel (Siegler, 1982; Holleman et al., 1994). In this atmosphere the patient's medical chart may be read by dozens, even hundreds, of individuals. In academic teaching centers where medical students train, the patient may be examined by a plethora of medical students and the patient's case is often discussed in the hallway, on elevators, and at large conferences. To protect patients and avoid misunderstandings in such situations, the primary physician should inform the patient of the nature of the facility, should ask the patient's permission for various members of the team, various medical students, and other trainees to examine the patient and to discuss the case.

For their part, medical personnel should refrain from discussing the case in hallways and elevators in a way that others can identify the patient. Persons attending case conferences should be reminded that the anonymity of the patient must be protected outside the confines of the conference room. If presenters or discussants plan to reveal the identity of the patient, pharmaceutical representatives and other persons without fiduciary obligations to protect confidentiality should be asked to leave the conference room before the case discussion begins.

CASE 12-4

J. S. is a college freshman who presented to the student health center complaining of headaches, a cough, and malaise. The physician, Dr. Velasco, told J. S. that it's probably "just a cold" and prescribes fluids, rest, aspirin, and a cough suppressant at bedtime. When J. S. returned 1 week later without any improvement and appeared distressed and dejected, Dr. Velasco noted that J. S. was facing his first college midterms and took a few minutes to ask J. S. about the stressors in his life. J. S. refused her offer of a referral to a psychiatrist but returned for weekly follow-up visits. J. S. appreciated Dr. Velasco's warm, motherly manner but the symptoms continued.

On the seventh week J. S. asked Dr. Velasco for a referral to a specialist and for a sickness excuse to allow him to take incompletes on two of his courses. Dr.

Velasco appeared shocked that the "cold" caused J. S. to miss so many classes. She signed the sickness excuse but recommended a thorough workup before opting for a referral. The cold agglutinin test was positive, indicating that J. S. had mycoplasma pneumonia. Dr. Velasco seemed embarrassed to have missed the diagnosis but told J. S. that he had an "atypical presentation" of "a rather rare illness" which is "extremely difficult to diagnose." She prescribed erythromycin and in 3 days the symptoms resolved completely.

Meanwhile, two of J. S.'s roommates have gone home for the winter holidays with "colds" and seen their local physicians, each of whom quickly diagnoses the problem as mycoplasma pneumonia.

TRUTH TELLING

Until recently, physicians routinely withheld the truth from their patients in a number of areas, such as a diagnosis of cancer, a poor prognosis, and any risks and side effects of treatment that might scare the patient from taking the treatment. Many physicians also hid their mistakes from their patients. Physicians believed that patients did not have the mental or emotional wherewithal to "take" the truth—at least when the truth hurt. In reality, it was the physician who felt uncomfortable with truth, particularly if the truth meant that the patient was dying or that the physician had failed the patient.

In Case 12-4, the physician makes a mistake that hampers a young student's college career. Dr. Velasco then makes a second mistake: She lies to the patient in an effort to cover the first mistake. Dr. Velasco's justification for the lie is that she does not want J. S., the patient, to lose confidence in her abilities. After all, confidence is an important ingredient in healing. The real reason, however, is that she feels guilty for the harm she has caused J. S. and much too embarrassed to reveal her shortcomings as a physician. She also fears that J. S. might become angry and that his parents might sue.

Now that J. S. and his family know that Dr. Velasco has lied, J. S. might indeed sue. After all, Dr. Velasco missed a diagnosis that most would have made, this mistake harmed the patient, and then Dr. Velasco lied to cover her mistake. Lying to clients is clearly a violation of the professional's fiduciary obligations to their clients. Like many physicians, Dr. Velasco underestimated the ability of her patients to accept her shortcomings, to forgive her mistakes, and to recognize that physicians are, after all, mere mortals. She underestimated her patient's ability to uncover the truth. She had a good relationship with J. S., yet, like many physicians and attorneys, underestimated the influence of that relationship in preventing litigation (Garr & Marsh, 1986).

And even if the patient's parents had sued, which they had every right to do, this would not in any way change the fact that the only morally decent thing to do is to disclose one's error to one's patient, to apologize, and, if possible, to make restitution (Peterson & Brennan, 1990). There may be exceptions, such as when the errors are minor or when the errors cause the patient no harm. When the errors are serious, patients have a right to know and physicians have an ethical obligation to tell them. Many attorneys will counsel otherwise, but their job is to tell you your minimal legal obligations, not to tell you the right or even the minimally decent thing to do. Nor is it their job to tell you how to be a good person or a virtuous physician. Most would agree that the minimally decent thing to *be* is to be honest.

An essential component of an effective physician–patient relationship—or of any successful relationship, for that matter—is trust. Relationships, both personal and professional, are built on the faith that the other can be trusted to tell the truth, to keep promises, to abide by agreed-on ways of doing things.

In the physician–patient relationship, honesty is essential. If the physician cannot trust the patient to tell the truth about symptoms, habits, and life-style, as well as willingness to follow the physician's recommendations and the side effects of treatment, the physician's best efforts will be stymied. If the patient cannot trust the physician to tell the truth about the nature of the illness or the risks and side effects of treatment, the patient will be less likely to follow the physician's recommendations. Also, an effective placebo will be wasted, as the patient will not place confidence in the healing powers of the physician (Brody, 1980).

Interestingly enough, the terms *confidence* and *confide* stem from the same root, *fidere*, which means trust or faith. To have confidence in a particular physician or healer, one must feel willing and able to confide in that healer. Patients are not likely to confide in persons they cannot trust, in persons they do not deem trust*worthy*. Healthcare professionals earn that confidence and trust through accumulating a steady track record of being honest with their patients. This requires resisting the temptation to avoid telling patients bad news. It requires resisting the temptation to mislead the patient by watering down the bad news.

COMBINING TRUTH WITH EMPATHY

It also requires, however, the art of telling the patient bad news in such a way that the patient does not abandon all hope. Physicians and healers who care deeply about their patients not only will want patients to understand the nature and severity of their illness but also will want them to sense that their physicians will not abandon them, that they will receive the best care possible, and that, although "hope" and "good outcome" may need to be redefined, there is always a basis for hope (Kubler-Ross, 1970). Good physicians recognize that patients need to hear the truth and that this might make them depressed. But the best physicians will assist the patients through the depression in such a way as to prevent their reaching a state of utter despair. The best physicians do not shirk from their responsibility to tell their patients the truth, nor do they blast out the bad news, leave the room, and leave the patients devastated by the truth. When the truth is told in a sensitive manner, the physician's voice can be an agent of healing even while the words themselves bring unpleasant news.

Combining truth with empathy is important for all types of physician–patient communications. If a patient with metastatic cancer asks you if she is going to die, you could simply say "yes" and fulfill your obligation to tell your patients the truth. But you would be shirking other responsibilities, such as the responsibility to be a healer and to ease suffering. Here's a better response: "I hope you live a long time, and I'm going to do what I can to help that happen. But I think you ought to know that most patients in your condition live for a shorter time, a few months. Either way, I'm going to be here to help. To help you live as long as you can, and when that's no longer in the cards, to help you be as comfortable as possible." For many patients, the fear of being abandoned is as great as the fear of dying. If the patient feels she can't trust her physician to tell her the truth, then she is unlikely to trust her to be there when she needs her.

Patients with diabetes mellitus, heart disease, and other chronic illnesses often become frustrated with the inconveniences, discomforts, and disabilities caused by their illness. A common defense mechanism is to deny the illness exists and to quit taking medications, or to take them sporadically. Physicians must be frank with these patients in pointing out that their illness is hidden but real and in confronting them regarding the outcome of not taking their medications. Even so, such bad news can be told in a caring manner. Begin by acknowledging their suffering: "I can't imagine the pain, the discomfort, the expense, the inconvenience, and the frustration of living with this disease." Continue by joining with them in their denial: "If I were in your situation I think I'd do just what you're doing. I'd try my damnedest to wish it away." Or: "As your physician and friend, I wish to goodness I could wave a wand and make this illness, this curse, go away. I've seen how it hurts my patients and I wish I could do more to help." Pause to listen to the patient's response. And truly listen: Don't pretend to listen while composing your next lines. In an indirect way, you've already addressed the patient's denial, and this may be sufficient to help the patient work through the denial. But a direct confrontation will often be necessary. "You're not going to like hearing this, but as your physician it's my responsibility to remind you that you've got a serious disease and it's going to kill you if you don't take your medications."

Sometimes physicians are reticent to discuss bad news because they aren't sure how extensively the patient wants to talk about "it." What commonly happens in these situations is that physicians, nurses, patients, and families do a very clumsy dance, dancing around "it." Nobody wants to give "it" a name. One way to break the ice is simply to acknowledge what is happening: "We could go on and on dancing around the truth, talking about 'it,' smoothing things over, or we could just come on out and say what we're thinking. My experience has been that, even though it's painful at first, most patients prefer to get things out in the open. They don't want me hiding things from them. I assume that this is how you feel too, is it?" Most studies show that physicians, not patients, are the ones who feel uncomfortable talking about death, cancer, and all the other "its" and who project this anxiety onto their patients (Edinger & Smucker, 1992). My experience has been that, despite the sting, patients feel relieved to finally know the truth and be able to begin dealing with it.

Many medical students feel uncomfortable talking with patients who have terminal illnesses or disabling injuries, or with parents whose children are found to have serious illness, mental retardation, or physical disability. A good way to break the ice is to greet the patient by naming the "it": "Good afternoon, Mrs. Shah. How is the cancer treating you today?" Another technique is to disclose the discomfort: "I feel uncomfortable asking you these questions so soon after you've heard some very disappointing news, but there are a few things we have to talk about if we are to provide the best care possible for your child."

WHEN THE PATIENT IS IN DENIAL

Sometimes the problem will not be that the physician has withheld the truth from the patient, but that the patient has not heard it. A common defense mechanism for dealing with devastating information is denial. This is a natural, healthy way to avert shock, to allow for time to process the information gradually (Weisman, 1972).

Except in emergency situations in which decisions must be made immediately, patient and family should be given time to absorb the information, to ask questions, and to get used to this new state of affairs. Treatment decisions can usually be delayed a few days, even weeks. During this time the patient might quite rationally seek a second opinion or a repeat of the diagnostic test. Physicians in this situation often feel that their expertise is being questioned or their authority undermined. Such a feeling reflects the physician's failure to recognize that cognitive denial is a normal, healthy reaction. Denial is a means of avoiding shock and reflects the patient's desire to maintain health and independence. It is also quite rational: X rays do get switched from time to time, physicians have been known to misread EKGs and EEGs, and many tests commonly produce false positives.

Rather than becoming angry with such patients or attempting to bludgeon them with the truth by insisting that the diagnosis is correct and that they must "take or leave" the recommended treatment, the physician should encourage the patient to seek a second opinion or, in some cases, a repeat of the test. Verifying the diagnosis is the first step toward accepting the reality of the illness and what must be done to treat it.

CASE 12-5

Mr. Martin Salgo presented to a surgeon, Dr. Frank Gerbode, appearing older than his 55 years and reporting leg cramps, hip pain, and pain in the lower right quadrant while walking and exercising. Dr. Gerbode concluded that Mr. Salgo had "probable occlusion of the abdominal aorta which had impaired blood supply to the legs and other areas and advanced arteriosclerosis." Dr. Gerbode recommended X rays of the GI tract and aortic angiography, the injection of a radiopaque dye into the aorta to visualize the plaque formation and confirm the diagnosis. Dr. Gerbode told Mr. Salgo that the procedure would be done under general anesthesia, but did not explain the possible complications of anesthesia or aortography. Mr. Salgo consented to the procedure. The day following the procedure Mr. Salgo awoke paralyzed in his lower extremities. The paralysis, caused by a hematoma pressing against the spine, proved to be permanent. (Salgo v. Leland Stanford, Jr. University Board of Trustees, 1957)

INFORMED CONSENT

When people get sick, they commonly experience a loss of control and feel that their privacy and personal integrity have been violated. This vulnerability is related to a number of factors, including the patient's weakness, the nature of hospitals and of medical and surgical tests and treatments, and the insensitivity of some caregivers. As students begin their medical training, it is important for them to appreciate the vulnerability of patients and the need to protect their right to self-determination as expressed through the principle of autonomy and guaranteed by the practice of informed consent to treatment.

For an informed consent to be valid the patient or his proxy must give consent. Yet there are times when the physician, for whatever reason, fails to obtain that consent. In Case 12-1, Ms. Ballard's oncologist and surgeon conspired with her daughter to have her breast amputated without her knowledge or consent. In past years some obstetricians tied the Fallopian tubes of indigent or mentally ill women without their consent, permanently sterilizing them. Sometimes burn patients have painful treatments forced on them (*Please Let Me Die*, 1974). Sometimes busy physicians *tell* their patients what they're going to do to them rather than offering their recommendation and awaiting the patient's consent before initiating treatment. Such actions are wrong, both legally and ethically, as indicated by a landmark ruling in 1914 by the New York Supreme Court: "Every human being of adult years and of sound mind has the right to determine what shall be done with his own body, and a surgeon who performs an operation without his patient's consent commits an assault for which he is liable in damages" (*Schloendorff v. Society of New York Hospital*, 1914).

In Case 12-5, Mr. Salgo clearly gave his consent, a point that Dr. Gerbode's attorneys felt sufficient to meet the legal requirements. Yet the jury awarded Mr. Salgo a large sum of money, ruling the consent invalid because Dr. Gerbode had failed to warn the patient of the risk of paralysis. Perhaps Dr. Gerbode considered the risk too minimal to mention. Perhaps he feared that Mr. Salgo might be frightened from going through with the procedure. Or perhaps Dr. Gerbode simply didn't feel he had any obligation to share this information with the patient. There certainly had been no legal precedent for doing so, at least not until then. The jury in this case established an important legal precedent in claiming that the physician must not only get the patient's consent but also that the consent must be an *informed* decision:

> A physician violates his duty to his patient and subjects himself to liability if he withholds any facts which are necessary to form the basis of an intelligent consent by the patients to the proposed treatment. Likewise the physician may not minimize the known dangers of a procedure or operation in order to induce his patient's consent. (*Salgo v. Leland Stanford, Jr. University Board of Trustees*, 1957)

ELEMENTS OF INFORMED CONSENT

For the consent to be truly *informed*, what information should be given the patient? First, the patient should be told the nature of his condition. Is it life-threatening? How will it affect his work, his life-style, his future? What pain, suffering, disability, or disfigurement might possibly result from this disease or injury? Second, the physician should describe the major recommended treatments for the patient's condition. What are the benefits of each treatment? What are the risks? What are the discomforts and other possible side effects? What are the costs? Third, the physician should describe the likely benefits, risks, discomforts, and side effects of nontreatment. A patient who refuses a Pap smear, for example, should be informed of her risk of cervical cancer and of the seriousness of that disease (*Truman v. Thomas*, 1980). These three elements are presented in Table 12.1.

EXCEPTIONS

There are, of course, a few exceptional situations in which the obligation to initiate a test or treatment is superseded by a more pressing obligation. In medical emergencies in which the patient's life or health is in danger and consent cannot be obtained from the patient or next of kin in a timely fashion, the physician should presume that the patient wishes to be treated aggressively. In situations in which children are in distress as a result of an injury or illness and the parents cannot be reached in a timely fashion, the physician

Table 12.1
Elements of Informed Consent

The nature of the patient's condition
    Whether the condition is life-threatening
    Anticipated pain, disability, disfigurement
Recommended treatment(s)
    Benefits
    Risks, discomforts, and other side effects
    Costs
Nontreatment
    Benefits
    Risks, discomforts, and other side effects
    Potential costs

---

should presume that the parents would want the condition treated in accordance with the standard of care rather than prolonging the suffering of the child. During public health emergencies, vaccines and quarantines may be required by law.

In some cases a patient may choose to waive her right to make an informed decision, turning the decision over to a relative or to her physician. Physicians should discourage this practice and should evaluate and address the underlying cause of the patient's unwillingness to decide for herself. The potential for abuse by paternalistic physicians and coercive family members makes this situation an ethical and legal quagmire. Physicians whose patients waive this right despite counseling should ask the patient to document the waiver in writing or should ask a colleague to witness the verbal waiver.

In the past some physicians have withheld information from patients by invoking the so-called therapeutic privilege. In these cases the physician believes the very attempt to gain informed consent will have serious health-related consequences for the patient. A commonly cited example involves a patient who is depressed, suicidal, and is found to have cancer. Oftentimes the issue is less a fear of suicide than fear that the patient will not choose the therapy the physician thinks the patient needs. The consensus among ethicists is that physicians should seldom, if ever, invoke therapeutic privilege, particularly if for paternalistic fears that the patient will not select the physician's recommendation. The reluctance to gain an informed consent usually reflects the physician's insecurity rather than the patient's and perhaps also unwillingness or incompetence to treat an underlying depression. Even in rare cases where, despite psychiatric treatment, the patient truly is at serious risk of suicide, the testing or treatment often can be delayed a few days or weeks until the patient is able to make an informed decision. In cases where the patient is incompetent to make an informed decision and unlikely to become competent in the near future, the physician should gain an informed consent from the patient's designated agent or next of kin (Faden & Beauchamp, 1986).

COMMON MISTAKES

Despite the wide ethical and legal acceptance of the patient's right to informed consent for tests and treatments, physicians often fail to respect this right. One of the most common mistakes is that the physician bypasses the competent patient and talks instead with the family. She may do this because she feels uncomfortable being with seriously ill or dying patients. Others lack the patience to communicate with feeble or confused patients who speak softly and slowly, or who may need to have information repeated several times.

Sometimes physicians fail to get a truly informed consent because they fail to explain the information in a way the patient can understand. Medical students can be particularly guilty of this mistake, as they are in the process of mastering a new vocabulary and forget that patients do not know the same jargon, nor do they have the same understanding of disease processes or treatment regimens. I advise students to imagine that the patient is a brother or grandfather or someone else whom one knows well, and to try to communicate the information to him in a way he'll understand. It is also best to ask the patient to explain to you, in his own words, what he hears you saying: what the options are, what the risks and benefits are, and what he wants to do to treat his illness.

Some physicians are guilty of "leading the witness." This occurs when a physician presents a biased version of the information that the patient will use to make her decision. For example, the physician omits or minimizes the risks of Treatment A and omits or minimizes the benefits of Treatment B. Or, the physician may include the pertinent information but may insinuate by voice inflection, word choice, or body language that the risks of Treatment B are more dangerous than the risks of Treatment A, when actually this is not the case: "Mrs. Mbiti, if you go with Treatment A, the only thing you have to worry about is a myocardial infarction, which most of our patients don't even get, but [lowering voice, speaking slower, and adopting a somber expression] if you choose Treatment B, I'm afraid there is a very real chance you'd develop AN IRREGULAR HEARTBEAT. During the first 2 weeks of treatment you might also break out with SOME VERY UNSIGHTLY RED AND WHITE SPLOTCHES ON YOUR FACE." The physician in this case should have explained the term *myocardial infarction* or used a familiar term, such as *heart attack*. The physician also should have given a more accurate impression of the relative odds and seriousness of each risk.

Some physicians are diligent in getting the patient's consent for the most invasive procedures but forget that every medication and every diagnostic test involves some discomforts and risks that ought to be explained to the patient. Some physicians mistakenly believe that getting the patient's signature on an informed consent form is all that is required. Actually, informed consent is a verbal communication between physician and patient. The patient's signature on the form is merely a legal record that the physician discussed the pertinent information with the patient, the patient understood it, and the patient freely decided to accept or refuse recommended tests or treatments.

Some physicians fail to inform patients of costs of recommended tests or treatments. Many prescriptions are never filled for this reason. Physicians often accuse these patients of being "noncompliant," but the real issue is that the patient was never given the opportunity to make an informed consent to treatment. Some physicians err by failing to inform patients of legitimate alternative treatments. For example, a patient with a back problem should be informed not only of the allopathic medical standards of care, but also of the legitimate chiropractic alternatives. Some physicians fail to inform their patients of the risks and benefits of nontreatment. For many years, Dr. Thomas recommended that Mrs. Cobbs have a Pap smear test. Each time she refused. After Mrs. Cobbs died of cervical cancer, her children sued, and won. The court ruled that the patient must be informed of "the risks of a decision *not* to undergo treatment" as well as the "risks inherent in the procedure . . . and the probability of a successful outcome of the treatment" (*Truman v. Thomas*, 1980) Having dealt with Pap smears every day, Dr. Thomas assumed incorrectly that most patients knew what they were and how they helped prevent deaths caused by cancer.

Physicians often falsely label certain types of patients as incompetent. We have already discussed one such type: the weak, feeble patient who talks slowly, barely audibly, and who may need to have information repeated two or three times before understanding it. Another type of patient often incorrectly labeled as incompetent is the person with disabilities. This is the result of the physician's inexperience with and prejudice toward persons who are blind, deaf and dumb, mildly retarded, or severely physically disabled.

Other patients often treated as incompetent include those who speak a foreign language or come from a culture with which the physician is unfamiliar. I recall one incident in which our medical team entered the room of a 95-year-old patient who had just been admitted from a local nursing home, heard him speaking "gibberish," and therefore assumed him to be incompetent to make medical decisions. Thus, the team did not attempt to inform him of the nature of his condition and the risks, benefits, and costs of treatment. Nor did they obtain his consent for treatment. Later the team learned that the patient was a Jewish immigrant from Russia. They also learned from a psychology consultant that in times of crisis patients often seek strength in the language of their youth or the language that bears religious significance for them. The patient may have been speaking Russian, Hebrew, Yiddish, or all three. Rather than the "gibberish" being an indication of incompetence, it may have indicated just the opposite: the patient's intelligence, his facility for many languages, and his ability, unlike that of the medical team, to have functioned throughout his life in multicultural settings and also to engage the religious as well as the medical meaning of suffering.

Physicians should presume that their patients are competent unless there is strong evidence to suggest otherwise. Patients who cannot communicate, who cannot understand basic facts, who cannot reason consistent with a personal value, who because of depression or anxiety cannot bring themselves to make any decisions, or who cannot stick with a decision are the types who may legitimately be viewed as incompetent. It should be emphasized that the definition of being unable to communicate is a narrow one: If a paralyzed patient can move her eyeballs once to indicate "yes" and twice to indicate "no," then she should not be considered unable to communicate. It should also be emphasized that patients who make decisions based on deeply held personal values should not be judged incompetent even if the physician dislikes those values. For example, a patient who refuses chemotherapy because he believes "the Lord will heal me" is not incompetent, nor is a patient who states that he believes in the healing power of "a strict macrobiotic diet." Even the patient who refuses chemotherapy because he doesn't want his hair to fall out may be deciding on the basis of a deeply held personal value.

On the other hand, the patient who refuses chemotherapy because he believes "the Viet Cong have poisoned all the medicines" is basing his decision on a psychotic delusion, not on a deeply held personal value, and such a patient should not be viewed as competent to make an informed decision. For such patients a proxy decision-maker should be identified. If the patient did not designate such a decision-maker prior to losing competence, then his spouse or partner, parents, adult children, siblings, or closest friends should be consulted.

CASE 12-6

Leon Jones, a 78-year-old man with advanced Alzheimer's disease, presented to Dr. Chen, his longtime physician, with cough, sore throat, and pneumonia. Dr.

Chen treated Mr. Jones with fluids and cough syrup but, in accordance with the wishes expressed by Mr. Jones prior to becoming demented, did not prescribe antibiotics. Dr. Chen then called a family conference at the nursing home where Mr. Jones lived.

Mr. Jones's oldest son demanded that his father be given antibiotics and admitted to the local hospital where he could be placed in an ICU and receive "the best care possible." Dr. Chen explained that Mr. Jones had asked to be allowed to die when his Alzheimer's reached an advanced stage. When the son continued to object, Dr. Chen showed him a copy of his father's Living Will and explained that as a physician he was legally bound to comply with this request. He explained that Mr. Jones no longer remembered who he was and that his condition was irreversible. Dr. Chen also explained that Mr. Jones had been concerned not to spend his wife and children's inheritance. Mrs. Jones affirmed that this had been her husband's wish and that she was ready to "let him go."

The second son said it was a disgrace that their father, who had once been such a friendly, outgoing member of the community, should be spending the last days of his life in an institutional setting. "Let's bring him home. If it's too much for mom to handle, we sons can rotate shifts to care for him 'round the clock." Dr. Chen acknowledged that many patients prefer to die at home but Mr. Jones had requested that once his Alzheimer's reached an advanced stage he wanted to stay in a nursing home where he could maintain as much anonymity as possible. "He wanted his friends to remember him the way he used to be," commented Mrs. Jones. "And he doesn't remember anything about the house or neighborhood anymore, or recognize who we are."

The youngest son, who had been closest to his father, asked whether some drug could be given to end his father's suffering: "I can't bear to see him this way." Dr. Chen and Mrs. Jones agreed that, as a devout Baptist, Mr. Jones probably viewed suicide as a sin. Dr. Chen explained that cough syrup and other medications could provide symptomatic relief and that he would give as much medicine as necessary to relieve pain, but that with advanced Alzheimer's Mr. Jones probably felt little pain. Moreover, Mr. Jones would most likely die very soon. Dr. Chen commented that the real pain was for those who had to watch him die. There was a long silence, then one by one family members held Mr. Jones' hand, cried, and recalled the good times they had had together.

Two days later Mr. Jones died in the nursing home, his youngest son holding his hand and his dog Pete at his side. The family asked Dr. Chen to read Mr. Jones's eulogy at the funeral, which was attended by hundreds of Mr. Jones's neighbors, coworkers, relatives, and friends, each of whom remembered Leon Jones as a friendly, outgoing member of the community.

—— DEATH, DYING, AND DECISION-MAKING ——

One of the most difficult areas of ethical decision-making for patients, physicians, and families involves serious illness and death. Pain, suffering, loss of control, fear of the unknown, anticipation of loss, grief, guilt, and the life review process all evoke strong feelings at a time when difficult decisions must be made. To help ease the decision-making process, the following framework may be useful.

Ethicists, like emergency room physicians, thrive on "three alarm" situations, but most of the more dramatic ethical dilemmas, like most medical emergencies, can and should be prevented. It is the physician's responsibility to help the patient anticipate and prepare for the future. The patient's primary care physician should ask her about her values and preferences regarding life, death, and end-of-life choices. These conversations should be documented in the chart and, where appropriate, shared with family members and close friends. The physician should also encourage the patient to consider writing an advance directive and assigning someone as a Durable Power of Attorney for Healthcare.

Advance directives, or living wills, give the patient an opportunity to express, in writing, his wishes regarding end-of-life treatment should the patient become terminally ill, incapacitated, and unable to express his preferences. Advance directives apply only to situations in which the patient has no reasonable hope of recovery; they do not apply to acute situations such as a car accident or bullet wound in which aggressive treatment might save the life of the patient and return him to good health. Physicians should encourage patients to indicate, verbally and in writing, any specific concerns. For example, some patients who do not want to be placed on respirators or given antibiotics may still wish, for religious or other reasons, to receive food and fluids. Once the advance directive is signed and witnessed, it is legally binding. Physicians should encourage patients to submit copies for their clinic and hospital charts and to give copies to close friends, relatives, and clergy.

Oftentimes family members ask physicians to continue providing curative treatments in violation of the expressed will of their loved one. Sometimes physicians feel uncomfortable complying with patients' requests for no heroic treatment. The purpose of the advance directive is to protect the patient from well-meaning but misdirected physicians and family members, such as Mr. Jones's sons.

Like the Durable Power of Attorney, which enables a person to assign someone as proxy for legal and financial decisions should he become incapacitated, the Durable Power of Attorney for Healthcare enables a patient to assign someone as a proxy for medical decisions. So many end-of-life decisions are difficult to anticipate, and the advance directive is so general that physicians should encourage patients to complete this document, even if they have also written an advance directive. This way the patient is assured that, if he should become incapacitated, his medical decisions will be made by someone who knows his values and preferences well. The physician should encourage the patient to discuss his values and preferences with his proxy decision-maker so that the proxy will indeed know what to do and will have the courage to make tough decisions if and when the time comes. The physician should also encourage the patient to assign a backup proxy; after all, the patient might outlive the proxy, or the proxy might be out of the country or for some other reason unavailable.

Whenever a patient is hospitalized or admitted to a nursing home, the physician and patient should discuss code status. This will be a stressful time for the patient, family, and physician, but careful attention to this matter can alleviate many future difficulties. Some patients, and some physicians as well, mistakenly believe that once aggressive treatments have been initiated, they must be continued until death. In the initial stages of a crisis, if there is uncertainty as to how to treat the patient, it is best to begin with aggressive treatment and then, as soon as an assessment is possible, to consider withdrawing treatment if it does not seem to be benefiting the patient or fitting the wishes of the patient.

STEP 2. CLARIFICATION

Most ethical problems can be avoided by careful attention to preventive ethics. Sometimes, however, there will be conflicts as a result of the intense emotions surrounding the suffering and death of a loved one. Mr. and Mrs. Jones and Dr. Chen did an excellent job of anticipating the debilitating effects of Alzheimer's, but they failed to communicate Mr. Jones's preferences to his sons. Perhaps the sons were not ready to face these issues.

When the conflicts arose, they had the potential to subvert Mr. Jones's plan of how to face death. They also had the potential to divide the family at a time when unity was most needed. Dr. Chen succeeded at averting these catastrophes by recognizing the misunderstandings and motives of each son, and clarifying each.

The first son misunderstood the terminal nature of advanced Alzheimer's disease, the second misunderstood his father's desire for privacy, and the third misunderstood the nature of his father's suffering and his religious values regarding suicide and euthanasia. Rather than engaging the sons in an argument or turning the decision-making process into a power struggle, Dr. Chen clarified the facts in a way that indicated respect for each son's feelings, a solid understanding of Mr. Jones's preferences, and careful preparation by physician, patient, and spouse for this difficult moment. Dr. Chen refrained from personalizing the conflict; by treating it as a series of factual misunderstandings, no one felt blame, shame, or bulldozed.

In my experience most ethical conflicts involve such misunderstandings. Sometimes the family and sometimes the caregiver jump to false conclusions. For example, the physician discovers that the parents are not giving their child the antibiotics the physician prescribed 2 days ago, and now the child is seriously ill. The physician concludes that the parents are guilty of abuse by neglect and asks for an emergency meeting of the ethics committee to consider asking a judge to remove the child from her parents' custody. The ethics committee meets with the parents and discovers that they misunderstood the physician's orders: They thought she wanted them to wait until the antihistamine prescription had run out before giving the child the new medicine. This problem could have been avoided, and with it all of the shaming associated with noncompliance and abuse, had the physician spent more time clarifying the facts of the case instead of hastily jumping to negative conclusions.

The other area requiring clarification is motives. Once Mr. Jones's sons understood their father's motives for his choices—to save money for his family, to be remembered well by friends and neighbors, and to remain faithful to his religious convictions—the sons could accept their father's decisions. And because Dr. Chen recognized that the sons' motives were good ones, he did not make the mistake of insulting them at this tender moment. Many physicians in this situation would have viewed the sons as obstreperous, would either have engaged them in a power struggle or capitulated to their demands, and would not have handled their complaints so adroitly.

STEP 3. REVIEW THE DECISION-MAKING PROCESS

If prevention and clarification fail, then the physician should review the decision-making process to see whether some point was overlooked or misapplied. The process we have recommended here involves attention to five basic concerns: beneficence, nonmaleficence, autonomy, justice, and values. In the case of assisted suicide or euthanasia, there is considerable debate among physicians, ethicists, and patients regarding: Whether these services constitute a benefit or a harm; whether the patient has a right to expect such a presumed benefit from the medical profession; whether legalization of such services would skid us down the slippery slope of genocide of the frail elderly and disabled, or at least create unjust pressures and incentives to eliminate those who cannot care for themselves; and whether assisting in suicide or euthanasia is consistent with the meaning and mission of the medical profession.

CONCLUSION

Far from focusing on rare or hypothetical situations, and far from being an exercise in semantics, abstract reasoning, or pondering questions that only lead to more questions, medical ethics addresses everyday clinical situations and helps provide practical, workable solutions. In this chapter I have offered a four-step process for clinical ethical problem-solving: (1) What benefits can I offer this patient, and what harms are also possible? (2) What are the patient's values and preferences? (3) What is fair in this situation? (4) Am I remaining faithful to my values and ideals, and to those of my profession? Careful attention to these four questions will usually result in ethically sound clinical decision-making. Should problems arise, the physician should clarify factual misunderstandings of the patient, family, or colleagues, as well as their motives. In most cases problems can be prevented by anticipating them and preparing for them.

In this chapter I have tried to focus on the areas in which ethical and legal consensus has been reached. Just as there are standards of care, say, in the treatment of an ear infection, there are ethical and legal standards regarding confidentiality, truth telling, and informed consent. Sometimes these standards will conflict with one another or with other important ethical and legal requirements, and sometimes physicians will disagree as to the best way to reconcile these conflicts, but the physician must make a conscientious effort to be as faithful as possible to each of these important standards of care. In so doing the physician will discover that fidelity to ethical standards of care is not just good ethics, it's good medicine.

CASES FOR DISCUSSION

CASE 1

A physician calls the home of a 15-year-old patient to tell her the results of her lab tests, which indicate that she has gonorrhea. Her mother, who is unaware of her daughter's problem, answers the phone and asks why the physician is calling her daughter. The physician states that it is a confidential matter between physician and patient. The mother states that she is the legal guardian of a minor, and has the right to know what's going on. Unsure what to do, the physician hangs up on the mother.

1. *What ethical considerations are most important in the treatment of a 15-year-old patient?*
2. *The physician could think of no better solution than hanging up. Can you think of a better way out of this embarrassing situation?*
3. *Now that the mother is suspicious, what should the physician do to ameliorate the situation?*
4. *How might this problem have been prevented?*

CASE 2

An 83-year-old woman presented to a family practice clinic with a large, deep ulceration on her lower leg and foot resulting from an injury from a dog chain that had denuded the skin 4 years previously. Grafting efforts had been only marginally successful. The patient had not been seen in the clinic for 2 years—she reported being treating by a cardiologist in Mexico—and since that time the ulceration had been reinjured, had worsened considerably, and osteomyelitis had set in. The physician admitted the patient to the hospital and requested an orthopedics consultation. The consultant felt that antibiotics were unlikely to help and recommended amputation within the next few days. The patient stated that she'd rather die than lose her foot.

1. *What options are available to the primary physician?*
2. *Should either physician try to persuade the patient to change her mind?*
3. *Is this patient incompetent? Why or why not?*
4. *Imagine that the orthopedist had "stolen" the patient from the family physician and was trying to coerce her to undergo surgery. What should the family physician do in such a situation? What should the family physician have done to prevent this from happening?*

CASE 3

During a routine preplacement examination, the patient volunteers that she smokes marijuana two or three times per month and asks whether the physician thinks she ought to quit. She also reports smoking a pack of cigarettes per day. In filing her report with the employer, the physician indicates that the patient is "fit for employment" but notes that the employee occasionally smokes marijuana.

One week later the patient returns to see the physician, angry because she has been fired from her job. The patient threatens to sue the physician for releasing confidential information to a third party.

1. *Was the physician correct in sharing this information with the employer? Why or why not?*
2. *Would this information be relevant if the patient were operating heavy machinery? working as a security guard?*
3. *What are the physician's obligations to the employer? What are the physician's obligations to the patient-employee?*
4. *What should the physician say to the angry patient? What should the physician do to rectify the situation?*
5. *If the woman had been a regular patient of this physician, would the physician's responsibilities be any different?*

CASE 4

Ron Stenberg, a 51-year-old geologist, has been a patient of Dr. Nardella's private practice for the past 12 years. One year ago he lost his job and with it his health insurance. He has been unsuccessful in finding other employment and recently lost his home through foreclosure. For the past few weeks he has lived on the streets and in shelters for the homeless. His only source of income is a few dollars per day from picking up aluminum cans.

He presents to Dr. Nardella today with depression and also with inflamed feet due to walking, worn-out shoes, and standing in lines. He worries that if his feet worsen, he will no longer be able to pick up cans. Dr. Nardella worries that if she refers Mr. Stenberg to the local public hospital, he will have difficulty getting transportation there, will not establish a close relationship with a primary care physician, and will not get the quality of care necessary to be healed of these problems.

1. *Is Mr. Stenberg still Dr. Nardella's patient?*
2. *What are Dr. Nardella's ethical responsibilities to Mr. Stenberg?*

3. *What are physicians' responsibilities to patients who cannot pay?*
4. *What are the public's responsibilities to patients who cannot pay?*

CASE 5

A 30-year-old patient, who has recently tested positive for HIV, expresses an unwillingness to tell his past sexual partners that they may have been exposed to the AIDS virus but states that he will always use a condom in the future. In accordance with the law, the physician has reported the positive test result to the local health department but still feels uneasy about the situation. The health department is backlogged and unlikely to work on the case for several months. At least two of the patient's recent partners are the physician's long-time patients.

1. *What are the physician's obligations to each of the affected individuals?*
2. *Would the physician be ethically justified in contacting individuals he believes to have been exposed to HIV? Are his obligations different to those individuals who are his patients?*
3. *Would the physician be justified in using persuasion to try to get the patient to change his mind? Coercion?*
4. *What responsibilities do patients have to physicians?*
5. *Under what circumstances might a physician legitimately "fire" a patient? Is this such a situation?*

RECOMMENDED READINGS

Beauchamp TL, Childress JF: *Principles of Biomedical Ethics*. London, Oxford University Press, 1989.

> The most widely used introduction to the foundations of medical ethics. Topics covered include utilitarian and deontological theories, autonomy, nonmaleficence, beneficence, justice, veracity and confidentiality, and ideals, virtues, and integrity.

Beauchamp TL, Walters L (eds): *Contemporary Issues in Bioethics*, ed 3. Belmont, Calif, Wadsworth Publishing Co, 1989.

> An anthology of the most influential scholarly essays and judicial decisions in the modern medical ethics, on topics ranging from abortion and euthanasia to the physician–patient relationship to research, health policy, and allocation of medical resources.

Brody H: *The Healer's Power*. New Haven, Yale University Press, 1992.

> The author, an ethicist and family physician, identifies the types of power that physicians bring to the physician–patient relationship and examines negative and positive ways of utilizing that power.

CHAPTER 13

B. Values

Health Policy and Economics

Ann C. Jobe and Christopher J. Mansfield

CASE 13-1

Mr. Olds, an Alzheimer's disease patient of Dr. Wellman, had a fall in the nursing home from what a nurse suggested might be a minor stroke. Dr. Wellman thought an MRI would be useful to confirm that possibility. He was advising Mr. Olds's daughter, Jane, about treatment options when she broke into tears. Jane stated that she is overwhelmed by problems in her life at the moment. Dr. Wellman had provided prenatal care and delivered her two children but had seen neither the children nor Jane in the last 4 years. In exploring the nature of her distress, he discovered that Jane divorced shortly after the birth of her last child. She has been working full time since then at the local minimart and "making do the best I can." Jane feels guilty that she can visit her father only on Sundays. She wants whatever is best for him but confesses she is more worried about her 6-year-old child who is having trouble in school and the 4-year-old who still suffers from earaches. Dr. Wellman asks her to make an appointment for herself. Jane says she probably should as she has worried about a lump in her breast for the past 6 months. She has postponed seeing a physician, however, because she doesn't have health insurance. Jane asks Dr. Wellman how much the visit will cost.

INTRODUCTION

One cannot begin to understand health policy without considering the economics of healthcare. Economic concerns accompany virtually all health policy issues. The control of healthcare costs has been on the agenda of every President's administration since 1969, when Richard Nixon called it a crisis (Starr, 1982). Healthcare financing has become an ongoing debate within the legislature of virtually every state.

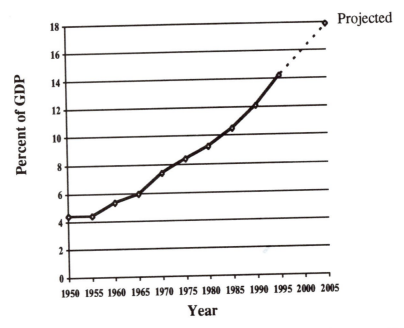

Figure 13.1. U.S. healthcare spending as a percentage of gross domestic product. Source: HIAA (1995); projection to 2005 from Burner and Waldo (1995).

Figure 13.1 plots the increase in healthcare spending since 1950. We spend more of our national wealth on healthcare each year and the trend is likely to continue. Of course, one might argue that health is important and that a nation as wealthy as the United States can afford to spend even more for health services than it does. Indeed, Engle's law (posited in the nineteenth century by the Prussian statistician) states that as income goes up, the proportion spent on food will decline, the proportion spent on housing will remain roughly constant, but the proportion spent on clothing, recreation, transportation, education, and medical care will increase. The United States enjoys a high standard of living, but it is clearly evident from Fig. 13.1 that the *rate of increase* in spending for health cannot continue indefinitely. Health services are a valuable commodity but money spent for health means less money available to purchase other, perhaps equally consequential, products and services. The amount we spend on health affects all other parts of the economy. As health insurance is an increasing expense of business, competitiveness of U.S. enterprise in the global economy is diminished. The annual rate of increase in spending has been about 10% since 1950. At that rate, spending doubles in 7 years. Healthcare services now account for more than we spend on either education or national defense—in fact, more than we spend on education and defense combined.

Spending for healthcare in the United States in 1995 was estimated to be $1 trillion, amounting to 14.2% of the nation's gross domestic product (GDP) (Burner & Waldo, 1995). As GDP is defined as the sum of all goods and services produced by a nation, this means that one of every seven dollars spent in the United States is for healthcare. U.S. health spending is divided among healthcare providers and institutions as shown in Fig. 13.2. The largest share (36%) is for hospital services, followed by physician services

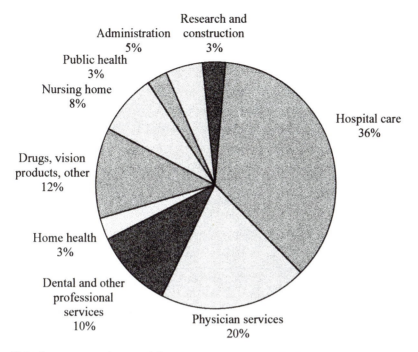

Figure 13.2. Components of national health expenditures—1995 ($1,007,600,000,000 estimated). Source: Burner and Waldo (1995).

(20%). The shares devoted to hospital and physician services have remained about the same over the years but the proportions of other components of the health system have changed. Since 1960, the relative portions spent on drugs and other products and research and construction have decreased by half. The nursing home and public health proportions have doubled. Chances are that the nursing home where Mr. Olds resides, Case 13-1, did not exist in 1960. Healthcare administration has a bigger piece of the spending pie today, and home healthcare is a burgeoning industry. The spending pie itself is more than 30 times larger than it was in 1960. Generally we can attribute its growth not only to increases in population but also to greater intensity of care, economywide inflation, and specific inflation in the price of medical care. Over the past 30 years, and particularly in the last decade, price inflation has accounted for more of the increase in expenditures than increases in either the intensity of care or growth in the population (Levit *et al.*, 1994).

Spending on medical care is also rising in other nations. No other country, however, spends as much on medical care as the United States, either in total or as a percentage of GDP. Figure 13.3 contrasts health expenditures as a proportion of GDP for the United States and seven other countries (Scheiber *et al.*, 1993). These data might make you wonder why other countries spend so much less and how they constrain the increase. You may have heard someone say, "Sure, the cost of healthcare is high in the United States, but we have the best medical care system in the world." And you might have heard that Americans live much longer than we used to. Life expectancy in the United States has increased from 47 years to 75 years since the turn of the century (Bureau of the Census, 1975, 1992). Figure 13.4 depicts the United States's spending for health as a proportion of

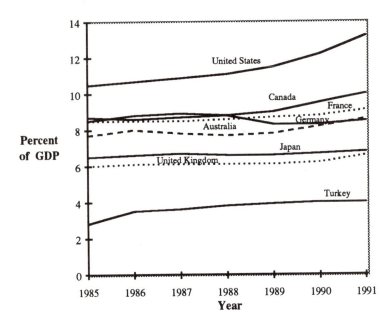

Figure 13.3. Health expenditures of selected countries as a percentage of gross domestic product. Source: Scheiber *et al.* (1993, Exhibit 1).

GDP along with increasing life expectancy. The slope of the life expectancy function portrayed is 0.30, about 1 year of life expectancy gained every 3 years.

You shouldn't jump to the conclusion that medical care is primarily responsible for this improvement, however. Much of the improvement occurred before the widespread use of antibiotics and the technology revolution in medicine during the 1950s and 1960s.

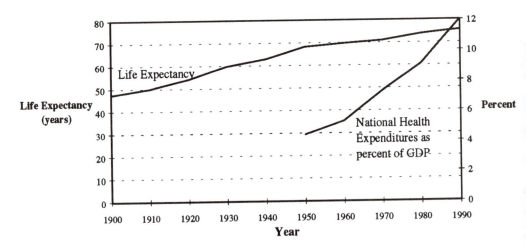

Figure 13.4. U.S. life expectancy and national health expenditures. Sources: Bureau of the Census (1975, 1992) and HIAA (1995).

A substantial portion of the gain attributable to medicine probably resulted from relatively inexpensive control of infectious disease, before large amounts of money were spent on "high-tech" diagnostic and treatment services for chronic disease. Finally, even though medicine's high-tech services improve diagnostic accuracy, often the results of such tests have little impact on the quantity of life. For example, though an MRI scan for Mr. Olds in Case 13-1 may help make the diagnosis of a minor stroke, such a diagnosis would not likely change Mr. Olds's treatment in a meaningful way.

The slopes of the two lines in Fig. 13.4 are not directly comparable (they measure different things) but they show that the positive correlation between spending and increased longevity in the United States is diminishing. Relative to other developed countries, high and continually increasing healthcare costs are unique to the United States; improvement in longevity is not unique. Life span has increased in all developed countries, but no country spends more for healthcare than the United States. Spending in the United States is 2.8 times more per person than in Britain, 1.5 times more than in Canada. When we compare the United States and other countries in terms of life expectancy, it is difficult to argue that the United States has the best medical care system. As is evident in Fig. 13.5, American men have shorter lives and American women die younger on average than in any of the comparison countries. Only in regard to life expectancy after 80 does the United States compare favorably. Infant mortality in the United States is higher than in all of the countries listed in Fig. 13.5, except Turkey.

The United States has more physicians per capita than all but two of the countries compared here (Table 13.1). There are fewer contacts per physician in the United States, however, and most countries use hospitals more than the United States. It is, of course, difficult to compare the quality of care. For those without financial barriers to care, the United States system offers a wide array of service, but opinion polls reveal that Ameri-

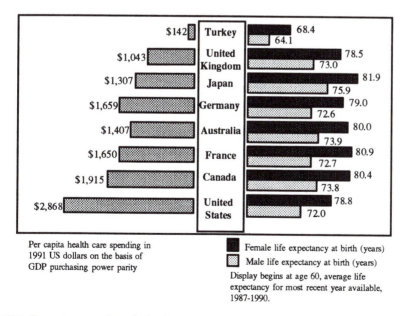

Per capita health care spending in 1991 US dollars on the basis of GDP purchasing power parity

■ Female life expectancy at birth (years)
▨ Male life expectancy at birth (years)
Display begins at age 60, average life expectancy for most recent year available, 1987–1990.

Figure 13.5. Per capita expenditure for healthcare versus life expectancy by country. Source: Scheiber *et al.* (1993), from OECD (1993).

Table 13.1

International Comparison of Medical Care Resources and Their Use—1990 (Selected Countries)[a]

	Hospital bed days per capita	Admission rate (percent of population)	Average days of stay	Physicians per 1000	Physician contacts per capita
Turkey	0.4	5.6	6.9	0.9	2.0
United Kingdom	2.0	15.9	14.5	1.4	5.7
Japan	4.1	8.3	50.5	1.6	12.9
Germany	3.3	20.9	12.9	2.0	8.8
France	2.9	23.3	12.3	2.7	7.2
Canada	2.0	14.1	13.9	2.2	6.9
United States	1.2	13.7	9.1	2.3	5.5

[a]Sources: Scheiber *et al.* (1993) and Organization for Economic Cooperation and Development (1993).

cans are less satisfied with their healthcare system than are Canadians (Blendon *et al.*, 1990).

CASE 13-2

Dr. Wellman has been pondering an MRI scan for Mr. Olds. He typically orders one for stroke patients. He knows it is expensive but figures that insurance will usually pay. On his way to the hospital board meeting, he thinks how ironic that Mr. Olds's daughter has not sought to have her breast lump examined.

On the agenda for the county hospital board that evening is the question of whether the hospital should purchase an MRI unit for its next expansion and renovation. The hospital contracts with Dr. Ray's private radiology group, which operates its own MRI, but Dr. Ray says she would be happy to recruit another radiologist to staff the hospital's unit. The MRI would be paid for by bonds guaranteed by the county. One of the board members who serves on the county board of supervisors questions whether the MRI is needed. She argues that one MRI ought to be enough and that with more patients enrolling in managed care insurance plans, revenues will be reduced. She reminds the board that the county is ultimately liable for the bonds and says the county needs a 100%-childhood immunization program more than another MRI. Dr. Wellman interrupts. He says that the two issues are completely unrelated and have different sources of financing. The board votes to include the MRI in the expansion plans and directs the administrator to negotiate with Dr. Ray for professional services.

ECONOMICS

Mastery of human biology and the science of medicine is an immense and worthy intellectual challenge. As Case 13-2 indicates, understanding the allocation of medical resources is also an important endeavor. Can we afford to provide *all* of the care that might be of benefit to everyone? If not, how might we choose which kinds of care, for whom? While philosophy and ethics help us understand the moral issues of rationing, economic concepts allow us to develop the specifics of health policy.

Economics is the study of how scarce resources are allocated. It offers concepts and tools to describe, predict, and optimize resource allocation.

> Economics is the study of how people and society end up *choosing*, with or without the use of money, to employ *scarce* productive resources that could have alternative uses—to *produce* various commodities and *distribute* them for consumption, now or in the future, among various persons and groups in society. Economics analyzes the costs and benefits of improving patterns of resource use. (Samuelson, 1980, p. 2)

It should be understood that economics is based on the fundamental assumption that people act rationally and make choices that maximize their self-interest; i.e., in making choices they maximize the *marginal utility* (incremental value) of each investment, production, or consumption decision. This assumption allows economists to construct theoretical models of human behavior. One of the most familiar models of behavior describes the two essential features of any market for goods or services—supply and demand.

FUNDAMENTAL CONCEPTS

Models of Supply and Demand

The less there is of a commodity, given a particular demand for it in an open market, the higher the price. Conversely, if its price is lowered, more of the commodity will be demanded. If the price goes up, consumers do with less and try to find substitutes for the good or service. This is the law of downward sloping *demand*, which is plotted as d–d in Fig. 13.6. *Supply* in relation to price and quantity can be similarly described. Amount supplied is plotted as the upward sloping curve, s–s. It describes the amount that producers are willing to supply at a given price. The slopes of supply and demand curves for different goods and services vary. Land is an example of a market operating according to the curves in Fig. 13.6. It describes the market for land such as might be available in a

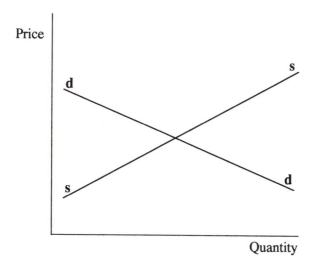

Figure 13.6. Supply and demand curves for land.

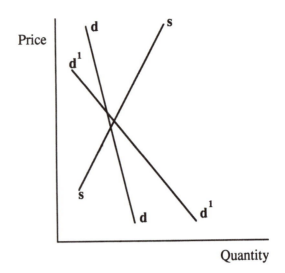

Figure 13.7. Supply and demand curves for medical care—with and without health insurance.

rural area where there is typically much choice on the part of both sellers and buyers about buying or selling a particular property at a given price.

In contrast, Fig. 13.7 portrays a simplified model of the market for medical services, where buyers (patients) have little choice of services to buy or substitute, and sellers have little competition. Much of medical care is perceived by the consumer to be necessity and price matters less than for optional commodities, but one's purchasing ability makes a difference. Two demand curves are shown in Fig. 13.7, depicting the demand of people with different purchasing ability. The more vertical one (d–d) applies to people like Mr. Olds who have health insurance. Having insurance makes the consumer even less sensitive to price, and the demand curve becomes steeper, i.e., less price elastic. The less vertical curve (d¹–d¹) applies to those in Jane's circumstance, who because they must pay out of pocket at the time of purchase are more sensitive to price. An increase or decrease in price has a larger effect on the volume of services demanded by those without health insurance than those with it. The supply–demand model is useful for understanding elementary markets where the elements of free enterprise operate with simplicity. Markets are said to reach equilibrium at the point supply and demand curves cross. If there is more product or service supplied, price will drop and consumers are inclined to buy more. Conversely, if consumers demand more, price will rise and suppliers will be inclined to sell more. Individuals and institutions will opportunistically seek to enter markets as suppliers where demand is high and supply will then increase to meet demand. At the point where supply and demand curves cross, an "equilibrium price" is established and the market "clears." There may be suppliers who would sell more if the price were higher and consumers who would buy more if the price were lower, but at the equilibrium or "going" price, the market is in balance. This is a theoretic model of behavior. It is supported by considerable empirical evidence in simple commodity markets, useful for considering important basic relationships in the challenge of allocating and distributing resources. It has been argued, and many believe, that the market alone is the most efficient way of allocating resources and government intervention is not necessary. This thesis is explored later in this chapter, but we must admit up front that the healthcare market is more complex and may not fit the theory of classic free enterprise. The demand curve in the healthcare market is an aggregate expression of the demand preferences of many kinds of consumers, for many kinds of products and services. The aggregate supply curve, likewise, is determined by the combined decisions and preferences of many kinds of suppliers, individuals, and institutions. Small subelements of the healthcare industry might fit the model, but there are many external considerations and reasons why classic, free-market theory may not be appropriate. Explore first, though, how medical care became an economic issue.

Monetarization of Medical Care

Before the turn of the century, there was not much medical care to purchase. Medicine offered the patient little hope or marginal utility, in the economists' vernacular. This began to change with the application of science to medicine. Yet until the 1940s most people paid for their healthcare out of their own pockets at the time of service or incurred a personal debt for their care. Most hospitals were voluntary, not-for-profit community institutions that originated out of philanthropy and depended heavily on local charity for capital as well as operating revenue (Stevens, 1989). Physicians were accustomed to providing charity care or discounting their fees according to a patient's financial circumstances. Proposals for nationally sponsored or compulsory health insurance were considered in the United States after Bismarck introduced it as a social reform in Germany in 1883. Such coverage has generally been opposed by organized medicine and others as being a form of socialism inappropriate for the United States (Starr, 1982).

Reasons for being admitted to a hospital increased as medicine became more effective, but widespread poverty during the Depression limited access. Thus, the need for hospital insurance increased and the Blue Cross movement began in the late 1930s. This voluntary, private insurance, which paid for hospital care, was followed by private insurance, Blue Shield, for physicians' services. A government ruling that exempted health insurance from wage and price controls during World War II set a precedent for exempting health insurance from income tax. The solid link between employment and health insurance was thus established. From a public finance point of view, employer-paid, private health insurance is subsidized by the government in the sense that tax revenues are foregone. This tax policy makes access to health insurance dependent on employment for most people.

With the proliferation of private insurance after the war, hospital revenues came principally from direct reimbursement by Blue Cross on a cost plus profit basis and from commercial indemnity insurance at 100% of charges. New capital came to the industry through the federal government's postwar Hill-Burton program for hospital construction. As a result of these developments, along with passage of Medicare insurance for the elderly and Medicaid for the poor in the mid-1960s, philanthropy became a smaller part of hospitals' budgets. Liberal reimbursement policies of public and private health insurance companies encouraged hospitals to expand services and invest in high technology with virtually no financial risk.

New money came also for the pursuit of science and its application to medicine. Billions of federal dollars were pumped into the National Institutes of Health to support the research enterprise of academic medical centers. Medical education became funded largely by state and federal tax dollars. Private and public insurance included payment for physicians' services, and physicians' incomes increased significantly in relation to the average worker's. These events provide partial explanation of how healthcare spending has grown to the point that it accounted for 14% of GDP in 1995. This trend was characterized by Eli Ginzberg (1984) as the "monetarization of medical care."

People are inclined to buy insurance when confronted with the possibility of expenses for which they cannot budget, or when they are averse to the risk of incurring expense. If their employer or the government offers it at a subsidized rate, it is even more attractive. Typical forms of health insurance provide an *indemnity benefit*, a *service benefit*, or a *prepaid benefit*. Indemnity insurance, often referred to as commercial insurance, reimburses the beneficiary for specified losses incurred. Typically this type of insurance has paid whatever the provider charges. Insurance providing a service benefit directly pays the provider a specified amount for each particular service, i.e., a *fee-for-service*. Sometimes the payment is a percentage of the cost involved (say 80%), with the insured person liable for the balance, referred to as *coinsurance*. Health maintenance organizations (HMOs) provide comprehensive benefits for a prepaid premium.

Indemnity and service-benefit insurance may require the insured first to spend some portion of her own money before any service is reimbursed. This is called a *deductible*. Typically, the deductible amount must be met each year before the insurance starts paying. Insurance plans may also require the insured to pay a portion of the cost of some or all specific services. The self-pay fraction is called a *copayment* or *coinsurance*. Some policies may include a *stop-loss* provision that sets a limit on the amount of the copayment. HMOs typically require no deductible and no copayments for most services, especially not for preventive and primary care services. Insurance policies may also have a *cap* on the amount of reimbursement for a specific service event or for lifetime benefits.

All insurance policies specify the range of services covered, called a *benefit plan*. The benefit plan may exclude specific services or kinds of providers. The *premium*, i.e., cost paid by the buyer, reflects the range of benefits, amount of deductible, copayment proportion, reimbursement limit, and the actuarial risk for the individual or group enrolled by the insurer.

The actuarial risk can reflect either the experience of the insured group or that of the entire community, *experience rating* versus *community rating*. Healthy groups use fewer services and may be offered lower rates. An essential concept of insurance is the *pooling of risk*, i.e., spreading it over a large population. When the risk is pooled, the cost of expensive but rare events is shared among many. This pooling of risk is the basis of all insurance. It is easy to see that experience-rated premiums for small groups could be greatly affected by *adverse selection;* i.e., if small groups are composed of older people or the less healthy, the premiums will have to be very high.

With experience rating, insurance companies are motivated to compete for the enrollment of healthy groups, leaving out the less healthy or offering insurance to them at very high premiums. The practice of selectively offering health insurance to healthier groups is referred to as *cherry picking*. Do you think a for-profit insurance company would be interested in having many enrollees like Mr. Olds or his daughter Jane?

Insurance companies may make individual business decisions that are at odds with the collective good of society. So also may the individual consumers, physicians, and other providers. The primary reason to have copayments and deductibles is to keep the individual patient involved in the economic calculus. The United States consumer is now only paying for about one-fifth of healthcare out of pocket (Health Insurance Association of America, 1995, Table 4.4). This proportion is greater than in most other countries, however (Scheiber *et al.*, 1992).

Not having a substantial and immediate financial stake can encourage patients to use preventive services but may lead to the problem called *moral hazard* (Pauly, 1968).

Having insurance with no copayment at the point of service, the individual is motivated to use as much service as may potentially be of benefit. Thinking of the supply and demand curves in Fig. 13.7, the slope of the demand curve for people like Mr. Olds in Case 13-1 is more vertical, *price inelastic*, than the one for those like his daughter who must pay out of pocket. As more people have such insurance, volume of services increases. If the demand curve shifts outward but the supply curve does not, the equilibrium price goes up if not regulated. The physician has little incentive to limit services and professional culture encourages doing all that may be of benefit for the patient, what Victor Fuchs has described as the *technological imperative* (Fuchs, 1990).

When there is no monetary cost to the patient at the point of service, the rational act is to take as much medical service as is perceived to be of benefit. The advice of physicians influences demand of course but it may also induce demand. The phenomenon of *physician-induced demand* is related to moral hazard. It happens when a physician orders more services than the patient would be willing to purchase if the patient knew as much as the physician. It may also occur when the physician has income expectations and reimbursement is assured. *Wallet biopsy* is the euphemistic term for the latter phenomena. The induced demand effect (Wilensky & Rossiter, 1983; Mitchell & Sunshine, 1992; Rice & Labelle, 1988) is similar to the increased volume of tests that occurs with defensive medicine and begs a distinction between consumer demand and clinical need. The *need* for medical or public health services may be more or less than expressed demand. Consider Jane's case and that of her father in Case 13-1. Medical need is a professional judgment; demand is consumer behavior. We may want to encourage the use of preventive services but our decisions should be guided by evidence, logic, and professional judgment.

Cost versus Benefit, Effectiveness, and Utility

Though only 20% of health expenditures are for physician services, about 80% of health expenditures are for services a physician has prescribed (Wilensky & Rossiter, 1983). How cost effective are those prescriptions? The graph of health expenditures and outcomes plotted in Fig. 13.4 suggests a diminishing relationship between the amount of medical care and longevity. Longevity is determined mostly by genetics, life-style, environment, and social factors beyond the realm of the medical model. There are many things modern medicine and public health services can provide to reduce morbidity and mortality, but each successive gain from medical intervention comes at an increasing cost, particularly in treating chronic disease. We are confronted not only by the limits of affordability, but by the point of diminishing returns as well. Physicians are accustomed to evaluating *risks* versus *benefits* objectively, but they frequently make very subjective judgments about *cost* versus *benefit*. Economic concepts help structure the discussion of cost versus benefit and make it more systematic. Consider the theoretical plot of cost against benefit in Fig. 13.8. Dollar values of medical expense and benefit are plotted against amount of service provided. The services could be diagnostic tests, physician visits, days in the hospital, physical therapy sessions, number of cosmetic surgeries, or other services. Cost increases are typically linear. Benefit is typically curvilinear, initially increasing and likely to have a much higher value than cost, but increasing at a diminishing rate. At some point, the benefit curve flattens and additional services produce less incremental benefit. At some point, more medical services may even begin to do harm.

Each increment in service should be prescribed in terms of expected incremental benefit and the incremental benefit weighed against the increment in cost. Economists call incremental cost *marginal cost* and measure it against *marginal benefit*. There is a much

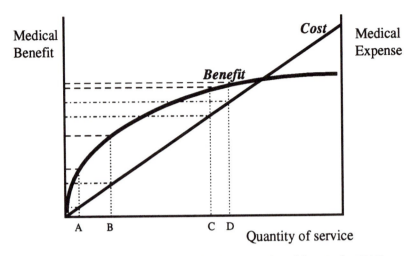

Figure 13.8. Medical cost versus medical benefit. Adapted from Fuchs (1990).

more favorable ratio of marginal benefit to marginal cost between points A and B than between points C and D. The economist's prescription is to continue providing service until the marginal benefit is equal to marginal cost. Most objective assessments would put the marginal benefit of Mr. Olds's MRI low relative to the cost, but high benefit versus cost for Jane's mammogram.

The health policy analyst uses these concepts in *cost–benefit analysis* (CBA) and its cousins, *cost-effectiveness analysis* and *cost–utility analysis*, to estimate the value of a new program or compare alternative programs, services, or therapies. CBA is applied to investments of capital, applications of new technologies, or making choices between alternative services. Case 13-2 is an example of where such an analysis is helpful. Dr. Wellman was correct when he said that the MRI unit and immunization were unrelated and funded by different income streams, but only from his or the hospital's point of view. The health policy analyst, taking a more global view, might well wish to compare the additional MRI unit to immunization services as alternative societal expenditures. CBA quantifies benefits and costs in dollar terms, measuring both direct and indirect costs and benefits. Intangible costs and benefits accruing to the patient or society, as well as the financial gain of a provider (pecuniary benefit), may also be identified. The focus of CBA is usually on long-term policies, programs, or capital commitments. Table 13.2 displays the elements of CBA for a childhood immunization program.

Though CBA is useful in policy analysis and forces the consideration of many nonclinical concerns, it is difficult to quantify all costs and benefits in monetary terms. It often asks for data that are not available or that force explicit statement of subjective values. What monetary value should be ascribed to a human life, to the potential life of an infant versus an octogenarian? What cost for suffering, the value to individuals of herd immunity? Cost-effectiveness analysis (CEA) and cost–utility analysis (CUA) avoid some of these problems. CEA can be used for evaluating specific clinical services and choosing between specific therapies or diagnostic procedures that have similar ends or purposes. Cost-effectiveness is a ratio of cost per unit of service or desired outcome; e.g., the net cost per death averted because of one intervention compared to another, the cost per vaccination, cost per life year saved, cost per disease occurrence or medical encounter averted, cost per surgical procedure, etc. CEA, applied to clinical trials or outcomes

Table 13.2
Elements of Cost–Benefit Analysis of Comprehensive Childhood Immunization Program

Costs	Benefits
Direct	Direct
Medical—Cost of vaccine, physician fees, nursing and other personnel costs, administration	Deaths averted, savings in life years
Nonmedical—Parents' time	Savings in future medical costs averted, morbidity and institutionalization avoided
Indirect	Indirect
Medical—Management of adverse reactions	Reduced loss of school days
Nonmedical—Loss of work for parents from adverse reaction	Reduced loss of work days
Intangible	Intangible
Incompatibility with values and religious beliefs of some citizens	Reduced suffering
Suffering and potential loss from adverse reactions	Level of herd immunity gained
	Protection afforded the nonimmunized
	Reduced loss of loved ones
	Pecuniary
	Fees and profits of manufacturers and providers

research, attaches dollar value to measures of clinical efficacy. It is useful in examining, for instance, the efficacy of coronary artery bypass graft surgery versus lipid-lowering pharmacological therapy, one pharmacologic agent versus another. It is used as a tool to guide expenditure and quality assessment decisions. When the denominator in the ratio can be expressed as well years (WYs) or quality-adjusted life years (QUALYs), CEA is called cost–utility analysis. QUALYs are the life years saved plus a factor for morbidity or pain reduced minus a factor for side effects.

These techniques are often used to compare unlike therapies or services, but such comparisons must be well structured beforehand and use the same assumptions and perspectives. If one wanted to compare the efficacy of therapies for otitis media (OM), for example, one should focus on a single type of OM, i.e., acute, chronic, or otitis media with effusion (OME). Using OME as an example, comparison of antibiotic therapy to tympanostomy is possible but difficult. The effect of surgery is likely to be confounded by antibiotics used in previous treatment and surgery is recommended only when OME has persisted for more than 3 months and bilateral hearing loss has been observed (AHCPR, 1994). Choosing between therapies of first resort, however, we could use CEA to compare different antibiotics with each other and with watchful waiting. Table 13.3 presents a hypothetical CEA of two antibiotics compared with a placebo. The comparison is limited to children aged 1 to 3 who have been diagnosed by reliable techniques as having OME for at least 6 weeks but less than 4 months, and who are otherwise healthy. Note that two cost-effectiveness ratios are given, one for a short-term outcome and one for a long-term outcome. In the short term, drug A appears to be twice as effective but less cost-effective than drug B. By 24 weeks, however, it was less effective and much less cost-effective (by a factor of three). Contrast both, however, to a choice of watchful waiting in this hypothetical situation.

With any of these techniques, it is necessary to identify the perspective of the analysis. Is it being done from the perspective of society (a population approach), the individual patient, a provider (clinical approach), or a payer (bottom-line approach)? The intervention must be carefully defined, as well as what it is being compared to. Is it to be compared to doing nothing, to a placebo, a similar intervention, different medical inter-

Table 13.3

(Hypothetical) Cost-Effectiveness Analysis of Two Antibiotics for Otitis Media with Effusion,
Compared to Placebo in Otherwise Healthy Children Aged 1–3 Years
Having Clearly Diagnosed OME of 6 to 16 Weeks' Duration[a]

Group	N	OME cases Clear at 3 wks	Clear at 24 wks	Direct cost Drug cost	Side effects Rashes, diarrhea	Unit cost	Future drug resistance proxy cost	Total net cost	Net cost per case cleared at 3 wks	Net cost per case cleared at 24 wks
Drug A	100	48	46	$2936	3	$150	$25	$3411	$71.06	$74.15
Drug B	100	24	52	524	6	125	25	1299	54.13	24.98
Control	100	18	42	0	0	0	0	0	0	0

[a]Synopsis of methods and materials:
1. Measurement of clearance of fluid from ear by otoscopic judgment and tympanometry
2. Confounding variables controlled by randomization and equivalent counseling to parents regarding environmental risk reduction
3. Cost effectiveness = Net cost per cases cleared
4. Net cost = Direct cost (total drug cost per treatment group) + Indirect cost ($25 for each side effect noted in chart, representing a cost to patient's parent for consultation) and $25 proxy for cost of potential future drug resistance is assumed
5. Price of antibiotic A to pharmacist: $5.24 for 10-day treatment; price of antibiotic B to pharmacist: $29.36 for 10-day treatment

vention, or to a form of primary prevention? Are the relevant costs and benefits specified and measured? These data often require techniques that are hard to come by. How valid are the measures chosen and the data employed? What assumptions are used in measuring the costs and benefits? Have uncertainties been accounted for by reporting the different results that occur when different assumptions and probability estimates are used? These techniques may be used by policymakers, payers, and physicians for different ends. For physicians, they are an aid to judgment about wise use of resources, not a substitute for clinical decision-making.

Free Enterprise and Competition

All nations must have some means for allocation and distribution of resources. The choices for constructing an economic system are found within the spectrum defined by free markets on one end and authority systems on the other (Smith, 1776; Marx, 1888; Lindblom, 1977). The United States has chosen a capitalistic system that relies mostly on free enterprise. No nation today relies completely on a centrally planned authority system.

The free-enterprise system is based first and foremost on the principle of private property—the right to have, use, and exchange it freely. Adam Smith's philosophy not only supported that right, but proposed that free markets were the most efficient way to allocate resources. The classical, free-enterprise system described by Smith is one of paramount simplicity, promising efficiency, equity, and dynamic flexibility. The appeal of a self-regulating social system, where equitable allocation and distribution occur without government interference, is strong. In the classic characterization of a free-market economy, efficient allocation of private goods occurs where the supply and demand curves cross. At this point, the amount desired and amount supplied are equal. In situations of perfect competition for private goods, the price system is an efficient way to allocate resources. *Allocation*, however, is not the same as *distribution*, and *private goods* must be distinguished from *public goods*. The market can allocate private goods efficiently, but does not necessarily distribute either private or public goods fairly.

Markets cannot allocate *public goods* efficiently. They do not always allocate private goods efficiently either. The market is particularly inefficient if all of the costs and benefits are not borne by the buyer and seller. All of society may gain from investments in education, highways, space exploration, biomedical research, the development of drugs and vaccines, etc. Individual economic transactions for things like immunization, family planning, preventive health services, the purchase of smoke detectors, even the purchase of health insurance, confer benefit to others. There may be significant societal advantage external to the immediate market decisions. Similarly, there may be external costs associated with private transactions and decisions, such as when irreplaceable natural resources are consumed, or when someone's environment is fouled, downwind or downstream of where the consumption occurs. Substantial external costs occur in healthcare too. Examples are public subsidy of medical education, hospitals purchasing expensive medical equipment benefiting few patients but enhancing physician income and increasing everyone's insurance premium, shifting the cost of graduate medical education to the hospital bills of patients. These are *externalities* in the economists' jargon.

Private goods are ones for which the benefits and costs of consumption are internalized, and consumption is rival (Musgrave & Musgrave, 1984, pp. 47–69). Markets will not allocate efficiently when consumption of a good is *nonrival, exclusion is not possible*, or when *benefits are not internalized*. If you buy and eat an ice cream cone, no one else can consume it (a rival good). Many may simultaneously enjoy a park, however, and a streetlight shines on all who walk beneath it (nonrival). Everyone benefits from national defense, police and fire protection, preservation of pure water sources, and pure food and drug regulation. For some goods and services, consumption may be rival, but exclusion may be neither possible nor good social policy, i.e., "free-riders" are allowed. Examples are libraries, public education, the Internet, public broadcasting, or treatment at the emergency room of a public hospital.

Medical care in the United States is by and large a private good, but we do not always exclude on the ability to pay. Medicaid is provided to selected categories of the poor; Medicare to all of the elderly, both rich and poor alike. The uninsured have limited access to care (albeit in *extremis*) at public hospital emergency departments and clinics. Many believe that medical care *should* be considered a public good, access to a basic minimum of which is a matter of democratic justice, and of benefit to all of society.

With medical care, the optimal efficiency promised by the market has not been achieved because public policy has not treated all medical care as a private good. Moreover, when it is treated as a private good, which is most of the time, the elements of competition may not be sufficiently present. Perfect competition requires the following elements: sufficient numbers of both buyers and sellers so that decisions of an individual cannot determine market price; complete knowledge of market conditions for both buyers and sellers; substitutability of products and services; and mobility of resources into and out of the market.

In many instances there are not enough sellers to afford the consumer choice of either provider or type of service. The consumer typically is at a disadvantage regarding knowledge of market conditions, the value of the service, or efficacy of substitutes. Licensing laws, accreditation, certificate of need laws, and the health professions' influence on education and workforce policy constrain mobility of resources into and out of the industry. Furthermore, professional practices have discouraged competition on the basis of price and quality.

When markets fail, government frequently intervenes. Electrical power, gas, water, sewer, taxis, rail and air travel, cable TV, and telephone services are common examples. In these cases, public policy has at times encouraged *monopolies* or a limited number of providers in the interest of efficient capital allocation. When monopolies are created, or free entry of providers discouraged, regulation of price and quality may be necessary for consumer protection. At one end of the spectrum of choices, government may step in to produce the good or service. At the other end, and depending perhaps on the degree of market failure, it may be more appropriate for government to restructure the market and provide incentives for it to work more efficiently.

In medical care, government has intervened in many ways. It has subsidized medical education. How many students could afford, or find loans for, the full cost of a medical education—approximately half a million dollars? Entry into the health professions has been both limited and subsidized, much more so than other professions. Health professions education has been treated as a public good, exempt from arbitrary imperatives of the market. To a large extent, the construction of hospitals and the conduct of biomedical research have also been treated as public goods. On the demand side of the market, government has subsidized health insurance for the four-fifths (or so) of the population lucky enough to have it. While improving allocation and distribution of resources in one way, however, government intervention may distort it in other ways. The exclusion of tax on employer-paid health insurance, the equivalent of a $90 billion subsidy in 1990 (Enthoven & Singer, 1995), and reimbursement policies for Medicare and Medicaid have caused the demand curve to become much less price elastic.

STRATEGIES TO CONTROL SPENDING

Failures of the market have contributed to the increasing national expenditures on healthcare but are not the sole cause. The amount we spend is a combination of the amount we buy and the price we pay, i.e., spending equals price times quantity. It is useful to separate the causes of increased spending into both price and volume issues. Contributing to greater volume are aging of the population, greater intensity of treatment, increasing income of the population, increasing consumer demand, less sensitivity of the consumer to price, provider-induced demand, and defensive medicine. Contributing to price increases are economywide inflation, oversupply of capital resources, increases in wages, professional salaries and profits, the costs of regulation, and increased administrative cost, much of which comes with the duplication and high overhead of having over 1000 insurance companies.

The options for controlling health spending lie within the authority system–market system continuum. This continuum is defined by government production of services, central planning and control on one end and an unfettered free market on the other. Cost-control strategies have varied across this spectrum but typically targeted single factors. The authority system (government) interventions are politically difficult to enact and implement but they are numerous. These strategies include: *Certificate of Need* laws to restrain investment in resources; price controls, rate regulation, and prospectively setting reimbursement rates for health services with *Diagnostic Related Group*s (DRGs) for hospitals and the *Resource-Based Relative Value Scales* (R-BRVS) for physicians; selective contracting and use of government's power as a large purchaser (*monopsony*) to elicit discounts; voluntary regional and state health planning; targeted subsidy of workforce training (e.g., primary care physicians and midwives); utilization review; malpractice law (tort) reform; control of provider fraud and abuse; increases in *copayments* and *deductibles* for Medicare and Medicaid; and support of technology assessment, *outcomes research*, and *clinical practice guidelines*.

Spending control strategies employed in the market system are easier to enact and quicker to implement. These private strategies have included raising consumer cost-sharing by increasing premiums, deductibles, and copayments; reducing benefits; excluding dependents from employer-paid coverage; requiring second opinions and purchase of generic drugs; worksite wellness programs; more prudent selection of health insurance carriers; corporate self-insurance; switching to HMOs; case management; and selective purchasing of services.

MANAGED CARE AND MANAGED COMPETITION

None of the public or private strategies described here provide a single answer to containing health spending. Some attempt to control price, others to control volume. Each has had limited success, but because they are piecemeal approaches, spending continues to escalate. Not all government strategies have taken a regulatory approach. There have been numerous attempts to harness market forces. The Nixon administration promoted managed care, an innovation of private enterprise. President Reagan also looked to the market to control spending as it sought to deregulate the healthcare industry in the 1980s. The Clinton proposal for health system reform relied on competitive market solutions as well. It specifically promoted managed care and proposed that government manage the competition among managed care plans. Private business strategies have, of course, supported the development of managed care all along.

There are many kinds of managed care organizations, and almost all insurance plans now have mechanisms to manage the utilization of care. All managed care organizations are not HMOs, however. An HMO is an organized system of health services delivery offering a comprehensive set of benefits to a defined population for fixed, prepaid fee. A health service organization that accepts a prepaid fee (*capitation*) has a strong incentive to manage care because they are directly at risk for the cost of it. With a prepaid fee for all care, it must limit utilization of expensive services by substituting more cost-effective forms and by providing preventive and primary care services that reduce the need for expensive chronic or acute care services. Administrators and the provider staff of organizations accepting financial risk for defined populations are guided daily by the concepts of cost-effectiveness portrayed in Fig. 13.8. Depending on the corporate motives of the organization, managed care is either a philosophy leading to good medicine or good business. Preventive services, improved continuity of care, and a focus on efficacy issues improve quality but may also improve profit margins.

Managed care organizations are distinguishable not only by profit motive but also by how much risk they assume and how they relate to their participating physicians. The distinctions are becoming increasingly blurred. At one end of the spectrum is the "managed" health insurance indemnity or service plan that simply employs utilization controls like preapproval and case management for certain high-cost services. Next would be the Preferred Provider Organization (PPO). Physicians in a PPO agree to abide by utilization management procedures and accept discounted payment rates for their PPO patients. Patients with this type of insurance may go to any physician but are encouraged by lower copayments or deductibles to go to the "preferred" physicians, hospitals, or other providers. PPO patients may be a small or large percentage of a physician's practice, depending on local market conditions.

Somewhere between the PPO and the HMO is the Point of Service (POS) plan. This plan is an HMO that offers the patient greater choice of physicians. In an HMO with the POS option, the patient is allowed to go to an out-of-plan, fee-for-service provider but pays a higher copayment or deductible. The managed indemnity plan, PPO, and POS plan accept increasing risk for managing within a fixed budget but have not nearly as much risk as the HMO. HMOs may be organized for profit or not-for-profit but they are also defined by how physicians participate in their governance and administration and how physicians share in the organization's financial performance. Typically, HMOs are described as a staff model, group model, or Independent Practice Association (IPA).

The staff model HMO employs a panel of salaried generalist physicians from which enrollees choose their primary care physician. The staff model may also employ some specialists but will contract with the less frequently needed specialists. The staff model HMO usually contracts for hospital care and other services. By these contracts, the staff model HMO organizes a (more or less) comprehensive and cost-effective delivery system for its enrollees. In addition to salary, physicians in some staff model HMOs may receive bonuses for achieving productivity targets or a share of profits. Such arrangements give physician staff a financial stake in the organization's success.

In the IPA and group model, the HMO is a separate entity that contracts with physicians in the IPA or medical group practice to care for its prepaid plan enrollees. Physicians are either self-employed (as in the IPA) or employed by the medical group, not by the HMO. In the IPA model, physicians join the IPA, which negotiates and manages their relationship with the HMO. In either the IPA or group model, physicians may have fee-for-service patients but accept the HMO's patients as capitated risk or at a discounted rate. The HMO may create networks of multiple groups and IPAs. The IPA and group model HMO don't control individual physicians as much as they control the system that serves its patients. These HMOs may, however, offer financial incentives to participating physicians to limit use of specialist or hospital services by holding back some percentage of reimbursement until an end-of-year review of the physicians' and plan's performance. The potential for conflict of interest exists whenever physicians have a financial stake in the utilization of health services, regardless of whether the HMO is a staff, IPA, or group model.

The shift of financial risk for care from the insurer to the provider is an important concept. It is greatest with the fully capitated plans. Managed care is fundamentally changing the way medicine is practiced and the market for indemnity health insurance is diminishing. HMOs accounted for 23% of enrollment in employer-sponsored health plans in 1994 (Foster Higgins, 1995), and growth is likely to continue irrespective of government policy. Managed care has given business control over its spending for health insurance; it restrains both price and volume. Relative to indemnity plans, HMOs have slightly lower hospitalization rates, substantially lower lengths of stay, less use of expensive tests and procedures, more physician visits and use of preventive services, somewhat less satisfaction with services, and greater satisfaction with cost (Miller & Luft, 1994).

There is great promise in managed care, but trade-offs must be considered. The consumer in particular must evaluate options in terms of comprehensiveness of benefits, the importance of preventive services, continuity of care, cost, and how much choice of provider is desired. Physicians will have to decide how to relate to managed care organizations and the extent to which they are willing to be gatekeepers for them. Society must determine how much oversight is needed. Managed care organizations have the same incentive as indemnity plans to avoid adverse risk selection, i.e., take the healthy patients and avoid the sick. To counteract this trend, government could play an important role. Government's role could be to promote fair competition among managed care organizations by ensuring a level playing field among all health insurance providers and managed care organizations. It could also, and may someday, choose to control the resources that are available to the healthcare system.

CLOSED VERSUS OPEN SYSTEMS

A fundamental aspect of an HMO is that for its enrollees it constitutes a closed system. It must operate within a fixed budget by closely estimating revenues and utilization and carefully managing utilization and costs. A big reason the cost of healthcare in the United States has been out of control is precisely that the system is so open. With so many different providers and types of insurance plans, so many unbundled and unmanaged services, so many people (41 million) not explicitly in the system, so many disjointed attempts to fix it, and so many interest groups trying to preserve their own stake in the system, control may remain elusive. Perhaps healthcare will remain an open pluralistic system because that is what Americans want. However, the essential feature that distinguishes our system from that of the Canadians and the British is the notion of a fixed budget. Once a budget is fixed and a commitment made to include all citizens in the care that budget will buy, there is a stronger requirement to manage the entire system. If the hospital in Case 13-2 were to become an HMO obligated to serve all people in its service area, do you think the Board would have voted to purchase the MRI unit?

CASE 13-3

Following the 1992 election, national health reform seemed inevitable—ready to be packaged and accomplished. The President placed health reform high on the agenda and an appointed Task Force analyzed and selected alternatives and delivered a complex legislative draft of proposals to the Congress. No substantial political constituency had been developed to support the open system "Managed Competition Clinton Plan" and legislators and staffers crafted their own versions, including closed-system models (Rep. McDermott's "Single Payer Plan"). Before proposals were brought before Congressional committees for discussion, special interest groups mobilized opposition. By the time of the fall 1994 elections no proposals had been approved.

——————— HEALTH POLICY ———————

Now that you have learned about the fundamental concepts related to health economics, it is time to place these concepts into the context of the policy-making process, as reflected by Case 13-3. Public policy-making, including the development of health policy, can be considered a set of processes, which includes the setting of the agenda, the specification of alternatives from which a choice can be made, an authoritative choice among the specified alternatives, and the implementation of the decision (Kingdon, 1984).

At any given time, the agenda is the list of subjects, concerns, problems, or issues to which governmental officials and people outside government are devoting time and attention. At any time there are numerous issues or problems; the agenda-setting process narrows these to the ones that become the focus of attention. Problems or concerns can be brought to prominence by systematic indicators (e.g., percentage of GDP spent on health-care, health workforce statistics), by a focusing event such as a crisis or disaster, or by feedback from current program operation. An agenda item has a higher likelihood of rising to prominence if it is congruent with the current national mood, has interest group support or lack of organized opposition, and fits the orientation of prevailing legislative coalitions and the current administration. A complex combination of factors usually is responsible for moving a given item into agenda prominence. In Case 13-3, healthcare reform became a focus of attention, high on the agenda, because of concern for the rising cost of healthcare and the number of individuals without health insurance. Healthcare reform was congruent with the national mood, fit the orientation of the current administration, especially that of the President, who had incorporated health reform as a campaign issue, and early on had interest group support.

After attention is focused on a specific issue such as healthcare reform, the next step in the process is to consider alternatives for governmental action. The process of specifying alternatives narrows the choices to proposals that will be most seriously considered and potentially become legislation. In Case 13-3, the cost of medical care was a prominent agenda item, as was the increasing number of individuals in the United States without health insurance. A number of alternatives, such as directly regulating hospital costs, managed competition, increased regulation of insurance companies, or comprehensive national health insurance, were considered. Proposals that are technically and budgetarily feasible, consistent with dominant values and the current national mood, and that have political support or lack organized opposition, have the highest likelihood of surviving long enough for serious consideration. In Case 13-3, so many alternatives were under consideration that few had enough political support to remain under consideration. More importantly, most of the alternatives had substantial organized opposition.

Various participants, including the President, the Congress, bureaucrats, and individuals and forces outside of government (e.g., media, interest groups, political parties, and the general public), can be sources of agenda items and alternatives. Frequently the agenda items and alternatives come from professional and special or consumer interest advocacy groups that make up the health policy community. The administration, including the President and his political appointees, is central to agenda setting, but has much less influence or control over the process of considering alternatives, and even less control over implementation. In Case 13-3, the President was able to focus attention on health reform, but was unable to bring forward a set of alternatives that survived long enough for serious consideration. Congress is central to both setting the agenda and specifying alternatives; legislators tend to have more impact on the agenda while their staffers concentrate more on the alternatives. During the 1994 Congressional session, staff of the major Congressional committees (e.g., Senate Finance, and Labor Human Resources; House Ways and Means) provided many alternatives that were brought into various committees for debate and revision. Outside of government, interest groups sometimes affect policy agendas and most often do so by devoting their efforts to negative, blocking activities. Interest group pressure can influence the government's agenda, and did so with increasing frequency in the scenario of Case 13-3. A group that mobilizes support by motivating its constituents to write letters and visit legislators, and stimulates its allies to do the same, can get the attention of government officials. In Case 13-3, strong opposition to the aspects of the President's plan that approximated a closed-system alternative and would have constrained the role of insurance companies was launched by the Health Insurance Association of America through an extensive media campaign. This campaign featured some very effective television advertisements featuring a young couple, "Harry and Louise," who communicated their fears and concerns about what would happen to them if the government became the sole agent for managing the delivery of healthcare services (Blumenthal, 1995). Interest groups such as the American Medical Association (AMA), the Association of American Medical Colleges (AAMC), and the American Hospital Association (AHA) mobilized their members, organizing letter-writing campaigns and Washington visits. Organized interests are heard more in the political process than are unorganized interests.

Mass media clearly affect the public opinion agenda, and this affects politicians. Media's role is to report and magnify events rather than originate them, but media can also serve as a venue for interest groups to express their support or opposition to alternatives. Public opinion through national surveys has a powerful impact on the policy-making process and can have either positive or negative effects. Some items become part of the governmental agenda because a sufficient number of voters interested in the issue make it popular for vote-seeking politicians. Consider, for example, the 1991 election of Harris Wofford as senator from Pennsylvania, winning over a strong opponent, because of his focus on healthcare reform issues. More often than not, public opinion constrains government action. In Case 13-3, numerous alternatives were debated through the fall of 1994. Public opinion contributed significantly to the failure to pass any legislation before the November election.

In a rational, comprehensive decision-making model, policymakers would first define their goals clearly and then set levels of achieving the goals that would satisfy them. They would then identify and study all alternatives that might achieve these goals. They would compare alternatives systematically, determining costs and benefits. After thorough analysis, they would choose alternatives that would meet the goals at the least cost. In practice, however, instead of considering each program or issue afresh, decision-makers take what they currently are doing as given and make small adjustments to what is currently being implemented. This is known as *incrementalism* and results in gradual policy changes. Incrementalism tends to characterize more the process of generating and selecting alternatives, while agenda setting or change seems to be nonincremental and can be quite abrupt. In Case 13-3, the election and the abrupt change in ideas about implementing comprehensive health reform that followed are examples of nonincremental change.

Incorporated within policy-making are three processes that develop and operate largely independently of one another, except at critical times. When these processes or streams are linked, policy is more likely to change. These processes are: problem recognition; the formation and refining of policy proposals; and the politics of enactment and implementation.

People recognize problems and then they generate proposals for policy change. They engage in political activities such as election campaigns and pressure group lobbying to further their agenda. Each participant mentioned here could be involved in any or all of these processes, and each participant can act as either an impetus or a constraint. The key to understanding policy change is the coupling of these processes. A problem is recognized, a solution is available, the political climate makes the time right for change, and the constraints do not prohibit action. For any of this to occur, there must be at least one significant policy entrepreneur. Policy entrepreneurs are advocates willing to invest their time, energy, reputation, and money to promote a position or attach a problem to a solution, joining problems, policies, and politics (Kingdon, 1984). They hook solutions to problems, proposals to political momentum, and political events to policy problems.

Governmental and nongovernmental agencies routinely monitor various activities and events. For example, the number of physicians produced and their specialty and location of employment are monitored by the government. Sometimes a focusing event, such as a crisis or disaster, or the personal experience of a policymaker, may call attention to a problem. Feedback is provided to governmental officials and decision-makers about the operations of existing programs. This feedback may indicate a problem in a program, that goals are not being met, that costs are higher than anticipated, or that there may be unanticipated consequences of a public policy. People must be convinced that change is needed for a specific condition to be defined as a problem. In Case 13-3, many people argued that indicators showed there was a large number of employed individuals who were unable to afford or obtain health insurance; others did not believe the feedback or indicators and were not willing to identify this as a problem requiring comprehensive health reform. To focus attention on a problem, participants will highlight indicators through press releases, speeches, or during hearings or committee testimony. Other strategies include associating with experiences of influential people and generating feedback in the form of letters, visits to decision-makers, and protest activity. The process of fixing attention on one problem rather than another is crucial to agenda setting. In Case 13-3, many problems related to healthcare were identified and competed for attention. Without focused attention and agreement as to the problem(s), identifying and choosing alternatives became impossible.

Specialists in policy communities, inside and outside government, generate alternatives and proposals, evaluate them, and collect evidence in support or opposition. This occurs simultaneously with lobbying and the mobilization of support or opposition by interest groups. Introducing bills and making speeches are used to test a proposal and gauge receptivity to an idea. For a proposal to survive, it must be technically feasible, compatible with the values of the policy community, have an acceptable cost, and be likely to be positively received among elected decision-makers and the public. As proposals are developed, they move through a long process of consideration, discussion, debate, revision, and testing. The process emphasizes persuasion and diffusion, and building coalitions, striking bargains, and providing concessions. The goal is to gain enough votes to pass the proposal out of committee and through the Congress.

Policy windows provide necessary opportunities for action on given initiatives to occur. They open for short periods for varying reasons. A window may open because of a change in the political stream, as in the change in administration that occurred in Case 13-3, or a redistribution of representation in Congress, as happened in the elections of November, 1994. It could also open because a new problem captures the attention of decision-makers and governmental officials. Problems may become more pressing (increasing cost of health insurance, number of employed individuals without health insurance, potential bankruptcy of Medicare Trust Fund, percentage of GDP spent on healthcare), creating an opportunity for advocates to attach their solutions to the problems. Policy windows present opportunities for problems, proposals, and politics to come together, and hence opportunities to move them up the decision agenda. In Case 13-3, the initial phases of the health reform debate caught the attention of the media, the public, and most legislators, creating a policy window. What did not occur during this process was the coupling of the identified problems, proposals, and political stream. There were many components to the Clinton proposal, and each seemed radical from some constituencies' point of view. The Clinton proposal, and other proposals drafted by various committees and legislators, all experienced high levels of opposition from special interest groups. Americans were not in the mood for a program that was characterized by the opposition as more big government. Consensus and commitment to reform became divided by disagreement between administrative and legislative branches and between and within the political parties in Congress. Additionally, the political impact of public opinion on the impending Congressional election and the massive special interest efforts brought the legislative debate on health reform to an impasse.

CONCLUSIONS

This overview of the policy-making process is not designed to make you an expert in either health economics or health policy but to provide a perspective of how the health policy that affects the delivery of healthcare services, research, and education is determined. As you can see, the process is complex, multifactorial, and dynamic. The principal issues are ones of economics, distributive justice, and control of the political decision-making process. Neither the quantity nor the quality of medical care provided to a population can be considered independent of cost. The questions of who shall receive care, the amount and kind, and how it shall be rationed cannot be avoided. They will be decided by either the market or the government. Government has the responsibility and authority to decide which, or what balance between the two basic systems to employ.

Policy will be determined in a political process. The key to understanding policy changes and the policy-making process is not where the idea came from, but what made it become a focus of attention and what sustained that focus. A prominent feature of the process is the combined effect of several converging factors. It is critical that health professionals, who are continually affected positively and negatively by the health policy-making process, understand the components of this coupled process and where their involvement can help develop effective and relevant health policies for the future.

As a physician, you must continue to remember the challenges of the Hippocratic oath (Relman, 1980; Relman & Reinhardt, 1986) regarding the role of the physician as a member of a profession and not a business enterprise, and maintain your primary interest in the welfare of your patients. As a member of a profession working to improve the healthcare status of individuals by participating in the policy-making process, you must remember that "the primary concern of professionals must not be the self-interest of the professional group or the corporation. If someday physicians and their organizations do become primarily self-interest groups, society—which has given them the privilege of being called professionals—will rise up and take that privilege away. And the profession will be no more!" (Lundberg, 1995). Your understanding of and involvement in the health policy-making process as a constructive contributor is essential in order to address the healthcare needs of the nation.

CASES FOR DISCUSSION

CASE 1

Mr. A. is a 54-year-old male who has had two coronary artery bypass graft (CABG) procedures for occluded coronary arteries. He is overweight, eats a high-fat diet, continues to smoke a pack of *cigarettes a day, and maintains a sedentary life-style. His response to your concern about his life-style choices and the impact on his heart disease is: "Gee, Doc, I can't imagine what the quality of my life would be like without my cigarettes, and I've tried to change my diet, that's too hard. Anyway, if those arteries block up again, my insurance will pay for the surgery." The cost for Mr. A's CABG is approximately $35,000, and the likelihood of reocclusion in 2–4 years is very high if risk factors are not modified.*

1. *Is there a difference in the value of a CABG for one individual versus utilizing the $35,000 for a free immunization program for the majority of children in the region? In this situation, would a cost-effectiveness analysis (CEA) assist in determining guidelines?*
2. *In Great Britain, an individual who refused to quit smoking was refused a second CABG. Is this an equitable allocation of resources? If so, how would health policy need to be developed that would accomplish this?*
3. *Does the calculus or result of the CEA change according to the perspective or interest of the analyst? How might the analysis be differently structured by the cardiothoracic surgeon, the cardiologist, general physician, patient, policy analyst, insurance company? In the example of otitis media with effusion, compare the perspectives of a pharmaceutical manufacturer, an otolaryngologist, a family physician, a parent, an indemnity health insurance company, an HMO.*

CASE 2

Medicare currently provides approximately $6.1 billion for graduate medical education (GME) to academic health centers (medical schools and teaching hospitals). Each year approximately 17,000 individuals graduate from U.S. allopathic and osteopathic medical schools and begin residency training. In 1993, 106,000 residents were in postgraduate training, and of those 25,000 were in first-year positions. More than 25% of all first-year slots were occupied by International Medical Graduates (IMGs—individuals who have graduated from medical schools outside of the United States). A large percentage of Medicare GME funds are directed to two northeastern states that each has 45–50% of its residency positions filled by IMGs. The cost of healthcare continues to rise each year and a significant proportion of that rise is Medicare-related expenditures, including funds for graduate medical education. The Congress is aware of the problem of escalating healthcare costs and is evaluating whether reducing the number of residency positions or the amount of GME funding through Medicare would move toward a balanced budget.

1. *What participants and/or special interest groups would be involved in responding to a proposal for legislation to reduce the number of residency positions? How might they position themselves, and what strategies might they utilize to support or oppose such a proposal? Are there special interest groups that might work together in these efforts?*

CASE 3

In 1994, cash and stock awards to the heads of the seven largest for-profit HMOs averaged $7 million. One chief executive officer received more than a $15.5 million package, including stock options worth $15.1 million. The large profits realized by these companies can be a result of cutting costs by reducing reimbursements to physicians and hospitals or by carefully controlling services and benefits available to patients.

1. *If patients are satisfied and the quality of care is not compromised, is the compensation justifiable and socially acceptable? If so, why? If not socially acceptable, what should be done?*
2. *Does this scenario represent an authority- or market system-based approach to health reform?*

3. Can the healthcare market reform itself or is government intervention needed? If government intervention is necessary in the context of the health policy-making process, how might this be accomplished?

CASE 4

Dr. R. and Dr. P. recently joined a Physician Organization (PO) and that soon will merge with a regional hospital to form a Physician Hospital Organization (PHO). The administrator of the hospital is eager to develop shared risk capitated agreements with several insurance companies moving into the region who want to develop a managed care integrated network and delivery system. In addition to being members of this network, Dr. R. and Dr. P. are being offered stock options and investment possibilities in the corporate entity of this network, whose stock will be traded on the stock exchange.

1. What are the implications of these agreements for Dr. R. and Dr. P.? for the hospital? for the insurance company?
2. Whose interests will be represented when Dr. R. and Dr. P. provide healthcare services for patients within this network? Is there a conflict of interest?
3. What might be some of the conflicts between the parties in this network?

CASE 5

County General Hospital (CGH), a 650-bed tertiary care center, is planning to form an integrated delivery network. It has half the hospital business in the region and an entrepreneurial CEO who wants to develop managed care plans before an insurance company or a physicians' group does. The new Regional Integrated Comprehensive Health System (RICHSys) would offer its own health insurance plan as an HMO and contract with Preferred Provider Organizations (PPOs) for some of the services. RICHSys could use the capital of CGH to underwrite the plan or find an insurance company partner to supply the capital. RICHSys is quietly negotiating with some of the primary care physicians to join the closed-panel HMO as salaried staff. Another group, called MicroMedManagement (MMM), is also planning to enter the managed care market in the region. It is seeking to contract with selected primary care providers and specialists in an IPA arrangement. It will negotiate a discount on each physician's fees on a yearly basis and offer a holdback that may be paid if the MMM plan performs well.

1. Should you contract with or join one of these organizations? If so, which one? Why?
2. What do you think is the hospital's interest in managed care?
3. Why do you think MMM is interested in bringing managed care to the region?
4. Why do you think the insurance company is interested in becoming a partner with RICHSys?
5. How do think RICHSys will control its costs? How do you think MMM will control its costs? Is either likely to market its product to the currently uninsured?

CASE 6

You decided to join the RICHSys as a salaried physician and have worked with them for 2 years. In the first year RICHSys lost money because of adverse selection and because it failed to control utilization well enough. In the second and third years it broke even, and now in the fourth year it looks as if the plan is going to have a surplus of about $1.5 million. The board of this nonprofit HMO wishes to bank half for facility improvement and expand benefits to enrollees with the other half. You have been put on the benefit analysis committee and are considering a number of options. The *committee is expected to recommend that more visits for alcohol abuse and mental health services without copayment be included in the plan. There is strong support also for providing free flu shots (at $8 per shot) to all enrollees over 55. The pediatricians would like to offer free infant and toddler car seats (about $50 each, with a useful life of 3 years) to all new parents as well as bike helmets at half-price (a $15 cost to RICHSys) to all elementary school children in the plan who take part in a Child Safety Day.*

1. *How should you present the analysis to the committee so they may make an informed decision?*
2. *What are some other options that the committee might consider?*

ACKNOWLEDGMENTS. The authors thank their colleagues: Jerri R. Harris, for her gracious and constructive editorial guidance, and Becky Mussat, for her cheerful and creative production of charts and graphs.

RECOMMENDED READINGS

Starr P: *The Social Transformation of American Medicine.* New York, Basic Books, 1982.

The thorough, award-winning scholarship in this book describes "the rise of a sovereign profession and the making of a vast industry." Paul Starr provides a very readable history interpreted through the conceptual framework of sociology. This work should help all medical students place the career they have chosen in the context of social systems and U.S. politics. In the first part of the book, Starr describes the rise of medical authority and its role in shaping the U.S. medical system. In taking the reader from the colonial United States to the turn of the century, he describes competing medical paradigms, how medical education and statute consolidated the authority of allopathic medicine, the roles of hospitals and public health, and the relationship of capitalism to medical practice. In the second part, he analyzes the relationships between physicians, the state, and the corporation. This is a primer for grasping the issues and politics of healthcare reform.

Enthoven A, Kronik R: A consumer-choice health plan for the 1990s. *N Engl J Med* (Part 1) 320(1):29–37. (Part 2) 320(2):94–101, 1989.

Professors Enthoven and Kronik set forth a proposal for universal health insurance that they argue is consistent with the pluralistic nature of U.S. society, the individualism of the U.S. psyche, and the incremental nature of U.S. politics. This consumer-choice health plan became the basis for the blend of competition and regulation advanced by the Jackson Hole Group in 1992, known as managed competition. This approach was incorporated into the Health Security Act proposed by President Clinton in 1993.

Himmelstein DU, Woolhandler S, *et al*: A national health program for the United States. *N Engl J Med* 320(2):102–108, 1989.

In this companion article, Drs. Himmelstein and Woolhandler, along with a writing group composed of over two dozen other physicians, called for an end to patchwork reforms and proposed a quite different approach, one similar to Canada's national healthcare system. Their proposal is for a comprehensive, single-payer system with a global budget for the operating expenses of hospitals and nursing homes, funding capital costs through a separate budget, and paying physicians on a salaried, fee-for-service, or capitation basis.

Kingdon JW: *Agendas, Alternatives, and Public Policies.* Boston, Little, Brown & Co 1984.

A very readable, concise description of how issues get on the political, policy-making agenda, who the government and nongovernment participants are, and what has to happen for action to occur.

CHAPTER 14

C. Special Problems

The Tobacco Pandemic

Alan Blum and Eric J. Solberg

CASE 14-1

Jane L., a 28-year-old graduate student, is waiting to see her family physician for her annual well-woman examination. She is concerned about an article in the **Women's Home Magazine** *that she has just read in the waiting room. The author warned of dangers associated with the use of oral contraceptives by women who smoke. Jane L. smokes one pack a day of Marlboro Lights 100s. Accordingly, she would like to stop taking the pill and get fitted for a diaphragm.*

Rather than simply acquiescing to the patient's request, the physician seized the opportunity to help the patient make the connection between health improvement and cessation of smoking, and to explain the relative risk of smoking compared to oral contraceptives. The patient expressed a desire to stop smoking and asked for help in doing so.

INTRODUCTION

As Case 14-1 illustrates, in only a few minutes there is much a physician can do to motivate patients to stop smoking. Such active interventions are more effective than relegating this task to ancillary personnel, a smoking cessation clinic, or a pamphlet off the shelf.

The biggest obstacle to tackling the tobacco problem is complacency—on the part of the public and health professionals alike—stemming from the belief that the war on smoking has been won (Blum, 1992). Although there is hardly a child or adult who has not heard that smoking is dangerous to health, the fact remains that the incidence of smoking has declined by less than 1% per year in the United States over the past decade. Moreover, women, teenagers, blue-collar workers, and minority groups in general are not appreciably reducing their cigarette consumption (Blum, 1993).

Cigarette smoking is the chief avoidable cause of death and disease in our society. Each year smoking is responsible for 18% of all deaths in the United States (Rakel & Blum, 1995). Approximately 40% of all deaths from cancer and 21% of deaths from cardiovascular disease are caused by smoking. Tobacco use contributes to more than 400,000 deaths annually in the United States, and more than 3 million annually worldwide (Centers for Disease Control, 1994a). Although cigarette smoking among adults declined from 42 to 27% in the United States during the 23 years following publication of the first Surgeon General's report on smoking and health in 1964, 28% of men and 24% of women continue to use tobacco regularly (Department of Health and Human Services, 1989; Rakel & Blum, 1995).

Ending the tobacco pandemic is not a *static* effort where health professionals educate the public about the adverse health effects of smoking in the hope that individuals will change their behavior, but rather a *dynamic* one where the tobacco industry changes its tactics to anticipate all efforts to discourage tobacco use (Blum & Solberg, 1992). As physicians and other health professionals work with their patients to end their smoking, cigarette companies continue to advertise their products, spending more than $5.2 billion on advertising each year, touting low-tar, implicitly "safer" cigarettes, with reduced prices and coupons for increased savings. Physicians should point out to smokers is that buying a $2 pack of cigarettes is a real "rip-off" as one costs less than 20 cents to manufacture. One patient, after smoking more than two packs a day for many years, realized he had "smoked a Porsche."

Concerns about smoking have long been raised in the scientific community. In 1928 Lombard and Doering reported a higher incidence of smoking among patients with cancer than among controls (Lombard & Doering, 1928). Ten years later, Pearl reported that persons who smoked heavily had a shorter life expectancy than those who did not smoke (Pearl, 1938). In 1939 Ochsner and DeBakey began reporting their observations on the relation between smoking and lung cancer (Ochsner & DeBakey, 1939). They and other outspoken opponents of smoking, such as Dwight Harkin and William Overholt, were met with derision by the medical profession, more than two-thirds of whom smoked.

Not until the epidemiological work in the 1950s of Doll and Hill (1956) in the United Kingdom and Hammond and Horn (1958) in the United States did the medical profession begin to take the problem seriously. Since that time, information about the health risks associated with smoking has been well publicized in the medical literature. The first U.S. Surgeon General's Report on Smoking and Health in 1964 concluded that cigarette smoking was the major cause of lung cancer in men. Besides lung cancer, smoking is a major cause of cancers of the larynx, oral cavity, and esophagus. It is a contributory factor in cancers of the pancreas, bladder, kidney, stomach, and cervix. Recent studies implicate smoking in leukemia, colon cancer, Graves' disease, depression, and renal disease in persons with diabetes mellitus (Blum, 1993). A dose–response relationship exists between smoking and all of these diseases.

Cigarette smoking is a primary risk factor for coronary heart disease (CHD). Overall, persons who smoke have a 70% greater CHD death rate, a two- to fourfold greater incidence of CHD, and a two- to fourfold greater risk for sudden death than nonsmokers (DHHS, 1982). The risk of stroke increases with the number of cigarettes smoked. The incidence of stroke among persons who smoke is 50% higher than among persons who do not smoke (Wolf *et al.*, 1988). Cigarette smoking is also the main cause of chronic obstructive pulmonary disease (COPD), which is the leading cause of disability in the United States.

More than 38 million Americans have stopped smoking cigarettes. Unfortunately, some 50 million Americans continue to smoke cigarettes, despite the consequences of smoking to their health (DHHS, 1990a). Smoking cessation has major and immediate health benefits for men and women of all ages. The 1990 Report of the Surgeon General outlines the benefits of smoking cessation. The report concludes that smoking cessation decreases the risk of lung cancer, other cancers, heart attack, stroke, and chronic lung disease. For example, after 10 years of abstinence, the risk of lung cancer is about 30 to 50% of the risk in people who continue to smoke, and after 15 years of abstinence, the risk of CHD is similar to that of persons who have never smoked.

CASE 14-2

Doctor Susan Murphy was asked to speak to a health class of junior high students in an urban area. She asked the students to recall images from the most familiar billboards in their neighborhoods depicting smoking. The students reported seeing blacks smoking menthol brands, such as Salem and Kool, on the billboards, white men smoking Marlboro and Camel, and women smoking thin, sleek cigarettes such as Virginia Slims, Misty, and Capri. Dr. Murphy then asked the students which brands of cigarettes their parents and grandparents smoked. The students were surprised to discover the effectiveness of the advertising and marketing efforts of the tobacco companies.

——————— WOMEN AND MINORITIES ———————

In 1964, at the time of the first Surgeon General's Report discussing the smoking epidemic, lung cancer was the leading cause of death due to cancer in men and the fifth leading cause of cancer mortality among women (Blum, 1993). This difference in lung cancer mortality between the genders, alluded to in Case 14-2, can be explained by the fact that until the 1920s, it was socially unacceptable—and in some states illegal—for women to smoke. Men had taken up cigarette smoking in large numbers toward the end of the nineteenth century—in part because antispitting ordinances to curtail the spread of tuberculosis had led the tobacco companies to switch from the promotion of chewing tobacco and cigars to the inhalation of tobacco smoke by means of the cigarette (Blum, 1993). Smoking did not take hold among women until the 1920s when the American Tobacco Company began a mass media advertising campaign with the slogan, "To keep a slender figure, reach for a Lucky instead of a sweet."

Because of the increase in smoking among women, lung cancer has surpassed breast cancer as the leading cause of cancer deaths among women. Cigarette smoking leads to other problems for women, especially during pregnancy. There is a confirmed association between maternal smoking and low-birth-weight infants, and there is an increased incidence of premature birth, spontaneous abortion, stillbirth, and neonatal death (Rakel & Blum, 1995).

Blacks and Hispanics have the highest rates of lung cancer and cardiovascular disease in the United States (DHHS, 1985). The disproportionately high rates of smoking-related diseases among ethnic minorities can be attributed to the successful marketing of tobacco products to minority communities (Blum, 1989). Billboards advertising cigarettes appear four to five times more often in inner-city neighborhoods than in middle-class suburbs (Scenic America, 1990). Cigarette advertising in black and Hispanic magazines and newspapers represents a major source of revenue for these publications. In more than 40 years of publication, the leading black-oriented magazine, *Ebony*, has carried few articles on smoking; not surprisingly, cigarette companies are a leading source of revenue (Blum, 1989).

The tobacco industry has been especially adept at exploiting racial identity in defining a profitable market among ethnic minorities. R.J. Reynolds Tobacco Company sponsors street fairs in Hispanic neighborhoods while simultaneously promoting their Camel and Salem cigarette brands. Brown and Williamson Tobacco Company has presented annual Kool Achiever awards to people who have improved the "quality of life in inner-city communities." Major black and Hispanic civic organizations, such as the NAACP, the Urban League, the United Negro College Fund, and La Raza, receive funding from tobacco companies; an exception is the National Coalition of Hispanic Health and Human Services Organizations.

The result of such successful marketing targeted to ethnic minorities is a higher rate of smoking among blacks and an increase in smoking among Hispanic women. Data from the 1987 National Health Interview Survey reveal that 32.9% of blacks smoke compared with 25% of the white middle-class population (DHHS, 1990b).

CASE 14-3

Billy J. is an 8-year-old who presents with a persistent cough. This is his third visit over the past 3 months, during which time he has missed several days of school. The principal has requested a physician's note to explain Billy's absences. Billy's parents are frustrated and believe that Billy is faking or exaggerating his symptoms to avoid school. Neither Billy nor his parents smoke, but the woman who takes care of him after school smokes in her house.

──── INVOLUNTARY OR PASSIVE SMOKING ────

Billy's parents should be aware that two-thirds of the smoke from a burning cigarette never reaches the lungs of the person who smokes, but instead goes directly into the air (DHHS, 1986). The 1986 Report of the Surgeon General, dedicated to a discussion of involuntary or passive smoking, defined environmental tobacco smoke (ETS)—also called secondhand smoke—as the combination of sidestream smoke that is emitted into the air from a burning cigarette between puffs and the fraction of mainstream smoke that is exhaled by one who smokes.

The effects of tobacco smoke on nonsmokers can be significant. An estimated 3000 nonsmokers die each year from secondhand smoke (National Institutes of Health, 1993). Fifteen percent of the U.S. public is allergic to cigarette smoke. An increasing number of studies have explored the health risks of the nonsmoker who is exposed to ETS. The toxic and carcinogenic effects of ETS are similar to those of tobacco smoke inhaled by active smokers. At least 14 studies have demonstrated a risk of lung cancer in nonsmoking wives exposed to the secondhand smoke of their husbands (Rakel & Blum, 1995). Passive smoking has been found to increase the risk of leukemia, lymphoma, and cancer of the breast and uterine cervix.

The risks of passive smoking extend beyond cancer. It is estimated that tobacco smoke in the home and workplace could be responsible for the deaths of 46,000 nonsmokers annually in the United States (NIH, 1993). Most of these, 32,000, are the result of heart disease, making passive smoking the third leading preventable cause of death after smoking and the consumption of alcohol.

Parents who smoke are more likely to have children who will smoke. The risk of a child smoking increases with each additional adult family member who smokes (Rakel & Blum, 1995). Over 50% of children under 5 years of age live in homes with at least one adult who smokes. Children of smoking parents are more likely to suffer from otitis media, bronchitis, and pneumonia. Numerous studies have shown that the increased incidence of cough, bronchitis, and pneumonia in children of smoking parents is proportional to the number of cigarettes smoked by the parents, particularly the mother (Rantakallio, 1978). Asthma is also more prevalent, and passive smoking has been linked to some instances of sudden infant death syndrome (Rantakallio, 1978).

CASE 14-4

Tim S. is a fourth-year medical student completing a dermatology elective. A patient he has seen for dry skin returned for a follow-up visit to get a renewal on a prescription for cortisone ointment. While she is waiting to speak with her physician, Tim recognizes her and asks if she has stopped smoking yet. She replies by saying she really did try, but that the stress at work and home have been unbearable, and she does not want to gain back the weight that she just lost. "I'm not ready to quit," she explains. However, she adds that she switched to a lower-tar brand and now actually smokes more cigarettes per day than ever before. Tim tells her that her smoking may contribute to her skin problem, and that if she doesn't stop she may not see much improvement. Tim tells her that her stress is just an excuse for not quitting, and warns her of the serious danger smoking is to her health.

───── SMOKING CESSATION ─────

Rather than scold his patient for not listening to him previously about the adverse health effects of smoking and the importance of stopping in Case 14-4, Tim should have used this opportunity to serve as a consumer advocate as much as a health nanny. Tim could have helped this patient not by remonstrating, but rather by suggesting that the stress she feels impelling her to light up a cigarette may in large measure reflect her dependence on nicotine and by correcting the myth that smoking low-tar cigarettes is safer.

LOW TAR MEANS LOW POISON

In the 1950s, confronted with declining cigarette sales after the publication of studies linking smoking to lung cancer, tobacco companies began producing filter-tipped brands and claimed that these filters removed certain components of smoke, which manufacturers have never acknowledged to be harmful (Miller, 1985). Brown and Williamson Tobacco Company purchased advertising space in the Medicine section of *Time* to claim that Viceroy cigarettes offered "double-barrel health protection," and advertisements for Liggett and Myers's filter L & Ms claimed they were "just what the doctor ordered." Until the 1960s tobacco companies promoted cigarettes at meetings of the American Medical

Association and other health organizations by means of scientific exhibits that sought to demonstrate the alleged benefits of one brand over another (Blum, 1992). Consumer demand soared. Currently, 97% of those who smoke buy filtered brands.

In the late 1960s, to allay public anxiety about cancer, tobacco companies began marketing brands with purportedly lower levels of "tar" and nicotine. Throughout the 1970s the American Cancer Society, the National Cancer Institute, and most major health organizations promoted the concept of a safer cigarette in the belief that most people who smoke cannot stop. Persons who switch to allegedly low-tar cigarettes have been found to employ compensatory smoking, whereby they inhale more frequently and more deeply to maintain a satisfying level of nicotine (Rickert, 1983; Miller, 1985). More simply, for the purpose of educating the patient who smokes, "low tar" can be translated as "low poison." Tar is a composite of more than 4000 separate solid poisons, including at least 43 known carcinogens. Cigarettes with reduced yields of tar, nicotine, and carbon monoxide are not safer. A recommendation to switch to such brands is misguided.

DEBUNKING COMMON MYTHS

An important myth surrounding smoking is that it relieves stress. This idea can be debunked by pointing out that the stress that is relieved is that which resulted from being dependent on nicotine—this is the essence of addiction. At the same time, deep breathing has a relaxing effect. The physician can suggest that the patient try to postpone for 5 minutes every time she intends to light up, then breathe slowly and deeply for 5 minutes, then reconsider whether the cigarette is important.

Another myth reinforced in advertisements for Virginia Slims and other cigarettes aimed at women and girls is that smoking keeps weight off. The woman who stops smoking need not gain weight if she relearns the joy of walking and other activities as much as one relearns the taste of food. By no means will all persons who stop smoking gain weight. Even among those who do, the average weight gain is less than 5 pounds (DHHS, 1990a).

Perhaps the biggest myth that has been encouraged in the medical literature is that the patient must be "ready to quit." Although common sense dictates that those who express a greater interest in smoking cessation will have a greater success rate, those patients who do not express an interest in smoking cessation symbolize the overall challenge to be faced in ending the pandemic. Setting a quit date, the essential element of the smoking cessation literature, may rationalize the continuation of an adverse health practice and may strengthen denial. It is helpful to remind patients that they can stop now.

CONSUMER ADVOCACY ROLE

Traditional office-based approaches begin by asking, "Do you smoke?" "How much do you smoke?" and "When did you start smoking?" Although this may provide the physician with relevant data for charting purposes, this approach is too often a signal for the patient to become defensive and resistant to further discussion, especially if the patient had no intention to stop smoking. There are alternative ways of obtaining information and at the same time piquing the patient's interest in the subject. By using and identifying with the vocabulary used by the consumer of cigarettes, the physician can adopt and be perceived in the role of consumer advocate as opposed to medical finger-wagger. The most important and nonthreatening questions to ask are, "What brand do you buy?" and "How much do you spend on cigarettes?" The patient is likely to be surprised and intrigued by these questions, which can be asked at any time in the course of the interview, because they appear to be nonjudgmental. They suggest that the physician is not a know-it-all and a polemicist. A question about the cost of cigarettes shows concern for the patient's financial well-being.

Promotions for various pharmacologic agents, mail-order gadgets, and clinics in smoking cessation reinforce the notion that cigarette smoking is primarily a medical problem with a simple, easy-to-prescribe, nonindividualized solution. When a patient requests a "drug that will help me stop smoking," the physician must confront the dilemma of not wanting to dash the patient's expectation while emphasizing that a drug or device is, at best, an adjunct and not a means of smoking cessation.

PERSONALIZE AND INDIVIDUALIZE

In addition to debunking common myths surrounding smoking, the physician can learn to personalize approaches to smoking cessation by carefully screening the pamphlets and other audiovisual aids available in the office. It is essential to scrutinize all such material, as one would with a new drug or medical device. Personally handing a brochure to a patient while pointing out and underlining certain passages or illustrations will provide an important reinforcing message.

Individualizing the message to the patient is the cornerstone of success in patient education. The same cigarette counseling method cannot be used for a high school girl, a construction worker, and an executive already showing signs of heart disease. In the case of a high school girl, the physician should not focus on such abstract concepts as emphysema and lung cancer, but rather emphasize the cosmetic unattractiveness of yellow teeth, bad breath, the loss of athletic ability, and the financial drain that results from buying cigarettes. As for the construction worker, the physician might suggest the likelihood of fewer lost paydays, greater physical strength, and even a lengthier sex life were he to stop smoking cigarettes.

In any event, such dialogue must be practiced over and over again like any medical procedure, and individualized to the patient. The counseling should be designed to call attention not only to the inevitable risks of smoking cigarettes but also to the chemically adulterated tobacco product itself, its inflated price, and the ubiquitous and ludicrous way in which the person's brand is promoted. In effect, the physician can shift the focus away from a resistant or guilt-ridden smoker and onto the product.

CASE 14-5

Dan Glatt, a fourth-year medical student and delegate to the American Medical Association's (AMA) Student Section, worked collaboratively with peers and colleagues to submit a resolution in 1992 for the AMA to adopt a policy stating that the AMA would no longer accept financial support from tobacco companies. A separate resolution submitted by another section of the AMA called for the AMA to "discourage all medical schools and their parent universities from accepting research funding from the tobacco industry."

——————— TOBACCO USE AND SOCIETY ———————

The ethical issues described in Case 14-5 arose primarily from a $250,000 grant that Fleischmann's Margarine gave the AMA for an anticholesterol campaign. Fleischmann's is owned by tobacco giant R.J. Reynolds. Similarly, the AMA received advertising revenue from tobacco company-owned products, such as Philip Morris-owned Kraft and R.J. Reynolds-owned Nabisco, for their cable television ventures. The AMA's acceptance of money from tobacco company "subsidiaries" was defended by members of the AMA's Board of Trustees through statements that public health programs may have to be cut if the AMA no longer received financial support from these companies.

Both proposals were referred to the Board of Trustees, as the AMA House of Delegates directed the Board to report back in 6 months with a "definition" of a tobacco company (Wolinsky & Brune, 1995). The resulting definition would thus apply to any AMA policy on nonacceptance of funds from tobacco companies and the AMA's encouragement of medical schools to end their acceptance of research support from the tobacco industry.

These proposals did not represent the first time that the AMA's ties with the tobacco industry were called into question. Nor was it the first time that medical students and residents were the originators of the debate. In 1979 a few resident physicians learned that the AMA's Members Retirement Fund owned $1.4 million in tobacco securities (Blum, 1983). In 1980, a handful of residents persuaded the AMA Resident Physicians Section to present a resolution to the House of Delegates declaring "the AMA fiduciary responsibility to the public is greater than its fiduciary responsibility to its investment portfolio," and asked for the divestment of the tobacco stock (Wolinsky & Brune, 1995). The AMA Board's finance committee chairman argued that the purpose of the pension fund was to make the biggest buck, not to make social statements. Other AMA officials attempted to minimize the issue by noting that tobacco companies were highly diversified and were involved in nontobacco industries.

The residents' resolution was defeated by the AMA, but after the resulting bad publicity the AMA received in national media for defeating the proposal, the portfolio managers sold the tobacco stock. In 1985, the AMA officially informed its investment brokers that tobacco securities could not be purchased without prior approval by the AMA Board or its finance committee (Wolinsky & Brune, 1995).

Dan Glatt in Case 14-5 and his colleagues in the Medical Student and Resident Physicians Sections of the AMA knew that their resolutions to end financial support of the AMA and medical schools by tobacco companies would not be well received by executives at the AMA, nor by the deans of medical schools and their parent universities. In June, 1993, the AMA Board unveiled its definition of the tobacco industry. The AMA defined the tobacco industry as "companies or corporate divisions that directly produce or market tobacco products along with their research and lobbying groups including the Council for Tobacco Research and the Tobacco Institute" (American Medical Association, 1993). The definition continued that "a company or corporate division that does not produce or market tobacco products, but that has a tobacco producing company as or among its owners not be considered a prohibited part of the tobacco industry." In other words, under the definition the AMA could not deal directly with tobacco companies, but could continue to trade with the companies' subsidiaries so long as they were not involved in the promotion of tobacco products, leaving the ethical question open for further debate.

CASE 14-6

Susan Evans, a first-year resident in family medicine, worked as a volunteer of the community-based health charity as part of the requirements for a preventive

medicine and health promotion curriculum of her residency program. The orga-
nization asked her to help them develop a curriculum for tobacco prevention to be
implemented in area schools.

331

MEDICAL
ACTIVISM:
BEYOND THE
EXAMINING
ROOM

Susan began her work by researching resources and other agencies that
work on the tobacco issue. In addition to the information she received from
traditional voluntary health agencies, primarily restricted to pamphlets about the
dangers of smoking, one organization called DOC (Doctors Ought to Care) pro-
vided her with materials developed for health professionals to present in the
school classroom. To Susan's credit, she did her homework. Rather than try to
reinvent the wheel, Susan discovered that much of the initial work and research
had already been done, and she simply needed to focus on implementation.

MEDICAL ACTIVISM: BEYOND THE EXAMINING ROOM

DOC, the example provided in Case 14-6, was founded in 1977 in order to educate the public, especially young people, about the major causes of poor health and high medical costs. One of DOC's primary objectives has been to tap the highest possible level of commitment from every health professional to combat the promotion of lethal life-styles in the mass media. Unfortunately, public health issues and health promotion do not receive the attention they should in U.S. medical schools and residency programs. Indeed, within the medical profession, incentives for health promotion have never been strong. Put in these challenging terms, there is understandable discomfort, skepticism, and even resistance by many physicians to health promotion efforts. Many physicians question why the responsibility, or onus, of health promotion should fall to the physician. To the busy practitioner, health promotion does not appear to be time-effective or cost-effective. For these reasons, a more concerted effort is needed to involve medical students, residents, and physicians in health promotion efforts.

To confront the tobacco pandemic, numerous strategies can be implemented in the clinic, classroom, and community (Blum, 1992). Some of the clinic strategies have already been described earlier in this chapter. But the messages imparted in the clinic must be reinforced outside the office. To this end, school-based programs must be made more engaging and enraging, placing an equal emphasis on what could be called the "three Ps": peer pressure, parental modeling, and propaganda. Too few educational programs in or out of the classroom, especially in primary schools, go beyond scare tactics and cognitive objectives about the dangers of smoking. By analyzing and satirizing the promotional techniques of tobacco companies and their media allies, students can delight in turning the tables on the firms that create cigarette advertisements. In studying the long arm of the tobacco industry around the world and making the connection between tobacco advertising and the deaths of family members and friends from tobacco-related diseases, students may learn to redirect their anger from teachers, parents, and health professionals to the authority figures in society who attempt to promote unhealthy products to children.

Physicians and other healthcare professionals can begin their own secondary education in this effort by learning more about the tobacco industry, its products, and the way tobacco is promoted in society. The three essential tools for such research are a map, a calendar, and a camera. With these tools, one can monitor the promotional strategies of the tobacco industry in one's own community and utilize the results as part of a larger school-based or community-based educational effort.

Legislation and policy initiatives, such as a ban on tobacco advertising and promotion, would also be helpful but lack sufficient support from Congress. On the other hand, enforcement by the U.S. attorney general of existing laws that regulate tobacco advertising could be a major step forward. For example, the Public Health Cigarette Smoking Act of 1969, which prohibits the promotion of cigarette brands on television, calls for a $10,000 fine for each violation of the law. If this law could be applied to national telecasts of tobacco-sponsored sporting events, levying fines of up to tens of millions of dollars per event—based on the hundreds of tobacco brand names shown on television during a tennis match or auto race—neither media corporations nor tobacco companies could afford to continue televising tobacco-sponsored sporting events (Blum, 1991).

Until such action is taken by federal agencies, it is important to counteract such promotions at the community level. By lampooning brand names as part of paid counter-advertising and sponsoring antismoking events, DOC has been instrumental in pointing out the vulnerability of the tobacco industry. Since 1978, DOC has used its version of the Virginia Slims Tennis Tournament—the Emphysema Slims, with the slogan "You've coughed up long enough, baby"—to counter cigarette advertising.

The passage of smoke-free indoor legislation has been the single major advance in the United States in terms of reducing cigarette consumption, thanks to the efforts of nonsmokers' rights groups. In simple terms, when adults learn of policies prohibiting smoking in public places and at work, they don't light up. Among teenagers, preventive measures should focus on demand reduction, encouraging young people not to *buy* these products and to save their money.

There is great need for a no-holds-barred revocabularization, i.e., a new set of terms, images, and other symbols with which to communicate to the public about tobacco products and manufacturers (Blum, 1980). A crucial phase in U.S. public health will be reached when the seven major tobacco companies in the United States are recognized as cancer's seven warning signs: Philip Morris (makers of Marlboro and Virginia Slims), RJR/Nabisco (R.J. Reynolds Tobacco Company: Winston, Salem, and Camel), Loews (Newport and Kent), Brown and Williamson (Kool and Barclay), American Tobacco (now owned by British American Tobacco: Carlton and Lucky Strike), Liggett and Myers (generics), and UST (United States Tobacco: Skoal and Copenhagen spitting tobaccos). Similarly, the leading preventable cause of death and disease in our society is not lung cancer, heart disease, or emphysema, but rather Marlboro, which is the leading brand among adults and adolescents.

To the physician, hard-hitting satirical counteradvertising that shifts the public focus away from the substance (tobacco, nicotine), the user (smoker), and the effects of the substance (lung cancer) to the manufactured product, the way in which it is promoted, and the promoters may seem overly political and at risk of invoking the wrath of the tobacco industry and its allies. This effect is precisely the intention. Cigarette sales have not been seriously damaged by warnings of the dangers of smoking, because danger has become part of the formula for selling cigarettes, especially to the fearless adolescent. Tobacco companies have blithely responded to thousands of research reports describing the dangers of smoking by funding hundreds more to seek further proof.

CONCLUSION

A concerted effort that includes physicians, researchers, nurses, dentists, pharmacists, and other health professionals is essential for ending the tobacco pandemic. By better understanding the opposition to this public health tragedy, with the knowledge that complacency plays a major role as a barrier to a well-coordinated effort, health professionals will gain the skills needed to become more effective in their efforts.

By studying and counteracting the tobacco industry like a parasitic disease, health professionals can begin to immunize children and change societal attitudes about smoking through humorous, positive health strategies implemented in the clinic, classroom, and community.

———————— CASES FOR DISCUSSION ————————

CASE 1

A resident, on completion of an oncology rotation, learns that one of the trustees on the board of the cancer center also serves on the board of a major tobacco company. The resident, who has just seen firsthand the toll that tobacco use takes on patients and their families, feels compelled to present this issue to the board of trustees by encouraging a colleague to introduce the problem through a faculty committee.

1. *Is it a conflict of interest for a trustee of the cancer center to also serve on the board of a tobacco company?*
2. *Is the resident acting appropriately by calling attention to this issue, or should this be left to those who set policy for the cancer center?*
3. *Should the resident alert others to this issue (i.e., the local news media)?*

CASE 2

A physician is approached by one of his patients to speak on her behalf to her employer who permits smoking throughout her worksite. The patient is allergic to tobacco smoke and, when exposed to it for long periods, experiences headaches, sneezing, and itchy, watery eyes.

1. *What obligation does the physician have for his patient's health and well-being?*
2. *Should the physician risk the alienation of his patient by her employer?*
3. *What information can the physician share with the employer without breaching the trust and confidentiality of his patient?*
4. *How could/should the physician approach his patient's employer?*

CASE 3

A prominent physician is invited to serve as the physician for his city's opera. As one who enjoys the performing arts, he feels this is a good opportunity to participate in civic activities and help promote his clinic. He reads in a newspaper report that the opera has just received a $150,000 grant from the nation's largest tobacco company, Philip Morris, which gives millions each year to support arts groups.

1. *Should the physician accept this position?*
2. *Should the physician question the support of the opera by the tobacco company?*
3. *Can the physician accept this position and then utilize the position to draw attention to the tobacco company's contribution?*

4. *Should the opera be concerned with the fact that they have received a grant from a tobacco company, since the company gives to so many other groups?*

CASE 4

A physician and faculty member at a leading medical school has accepted the position of associate editor for a regional medical journal. In considering manuscripts for an upcoming issue devoted to lung disorders, he is informed by a reviewer that one manuscript was submitted by researchers whose study may have been funded by the Council for Tobacco Research.

1. *Is it appropriate for the editor to ask the researchers who funded their study?*
2. *Should the editor reject the manuscript solely based on the source of funding provided for the study?*
3. *Should the editor compare this situation to the acceptance of a manuscript whose researchers received funding from a pharmaceutical company?*
4. *Understanding that millions of dollars are spent by the Council for Tobacco Research each year to fund biomedical research, should journals develop policies regarding their publication of manuscripts submitted by researchers who have accepted research support from the tobacco industry?*

———————— RECOMMENDED READINGS ————————

Blum A (ed): *The Cigarette Underworld.* Secaucus, NJ, Lyle Stuart, 1985.

This book was published as a second printing of the December, 1983, issue of the *New York State Journal of Medicine* (Vol. 83, No. 13), the first medical journal ever to devote an entire issue to a consideration of the world tobacco pandemic. Rather than a discussion of the adverse health effects associated with smoking, this book focuses on the social and political history of the leading cause of death in the twentieth century, namely, the tobacco industry.

Wolinsky H, Brune T: *The Serpent on the Staff: The Unhealthy Politics of the American Medical Association.* New York, Tarcher/Purman, 1995.

In this book, Wolinsky and Brune provide an inside look at some of the policies developed within the American Medical Association, whose political intentions often conflict with the organization's stated public health mission.

Smith S, Smith J (eds): *Medical Activism: DOC's Approach to Countering the Tobacco Pandemic.* Houston, TX, DOC (Doctors Ought to Care), 1992.

Outlined in this guide is a blueprint for health professionals to become more active in counteracting tobacco use and promotion. Strategies designed for the clinic, classroom, and community are highlighted, and successful examples are shared.

CHAPTER 15

C. Special Problems

Alcohol and Drug Abuse

Kristen Lawton Barry

CASE 15-1

Frank Jones is a 38-year-old married auto mechanic who came to see Dr. Smith today for a follow-up visit to assess his hypertension. Dr. Smith has been working with Mr. Jones for 1 year and his hypertension has remained labile despite varying medication regimes. At this visit, Mr. Jones mentioned that he has also had pains in his stomach for the last month and attributed it to arguments with his wife. When asked, he said that he doesn't drink much—just a few beers a day.

INTRODUCTION

Alcohol and drug disorders are among the most common medical problems primary care physicians encounter in their practices (Brown, 1992). Mr. Jones in Case 15-1 and many other patients present us with opportunities to intervene before alcohol and drug problems have advanced to the most serious consequences.

Working with patients around issues of alcohol and drug abuse is commonly perceived as a "can of worms" best left unopened. Once the worms are wriggling all over the office, it's difficult to get them back in the can, especially during a standard 15- to 30-minute office visit. The purpose of this chapter is to provide readers with: (1) the background to understand the extent of the problem, (2) the role physician attitudes play in the recognition and treatment of these problems in the office, (3) strategies to screen and assess alcohol and drug problems, (4) strategies to provide brief interventions, and (5) strategies to determine who and how to refer in the context of the time constraints of medical practice.

PREVALENCE

DEFINITIONS AND TERMS

The terms presented in this chapter are derived from both the clinical and research expertise of professionals in the field of addiction medicine (Fleming & Barry, 1992). The term *addictive disorders* includes the clinical problems of alcohol and drug dependence as well as other disorders that have often been classified as addictions, such as eating and gambling disorders. *Alcohol or drug disorder* is often used to describe the spectrum of problems associated with the negative consequences of mood-altering drugs. *Substance abuse* and *substance dependence* (alcohol or drug dependence) are terms based on standardized alcohol and drug criteria such as those from the *Diagnostic and Statistical Manual of Mental Disorders* fourth edition (DSM-IV) (American Psychiatric Association, 1994). These terms are often used for insurance reimbursement and are generally accepted by the medical community.

To diagnose alcohol and drug disorders clinicians look for behavioral factors such as the inability to cut down or stop, social and emotional consequences such as family problems or work and school problems, and physiological symptoms such as insomnia, gastrointestinal pain, liver toxicity, tolerance (over time it takes more of the substance to feel an effect), and withdrawal. One of the limitations in the alcohol and drug field is that, unlike many other medical problems, there are no laboratory tests to make a definitive diagnosis of alcohol or drug abuse or dependence. Liver function and other laboratory tests detect end organ damage but do not detect the primary disorder. Only about 20% of people with alcohol abuse or dependence have elevated serum gamma-glutamyl transferase (GGT) (Babor *et al.*, 1989). Numerous studies indicate that increased alcohol consumption is related to increased health risk for various cancers and heart disease. Figure 15.1 depicts the relationship between levels of drinking and severity of alcohol-related problems.

Psychoactive drugs may be sanctioned medically to modify or control moods. However, any use of a psychoactive substance to change the state of mind that is harmful to oneself or others is considered abuse. *Abuse* and *dependence* pertain to both alcohol and drugs. Definitions regarding low-risk, at-risk, and problem use focus primarily, but not exclusively, on alcohol.

CASE 15-2

Josh Sanderson is a 28-year-old married car salesman with two small children and no family history of alcohol-related problems. He got drunk a few times in college but did not like the aftereffect. Since he married and had children, most of his activities have centered around his family and other friends with small children. Alcohol is not often a part of family activities. Mr. Jones generally drinks one or two beers twice a week.

LOW-RISK USE

Psychoactive substance use as in Case 15-2 that does not lead to problems is called *low-risk use*. Persons in this category can set reasonable limits on alcohol consumption and do not drink when pregnant or trying to conceive, driving a car or boat, operating heavy machinery, or using contraindicated medications. They do not engage in binge

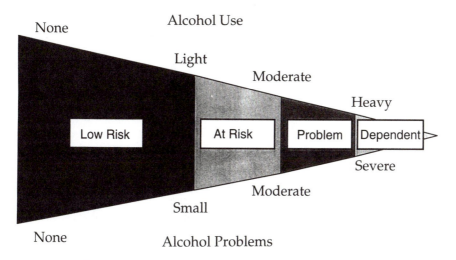

Figure 15.1. Levels of drinking and severity of alcohol problems.

drinking—more than 2 or 4 drinks per occasion for women and men, respectively—or in excessive regular drinking—more than 7 drinks a week for women or 14 drinks a week for men (NIAAA Guide, 1995). Low-risk use of medications/drugs would include using an antianxiety medication for an acute anxiety state following the physician's prescription (Trachtenberg & Fleming, 1994).

CASE 15-3

Maria Adelman is a 26-year-old single graduate student who drinks three or four beers two or three times a week, mostly on the weekends. She smokes marijuana about once a month when she gets together with an old friend from college. She has no family history of alcoholism. She usually drives home after drinking with friends but has had no accidents. She reports that she does not always practice safe sex when she has been drinking but has no other consequences of alcohol or drug use.

AT-RISK USE

At-risk use is use that increases the chances that a person will develop problems and complications related to the use of alcohol as in Case 15-3. These individuals will consume more than 7 or 14 drinks per week for women and men, respectively, or they will drink in risky situations. They do *not* currently have a health problem caused by alcohol, but if this drinking pattern continues over time problems might result.

CASE 15-4

Mark Lorenzo is a 51-year-old executive with a large marketing firm. He has had an alcohol and tobacco problem for many years resulting in abdominal pain, hypertension, and one auto accident while driving under the influence. He stopped using both substances 3 years ago after much discussion with his physician, family, and employer who explained the risks to his health, family life, and career. He reported that the major problems associated with his alcohol use were continuing. Once he made up his mind to stop, he did so without withdrawal symptoms and has remained abstinent for 3 years.

PROBLEM USE

Problem use refers to a level of use that has already resulted in adverse medical, psychological, or social consequences as in Case 15-4. Potential consequences include accidents and injuries, legal problems, and sexual behavior that increases the risk of HIV infection. Although most problem drinkers consume more than the low-risk limits, some people who drink smaller amounts may experience alcohol-related problems, such as the elderly and persons with severe medical or psychiatric problems.

CASE 15-5

Karen Crawford is a 36-year-old single physician who was discovered using intravenous fentanyl while on call in the second year of her residency. She said she was only experimenting. Although she used alcohol and marijuana in college, she reported no blackouts and said she was always able to stop using alcohol and marijuana. Both her family and the residency director intervened with her and she entered an intensive inpatient treatment program. The urine drug screen taken when she entered treatment revealed she had also been using cocaine and marijuana. After she completed the treatment program, her urine drug screens were negative and she remained abstinent at 6-year follow-up.

CASE 15-6

Samuel Jackson is a 52-year-old construction worker. He has had chronic abdominal pain and unresolved hypertension for the past 8 years. Two years ago, after experiencing withdrawal symptoms during a hospital admission for a work-related injury, he entered an alcohol treatment program. After 1 year of abstinence, Mr. Jackson began drinking again. He now drinks approximately eight beers a day plus some additional liquor once a week. His physician is aware that this is a chronic relapsing disorder and continues to work with Mr. Jackson to help him stabilize his medical conditions and find longer-term help for his primary alcohol dependence.

DRUG AND ALCOHOL DEPENDENCE

Those who use at the level of *alcohol or drug dependence* have a medical disorder characterized by loss of control, preoccupation with alcohol or drugs, continue to use despite adverse consequences, and suffer physiological symptoms such as tolerance and withdrawal as in Cases 15-5 and 15-6 (American Psychiatric Association, 1994). A wide range of legal and illegal substances can be addictive.

Kathryn Sampson is a 65-year-old widow living alone in an apartment in a housing project. She broke her ankle a month ago and has been cared for since then by a visiting nurse. She came to the clinic for routine follow-up for her ankle. When asked by the physician to talk about how the accident happened, she was evasive. The physician then asked some questions about her general health and Mrs. Sampson reported, "I'm so tired all the time and I don't sleep well. I must need stronger sleeping pills. I've been taking the kind I can buy myself in the drugstore. I've been taking that medicine [Zantac] for my stomach, but things don't seem much better." Since the effect of alcohol is exacerbated both by age and by the use of Zantac and over-the-counter sleeping pills, her physician discussed with her the potential problems of mixing some medications with alcohol and her desires to remain as independent as possible. She generally drank one glass of wine a day before dinner just as she and her husband did when they were younger. The physician encouraged her to work with the community services available to find outside activities and to stop the use of alcohol. She felt that she would be able to follow her physician's recommendations.

SPECIAL POPULATION: OLDER ADULTS

The elderly pose special concerns when setting drinking and medication use criteria. Compared with younger people, older adults have an increased sensitivity to alcohol and over-the-counter and prescription medications. There is an age-related decrease in lean body mass versus total volume of fat, and the resultant decrease in total body volume increases the total distribution of alcohol and other mood-altering chemicals in the body. Liver enzymes that metabolize alcohol and certain other drugs are less efficient with age and central nervous system sensitivity increases with age.

Of particular concern in this age group is the potential interaction of medication and alcohol. For some patients, any alcohol use, coupled with the use of specific over-the-counter or prescription medications, can be problematic as in Case 15-7. Alcohol use recommendations in this age group are generally made on a case-by-case basis and are generally lower than those set for adults under 65.

SPECIAL POPULATION: ADOLESCENTS

Children and teens are especially susceptible to influences that encourage risk-taking and experimentation with substances. The age at which adolescents begin to use alcohol and illicit drugs, particularly if it is before the age of 15, is a strong predictor of later problems with substances (Institute for Health Policy, 1993). The incidence of binge drinking five or more drinks in a row for teens was at an all-time high of 41% in the early 1980s and decreased to 29.8% in 1995. Although there was a downward trend in the use of illicit drugs by teens, use increased significantly between 1992 and 1993. The lifetime prevalence of any illicit drug use is 42.9% while prevalence in the previous year before sampling is 31% (*HHS News*, January 31, 1994). Alcohol and tobacco are often referred to as "gateway" drugs because teens who progress to substance abuse often start with these two drugs. Two-thirds of tobacco smokers aged 12 to 17 have also used an illegal drug (Morrison, 1990). From a clinical perspective, it is important to ask all adolescents about tobacco, alcohol, and other use. Statistics indicate that those who use tobacco are at risk for other substance use. Framing initial questions to ask about use at their school and friends' use can be lead-ins to questions about their own behavior. Sports physicals are also a good time to address these issues.

NATIONAL PREVALENCE DATA

Prevalence data are important since clinicians in primary care can expect that about 15 to 20% of their adult patients have past problems with alcohol or other medications and drugs and about 8 to 10% have current problems. Prevalence in the United States is often measured through national telephone surveys, face-to-face large-scale clinical surveys, and tax receipts. Figure 15.2 plots data collected from 1977 to 1990 on trends in alcohol, tobacco, cocaine, amphetamine, and marijuana use in a series of annual telephone surveys based on national probability samples. The data presented only include subjects between 18 and 25 years old, but changes in other age groups reflect similar trends.

The Epidemiological Catchment Area (ECA) Study (Regier & Robins, 1991) is a landmark study conducted in five sites in the 1980s. It used face-to-face interviews based on DSM-III criteria for substance abuse or dependence. In this community-based sample of 20,291 adults, approximately 16.7% of the persons sampled had a lifetime substance abuse disorder, 6.1% had problems in the previous 6 months, and 3.8% reported problems in the last month.

National data on alcohol use are based on tax receipt reports per capita consumption. "Apparent per capita consumption" is determined by dividing the total quantity of alcohol sold by the total population aged 14 and older (Williams *et al.*, 1991). These estimates attribute average consumption to all members of the population; they do not consider

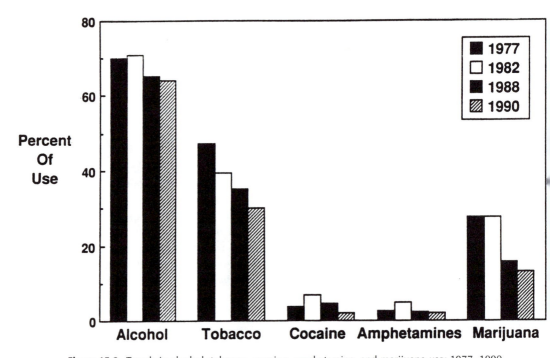

Figure 15.2. Trends in alcohol, tobacco, cocaine, amphetamine, and marijuana use: 1977–1990.

actual individual consumption. Per capita consumption is measured in gallons of pure alcohol. Although the per capita alcohol consumption is down to its lowest level since 1976, it is still high at 2.43 gallons of pure alcohol per person. This translates to approximately 576 twelve-ounce cans of beer. The number of abstainers has increased slightly. The Behavioral Risk Factors Study (BRFS), which is conducted in most states in coordination with the Centers for Disease Control, is used to obtain data on abstinence by state. In this survey, people aged 18 and over are asked to report alcohol consumption in the last month. The District of Columbia, Alaska, and Wisconsin have the highest rates of per capita consumption (3.28, 4.23, and 2.97 gallons, respectively), while Wisconsin has the lowest percentage of abstainers (30.1%).

PRIMARY CARE PREVALENCE DATA

Studies that address the prevalence of alcohol and drug problems in primary care practices are important because they provide an estimate of the extent of these problems. Using methods similar to those used in the ECA study, Fleming and Barry (1991) estimated lifetime and 12-month prevalence of alcohol and drug disorders in five family medicine clinics in three counties in Wisconsin in 1988. Lifetime prevalence ranged from 16 to 28% in the five clinics. The 12-month prevalence ranged from 9 to 15%. The lifetime prevalence of drug disorders was 7 to 9%. Three percent of the sample had drug problems in the previous year.

Although 12-month prevalence of alcohol disorders is high, there is an even larger group of patients in primary care practices who are problem drinkers. As part of a large clinical trial testing the effectiveness of brief physician advice with problem drinkers, Fleming and Barry screened approximately 20,000 adults in primary care practices in Wisconsin. Preliminary findings from the survey indicate that the prevalence of problem drinking is age dependent and ranges from 15 to 20% for men and from 8 to 10% for women. Approximately one-fifth of the men have more than 15 drinks a week and 1 in 8 have 3 or more drinks a day. Women engage in problem drinking less often than men.

Clinicians who are finding fewer cases of problem drinking and alcohol or drug disorders in their own practices may want to begin screening programs. Because patients with a previous history of problems with alcohol or other drugs are at risk for relapse, establishing a history of use can provide important clues for future problems.

CASE 15-8

Carlotta Brown is a 26-year-old woman who grew up in the inner city of a large metropolitan area. She has a 2-year-old son and is living with her mother. She has been unable to work and is insured by Medicaid. Ms. Brown was in the emergency department last night reporting chronic headaches and fatigue and asking for some pain medication for her headaches. She was given a prescription for one night and told to visit her regular physician, Dr. Jones, today. He knows that she is under a lot of stress but is unsure if she is drug seeking and suggests some alternatives to medications. Further probing about her current use of drugs and alcohol angers her. As she leaves she states that Dr. Jones is "just like those other doctors who think I'm an addict and don't care if I hurt."

Jane Morrow is a 46-year-old housewife married to an insurance executive in the community. She has two children, both boys, who are 20 and 18. She has been a patient in this particular practice for 10 years. She comes to the clinic today with abdominal pain and headaches. She has been taking Fiorinal for headaches during the last year. When asked about any stress or changes in her life she mentioned that her sons were both off at school and her husband was so busy that she felt very lonely. Mrs. Morrow said, however, that her bridge club and other groups help her to forget some of her loneliness and that they all take turns finding exotic food and drinks to serve. She is a well-known hostess and active volunteer in civic causes.

PHYSICIAN ATTITUDES

Implementing practice procedures to detect alcohol and drug disorders can be hampered by a variety of factors, including screening administration, lack of standardized follow-up procedures, and personal concerns of physicians and staff. The role of personal attitudes is illustrated in this section.

Societal stereotypes about people who have alcohol and drug problems can be misleading since alcohol and drug problems are shared by every class, race, and religion. A number of factors in addition to basic societal stereotypes affect clinician attitudes about substance abuse. All of these factors can, in turn, affect the quality of care provided to patients with alcohol and drug disorders. The failure to diagnose and treat alcohol and drug disorders may result from inadequate training, a sense of futility about the effectiveness of treatment, and denial stemming from the physician's own family history (Waller & Casey, 1990).

Until the last decade medical schools and residencies devoted little curriculum time to issues of substance abuse. In a review of changes in medical education about substance abuse in six clinical departments (psychiatry, family medicine, internal medicine, pediatrics, emergency medicine, and obstetrics-gynecology) in the 126 U.S. medical schools from 1976 to 1992, Fleming *et al.* (1994) found significant increases in the numbers of required and elective curriculum units for medical students between 1986–1987 and 1991–1992. The number of medical schools requiring courses in substance abuse treatment increased from five to eight in that same time period. There were significant increases in the number of curriculum units for residents in family medicine and pediatrics. The average number of faculty in the 116 medical schools that reported units on substance abuse was 4.1. There were 45 fellowships in addiction medicine identified in 1991–1992, with a total of 61 fellows in training. While these findings confirm positive changes, 118 of 126 programs still do not require such courses. Curriculum time and number of faculty with expertise in this field does not compare well with other areas with similar prevalence, such as cancer and heart disease. Training for primary care physicians in the recognition, diagnosis, treatment, and referral of alcohol and other drug problems still remains a concern.

The sense of futility physicians sometimes feel in the treatment of alcohol and drug problems often begins early in medical school. Rotations on medical services and in the emergency department often expose students to patients suffering from severe complications of alcohol and drug disorders. Students seldom work with patients at earlier stages of the problem when brief interventions are most effective and the results of the professional's efforts are more readily apparent. Medical students are more likely to see drug seeking patients such as Carlotta Brown in Case 15-8 on rotations in the emergency department than they are to see patients like Jane Morrow in Case 15-9 whose symptoms are less apparent in part because we are less likely to look for symptoms in patients who have better coping skills and support systems in the community.

In addition, in inpatient and emergency situations, students seldom have the opportunity for longer-term follow-up that would allow them to see the positive results of their efforts. Classes and clinical rotations with primary care physicians who understand addictions are beginning to provide learners with a more balanced picture of these disorders and will hopefully change attitudes and behaviors in the process. Recent research indicates that physicians who have a special interest and some experience with addictions regard patients with a substance abuse diagnosis as much less difficult to manage than do their colleagues with less interest and training (Farrell & Lewis, 1990).

Many of the newer innovative programs designed to teach medical students, residents, and practicing physicians about alcohol and other drug disorders work not only to change attitudes but also to change behaviors. Research has indicated that a change in attitude toward the treatment of alcohol and drug disorders does *not* necessarily lead to a change in actual practice behavior. Useful practice experiences seem to have the greatest impact on future behavior. Practice experience can come through working with primary physicians with alcohol and other drug abuse expertise, attending open Alcoholics Anonymous meetings and talking to members, spending time at a treatment center, and role-playing situations with patients when alcohol and drug questions need to be addressed.

Finally, a personal or family history of alcohol or drug problems can affect a physician's ability to adequately treat patients with symptoms of these disorders. With the increasing national awareness of the effects of alcohol and drug problems, medical schools are beginning to institute student assistance programs to help medical students deal with personal concerns that have an impact on their education and future careers. An awareness of the impact that alcohol and drugs have had in any of our lives is the first step toward confronting the issues from both a personal and a professional perspective.

CASE 15-10

Larry Simmons is a 45-year-old marketing analyst who lost his job 5 months ago during corporate layoffs. He has been treated by Dr. Adams for the last 8 years. Dr. Adams has worked with him in the past to cut back or stop his use of alcohol but he continues to have six to seven mixed drinks a day during the week with more on weekends. He has a history of chronic hypertension and has been unable to stop smoking. Mr. Simmons was recently hospitalized for acute pancreatitis related to his alcohol use. While in the hospital he was referred to an alcohol and drug program for evaluation. Dr. Adams is continuing to help him stabilize his medical conditions and is working with the alcohol and drug program to help him obtain longer-term help for his primary alcohol and nicotine dependence.

————— MORBIDITY AND MORTALITY —————

Excessive alcohol consumption and drug use can affect every organ system in the body depending on the individual's genetic predisposition and the amount, length, and pattern of use. The presence of other diseases are also cofactors that can increase risk. With regard to physical harm, alcohol is a risk factor for coronary heart disease, cancers (particularly of the female breast), and overall mortality. Morbidity and mortality reports regarding illicit drugs often do not include HIV/AIDS statistics for intravenous drug users. Death rates almost double when this group is included in the analysis.

This section will briefly review the most salient findings regarding alcohol and drugs and health risk. For more complete reviews, see Anderson *et al.* (1993) and the Eighth Special Report to the U.S. Congress on Alcohol and Health (1993).

ALCOHOL-INDUCED LIVER CIRRHOSIS

In the past alcohol-induced liver cirrhosis was thought to come from nutritional deficiencies common in heavy drinkers, but now the evidence suggests that alcohol itself is toxic. Nutritional deficiencies do still play a role in alcoholic liver damage. One of the crucial factors in the development of cirrhosis is the quantity of alcohol consumed. Prospective studies indicate that the risk of cirrhosis becomes significant when intake is, on average, above 80 g/day (6.2 ounces) for men or 20 g/day (1.55 ounces) for women (Grant *et al.*, 1988). The average duration of heavy drinking for cirrhotic patients is between 10 and 20 years.

Gender increases susceptibility to alcohol-induced liver damage. More serious forms of alcoholic liver disease are seen in women at lower levels of consumption than are seen in men. One study found liver damage in women consuming 21 to 40 g/day (Pequignot *et al.*, 1978). It also appears that women suffer damage after drinking heavily for much shorter periods of time than men. The higher risk for women may occur because they have higher peak blood alcohol levels and a slightly higher rate of hepatic metabolism of alcohol resulting in a higher production of acetaldehyde, which may play a part in alcohol-induced liver injury. Another possible link is found in the hypoxia hypothesis (Saltatos & Soranno, 1991), which predicts that women are more susceptible to alcoholic liver damage because they have lower hematocrits, lower hemoglobin levels, and a higher prevalence of anemia.

PANCREATITIS

The effects of alcohol on the pancreas are well established. Approximately 65% of all cases of pancreatitis are alcohol-related (Balart & Ferrante, 1982). The greater susceptibility of women to tissue damage from alcohol is not just limited to the liver. Women are also more likely to have pancreatitis with a shorter duration of heavy alcohol use than men.

CARDIOVASCULAR DISEASE

Alcohol-related cardiovascular disease includes raised blood pressure, cerebrovascular hemorrhage (stroke), arrhythmias (disturbances in heart rhythm), cardiomyopathy (heart muscle disease), and coronary heart disease, including sudden coronary death. While there is increasing evidence that light to moderate alcohol consumption decreases the risk of death from coronary artery disease (CAD), chronic heavy drinking is associated with many of the other cardiovascular diseases (Lands & Zakhari, 1990). Even though there has been a decrease in mortality from these diseases because of public awareness of risk factors associated with lifestyle, cardiovascular disorders continue to be the leading cause of death in the United States (Eighth Special Report, 1993).

A number of studies have shown a lower risk for CAD for light to moderate drinkers, generally one to two drinks a day, compared with abstainers (Anderson *et al.*, 1993). There is a "J"-shaped curve wherein nondrinkers have a slightly higher rate of CAD than light drinkers, with risk increasing as consumption increases (Rosenberg *et al.*, 1981; Stampfer *et al.*, 1988). On the other hand, some critics have argued that the higher mortality among abstainers was related to people in that category who stopped drinking because of ill health (Marmot & Brunner, 1991). Recent studies have shown that "sick quitters" do not completely explain the protective effect of light alcohol use against CAD (Anderson *et al.*, 1993). The findings regarding CAD need to be weighed against the risk of other diseases associated with alcohol use for both men and women, such as hypertension, cardiomyopathy, stroke, and some cancers.

Cocaine abuse can lead to serious cardiac complications (Bunn & Giannini, 1993), including myocardial ischemia and infarction, myocarditis, cardiomyopathy, and arrhythmias. Hepatic transformation from the use of alcohol and cocaine together can produce cocaethylene, now thought to be primarily responsible for many cocaine abuser deaths. Treatment of cardiovascular complications has focused on cocaine-induced ischemia, hypertension, and arrhythmias. Thrombolytic agents have been used in the treatment of myocardial infarction but their use with this population remains controversial.

CANCERS

Alcohol and the risk of cancer has been comprehensively reviewed (Anderson *et al.*, 1993; Eighth Special Report, 1993). The International Agency for Research on Cancer's monograph reviewed cancers and alcohol risk and concluded that alcohol is causally related to cancers of the oral cavity, pharynx, larynx, esophagus, and liver. Recent compelling research has suggested that breast cancer should be added to the list of cancers linked to alcohol.

The role of alcohol in cancers of the gastrointestinal tract is still controversial. There is less evidence of elevated risk of stomach, pancreatic, and colon cancer (Bouchardy *et al.*, 1990; Ferraroni *et al.*, 1989; Nomura *et al.*, 1990), and more evidence for a link between alcohol and rectal carcinoma (Stemmerman *et al.*, 1990).

As expected, alcohol abuse plays an important role in the development of primary liver cancer. Some research has indicated that hepatitis B viral infection is an important risk factor in the development of primary liver cancer, while other research shows that heavy alcohol use, even without hepatitis B, is causally linked to liver cancer (Ohnishi *et al*, 1987).

Of the 17 studies of breast cancer in women reviewed by Anderson *et al.* (1993), 11 showed a significant positive association with alcohol consumption, including all 5 of the cohort studies in their sample. The consistency of the 5 large cohort studies is compelling evidence to counsel women to limit their use of alcohol. Several of the studies indicate that risk increases slightly with an intake above one drink a day. Alcohol has not been implicated in other female cancers such as endometrial or cervical cancer.

HIV/AIDS

Sharing of contaminated injection equipment is the primary means of HIV transmission among intravenous drug users. Recent reports indicate that the drug use in this population has changed to include widespread use of cocaine. In the United States, approximately 34% of all cases of AIDS in adults have occurred either in injection drug users or in their sexual partners (O'Connor *et al.*, 1994). When HIV/AIDS is included in the statistics for illicit drug mortality, the numbers double. In 1990, roughly 20,000 deaths were attributed to the use of illicit drugs, with 9000 HIV-related (DesJarlais *et al.*, 1992).

Of particular importance to the medical community is the documented observation that HIV-related complications among injection drug users differ somewhat from those of other HIV-infected population groups. Physicians treating these individuals need to address clinical and psychosocial issues related to both drug dependence and HIV infection. These patients are more likely than other HIV patients to have frequent occurrences of pyogenic bacterial infections, particularly pneumonia, endocarditis, and septis, HIV-related tuberculosis, and sexually transmitted diseases such as syphilis and human papilloma virus. They are also more likely to have hepatitis, other retroviral infections, and cancer, such as lung and cervix. The 1992 revised AIDS case definition of the Centers for Disease Control and Prevention includes recurrent bacterial pneumonia, pulmonary tuberculosis, and cervical carcinoma as AIDS-defining illnesses in patients with HIV infection (1993 Revised Classification, *Morbidity and Mortality Weekly Report*, 1992f; 41) (no. RR0-17). This change should provide better epidemiological data on HIV by more accurately reflecting the illnesses seen in drug users and women.

OTHER

Fetal Problems

Cocaine use during pregnancy has been associated with fetal problems, including intracerebral hemorrhage and vascular spasm (Brown *et al.*, 1992) as well as premature rupture of membranes, spontaneous abortion, pregnancy-induced hypertension, and precipitate delivery (Slutsker, 1992). The interpretation of data from epidemiologic studies to assess the association between adverse pregnancy outcomes and cocaine use are limited by misclassification of users, reporting bias confounded by socioeconomic factors, and inaccurate measurement of cocaine use.

Brain

Although chronic alcohol dependence is associated with reduced cerebral blood flow (CBF), changes in CBF after marijuana smoking are variable, increases and decreases having been reported (Mathew & Wilson, 1991). Chronic use of marijuana, however, seems to reduce CBF. Most inhalants and solvents are vasodilators, with chronic abuse also showing a decrease in CBF. These decreases are at least partially reversible with abstinence.

CASE 15-11

Jeanine Jefferson is an eighth-grade student in a suburban middle school. She is an athlete on the soccer and basketball teams. She and her friends enjoy sports in general and meet to watch sporting events on television. While watching the women's soccer playoffs they noticed a really great ad featuring a new type of beer. The music and slogans were very attractive and appealed to young women in particular. One of the girls mentioned that her older sister in college had some of the beer at home and maybe they could try it.

Because the use of addictive substances typically begins at an early age, and because early onset of use is one of the predictors of later health problems, society's role in the problem is an important consideration. Although this chapter and numerous articles address the alarming statistics regarding the economic, social, and emotional costs of alcohol problems, the alcohol industry insists that its marketing techniques do not influence those under the legal drinking limit. Studies in the United States and other countries indicate the powerful potential of alcohol advertising. Grube and Wallack (1994) tested fifth- and sixth-graders' awareness of beer advertising and their retention of information contained in the advertisements. They found that awareness and retention of the information influenced the children's beliefs, knowledge, and intentions regarding the use of alcohol. The children who were more familiar with specific advertisements were more likely to have positive attitudes about alcohol. In a second study, Madden and Grube (1994) analyzed the number of alcohol and tobacco advertisements included in a random sample of televised sports events. They included the appearance of stadium billboards, on-site promotions, and product sponsorship announcements and advertisements. These programs primarily aired beer commercials with a number of the ads portraying activities with high trauma risk such as water sports while drinking.

Studies commissioned by the Surgeon General in 1991 revealed that young people were inaccurately informed about alcohol, found the packaging of alcohol confusing, and were attracted to wine coolers and beer, which are packaged and advertised to be attractive to this age group. The main conclusion of these and other studies is that the most important effect of alcohol advertisement is not on immediate use but in its pervasive influence on society's view of alcohol. Alcohol is associated with some of our most important life events, yet the negative potential of the drug is not discussed.

The only programs that have been found to be successful in working with societal impressions of alcohol have been social influence programs that include information, decision-making, and resistance skills training. The techniques are used in programs with children and adolescents and have also been successfully used in brief advice protocols in primary care settings. Prevention and brief intervention strategies in primary care settings can play a crucial part in a public health effort to address these problems throughout the life span.

CASE 15-12

Judy Field is a 35-year-old patient of Dr. Martin. She is married and has two daughters, aged 9 and 7. Ms. Field has been Dr. Martin's patient for 10 years since moving to this community. During an annual physical examination Dr. Martin asked her to complete a short questionnaire about her health habits regarding nutrition, exercise, smoking, alcohol, and other drug/medication use. Ms. Field reported that she drank two glasses of wine every day of the week and two additional cocktails on the weekend. Because she met the criteria for at-risk drinking, Dr. Martin asked further questions to assess use and discovered that Ms. Field had been under more stress at work, was experiencing some new gastric distress, and was not sleeping well. Her alcohol use had increased as the work problems increased in the last year. Dr. Martin and her nurse, Melissa Enders, worked with Ms. Field to cut back on her drinking using a brief intervention model. Her gastric distress improved. At the end of 1 year, she was consuming approximately one drink 3 days a week, was sleeping better, and was better able to handle the changes on her job.

THE PHYSICIAN'S ROLE IN TREATMENT AND PREVENTION

The link between substance use and health risk naturally leads to an examination of the role of primary care practitioners in the detection and treatment of people with these disorders. As the statistics in the prevalence section of this chapter suggest, detecting at-risk and problem drinkers is as important as recognizing patients who are alcohol dependent. In fact, the majority of people experiencing health problems secondary to their alcohol or other drug use are at-risk users rather than alcohol or drug dependent. Intervention at this stage has the potential to prevent longer-term medical, social, and psychological consequences. *This means that primary care physicians have a crucial role in the prevention and early intervention of alcohol and drug problems in their patients* (Saunders *et al.*, 1993).

SCREENING/ASKING THE FIRST QUESTIONS

To be able to practice prevention and early intervention with patients, clinicians need to screen for alcohol and drug problems. Screening can be done as part of a routine health examination and updated annually, before prescribing medications, or in response to problems that may be alcohol or drug related.

The common signs and symptoms of alcohol problems seen in primary care settings are listed in Table 15.1.

As mentioned earlier, *any current use of tobacco or illicit drugs is considered at-risk*

Table 15.1
Signs and Symptoms of Alcohol Problems

Medical signs
- Stomach/abdominal pain
- Elevated blood pressure
- Chronic tension headaches
- Insomnia (accompanied by a medication request)
- Sexually transmitted diseases
- Frequent accidents and trauma
- Fatigue
- Chronic depression
- Chronic diarrhea
- Memory loss

Family patterns
- Frequent visits by other family members
- Unexplained symptoms, such as headaches or abdominal pain in a child
- Trauma secondary to physical abuse
- School problems in a child
- Depression or anxiety disorders in a family member

Table 15.2
Specific Recommended Questions for Alcohol Screening
(Often Asked in the Context of a Series of Health Behaviors)

- Do you drink alcohol? (If no, is that a change?) If yes:
- About how many days a week do you drink alcohol?
- On a day when you drink, how much do you drink?
- How many days a month do you have four or more drinks?
  Screening is positive for men drinking more than 14 drinks a week, for
  women drinking more than 7 drinks a week, and for men or women
  who report *any* single occasion when they have consumed more than 4
  drinks in the past month.

behavior. The initial screening questions listed in Table 15.2 for alcohol can be used for other drugs with any positive responses indicating risk (see also Table 15.3).

However, because of the relationship between alcohol consumption and health problems, questions about consumption (quantity and frequency of use) provide a method to categorize patients into levels of risk for alcohol use. The traditional assumption that all patients who drink have a tendency to underreport their alcohol use is not supported by research (Babor *et al.*, 1989). People who are not alcohol dependent often give accurate information.

Physicians can get more accurate histories by asking questions about the recent past; embedding the alcohol use questions in the context of other health behaviors (e.g., exercise, weight, smoking, alcohol use); and paying attention to nonverbal cues that suggest the patient is minimizing use (e.g., blushing, turning away, fidgeting, looking at the floor, change in breathing pattern).

Screening questions can be asked by verbal interview, by paper-and-pencil questionnaire, or by computerized questionnaire. All three methods have equivalent reliability and validity (Greist *et al.*, 1987; Barry & Fleming, 1990). Any positive responses can lead to further questions about consequences. *To successfully incorporate alcohol (and other drug) screening into your practice, it should be simple and consistent with other screening procedures already in place.*

ASSESSING/WHAT TO ASK NEXT?

Assessment helps the clinician to determine the severity of the alcohol problem—whether or not the patient is an at-risk drinker, a problem drinker, or alcohol dependent.

Table 15.3
Specific Recommended Questions for Drug Screening

- Do you :
  - a. use prescribed or over-the-counter drugs in excess of the directions?
  - b. use any nonmedical drugs?
  - (If no, is that a change?) If yes:
- What medications/drugs are you using?
  Screening is positive if any use of prescription or over-the-counter drugs in excess of the directions is present, and if there is any use of nonmedical drugs.

Table 15.4
The CAGE Questions*a*

- Have you ever felt you should cut down or stop drinking/drug use?
- Have people annoyed you by criticizing your drinking/drug use?
- Have you ever felt bad or guilty about your drinking/drug use?
- Have you ever had a drink /drug first thing in the morning or after rising to steady your nerves or get over a hangover (eye-opener)?

Additional Question

- Has your drinking/drug use ever caused you problems (for example, problems with family, work, school, sleep, accidents, or injuries)?

*a*Adapted from the CAGE/AID, Brown (1992).

The following are some general guidelines for clinicians to adapt to each particular patient and situation. Physicians can follow questions about consumption with the CAGE questions (Ewing, 1984) adapted to include drugs of abuse (Brown, 1992) plus a question on the consequences of alcohol use (Table 15.4).

Screening and assessment can be completed during a standard 15-minute office visit.

It is appropriate to conduct laboratory tests such as liver function tests on patients who are heavy drinkers. The sensitivity of GGT tests is about 20 to 60%, depending on the chronicity and severity of the alcohol problems (Beresford *et al.*, 1990; Cushman *et al.*, 1984). In these patients, physical findings such as elevated laboratory values can be a powerful motivator to change behavior. GGTs can also be used to monitor compliance with a treatment program.

To assess *dependence* in patients who report alcohol-related problems, have a history of failed attempts to stop or cut back, or report withdrawal symptoms such as tremors, the questions in Table 15.5 may be helpful. *These questions can also be adapted to other drugs.*

Physicians should refer any patient thought to be alcohol or drug dependent for a diagnostic evaluation and possible specialized alcohol and other drug treatment.

Assessing the use of other drugs includes asking the patient about prescriptions, particularly antidepressants, benzodiazepines, and codeine; over-the-counter drugs; and illicit drugs (particularly marijuana, cocaine, and heroin). If there is evidence for either prescription drug abuse or illicit drug use, the patient should be referred to a specialist for a diagnostic assessment and possible specialized treatment. For a more comprehensive discussion of the diagnosis and treatment specifically of *drug abuse* in primary care, see Trachtenberg and Fleming (1994).

Table 15.5
Dependence Questions

- Are you ever unable to stop drinking once you start?
- How many drinks does it take to get high? Does it take more drinks than it used to to get high?
- Do you drink in the morning to get over a hangover or stop the shakes?
- Do you have strong urges to drink? Do many of your everyday activities revolve around drinking?

Although traditional approaches to alcohol and other drug problems have focused on long-term counseling, there is increasing evidence that brief intervention, delivered by a physician, can effectively reduce drinking in at-risk and problem drinkers, persons who are not alcohol dependent. The clinical trials of brief advice with at-risk drinkers have been based, in part, on the original "stop smoking" trials. Studies in Europe and elsewhere have demonstrated a significant (10 to 20%) reduction in drinking by persons in the experimental groups when compared with control groups that did not receive the advice (Kristenson *et al.*, 1983; Saunders *et al.*, 1993; Fleming & Barry, 1995). These findings are consistent across more than ten trials. The effectiveness rates are similar to those found with at-risk and problem drinkers in traditional alcohol treatment. There have been no clinical trials of brief advice with marijuana use to date.

In providing brief advice or intervention, the physician offers clear advice to cut down or stop drinking, often in the context of a health, social, or family problem:

> I'm concerned about your [particular symptom(s), e.g., high blood pressure, sleep problem, abdominal pain] and I think your alcohol use may be a part of the problem.

Based on clinical judgment regarding the seriousness of the alcohol problem, the clinician will decide if the patient should cut down or be abstinent. The physician may say,

> I want you to stop drinking any alcohol for the next month so we can see if your abdominal pain decreases.

or

> I want you to cut back your drinking to no more than one drink every other day. How do you feel about that?

This last statement provides the opportunity to negotiate and empowers the patient to be a part of the decision-making process. These approaches can also be tests to determine the seriousness of the patient's alcohol problem. If the patient cannot abstain or cut down, it suggests a more serious problem that requires referral and follow-up.

Brief interventions often include the use of a behavior modification pamphlet or self-help book that includes levels of drinking in the general population, a discussion of consequences, an agreement to cut back, a discussion of risky situations, ways to cope with setbacks, and ways for the patient to reward herself for success. A follow-up phone call 2 weeks after the office visit to determine if the patient is able to keep the agreement and follow-up office visits (at 1-month intervals) are often beneficial. *Brief interventions can be completed during a standard 15-minute office visits.*

SPECIALIZED TREATMENT

Brief advice is not appropriate for all patients with alcohol problems. Those who are alcohol dependent or for whom brief advice has been unsuccessful need specialized treatment. Successful treatment of alcohol and drug dependence began in 1935 with the development of Alcoholics Anonymous (AA), the first of the 12-step self-help groups.

Programs like the Minnesota model of alcoholism treatment, which includes an abstinence-oriented treatment program with education, individual and group therapy, and participation in AA, have been the mainstay of alcoholism treatment in the United States (Cook, 1988) but have only been tested in controlled clinical trials recently (Keso & Salaspuro, 1991). In a comparison between the Minnesota model and a traditional model based on individual, group, family, and work therapy without AA or a goal of abstinence, 26% of the patients in the Minnesota model were abstinent at the end of 1 year compared with 10% in the traditional model.

In the last decade, the alcohol and other drug abuse (AODA) field has moved away from 28-day inpatient programs to outpatient programs and several other models of treatment. These treatment models include cognitive behavioral therapy, cue therapy, and motivational enhancement techniques. Trends in AODA treatment reflect more freedom to choose programs that will best meet the needs of individual patients. The choice of treatment depends on motivation to change, co-occurring medical and psychiatric problems, and family issues to be resolved, as well as what treatment options are available in the community. Studies of treatment matching are under way to determine characteristics of patients who benefit from each of the types of treatment modalities.

USE OF ALCOHOL-SENSITIZING AGENTS

Medications with alcohol-sensitizing effects, like disulfiram (Antabuse), have been used to stop patients' alcohol use during treatment. The disulfiram–alcohol reaction includes flushing, nausea, vomiting, and cardiovascular changes (Wright & Moore, 1989). Treatment programs and practitioners show great variability in prescribing disulfiram. This variability often depends on philosophy and administrative approaches (Eighth Special Report, 1993, p. 333) rather than on patient characteristics or treatment setting. Fuller *et al.* (1986), in a controlled clinical trial, found that disulfiram had no long-term effect on abstinence but that patients who received 250 mg/day had fewer drinking days than those on smaller doses or on placebo.

It should be noted that disulfiram may not benefit patients who have difficulty following medication regimens and that there is continued concern about the side effects and toxicity (Christensen *et al.*, 1991; Wright & Moore, 1989). Because of this concern, other aversive agents, such as calcium carbamide, which does not have the drowsiness and lethargy associated with disulfiram (Peachey *et al.*, 1989), are being tested. Calcium carbamide, however, is not approved for use in the United States and is contraindicated for patients with thyroid disease. Disulfiram should not be used in the absence of an ongoing treatment and monitoring program.

REFERRAL

Identifying the particular expertise of specialists in the community is important if treatment matching (matching the needs of the patient with the available programs) is to occur. Physicians may use the following steps to determine their community resources (Barry & Fleming, 1994): (1) Ask colleagues for names of treatment programs or individual providers; (2) contact an AODA treatment program or specialist, mental health center, or hospital for consultation about a specific patient problem; (3) call the state alcohol and drug abuse agency for the names of publicly and privately funded treatment programs; (4) call employee assistance programs in the area; and (5) complete the Community Alcohol and Drug Treatment Resource Guide (Table 15.6) including telephone numbers of key professionals in the community, and post the guide in the nursing station, reception area, or exam room.

Table 15.6
Community Alcohol/Drug Treatment Resources

---

1. Alcohol and drug specialist:

Name _____ Phone _____

Name _____ Phone _____

2. Physician with expertise in alcohol and drug disorders:

Name _____ Phone _____

3. AA phone numbers _____

_____

4. Community substance abuse services (publicly funded):

Name _____ Phone_____

Contact person _____

Type of facility (circle): residential/outpatient/evening/adolescent/adult

Specialized program _____

5. Other treatment programs:

Name _____ Phone _____

Hours _____ Contact person _____

Type of facility (circle): residential/outpatient/evening/adolescent/adult

Specialized program _____

Name _____ Phone _____

Hours _____ Contact person _____

Type of facility (circle): residential/outpatient/evening/adolescent/adult

Specialized program _____

When referring patients to a specialist, it helps to tell the patient that a second opinion from a specialist is needed, to make telephone calls to the AODA specialist to set up the assessment while the patient is in the office, and to ask the specialist to call once she has completed the evaluation. This allows the physician to participate in long-term follow-up and provides continuity of care to patients who are in need of ongoing support.

Sometimes patients refuse to see specialists or do not have the financial or family resources to go into treatment, e.g., childcare is unavailable, older adults are afraid to leave home for treatment because they might not be able to go back to their home again. When this happens, physicians can take two steps to help these patients. First, they can identify recovering alcoholics in their own practices who are willing to meet with persons with AODA problems to discuss ways to change drinking behavior. Second, they can ask the patient to attend self-help groups such as AA. The patient may need to attend more than one group to find one that is comfortable, e.g., smoking versus nonsmoking groups. Two types of group meetings that do not follow a 12-step model are Rational Recovery and Women for Sobriety. These groups are most often found in midsized and larger cities.

As mentioned earlier, the majority of persons who drink suffer no adverse consequences. For those patients who do not drink above the at-risk cutoffs, do not abuse prescription drugs, and do not use illicit drugs, a clear positive message reinforcing that behavior is appropriate:

> Our goal is to prevent future health problems. Your exercise program looks good and your weight has remained stable. Since you have no family history of alcohol or drug problems and are taking no medication to interfere with alcohol, not exceeding a glass of wine once or twice a week should not cause any additional medical problems for you.

It is often easier to remember to intervene with problems than to provide verbal support for healthful behaviors. There are few opportunities in clinical medicine to make significant long-lasting changes in the lives of patients. Helping a patient to avoid the consequences of an alcohol or drug disorder is one such opportunity. Treatment programs that focus on recovering professionals report 5-year success rates of over 80%. No other chronic condition has such a high potential cure rate. Models for screening, assessment, brief advice, and referral are now available (NIAAA, Physician's Guide to Helping Patients with Alcohol Problems, 1995).

CONCLUSION

This chapter provides background data concerning the importance of prevention and early intervention in the area of alcohol and other drug problems, effective screening procedures for at-risk drinkers and drug users, a brief intervention protocol to be used with patients who are not alcohol or drug dependent, and steps to establish a referral network for patients who need specialized treatment. As healthcare in the United States changes, the role of primary care physicians in the prevention and treatment of alcohol and other drug problems will broaden.

CASES FOR DISCUSSION

CASE 1

George Williams is a 63-year-old white school custodian whom you have seen a few times in the last 3 years after his previous physician, Dr. James, retired. You admitted him to the hospital for pneumonia last year and found that he had mild emphysema from a long history of smoking. He had been treated for hypertension for 5 years. His blood pressure was stable in the hospital, so you discontinued the medication and advised him to avoid salt in his diet. He came to the office last week for a yearly physical, the results of which were within normal limits except for the mild emphysema and an elevated blood pressure of 160/105 mm Hg. At his insistence you continued Dr. James's prescription for triazolam 0.125 hs, prn (at bedtime as needed) for insomnia. You asked him to return in 1 week (today) for a blood pressure recheck and planned to spend more time discussing his smoking. His laboratory tests came back today and you discovered that he has an elevated GGT and an MCV of 98 (normal = 80 to 96). During the physical examination he stated that he drinks a few days a week with his friends at the corner bar. You are also concerned that he has been calling for prescription renewals increasingly early in the last 3 months.

1. What additional screening questions will you ask him?
2. What areas should be assessed for more severe alcohol or other drug problems?
3. Do you think he will be a candidate for brief advice?
4. If you think Mr. Williams needs an assessment by an AODA specialist, how will you approach the subject with him?

CASE 2

Dr. Pendleton is a 48-year-old primary care physician who has been the medical director of a clinic in a small rural community in the Midwest for the last 3 years. He grew up in a large city and moved to a smaller community for his residency program. He engaged in binge drinking in college with his fraternity brothers, used marijuana regularly, and experimented with cocaine a few times. During his residency program he and the other residents had in-home parties every few weeks. He noticed that he was able to drink more than anyone else and was a little irritated that none of them seemed to want to go out drinking as often as he did. His use of marijuana and cocaine stopped during his years in the residency program. After completing his residency, his drinking also tapered off because he was so busy with his new practice and young family. During the last 3 years Dr. Pendleton's binge drinking has increased but has generally been confined to evenings although his nurse has noticed changes in his personality and has smelled alcohol on his breath during working hours on one occasion. His wife recently filed for divorce. He had three instances of being intoxicated while on call in the last few months, one of which you and another junior colleague noticed. You were uncertain if you should report this or talk to him yourselves. After checking into what help was available, you decided to get some help from the impaired physicians program of the state medical society. The physician intervenors assured you that the information you both provided would be kept confidential and that they would work with Dr. Pendleton. They met with Dr. Pendleton and explained that there were reports of alcohol-related problems in his job performance. Although he initially denied problems related to his drinking, the committee arranged for an alcohol and drug assessment as well as a urine drug screen. In addition to binge drinking, Dr. Pendleton was using benzodiazepines on a regular basis. He entered a treatment program for professionals and was clean and sober at 1 year posttreatment.

1. Would you have confronted Dr. Pendleton yourself first? If yes, what would you say? If no, why not?
2. Would you have confronted someone who was a colleague without seniority or a subordinate? If yes, what would you say? If no, why not?
3. How could an impaired physicians program help a physician such as Dr. Pendleton?
4. How can you find out about an impaired physicians program in your area?

CASE 3

Sal Franco is a 74-year-old man living alone in an apartment in a complex for older adults. He owned a grocery store with his wife Mary for 44 years. He and Mary sold the business to their son Dominique when Sal was 70 with plans to travel and enjoy their remaining years together. Shortly after their retirement, Mary was diagnosed with bone cancer and died within 6 months of the diagnosis. Mr. Franco has been alone for the last 3 years. Although he was a "hard drinker" as he described it in his 20s and 30s, because of gastritis and high blood pressure, his use of alcohol was limited to his weekly poker games and Sunday family meals for many years. Because Sal and Mary spent most of their time working at the grocery store and involved in family activities, there was little time left for friends. Now he has time on his hands and uses alcohol to alleviate some of the pain and stress of his loneliness, generally having three drinks a day. He has developed few outside interests and doesn't know where to start. He came to the clinic for follow-up of his labile hypertension and gastritis. You asked Mr. Franco how he was feeling and received this response, "Oh, Doctor, I guess I'm OK for an old widower. I sometimes think it really doesn't matter how I feel at this age." You followed up with some questions about what Sal does with his time and discovered that he uses alcohol to excess along with taking over-the-counter medication to sleep.

1. What assessment questions would you ask to determine the extent of the problem?
2. How would you work with Mr. Franco to cut back or stop his use of alcohol?
3. What outside agencies and activities might be useful to Mr. Franco, who is spending most of his time alone? What would you suggest to him?
4. How would you help him get connected with programs or agencies in the community that could provide some interests in life for him? Are there other professionals in your clinic who could be of assistance with this issue?

CASE 4

Josh Kendrick is an 18-year-old high school senior who is graduating this year. He came to the office for his physical examination before he leaves to be a camp counselor for the summer and attends a local university in the fall. He was on the wrestling and baseball teams all 4 years of high school and has been active in extracurricular activities sponsored by the school. His grades have been good, mostly Bs and a few As. As part of your routine physical examination you ask questions about alcohol and drug use. Josh reports that he drinks about once a month at parties and uses marijuana at least once a week with friends.

1. What other questions would you ask about his use of alcohol and drugs?
2. If he was not so forthcoming about his use, what types of questions would be a good lead-in to questions about his use?
3. Is Josh's use problematic at this time? If yes, what would you do next? If no, what will you say next?
4. What prevention messages would you give him as he goes off to college?

CASE 5

Mandy Quist is a 25-year old married computer programmer who has been in your practice for 3 years. At her last physical she indicated that she drank a glass of wine three times a week. She experimented with marijuana in college but has not used any illicit drugs in the last 2 years. She exercises three times a week in an aerobics class at the YWCA, does not smoke, and her weight has remained stable since she entered your practice. Mrs. Quist has been trying to conceive and is here for a pregnancy test.

1. What advice will you give her regarding the use of alcohol, medications, and drugs?
2. What prevention messages will you give her about her other health behaviors?
3. What advice would you give her regarding her health behaviors during pregnancy?

——————— RECOMMENDED READINGS ———————

Eighth Special Report to the U.S. Congress on Alcohol and Health: U.S. Department of Health and Human Services, Public Health Service, National Institutes of Health, National Institute of Alcohol Abuse and Alcoholism, ADM-281-91-0003, 1993.

This state-of-the-art publication is a very useful reference covering the effects of alcohol on health in a variety of areas. It includes sections on the nature and extent of alcohol use and alcohol-related problems, causes of alcohol abuse and alcohol dependence, consequences of use, abuse, and dependence, prevention and early intervention, and treatment approaches.

Fleming MF, Barry KL (eds): *Addictive Disorders.* St. Louis, MO: Mosby Yearbook Medical Publishers, 1992.

This is a practical clinical guide to the recognition, assessment, and treatment of alcohol-related problems in primary care settings. Topics include identification and treatment of primary addictions, treatment of medical problems associated with alcohol and drug disorders, clinical approaches to specific populations such as adolescents, women, and older adults, and related medical problems such as eating disorders, mental health disorders, HIV/AIDS, and gambling disorders. The book is presented in outline format to provide easy access to the material for use in the office.

National Institute of Alcohol Abuse and Alcoholism: NIAAA Physician Intervention Guide, 1995. For development information contact Francis Cotter, MPH, NIAAA, Willco Building, 600 Executive Blvd, Rockville, Md 20892-7003.

The NIAAA with the cooperation and help of experts in the alcohol field from around the United States have developed a physician intervention guide to aid the identification, assessment, and treatment of persons with alcohol-related problems in the office setting.

CHAPTER 16

C. Special Problems

Violence

L. Kevin Hamberger and Bruce Ambuel

Betty is 23 years old and bringing her newborn son to the office for a well-baby check and postpartum exam. She has a large hickey on her neck. The baby is healthy and Betty says that both she and Joe (the father) are very happy with the baby. The baby sleeps well, has a good appetite, and mostly has a good disposition.

Betty is somewhat concerned that the baby has "spells" when he just seems to cry and cry. During these "spells" Betty reports feeling somewhat tense and uncertain about what to do. Putting him in his crib and shutting his door helps somewhat. She states that Joe sometimes wonders why the child "won't mind" and "just be a good boy, like he's supposed to." She accepts information on child development and assures the physician that the baby is in no danger of being abused. She states that both she and Joe "went through that as kids" and have no intention of putting their kids through it. She does express openness, however, to being contacted by someone from the county Home Aid office for a little extra help and learning some parenting tips. Betty is not sure, however, whether Joe will go along with the idea.

With this last comment, the physician, referring to Betty's hickey, noted half-jokingly, "I thought I instructed 'no sex' for at least a month after the birth." Betty, looking to the floor, quietly replied, "I guess Joe couldn't wait." Betty's exam was essentially negative, and she was healing as expected. Betty was scheduled for another well-baby check in 6 months.

The physician had an uneasy feeling about Betty and Joe, but was uncertain about the precise nature of those concerns and how to go about evaluating them. The following history was collected about Betty during her prenatal course. Betty completed the 11th grade, having left school because of pregnancy, though she later miscarried. Throughout her most recent obstetrical course, Betty was reasonably compliant with her diet and nutrition and showed adequate weight gain and appropriate interest in her pregnancy. Both Betty and Joe smoke, although

Betty gave it up during her pregnancy, and has not yet resumed the habit. She noted during her pregnancy that she was going to try to quit permanently. She reported that her relationship with Joe was stable and that he was looking forward to the baby's arrival. She has lived with Joe for 3 years.

Joe is 24 years old and completed the 11th grade. For the past 3 years, he has been self-employed in a tree removal business. Betty moved in with Joe 3 years ago because she "couldn't take" living with her previous partner. She reported that Joe works hard trying to make his business succeed. Joe came to a couple of the OB visits but was very quiet and did not disclose much about himself. He participated in the prenatal classes and the birth of their son.

INTRODUCTION

The physician's uneasy but unarticulated feelings about Betty and Joe in Case 16-1 are justified by their history, if it were known. As a child, Betty was sexually abused by her grandfather, who lived with her family. Because of limits of physical space, Betty had to sleep in a room in the basement. Her grandfather made many late-night "trips" downstairs, when he would fondle her vaginal area and have her perform oral sex. This began when Betty was 5 years old. When Betty was 12, her grandfather had intercourse with her for the first time. Although she was threatened that she would be hurt if she ever told anyone of the abuse, Betty tried to tell her mother. Betty's mother, however, spanked and slapped her for "saying such things" about her grandfather, and warned her never to "say such things again."

At age 15, Betty moved out of the house and in with her 17-year-old boyfriend. He rarely worked and, although Betty continued to go to school, both "partied" a great deal, drinking alcohol and experimenting with drugs. He was very violent with Betty, beating her with his fists, throwing dishes at her, and, on one occasion, trying to drown her in the bathtub. On one occasion she tried to return home, but her parents told her, "You made your bed, now lie in it." She became pregnant during this time. She then decided to drop out of school and prepare to give birth. At 26 weeks she miscarried but did not return to school because "I just didn't feel like going back." Her boyfriend blamed her for losing the baby and beat her as punishment. She escaped to a battered women's shelter and ended the relationship.

Betty met Joe and was attracted to him because he treated her well and was a hard worker. Betty told Joe about her prior abusive relationship, and he promised never to hurt her or do anything to make her afraid. He was going to "take care of her." Six months into their relationship, however, they had a big fight over Joe's drinking and he slapped her. Following the fight, Joe felt remorse and expressed fear that Betty would leave him. He mentioned that he ought to just kill himself now and get it over with, if he couldn't have her. Betty felt afraid of being responsible for Joe's death if she left and he killed himself. She stayed. Three months later Joe wanted to have sex, Betty refused, and Joe became incensed. He grabbed her breasts and pushed against her with his body, telling her "You're mine and I'll have you if I want." At other times, Joe would "remind" Betty that he "could" do to her what her ex-boyfriend used to do. This type of statement would gain her compliance without having to resort to physical violence.

Joe grew up the oldest of three children, with a younger brother and sister. Joe's father was a construction worker who traveled the country to follow jobs. His mother was a waitress when she could find work outside the house. Joe's father was violent to his mother, beating her physically or "tearing up the house" after a night of heavy drinking. Joe recalls staying awake nights, fearful that his father would come home and hurt someone and fearful that he wouldn't come home at all. At times his father would round all the children up in the middle of the night to make them watch as he beat one of them with an extension cord for some rule infraction. They were made to watch so all of them could "learn a lesson." Once when Joe was 11 years old, his father took him hunting in the woods. At one point, Joe's father made him kneel down and placed the shotgun to his mouth, asking Joe if he "trusted" his father. Joe never told anyone of the incident. At age 15, Joe ran away from home and moved across the country, living in the streets and surviving on side jobs he picked up along the way. Prior to meeting Betty, Joe socialized mostly in bars, getting into barfights several times a week. On one occasion he was shot, sustaining a flesh wound, while trying to help a friend in a fight.

The story of Betty and Joe is fairly typical. Many men who batter their partners were themselves victims of child abuse and witnessed abuse in the family of origin (Hamberger & Hastings, 1986). Children who are abused are at risk for becoming violent offenders as adults. Further, many men who abuse their partners are also violent outside of their immediate relationship (Saunders, 1992). Hence, it is not surprising that Joe often fought in bars and was himself the victim of violence in such settings.

In Betty's case, child sexual abuse is not viewed as a "cause" of her victimization as an adult. However, the degradation and hopelessness she experienced in a nonsupportive family limited her choices and led directly to her decision to leave home early. Her lack of preparation for independent living and the effect of the sexual abuse on her self image left her vulnerable to involvement in relationships with men who abused her.

This case also illustrates that, even though an individual or couple may present with one particular "type" of violence issue at any given time, both victims and perpetrators often exhibit complex histories. If these histories are not known or well understood, our patients may do things that seem pathological, inexplicable, or "proof" of noncompliance. Such misunderstanding can lead to victim-blaming and assignment of pejorative diagnostic labels, such as "hysterical" or "borderline personality."

Another problem that can arise from such misunderstanding is the application of inappropriate or inadequate interventions. For example, a friendly pat on the back with a survivor of childhood sexual abuse may seem innocuous to a healthcare provider but may be emotionally overwhelming to the survivor. A doctorly scolding may be therapeutic to some individuals to enhance compliance, but a man who learned to distrust authority through beatings and abuse may react by leaving the practice and rejecting all encouragement to seek help.

To understand how violence affects patients such as Betty and Joe and what physicians should do to help them, this chapter will present the following information. First, we will consider the nature and prevalence of violence: what is violence? what are the various types of violence? what function does violence serve in families and society? how do family and stranger violence differ from each other? how prevalent are the various types of violence? how prevalent is violence in medical settings? Next, we examine the attitudes of physicians toward victims and perpetrators of violence and consider their therapeutic value. Third, we consider the impact of violence on the health of victims, perpetrators, family, and society. Fourth, we ask why violence is so prevalent and consider ways that criminal justice systems, social service systems, and religious and other institutions can best address this problem. Finally, we consider ways that physicians can intervene to prevent and curb violence. On completing the chapter, the reader will understand: the impact on patients of societal-generated violence, including that caused by family members and strangers; the dynamics that characterize violent and abusive relationships; and the physician's role in assisting patients who are affected by violence and in preventing violence through individual and societal-level interventions.

CASE 16-2

D. J., a healthy, active 9-year-old, was spending the beautiful Saturday afternoon at his neighborhood park, hanging out with his friends and watching some older men play basketball. A heated argument broke out on the court, and one of the men involved in the game pulled out a gun. He repeatedly fired the gun, clearing the area around the basketball court. When the immediate excitement had subsided, D. J. was seen lying with his head in a pool of blood. He was dead, killed by a bullet wound to the head. That evening, some neighborhood leaders called for the closing of that park. The next day, a team of counselors was dispatched to D. J.'s school to talk with his friends and classmates. Many spoke of their fears of being harmed and of not feeling safe anywhere, including their own homes.

THE NATURE AND PREVALENCE OF VIOLENCE

WHAT IS VIOLENCE?

Violence is "the threatened or actual use of physical force or power against oneself or against a group or community which either results in, or has a high likelihood of resulting in injury, death or deprivation" (Rosenberg, 1994). Violence is functional, intended to dominate, punish, or control another individual, group, or community. The concept of violence usually brings to mind images of extreme destructive acts such as a recent case in which a man bludgeoned his wife with a sledgehammer and watched her die over a 6-hour period, or the serial killer who cut up and cannibalized his victims. Violence actually is multidimensional, consisting of acts that vary according to type, severity, frequency, and impact. Violence can be considered legitimate, as when a law enforcement officer subdues and neutralizes a dangerous criminal with a nightstick. Violence can also be considered illegitimate, as when an angry husband kicks down a door that his wife is hiding behind for safety or when a police officer uses excessive force.

Within the field of spouse abuse, Anne Ganley (1989) has identified and defined four basic types of violence. Although developed primarily for understanding partner violence, this typology can serve as a heuristic for understanding virtually any type of interpersonal violence.

DIMENSIONS OF VIOLENCE

The first type of violence is actual physical violence, and it involves direct physical attacks on the victim's body. Physical violence includes a wide range of actions from grabbing and restraining to pushing and shoving to slapping, punching, kicking, clubbing, choking, drowning, burning, stabbing, and shooting. Note that physical violence constitutes a continuum of actions ranging from apparently less severe behaviors (such as pushing and shoving) to more severe and even life-threatening behaviors, such as using a

knife or a gun. Even less severe violent behaviors, however, can have great injury potential. One of us (L.K.H.) has conducted over 1000 assessments of domestically violent
offenders, many of whom insisted that they "only" pushed their partners. In-depth assessment of these "pushing" incidents has frequently indicated that the impact has been
severe. For example, one offender who reported he had "only pushed her" later admitted,
when asked, that he tried to push his partner out of a closed second-floor window. Another
reported succeeding in pushing his partner off a second-floor balcony, resulting in multiple fractures. Still another reported shoving his partner down a flight of concrete steps,
causing her serious head injuries. Hence, although an offender may report using seemingly
less severe violence in an assaultive act, it is important to assess carefully the context and
consequences of the violence.

A second form of violence is sexual. Sexual violence involves any actual or threatened assault of a sexual nature against a victim's body. This can range from unwanted
fondling or touching of sexual areas to forced sexual acts. Sexual violence also includes
coercive, threatening statements, exposure, and other actions that induce fear in the victim
for purposes of sexual gratification and control in the perpetrator. This could include
threatening to carry out sexual acts against the victim's wishes or threatening violence if
sex is not provided. With children, in particular, sexual violence can include exposure to
pornography, taking pictures for adult gratification, exposure to genitals, or adult sexual
contact.

As with physical violence, sexual violence usually involves direct action against a
victim's body and constitutes a continuum of acts. As with physical violence, however, it
is important not to assume that so-called minor acts of sexual violence are not serious. For
example, many battered women report feeling degraded and humiliated after being coer-
cively touched and fondled by their partners. Likewise, victims of sexual harassment are
not always directly physically assaulted. Nevertheless, such victims often report experiencing intense emotional distress.

A third form of violence is property and animal destruction. This type of violence
typically does not involve direct physical attacks against a victim's body but is nevertheless directed toward a victim. Examples include breaking down doors or windows or
destroying cars, household items, and favorite personal possessions. Violence toward
animals includes injuring and killing of pets, which may be displayed prominently in the
victim's view. These actions communicate the perpetrator's destructive power and willingness to use violence to accomplish some goal, while terrorizing the victim.

The fourth type of violence is psychological violence. Psychological violence includes a wide range of behaviors, such as name-calling and insults, following and stalking,
forcing someone to do degrading things, and controlling the victim's movements and
relationships within the community. In domestic violence situations, controlling economic
resources and manipulating children is also part of psychological violence.

THE FUNCTION OF VIOLENCE

Violent behavior is functional. That is, people use violence intentionally to achieve
certain outcomes that have value to the perpetrator. The outcomes are reinforcing and thus
increase the probability that violence will be used again in subsequent similar situations.
One key to preventing violence is to determine how it functions to reinforce, then change,
the value of the reinforcers. For example, in the field of partner violence, Ganley (1989)
suggests that violence functions to dominate, control, or punish one's partner. In Case
16-1, Joe indicated he battered Betty in an effort to get her to "quit bugging him" when he

came home from work tired. On other occasions he threatened to hit her (psychological battery) to keep her from associating with her friend in the neighborhood. Although Joe never actually said the words "dominate and control" in describing how violence worked for him, the themes in his explanations clearly indicated the dominating and controlling functions of violence for him.

From a societal level, violence may function to dominate or oppress an entire class of people. Violence toward women, for example, can be analyzed as part of a larger, historical pattern of male domination of women, through the development, by males, of social systems that favor men and oppress women (Martin, 1985). In the home, women perform a disproportionate amount of childcare and "domestic" duties, and our society provides few resources for childcare (Mederos, 1987). In the workplace, women occupy a disproportionate number of lower-paying, lower-status jobs, and experience greater difficulty being promoted to higher-level management jobs than men. In divorce cases, women typically experience a greater drop in standard of living than do men. This creates societally sanctioned disincentives for women to leave abusive partners, thus maintaining the cycle of violence. Physical and sexual violence, or the threat of such violence, also reinforce the broader social-level inequities (Pagelow, 1984). Thus, domestic violence, together with societal maintaining factors, disenfranchises and devalues women, not only affecting battered women, but also functioning to oppress the entire group.

Sometimes violence has a protective function. In our work with battered women, we have learned that many women use physical force to resist the violence and coercion of their abusive partners. A recent study comparing male and female perpetrators' reasons for using violence showed that over two-thirds of the men reported reasons related to domination, control, or punishment. In contrast, about two-thirds of the women reported using violence to defend against an attack or retaliate for a previous attack against them (Hamberger, 1994). Hence, as with understanding the type and outcome of violence, discussed in this section, it is important to assess carefully the function of violence for a particular patient prior to developing conclusions about its meaning.

FAMILY VERSUS STRANGER VIOLENCE

Although the topography or specific forms of violent behaviors may appear similar when directed toward strangers or family members, actually there are significant differences between violent crimes involving strangers and violent crimes within the family. These differences may affect how individual actors may react and how the system, including healthcare providers, may react.

Contrary to popular belief, most violence occurs between people who know each other, not between strangers. For example, a woman is more likely to be raped by an acquaintance, friend, or partner than by a stranger (American Medical Association, 1992). Child abuse is primarily a problem of parents or caretakers hurting the children under their care. Contrary to the idea that child sexual abuse is perpetrated by strangers, most is perpetrated by family or caretaking adults and older children (Haugaard & Reppucci, 1988). Elder abuse is also more likely to be committed by an adult child than by a stranger (Costa & Anetzberger, in press).

Stranger violence may have the effect of damaging or destroying, within the victim, the notion that the world is basically a safe place. Stranger violence, even to someone not directly affected, may result in a decreased sense of security and the adoption of behaviors designed to reduce a sense of risk. Family violence, however, destroys or undermines any sense of safety and trust within life's most intimate relationships. Survivors of stranger violence *may* be able to avoid the scene of their victimization. They may also be willing to cooperate in criminal justice and prosecution efforts to bring the offender to justice. For victims of family violence, however, leaving the offender or the household may not be an option, at least immediately.

A child victim may tell another parent or adult, only to be met with disbelief or, worse, punishment for "causing trouble." Child victims may be told that if they report the violence, it will be their fault if the offensive family member is incarcerated or put out of the family. Child victims are often threatened with more violence if they disclose the abuse. In addition to being dependent on and frightened of their abuser, child victims may also love the abuser, creating tremendous conflict about disclosing abuse. They may also have been blamed for the abuse, which was characterized by the abuser as "discipline" and "for your own good."

Similarly, victims of elder abuse and partner violence face many obstacles to reporting the violence or leaving the violent offender. These obstacles include financial and emotional dependency, acceptance of blame for the abuse, fear of retribution for efforts to end the abuse, and fear of death at the hands of the offender. Many family violence victims have been threatened with death if the abuse is reported or if they try to leave the perpetrator. Because past threats have been backed up by the offender, the victim may legitimately fear for her life when contemplating leaving. As with child victims, victims of elder and partner violence may love the offender and be hopeful that the violence will end. Sometimes, particularly with elders, physical infirmities preclude the option of leaving an abuser.

Because of the complexities of family violence, it is important to withhold judgment and prescriptive advice prior to conducting a thorough assessment of dangerousness and resources. Providing advice to victims of family violence on the basis of principles appropriate to stranger violence could further victimize the patient, particularly in the area of leaving the offender. Research has shown that the most dangerous time in a victim's life is when she attempts to end the relationship with her abuser (Rasche, 1988). Methods for asking about child maltreatment and partner violence are summarized in Tables 16.1 to 16.3.

PREVALENCE OF VIOLENCE IN SOCIETY

Violence is difficult to measure. Many studies rely on official statistics, gathered through government agencies (Gaquin, 1977–78). These data often use narrow definitions of violence and provide information only on cases brought to the attention of authorities. Thus, such studies underestimate true incidence and prevalence rates. Other studies (Straus & Gelles, 1986) utilize random samples recruited from the community. Such studies may be more representative than studies based on official statistics but may also suffer from underreporting because survey participants may not want to tell someone that they have been victimized or have perpetrated violence. Violence is also difficult to define. In the field of child sexual abuse, for example, there are differences between studies in the operational definitions used, particularly in some of the "borderline" cases. There is wide agreement between researchers that forced intercourse constitutes abuse. On the other hand, there may be less agreement about whether, say, a parent taking nude photographs of his children constitutes abuse. In spite of these inherent difficulties with conducting research on incidence and prevalence of violence, a number of studies have informed us as to the amount of violence in our society.

Table 16.1

Identifying Child Abuse or Neglect: General Signs and Symptoms

1. General signs of distress in a child that warrant further assessment
   - Symptoms of anxiety or depression
   - Social withdrawal
   - Aggressive, mean, or violent behavior toward others
   - Low self-esteem
   - Attention problems, failure to learn, or developmental delay
   - Extreme perfectionism, fearfulness, or intolerance of own mistakes
   - Extreme need for attention
   - Regressive or childlike behavior
   - Inappropriate hygiene
   - Parental child: child takes parental role with siblings or has excessive domestic responsibilities
   - Sudden change in behavior or school performance
   - In late childhood and adolescence: eating disorders; sexually active before age 15, or multiple partners; pregnancy; self-mutilation; attempted suicide; running away
2. Action (when you observe general signs of distress):
   - Interview the parent(s) and child
   - Document in the chart
     S: What the child and parent(s) said. Use quotation marks to document exact words
     O: What behavior, signs, and symptoms you observed
     A: Your assessment of stress-related problems
     P: Describe follow-up plans
   - Schedule follow-up appointments to assess changes over time
   - Refer to a mental health professional with training in child development and request a report
   - Consult schoolteacher or counselor

© B. Ambuel, Family Peace Project, Family & Community Medicine, Medical College of Wisconsin, 210 NW Barstow, #201, Waukesha, Wisc 53188, (414) 548-6903. Reprinted with permission of the author.

Child Physical and Sexual Abuse

Based on national surveys, 11% of children are physically assaulted by a parent each year. Such assaults include kicking, biting, hitting, or more severe physical violence (Gelles & Straus, 1988). Further, 2% of children are estimated to experience severe physical assault by a parent—beating, striking with an object, threatening, or assaulting with a weapon (Gelles & Straus, 1988). Based on retrospective studies with adults, it is estimated that at least 20% of girls and 5 to 10% of boys experience sexual abuse before age 18 (Finkelhor, 1994).

Partner Violence

Two national studies of prevalence of partner violence among heterosexuals have estimated that each year about 16.1% of married women are assaulted by their husbands (Straus *et al.*, 1980; Straus & Gelles, 1986). Similar rates have been found among nonmarried couples (Makepeace, 1981). Although gay and lesbian couples have been more difficult to study, available data suggest that rates of violence among gay and lesbian couples are about the same as those for heterosexuals (Island & Letellier, 1991).

Elder Abuse

Little data exist on incidence and prevalence of elder abuse. Nevertheless, it is estimated that each year between 300,000 and 1.5 million elders are abused. The most

Table 16.2
Identifying Child Abuse or Neglect: Specific Signs and Symptoms

1. Specific signs and symptoms of child abuse and neglect that warrant action:
   • Unusual or suspicious bruises, burns, rectal or genital pain or bleeding, or injury inconsistent with reported event
   • Sexually explicit play with dolls or other children, including play with dolls or other children that illustrates intercourse, oral intercourse, or anal intercourse (Distinguish from normal self-exploration and masturbation)
   • Inappropriate touching of other children's private areas (buttocks, genital area)
   • Specific comments or complaints about being maltreated, neglected or sexually touched
   • Lack of basic needs (e.g., food, clothing, medical and dental care)
   • Grossly inappropriate hygiene
   • A child left unsupervised for long periods of time
   • In your professional opinion, you suspect the child is being abused or neglected
2. Action (when you observe specific signs of abuse or neglect):
   • *Immediately* file a report with child protective services (CPS) and engage your clinic's protocol. Involve parents in filing the report when this does not place the child at risk
   • Hospitalize the child when necessary to treat injuries or place the child in safe environment
   • Document the nature of injury and observations carefully in the child's chart
     S: What the child and parent(s) said. Use quotation marks to document exact words
     O: What behavior and injuries you observed. Drawings and photographs describe location and quality of injuries. Include a ruler in photos for scale, and victim's face for identity
     A: Your assessment of potential child abuse
     P: Describe any safety and follow-up plans
   • If you are unsure about reporting, consult a trusted colleague, a local expert, or a child abuse caseworker at child protective services. Discuss a hypothetical situation to maintain confidentiality. Trust your own professional judgment
   • Develop a treatment plan for the child and family that engages clinic and community resources

© B. Ambuel, Family Peace Project, Family & Community Medicine, Medical College of Wisconsin, 210 NW Barstow, #201, Waukesha, Wisc 53188, (414) 548-6903. Reprinted with permission of the author.

common form of elder abuse is self-neglect, in which the elder stops caring for himself, but the family or significant support group fails to provide needed support (Tatara, 1993).

Sexual Assault

Sexual assault of women is believed to be a highly underreported form of violence. Official FBI statistics show that, in 1988, over 92,000 rapes were reported to police, but experts estimate that 90% of sexual assaults go unreported (Bryant, 1990). Epidemiological studies indicate that about 20% of adult women and 15% of college women report being sexually assaulted during their lifetime (Koss, 1993). Rates of sexual assault are believed to be higher among women of color (Koss, 1993).

Firearm Violence

Violence involving firearms deserves special attention because firearms are such a lethal mechanism of injury. A number of recent surveys have reported on use of firearms, particularly handguns, in perpetrating violence. Callahan and Rivara (1993) found that 33% of high school handgun owners reported having shot at someone. Over 9% of female students reported involvement of firearms in the suicide or homicide of family members. Six percent of male high school students reported carrying a gun to school at some time. Fingerhut *et al.* (1992) studied rates of firearm homicide among youth in both rural and

Table 16.3

Screening and Case Finding for Relationship Violence: Summary of Interview Strategies

A. Screening for current partner violence
- "Are you in any relationships where you are afraid for your personal safety, or where someone is hurting you, threatening you, forcing sexual contact, or trying to control your life?"

B. Screening for past violence
- "As an adult, have you ever been a victim of violence, such as assault or sexual assault?"
- "Have you ever been in a relationship where your partner hurt you, threatened you, forced sexual contact, or tried to control your life?"
- "When you were a child or adolescent, did anyone ever physically hurt you, force sexual contact, or hurt you psychologically (for example, by telling you that you were worthless or unwanted)?"

C. Case finding with general signs of distress
- "In my experience, these types of symptoms are sometimes caused or made worse by stress. Are there any sources of stress in your personal life, family life, or at work?"
- Screen for current violence (A) and past violence (B)
- Screen for other causes of distress (positive and negative life events; family problems; depression or anxiety, etc.)

D. Case finding with specific signs of violence
- "In my experience, this type of injury is sometimes caused by other people's actions. Are you safe? Is anyone hurting or threatening you?"
- Screen for current violence (A)

E. When you suspect abuse but the patient denies abuse
- "I'm concerned about your safety and would like to tell you about several community resources you can use if you ever need them."
- Describe resources, offer follow-up, and document as in protocol
- Do not confront or challenge the patient

© B. Ambuel and L.K. Hamberger, Family Peace Project, Family & Community Medicine, Medical College of Wisconsin, 210 NW Barstow, #201, Waukesha, Wisc 53188, (414) 548-6903. Reprinted with permission of the authors.

urban areas. Among urban youth, the firearm-related homicide rate was 13.7 per 100,000. Among rural youth, the firearm homicide rate was 2.9 per 100,000. Black youths had the highest rates of death from firearms. Further, Fingerhut *et al.* found that between 1979 through 1987 rates of firearm homicides increased dramatically. In contrast, during the same time period non-firearm-related homicides decreased or remained stable. Most intentional firearm violence occurs between people who know each other (Kellerman *et al.*, 1993) or is self-inflicted (Goldberg, in press). In addition, for every firearm homicide, there are approximately 7.5 nonfatal firearm-related injuries (Rice & McKenzie, 1989).

Witnessing Violence

Although physical violence directly claims many victims, there are also many indirect victims. Indirect victims are those who have witnessed violence or are somehow associated with victims of violence. Such individuals include child observers of parental violence, relatives of violence and homicide victims, or victims of other forms of violence. According to the American Psychological Association (1993), for example, 73% of eighth-graders surveyed in Chicago had seen someone shot, stabbed, robbed, or killed. Untold thousands of children observe parental violence. Such witnessing of violence can have profound effects on the mental well-being of the observer, including posttraumatic stress.

A number of studies have assessed rates of victimization among patients attending hospital emergency rooms and outpatient primary care and specialty clinics. For example, Koss *et al.* (1991) found that 57% of women attending a health maintenance organization had been victims of crime, including rape, physical assault, and noncontact crimes. Greenwood *et al.* (1990) found that 5% of male and female patients at a multispecialty clinic reported having been physically abused as children. Among female patients, 16.9% reported child sexual abuse. No men reported childhood sexual abuse. Drossman *et al.* (1990) studied violence in the backgrounds of women attending a gastrointestinal disorders clinic. The authors found that 44% of the women reported physical or sexual abuse in either childhood or adulthood. Women are frequently victims of partner violence during pregnancy. One study (Hillard, 1985) found that 10.9% of women in an obstetrical clinic reported being battered. Helton *et al.* (1987) observed violence occurring in the lives of 8% of women during their pregnancy. In a family practice setting, it was found that about 23% of women reported being assaulted by a partner in the past year. Nearly 40% reported assault at some time in a relationship during their adult life (Hamberger *et al.*, 1992).

Based on the review above, there is little question that violence is a prevalent reality in the United States. Victims and perpetrators of violence are all around us, both in our communities and in our healthcare settings. In addition to routine health concerns, they seek medical treatment for injuries sustained from violence and for stress-related health concerns that follow victimization. Further, victims also often carry the emotional scars of violence, both directly experienced and observed, in other areas of their lives. Hence, physicians can expect to encounter numerous victims and perpetrators of violence in their practice.

Patients are not the only victims or survivors of violence. Physicians themselves may suffer the burdens of violence in their own lives. These personal experiences and knowledge can affect the attitudes and practices of physicians in treating victims and perpetrators.

CASE 16-3

Judy, 23 years old, came to the clinic for her first OB visit. She has two other children, all with the same partner. Though not married, Judy and Bill have cohabited for 5 years. While taking her vitals, the nurse noticed a handprint bruise on her right bicep. She subsequently notified the physician of her concern that Judy might have been "roughed up" by someone. On completion of the physical portion of the exam, the following exchange took place:

DOCTOR: *How are things going with Bill?*

JUDY: *Good.*

DOCTOR: *How does he feel about the pregnancy?*

JUDY: *He's not real excited.*

DOCTOR: *Oh, why is that?*

JUDY: *He blames me for getting pregnant.*

DOCTOR: *Well, just tell him it takes two to tango!*

JUDY: *I'll say!*

DOCTOR: *How did you get that bruise on your right arm?*

JUDY: *We tangoed the other night.*

DOCTOR: *Well, you've got to be careful now. After all, you're going to have a baby. We'll see you next month.*

PHYSICIANS' ATTITUDES TOWARD —— VICTIMS AND PERPETRATORS —— OF VIOLENCE

In Case 16-3, Judy provided two very powerful signs that she might be battered—the bruise and the "tango" quip—yet the physician never responded directly to these signs. When the opportunity presented itself, Judy instead got a patronizing lecture. Why didn't the physician delve more deeply into the violence in Judy's life?

First, it is important to know that Judy is not alone in not being asked about violence by her physician. Hamberger *et al.* (1992) found that only 1.7% of women in a family practice center were asked by their physician about violence. Other studies have found similar low physician inquiry rates in ambulatory settings (Rath *et al.*, 1989) and emergency settings (Stark *et al.*, 1979).

There are several reasons why physicians do not ask about violence in their patients' lives, even when clear indications of violence are evident. Common reasons for not asking about violence include fear of "opening Pandora's box," or being overwhelmed with what they may be told. In addition, not having enough time to deal with a victim in crisis is another reason frequently given for not asking about violence. Some physicians do not believe that domestic violence is a true "medical" issue. Other physicians express some desire to ask about violence but do not do so because of lack of knowledge of what subsequent steps to take if battering is disclosed. Still others believe that there are no victims or perpetrators of partner violence in their practices. Finally, in our experience, many physicians and other healthcare professionals do not know how to ask about violence, or else fear angering their patients for being "too intrusive."

CASE 16-4

Jill came to her physician's office because of right rib pain. She told the physician that her husband had punched her several times three nights ago and might have cracked her ribs. The physician offhandedly mentioned that she "should either take up boxing or else learn to be a better wife." Jill felt humiliated and decided it was simply not safe to talk about violence with a physician.

CASE 16-5

Sue had a slightly different experience. After telling her physician about being battered, she initially felt supported by his empathy. Some time after Sue left the office, the physician called Sue's husband and "counseled" him to stop hurting her. Three days later, she came into the emergency room with a broken nose. Sue's husband punished her for telling the physician.

COUNTERTHERAPEUTIC REACTIONS TO VICTIMIZATION

371

PHYSICIANS'
ATTITUDES
TOWARD
VICTIMS AND
PERPETRATORS
OF VIOLENCE

In Case 16-3, the physician felt uncomfortable and chose to avoid the issue by making an inappropriate comment rather than asking direct questions to gather more information. Cases 16-4 and 16-5 illustrate that some well-meaning actions can be very inappropriate and detrimental to the safety of the victim. Other inappropriate actions include medically treating symptoms without working to end the violence. Examples include medicating anxiety or depression symptoms or suturing a wound, but failing to provide resource information or to conduct safety planning.

CASE 16-6

Jackson is a 25-year-old steelworker who came to the clinic for evaluation of a back injury. The physician noticed alcohol on his breath, so as part of the evaluation, alcohol abuse was also assessed. Because the physician had read that alcohol abuse is often associated with domestic violence, the following exchange took place:

DOCTOR: *How does your drinking affect your relationship with Barb [his wife]?*

JACKSON: *Well, she gets on my case when I've had a few, sometimes.*

DOCTOR: *When she gets on your case, how do you react?*

JACKSON: *It depends. If I get tired of it and don't want to hear any more of her lip, I might let her know.*

DOCTOR: *Do you ever let her know by, say, yelling at her?*

JACKSON: *Sometimes. After all, if she yells at me, I can yell at her, can't I?*

DOCTOR: *I suppose we all need a good scolding now and then. Tell me, do you ever lay a hand on her when you two are arguing?*

JACKSON: *Sometimes she gets right up in my face or stands in my way when I want to leave, so I have to move her out of the way.*

DOCTOR: *Well, it's easy to see why you'd get upset with someone getting in your space during a dispute.*

PERPETRATORS

As with victims of violence, perpetrators often remain invisible in medical settings. Sometimes physicians collude with perpetrators by providing tacit support for the violence, as in Case 16-6. Although reports of violence were elicited, the physician failed to respond appropriately to the findings. Twice the physician responded to reports of abusive behavior with "understanding" and supportive comments, rather than therapeutically confronting the violence. To Jackson's report of yelling at his partner, the physician acknowledged the occasional need for a "scolding." Later, in response to Jackson's report of using physical force, the physician excused Jackson for being upset, did not mention his use of force, and placed responsibility for Jackson's behavior on his partner for "getting in [his] space." Rather than therapeutically confronting Jackson's aggressive and controlling behavior, the physician's actions actually provided Jackson emotional support and justification. Hence, the violence was minimized as the primary problem, and his partner's "negative" behavior became the focus and reason for Jackson's aggression.

Sometimes failure to confront violence results from fear that such confrontation might result in aggression from the patient. Violence evokes painful and fearful images, even among healthcare providers. The thought of confronting someone who batters his partner or is violent on the street may be accompanied by fears that the healthcare provider will also be assaulted. A natural defense against such fear is to avoid asking about or confronting a patient with the wrongfulness of his violent behavior. In the authors' experience in a typical outpatient setting with nondelusional or nonpsychotic patients, the risk of assault is low.

Still other inappropriate physician responses include becoming overly moralistic or righteously indignant with a perpetrator. Violence as a social problem is rightly viewed as an evil that destroys families and individual lives. Further, all concerned citizens should be angry about it and work to end violence. However, angry or moralistic pronouncements to an offending patient will usually bring denial, loss from the practice, and possible renewed violence toward his partner. A more appropriate and effective approach is to deal with violence issues in a matter-of-fact, collaborative, and concerned manner. The concern is for all involved, including the perpetrator, his partner, and his children. By getting a perpetrator to realize the damage he does to his entire family, he is more likely to consider the need to change. By helping a perpetrator focus on his need to change, the physician can motivate him and provide appropriate referral information for abuse abatement counseling (Chelmowski & Hamberger, 1994).

CASE 16-7

Jimmy is 19 years old. He has been a member of the Scorpions, a street gang, for as long as he can remember. His parents were never married, and Jimmy can't remember the last time he saw his father, who is in prison for armed robbery. Jimmy had three older brothers, but the next oldest was killed in a gang-related shooting 3 years ago. Jimmy never completed the eighth grade because of fighting and truancy. Since that time he has survived on the streets, hustling odd jobs, selling drugs, and assaulting people for pay.

Tonight, Jimmy comes to the emergency room with a gunshot wound that shattered his lower spine, and another that penetrated his left brain. He was shot when he and his friends encountered a rival gang in an area on the border of their turf. Three years ago, Jimmy sustained a flesh wound in another fight. He bragged that he was invincible. Tonight's wound will leave him paralyzed. In addition to being confined to a wheelchair, he will experience chronic pain and require the use of a colostomy bag. His head wound will result in loss of use of his right arm and compromise visual–spatial abilities. He will require about a year to rehabilitate, and another 6 months for assisted independent living.

—— WHY IS VIOLENCE A HEALTH PROBLEM? ——

Intuitively, violence appears primarily to be purely a social problem or, at least, a problem affecting a few individuals and families. For many, violence seems to be something that happens "out there," affecting someone else. Recalling the statistics above, however, it is clear that violence is pervasive and epidemic. Moreover, no group is immune from violence. Research indicates that violence is responsible for both injuries (Saltzman *et al.*,

1992) and death (Fingerhut *et al.*, 1992). Therefore, physicians and other healthcare providers have begun to consider violence to be a health problem that is a significant cause of morbidity and mortality among their patients, as illustrated in Case 16-7.

Throughout this ordeal, Jimmy in Case 16-7 will require the services of a neurosurgeon, neurologist, internist, specialized nursing staff, medical assistants and home health aids, rehabilitation psychologists, transportation aids, and vocational rehabilitation specialists. Following rehabilitation, Jimmy will require lifetime care of his colostomy, medication and rehabilitation for chronic pain, and disability support because of his limited prospects for vocational rehabilitation. He is at risk of infections, decubitus ulcers, drug addiction (to pain medications), depression, and numerous other complications secondary to the paralysis and brain injury.

Violence, in all of its forms, affects both the medical and emotional status of those who are victimized. Sometimes physical wounds heal, but as illustrated in Case 16-7, sometimes they lead to substantial disability, other medical problems, and even death. The psychological wounds of violence also often continue long after the violence. Research by Koss *et al.* (1990) with women crime victims showed that, compared with nonvictims, victims of violent crime rated their health status lower and made more physician visits over a 1-year period following the crime. Hence, violence has a significant effect on morbidity, mortality, and quality of life.

These effects of violence accrue not only to those directly victimized, but also to the patient's family. For example, Jimmy has a baby daughter whom he will not be able to swing over his head anymore. Although he receives disability checks, Jimmy has limited earning potential. Society loses out because of Jimmy's injury, as a result of his loss of productivity, and the demands his disabilities place on the healthcare and social welfare systems. The death of Jimmy's brother 3 years earlier also removed a potentially productive citizen from society.

CASE 16-8

Bill and Joy were high school sweethearts. They have been married for 8 years and have three children, aged 2, 3, and 7. Bill works as a sales representative for a sporting goods wholesaler. Joy is a homemaker. After marriage, Bill insisted that Joy stay home and "keep the home fires burning." He frequently stated proudly that Joy would "never have to work as long as he was the man of the house." She has no marketable job skills.

Shortly after marriage, Bill punched Joy in the nose and ribs during an argument. She called the police, but they did not arrest Bill, stating that if Joy wanted to press charges, she would have to go down to the courthouse the next day to press charges herself. She decided against pressing charges this time but brought the matter to the attention of her mother during a get-together a week later. Her mother instructed Joy not to bother her with such complaints, since Joy "made her bed and now she has to lie in it."

Three months later, Bill pulled Joy's hair, kicked her in the leg, and threw her onto the floor. This time, Joy went to the DA's office to press charges, just as the police instructed her. The assistant DA who took her complaint told Joy that she had better not "crap out" on him by dropping charges, like so many battered women do.

One year later, following another beating in which Bill broke Joy's nose, she went to the emergency room for medical attention. The ER physician expressed indignation that "couples these days can't seem to solve their problems without violence." He further advised her to get away from Bill, if she knew what was good for her.

Five months later, Bill blackened both of Joy's eyes. She went to speak with her pastor about the abuse. The pastor encouraged her to keep the faith, pray for the strength to forgive her husband, and try to be the best wife and mother she could.

One year later, Joy did attempt to leave Bill. Because all of the assets were in his name, however, she was unable to take more than the weekly $75 grocery money with her. She applied for food stamps and welfare benefits but because she was still married and the family income was too high, she didn't qualify for assistance. She did not have a work history or job skills to qualify for any but the most basic employment—insufficient to support her and her children.

Joy returned home, and 2 months later, suffered a back injury after Bill threw her to the floor. The examining physician was familiar with her case and that she had left Bill before, only to return. The physician concluded that she had a masochistic personality and recorded this in her chart. There was no discussion about safety planning or provision of information about battered women's advocacy services. Joy returned home once again.

WHY DOES THE PROBLEM EXIST?

Why was Bill able to use violence with impunity in Case 16-8? The easy answer is that no one told Bill he was responsible for the violence and had to stop it. Wherever Joy went for help, she was told that the violence was her responsibility. Although states differ in the legalities and criminal justice procedures for confronting partner violence, in many ways the dynamics described in case 16-8 are fairly typical of the experience of many battered women. Joy's family did not support her. The criminal justice system created barriers to arrest and prosecution. The medical system failed to provide safety assistance and negatively labeled Joy when she "failed" to do the "right" thing and leave Bill. Her religious institution encouraged her to endure the battering while suggesting that she was responsible and could control the violence. The social welfare system presented technical, bureaucratic obstacles to Joy's living independently of Bill.

In a more general sense, violence is supported by societal structures and practices that either value violence or promote the oppression of certain groups. In the case of partner violence, such oppression takes the form of sexism. Joy grew up in a society that taught her that it is her responsibility to "keep the home fires burning," care for children, and define herself as dependent on a man for support. For elder abuse, ageism is a factor. Gang and youth violence are often related to racism and classism. Violence toward sexual minorities is related to heterosexism and homophobia.

U.S. society glorifies violence in many ways, including violence-based entertainment. A report by the American Psychological Association (1993) noted that our children watch an average of 23 to 28 hours of television per week. During prime-time viewing, they see an average of 5 to 6 violent episodes per hour. During Saturday morning viewing, children see 20 to 25 violent incidents per hour.

Other social and cultural factors play a role in promoting or maintaining violence. Ready availability of handguns, high unemployment of young men, especially minorities, and urban decay, together with decreased resources for coping and conflict resolution, may all impact violence.

SOCIETAL INTERVENTIONS

A number of social-level interventions can be brought to bear on the problem of violence. The case of partner violence above serves as a heuristic for understanding factors that support and maintain violence. It also gives clear ideas for societal-level interventions to stop violence. Although other forms of violence may require unique interventions, the process of working in the community at various levels is similar.

The Criminal Justice System

A major social-level intervention involves development and implementation of criminal justice policies that include unequivocal and consistent responses that hold offenders responsible. This includes arrest, prosecution, and penalties that clearly communicate that violence is unacceptable and will not be tolerated in society. Hence, police must be expected and supported in enforcing the law. Prosecutors must pursue litigation and judges must hand down reasonable sentences. If probation is part of the sentence, probation agencies must provide adequate supervision.

The Social Services System

Many victims of violence depend on components of the social welfare and service system for assistance in surviving and escaping violence. Unfortunately, such systems often seem to operate as large, impersonal bureaucracies, with intricate, contradictory rules impossible for a person in crisis to negotiate. Although many victims would benefit from social services, they may be unaware of their options or may fail to qualify on the basis of technicalities. Social service systems can be made more "user friendly." Alternatively, a system of advocates can be developed to assist victims in accessing needed services and benefits.

Community Programs

Communities can develop prevention systems for victims of violence or high-risk families. Examples include providing respite services to caregivers of children and frail elderly. Such services and programs can support families at risk to reduce pressures and risk of violence. Further, other services and programs such as community-based recreational programs and job training programs can help people find meaning and a sense of purpose in their lives to reduce risk. Moreover, learning job skills and having employment opportunities can provide individuals with resources to escape violent situations in which they are often trapped by poverty and lack of skills.

Religious Institutions

Matters of spirituality and faith are often intertwined with violence. Those who commit violence may feel desperation, ennui, or nihilism. Victims of violence often rely on their faith, question their faith, or have their faith questioned by others. Religious and spiritual community leaders can be called on to provide healing for victims and survivors through absolution from responsibility for the violence. The healing process for offenders can be facilitated through identifying their violence as wrong and offering resources to change. Those at risk can be identified in religious settings and provided with activities and opportunities that steer them away from violence. Research has shown that youth, in particular, who identified with and were involved in church groups were less likely to be involved in gang activities (Zimmerman & Maton, 1992).

The Medical System

Because the medical system is often in the "front lines" of violence intervention in the form of trauma and emergency medicine, physicians and other healthcare providers are in a prime position to begin providing preventive care to those at risk of perpetrating and victimization. Through screening potential victims, providing patient education to all patients about ways to avoid violence, and actively supporting potential perpetrators in nonviolent life-styles, physicians can begin to make an impact. Further, physicians can influence clinic policies and protocol for identifying and assisting victims. Clinics and hospitals can provide clear public messages that they are safe places for anyone needing to escape violence.

The Education System

The education system also plays an important role in violence prevention and intervention. Guidance and health curricula can include programs for prevention of violence through respectful conflict containment and peer mediation. Children identified as at risk for violence exposure can be provided guidance-based programming to address issues related to violence in the home or neighborhood. Finally, schools can implement policies and procedures that support teachers in filing reports of child abuse and neglect.

CASE 16-9

Sue is a 16-year-old high school sophomore who comes to the clinic for her athletic physical for basketball. Her family is well known to clinic physicians. Her father is an alcoholic and her mother has struggled with depression for several years. There has been some concern that Sue's father abused her mother, but nothing was ever confirmed. Last year, Sue came to the emergency room for acute alcohol intoxication and was encouraged to see a counselor. She comments to the physician that, for the past 6 months, she has been dating Chuck. She likes him, but feels that he is too possessive and won't give her any space. She denies that she is sexually active but reports that Chuck has been putting heavy pressure on her lately.

CASE 16-10

Bill is a 76-year-old widower who lives with his 52-year-old unmarried son, Jake. Bill has been coming to the clinic for several years for monitoring of his heart medication and arthritis. Jake, an unemployed factory worker, usually brings Bill and accompanies him to the examination. Today, Bill has several bruises on his right arm and shoulder. When asked how it happened, Jake answered that he fell in the garage. The physician believes that the explanation for the injury is not consistent with the pattern of bruising. Furthermore, there were several other bruises on other parts of Bill's body in various stages of healing.

WHAT PHYSICIANS CAN DO: PREVENTION AND INTERVENTION

Sue's case, 16-9, presents many opportunities for preventive action. First, since athletic physicals are the primary types of visits for healthy adolescents, the setting alone provides an opportunity to ask about Sue's concerns for her safety, at home, in her relationship with Chuck, and at school. Although Sue might deny any concerns at present, she will appreciate being asked and will identify the physician's office as a resource for safety information if she ever needs it. Her decision-making about sex with Chuck can be validated and reinforced. She can be asked about her drinking as it relates to other high-risk activities (violence, sexual activity), and reinforced for making healthy choices in that part of her life as well. Finally, the physician may consider talking with Sue's mother during her next appointment about safety in the home.

In Case 16-10, the physician's role is intervention rather than prevention. Intervention first involves separating Bill and Jake and talking to Bill alone with reassurances that his disclosures are confidential. If there are mandatory reporting laws for elder abuse, these must be acknowledged and complied with. In every case, such disclosure should be done in collaboration with the elder, particularly if he is competent. Social service resources for assisting elder victims and families or caregiver perpetrators should be accessed. Once the abuse is acknowledged and out in the open, family-level interventions may be feasible, if all members are amenable and the perpetrator acknowledges the abuse. Part of the intervention might be to help Jake find respite care for Bill to reduce the pressure and isolation Jake feels in caring full-time for his father with no outside help. If Jake has a drinking problem, alcohol abuse counseling can also be offered. If Bill is competent to handle his own finances, he can be given anticipatory guidance about selecting an appropriate guardian and durable power of attorney, if Jake is not appropriate for the task. The physician can also advocate for Bill with social agencies to ensure that he receives adequate services to enable independent living for as long as he is able and willing. Such resources include visiting nurses, home health aids, senior center accessibility, mobile meals, and so on. Speaking out on behalf of elderly citizens to community groups, legislators, and policymakers is another way physicians can intervene on a social level.

CONCLUSIONS

Violence is a complex phenomenon that includes psychosocial, political, and medical issues. Traditionally, medical practitioners have treated primarily the biomedical sequelae of violence. The reluctance to intervene at psychosocial and political levels has been rooted in traditions that emphasize pathophysiology and biophysical mechanics of injury and rehabilitation. Etiology of violence-produced injuries has often been ignored or dismissed as outside the domain of "true" medical practice (Warshaw & Poirier, 1991). As a result, injuries have been examined outside the context of their cause. Further, medical treatments have been administered and documented in ways that dissociate the injuries from the violence that caused them.

More recently, epidemiological surveys have begun to illuminate the high incidence and prevalence of many forms of violence. These studies demonstrate that violence is not rare or aberrant in our society but is a major epidemic with profound implications for the well-being of our society. Medical implications include morbidity and mortality, which have personal, familial, and communitywide implications. These include decreased quality of life, increased stress, and economic factors such as loss of productivity, costs of medical treatment, and costs for law enforcement and justice-making.

Increased attention to violence as a social problem allows the development of a public health perspective and thus a role for the practicing physician (Hamberger, 1993). On the level of the patient and family, physicians can make violence screening a routine practice. Given the prevalence of violence in our society, there is little doubt that such screening will prove beneficial. Interventions include empathic and supportive listening and providing information about violence risks and resources for help. Intervention also includes appropriate follow-up with patients around violence issues and documentation.

Physicians can and should become involved in community and societal-level violence prevention initiatives. Such initiatives include community task forces on violence prevention and setting policy to prevent violence. One model of such an initiative is the Family Peace Project (Ambuel *et al.*, 1994). The Family Peace Project is an interdisciplinary initiative to provide healthcare professionals with the knowledge, skills, and attitudes to work with patients who are struggling with violence issues. The Project provides intensive didactic training, which includes direct contact with victim survivors and various agencies that deliver services to victims and perpetrators of violence. Physicians bring to such projects expertise and credibility as community leaders. These contributions facilitate violence prevention efforts to enhance safety for vulnerable societal members.

CASES FOR DISCUSSION

CASE 1

John is a 22-year-old drywall contractor who is coming to the office for referral for an alcohol assessment. He has a number of tattoos, including the letters L-O-V-E on his right fingers and H-A-T-E on his left fingers. He wears a large knife on his belt. His attire is consistent with someone who belongs to a motorcycle club. While giving him a "once over" the physician notices that the knuckles of both hands are scraped and scabbed. He makes numerous references to "partying" and "rock 'n rolling" in bars and with his "old lady."

1. *Has John given any hints that he may be involved in violent behavior? Explain.*
2. *How would you ask about John's use of violence?*
3. *How would John's cultural context support his use of violence?*
4. *What community resources might be helpful to John?*

CASE 2

Jenny is a 24-year-old single mother who is bringing her 13-month-old son, Jason, for a well-child check. Jenny lives with her mother and works as a waitress at the local truck stop. Jason's father is out of the picture, providing no support or visitation. During the exam, Jenny begins to talk about how Jason frequently "drives me nuts" with his "bad behavior." She reports feeling extremely tense during those episodes and copes by screaming at him and locking him in his room. Her mother, who is divorced, works and is reluctant to use her spare time watching Jason since she feels she is helpful enough by giving Jenny and Jason a place to live. As Jenny talks about her stress she begins to cry and states "I hope I don't end up doing to Jason what my mother did to me."

1. Should this mother be reported to Child Protective Services? Why or why not?
2. What community supports are needed to help Jenny cope with her situation?
3. What family interventions would facilitate Jenny's efforts to cope?
4. How would you ask Jenny about possible abuse of Jason?

CASE 3

Marie is 40 years old and is seeking medicine for "stress." She describes symptoms of anxiety that she relates to problems at work and at home. She relates that she and her husband argue a lot about sex and that he frequently calls her "frigid." These arguments last into the night, resulting in fatigue and reduced job performance the next day. In describing the problem briefly, Marie notes that sex is painful and that her husband criticizes her for not wanting sex. She adds that he states, "I don't care if you want it or not, I'm just gonna take it!"

1. Does this couple need sexual dysfunction counseling?
2. Would you prescribe antianxiety medications to Marie?
3. Would it be proper to assess Marie for a history of child sexual abuse?
4. To which community resources would you direct Marie?

CASE 4

Josh is a 29-year-old engineer coming to the clinic for help with depression and sleep disturbances. He relates that he hasn't eaten well for 2 weeks and has lost about 10 pounds. Josh further states that 2 weeks ago, his wife, Melinda, to whom he has been married for 10 years, filed for divorce. They have three children, aged 8, 6, and 3. During the discussion, Josh mentions that "I've given her everything, and now she is taking it all away." Later on he states, "I don't think I can live with this. I'm gonna have to do something to make it right."

1. Is Josh suicidal? Is it appropriate to assess suicide in this case?
2. Is Josh homicidal? If so, who could be a foreseeable target?
3. Should Josh be hospitalized?
4. Should the police be contacted?
5. Is antidepressant medication indicated?
6. Should Josh's estranged wife be warned about risks to her safety?

CASE 5

Ben is 14 years old and lives with his mother and two older sisters in an economically depressed part of town. His mother works two jobs to support the family. Ben is going to school and wants to go to college some day. The area around school and the school itself is divided by two gangs that frequently fight. Ben does not belong to any gang, but lately has been receiving a lot of pressure to join one. He is hassled on the way to school, pushed around at school, and 2 weeks ago someone threw a rock through a window of his house while his mother was at work. He is coming to the office today for an athletic physical.

1. What community resources can help support Ben's efforts to avoid gang involvement?

2. Does Ben's mother need to spend more time with him?

3. How should Ben be counseled to cope with being assaulted?

─────── RECOMMENDED READINGS ───────

American Medical Association: *JAMA* 267(22):2985–3108, 1992.

> This special issue of *JAMA* provides several empirical studies and essays on societal violence. A major focus is on firearms as a primary cause of violence.

American Medical Association: *JAMA* 267(23):3109–3240, 1992.

> This issue of *JAMA* is largely devoted to violence against women and children. Ethical and value considerations for physician involvement in violence prevention are also discussed.

American Psychological Association: *Violence and Youth: Psychology's Response*. Washington, DC: American Psychological Association, 1993.

> This report provides a comprehensive overview of the causes of violence and experiences of victims of violence. Recommendations for research and public policy are presented.

Hendricks-Matthews M, Costa AJ (eds): *Family Violence. Report of the First Ross Roundtable on Critical Issues in Family Medicine*. Columbus, OH, Ross Laboratories, 1993.

> This work provides an in-depth overview on the different types of family violence. The physician's role in violence prevention is also described.

CHAPTER 17

C. Special Problems

Mental Illness

Frank Verloin deGruy III

CASE 17-1

Louise Davis is a 35-year-old bank teller who is in Dr. Abel's office, sobbing uncontrollably. Her troubles started about 3 months ago, when she began having problems with sleep. She falls asleep at about 11 o'clock at night, but awakens at 3 or 4 AM, unable to return to sleep. Now she always feels exhausted, and has begun having difficulty concentrating at work. She notices that she frequently forgets to follow through on tasks, and has made calculation errors, something she never did previously. She has lost interest in all her hobbies, has stopped going to church, and has stopped visiting her friends. She wonders if she should be replaced at work by someone more valuable to the company.

INTRODUCTION

Mental illness is now recognized as an important health problem in this country: Mental disorders are common, they cause significant distress and impairment, and they are frequently overlooked and undertreated (Higgins, 1994). This chapter will describe the extent of diagnosable mental illness in the United States, list the most common mental disorders and the health consequences of each, describe the sources of care for people with mental illness, and describe the adequacy of care for patients with mental illness.

DEFINITION OF MENTAL ILLNESS

All proposed definitions of mental illness and mental disorder have limitations and do not work well in all circumstances. Moreover, there are fundamental disagreements over whether certain conditions should be regarded as mental illness and whether the basic problem is best understood as within the individual or within the system of relationships in which the individual is located. This disagreement has very important implications. For example, a woman who is experiencing severe abuse from her husband may well exhibit criterion symptoms for major depression. While one may define the problem as depression, an assessment at the level of the family system might yield a diagnosis such as Severe Interpersonal Conflict with Physical Abuse of an Adult; in this instance the depressive symptoms might be viewed as a normal response to an abnormal situation. These two formulations have drastically different management implications.

With these caveats in mind, I will offer the definition of mental illness given in the American Psychiatric Association's *Diagnostic and Statistical Manual of Mental Disorders*, fourth edition (DSM-IV) (American Psychiatric Association, 1994). This definition is widely accepted, and quite useful. A mental disorder is a distinct psychological or behavioral syndrome or pattern that is associated with *distress* or *impaired function*, or the *risk* of pain, disability, loss of freedom, or death. The syndrome must not be an expectable response to a traumatic event. Deviant behavior *per se*, and conflicts between an individual and society, are not considered mental disorders unless the deviance or conflict is a symptom of a dysfunction within the individual.

MIND–BODY DUALISM AND THE BIOPSYCHOSOCIAL MODEL

While it is convenient and useful to think of mental disorders as "real" entities, this convention can mislead the clinician into fundamentally misunderstanding the patient's predicament and thereby making serious management mistakes. In 1641, Rene Descartes published *Meditations on First Philosophy*, in which he postulated a dualistic reality: the external physical world and the internal mental world. Much of what we know as science rests on this formulation, and much of what we know in medicine rests on science. Nevertheless, this separation of mind from body seduces us into overlooking the deep, extensive, and inherent connections between these two domains. Mental disorders always feature physical symptoms, and physical disorders always feature mental symptoms. The two simply cannot be separated, and we do so here for heuristic purposes only. Thus, it must be kept always in mind that mental illness is an *inherently* incomplete construct—a mental diagnosis can only partly describe the condition of a person so afflicted. The clinician who desires a more comprehensive perspective will be better served by a biopsychosocial formulation, in which physical, psychological, and social domains are systemically assessed and integrated (Engel, 1977). Some would add a fourth dimension, the spiritual, to this model.

DIAGNOSTIC VARIABILITY AND CULTURAL CONSIDERATIONS

In the United States most of the mental health community has agreed to codify mental illnesses by the conventions established in the DSM-IV. In fact, the DSM-IV diagnostic conventions have enjoyed worldwide acceptance. However, a number of authors have voiced reservations about the assumptions and implications of the DSM diagnostic system (Denton, 1996; Klerman *et al.*, 1984; Ritchie, 1989); I would encourage the reader to review one or more of these critiques for a broader perspective on our practice of making mental diagnoses. A DSM-IV diagnostic entity generally consists of a list of criterion symptoms; the patient must exhibit or admit to a specified number of them. One might infer from this that mental illness manifests identically, or at least similarly, in all people, from all cultures. While certain cores symptoms of a given disorder do seem to occur across cultures, there is much transcultural variation in the manifestations of mental illness (Kleinman, 1980). For example, certain Chinese and Latina groups tend to "somatize" their distress, such that the presenting complaints of mental disorders are more likely physical symptoms (Escobar, 1987; Lin *et al.*, 1985). Moreover, some syndromes are limited to one or a few cultural settings. An example of this might be *susto*, an illness that occurs in Latina peoples. It is said to be an illness caused by intensive fright, which dislodges the soul from the body. Symptoms include insomnia, irritability, fatigue, anorexia, weight loss, restlessness, and outbursts of hysteria and fainting (Trotter, 1985).

383

PREVALENCE AND
INCIDENCE OF
MENTAL
DISORDERS IN
THE UNITED
STATES

CASE 17-2

Dr. James Ray is a family physician in a small town in the Midwest. The first six patients on his visit list this morning were:

Terry Lopez, a 4-year-old boy returning for an ear check after 10 days of antibiotics for otitis media.

Marvin Simon, a 37-year-old plumber with shoulder pain, probably the result of a rotator cuff injury.

Tonya Tolliver, a 49-year-old secretary who returns with abdominal pain. She feels overwhelmed at work and has an adolescent son who was arrested last week.

Jerry Davis, a 50-year-old salesman who came in to get a prescription for insomnia. He drinks about 12 beers a night while he is on the road, which is four or five nights a week.

Angela Barnes, an 80-year-old woman who complains of constipation. Her son, with whom she lives, reports that she has worsening forgetfulness, disorientation, and crying spells.

Chelsea McGovern, a 25-year-old physical therapist who came in for a Pap smear and oral contraceptives.

PREVALENCE AND INCIDENCE OF MENTAL DISORDERS IN THE UNITED STATES

Of the six patients in Case 17-2, two (Jerry Davis and Angela Barnes) have strong evidence for a mental diagnosis, and another (Tonya Tolliver) has a physical symptom that seems related to her mental distress. This would be a fairly typical clinical experience for a primary care physician, and reflects the frequency with which mental illness and symptoms appear in the population that primary physicians serve.

THE EPIDEMIOLOGIC STUDIES

The ECA Study

The edifice of knowledge in medicine is uneven, and in some places entirely absent. Happily, this situation does not apply to our knowledge of the nature and extent of mental disorders in the United States. Thanks to an extraordinary study—the Epidemiological Catchment Area (ECA) Study—we know a great deal about the mental illnesses that affect our citizenry, which subgroups are particularly affected, who receives services for these disorders, and where these services are rendered (Robins & Regier, 1991). This study was conducted in the 1980s, and consisted of careful diagnostic interviews with over 20,000 subjects randomly selected from five sites. One of the most important general findings from this study was that 32% of Americans had experienced a mental disorder at some time in their lives, and 20% had an active disorder. Thus, this is a problem of enormous magnitude—which is why mental health care education, research, and provision of services have become national priorities.

In the ECA Study there were important differences in prevalence by site, from a high of 41% lifetime and 27% current diagnosis rate in Baltimore, to a low of 28% lifetime and 18% current in New Haven. From this and other epidemiologic studies we also learned that most people seeking care for mental disorders do so in a primary care, rather than a mental health care, setting.

There are quite a lot of population-based data on specific mental disorders, or particular aspects of specific disorders, that augment and corroborate the ECA data set and that sometimes address important issues not dealt with in the ECA Study. I have largely ignored this literature, electing instead the path of parsimony and simplicity: The reader can find most of the salient findings of the ECA Study collected under one volume, to which I have made extensive reference (Robins & Regier, 1991).

The MOS Study

The ECA Study was population-based and selected subjects at their homes. An equally ambitious study (or set of studies) has been conducted with *patients*—people who were selected from the waiting rooms of physicians' offices in three cities—to learn about their illnesses and symptoms. This study, the Medical Outcomes Study (MOS), was not concerned specifically with mental disorders, but assessed patients with certain tracer conditions: hypertension, coronary artery disease, diabetes, chronic lung disease, and depression (Wells *et al.*, 1988). The MOS contains much detail about the functional consequences of these conditions and the adequacy of care rendered for patients with these conditions. This was the first study to show, for example, that depression was a serious medical illness, with impairment equal to or exceeding other chronic medical conditions (Wells *et al.*, 1989).

The PRIME-MD 1000 Study

This study, which was undertaken in four U.S. primary care practices, aimed to develop and validate an instrument for making rapid and accurate mental diagnoses in primary care settings (Spitzer *et al.*, 1994). The PRIME-MD study documented the incidence and profiled the characteristics of patients in this setting with any of 24 mental diagnoses. This study measured the extent of comorbidity between diagnoses, and compared the impairment associated with these disorders with that of common physical disorders. One of the principal findings of this study was that 26% of primary care patients currently suffer from a mental disorder, and another 13% qualify for a "subthreshold" diagnosis, not sufficient to meet DSM-III-R (or DSM-IV) criteria, but sufficient to show significant functional impairment. It is noteworthy that there was considerable variation across sites—the site range for any PRIME-MD diagnosis was 30–52%. Another important finding from this study was the demonstration that functional impairments and disability in primary care patients were much more strongly related to mental disorders than physical diagnoses (Spitzer *et al.*, 1995).

Much work from the international perspective has been directed by the World Health Organization; for example, their recently completed Collaborative Study on Psychological Problems in General Health Care detailed the relative prevalence and functional consequences of mental illnesses in primary health care facilities in 14 cities around the world (Ormel *et al.*, 1994). This study, which included over 5000 patients, showed an overall incidence of current mental disorder of 21%, with a dramatic range across sites, from a high of 53% for patients in Santiago, to a low of 8% for patients in Shanghai.

CASE 17-3

Peter Bosarge is a 41-year-old evangelical preacher who came to the emergency room because of chest pain. For the last month, every time he begins to preach, he has developed a sharp left-sided chest pain, a feeling of breathlessness, diaphoresis, and an overwhelming fear that he is going to die. Immediately thereafter he develops diarrhea, and the episode passes. Early this morning he was awakened from a sound sleep with another attack. His father, also a preacher, died of a heart attack at age 41. He has undergone exhaustive cardiac evaluation, including two catheterizations, and no heart disease is present. He has become so fearful of another attack that he has stopped preaching.

THE DIAGNOSTIC ENTITIES

THE DISORDERS

There are over 250 mental disorders listed in the DSM-IV manual. Most of these diagnoses have a relatively large medical literature associated with them. It is far beyond the scope of this chapter to even mention all of these illnesses, let alone describe them. Our purposes will be better served by simply grouping mental illnesses into general categories and describing a few selected disorders within these categories. I will therefore attempt to describe only those mental diagnoses that, because of their frequency, seriousness, or impact on medical or mental health practice, are of the most consequence to the health of our nation.

CASE 17-4

Jerry Baker was 39 years old when he finally made an appointment to see his wife's family physician. He had been extremely successful in his business career, having acquired and successfully run almost a dozen companies. He had always been an exceptionally hardworking man—his wife described him as obsessed with work—but for the past 6 months he had experienced progressively more difficulty doing his work. He described two problems: loss of motivation and difficulty actually attending to the details of his work. His mind would drift, and he began forgetting to do things. His motivation became so impaired that he refused to go to work for an entire week, a behavior that cost one of his companies several hundred thousand dollars. This precipitated his visit to the physician. He described himself as a "shell" of his former self: He didn't enjoy work any more. He didn't enjoy anything any more; even his passion for good food had disappeared. He had begun sleeping up to 14 hours a day, and still was fatigued. He had actually begun thinking that he and his family would be better off if he were dead.

His physician conducted a thorough physical evaluation, and discovered no abnormalities, other than profound sadness and slowing of thought and movement in this previously energetic, optimistic man.

Depression and Other Mood Disorders

More people are afflicted by mood disorders than any other category of mental illness. We will concern ourselves here with three diagnoses within this general category: major depression, dysthymia, and bipolar disorder. What are these disorders? What do people who have them look like? Case 17-1, which opened this chapter, and Case 17-4, just above, describe people who are suffering from a major depressive episode. The salient symptoms are a loss of interest in previously enjoyable activities, insomnia or hypersomnia, fatigue, psychomotor retardation (or agitation), diminished ability to concentrate, and feelings of worthlessness, including suicidal thoughts. In the general medical setting, about 25% of adults are suffering from a mood disorder (Spitzer *et al.*, 1994). The distribution of diagnoses within this category and the general demographic breakdown parallel that of the general population.

While symptoms must have been present for only 2 weeks for a major depressive episode, the diagnostic criteria for dysthymic disorder require the presence of symptoms most of the time for at least 2 years. During this time, the person must have had a depressed mood and at least two other symptoms such as poor appetite (or overeating), insomnia (or hypersomnia), fatigue, difficulty concentrating, poor self-esteem, or feelings of hopelessness.

Bipolar disorder is characterized by episodes of mania or hypomania, usually also interspersed with depressive episodes. A manic episode is dramatic to behold and terrible to experience; it consists of at least 1 week of elevated, expansive, or irritable mood, in conjunction with grandiosity, decreased need for sleep, pressure of speech, racing thoughts and flight of ideas, easy distractibility, and excessive pursuit of pleasurable, often risky, behavior. People experiencing a manic episode often feel invulnerable and cannot be persuaded that their behavior is inappropriate; therefore, treatment is difficult to initiate.

In the U.S. population, about 8% of adults have met criteria for one of the mood diagnoses in their lifetimes: 5% have suffered a major depressive episode, 3% meet criteria for dysthymia, and less than 1% have ever experienced a manic episode. In the general population, women are affected by mood disorders at about twice the rate as men; diagnostic rates tend to decrease with age, and are roughly comparable across racial and ethnic categories (Robins & Regier, 1991). There is some evidence for a genetic predisposition, particularly for the bipolar disorders; divorce and unemployment seem to be risk factors for depression (American Psychiatric Association, 1994). People with bipolar and major depressive disorders use far more health services, both psychiatric and medical, than their unaffected counterparts (Leaf, 1994).

Miriam Welch had shredded three tissues in the first 3 minutes of her office visit. She was so fidgety that her physician was beginning to feel nervous just being in the room with her. Miriam was 29 years old and on the verge of remarrying. She came in for a contraception examination, but it was clear she had something else on her mind: "I have always been a worrier, but this has gotten ridiculous. For the last year or two, I have stayed on edge about everything. Everything worries me now. My new marriage might not work out. I probably will get laid off when our company reorganizes, then I won't make my rent and will get evicted, and on and on. I get headaches all the time, and I've gotten to where I can't keep my mind on anything more than a minute. I can't even read the newspaper any more, for being so distracted. I just feel so tired and irritable and on edge!"

Anxiety Disorders

The anxiety disorders encompass panic disorder, phobias, obsessive–compulsive disorder, posttraumatic stress disorder, acute stress disorder, and generalized anxiety disorder. As a group, these disorders are almost as common as the mood disorders. Each condition has its own characteristic clinical presentation; the most common ones will be summarized briefly here.

Peter Bosarge, described in Case 17-3, is suffering from panic disorder and is developing secondary phobias. Note the sudden appearance of intense fear and discomfort. This patient's panic attacks were associated with cardiac symptoms, but the symptoms can also be gastrointestinal (diarrhea, nausea), neurological (numbness, dizziness), or psychological (fear of dying or going crazy). The person must have either recurrent attacks or a persistent fear of recurrence. One of the most problematic complications of panic attacks is the development of avoidance behaviors, or phobias. This is a fear of being in a place or situation in which help might not be available or escape might be difficult in case of a panic attack. Such phobias can severely limit a person's ability to carry on a normal life—people with severe phobias may become completely homebound. About 2–3% of people have at some time qualified for panic disorder, and about half of them have an associated agoraphobia (Robins & Regier, 1991). Like depression, the disorder is found in about twice as many women as men.

People with obsessive–compulsive disorder are burdened with either recurrent obsessions or compulsions that are time-consuming or cause significant distress or impairment. The affected person can see that this is unreasonable, but is unable to prevent the intrusive thoughts or behaviors. Obsessions are persistent thoughts or impulses, usually unrelated to a real-life problem, such as concern over contamination from shaking hands, or fear that one has left the door unlocked or the stove on, or sexual imagery or aggressive impulses. These thoughts or impulses cause distress. Compulsions are repetitive behaviors (e.g., repetitive hand washing) or mental acts (e.g., counting, repeating words) employed to reduce the distress. The ECA data suggest a lifetime incidence of 2.6% for obsessive–compulsive disorder, which is surprisingly high in light of the much lower incidence measured in mental health and general medical settings. This suggests that many people with obsessive–compulsive disorder do not seek help for their condition, at least from a medical or mental health professional. This condition is equally common in males and females, and usually begins in adolescence or early adulthood.

Acute stress disorder and posttraumatic stress disorder (PTSD) can be thought of as essentially the same disorder at different points in time. After an extremely traumatic stressor, such as witnessing a murder, or being raped or tortured, or learning of the unexpected or violent death of a family member, a person may develop a characteristic set of symptoms. These symptoms involve flashbacks or dreams about the event; avoidance behavior or numbing of feelings associated with the trauma; and symptoms of agitation, insomnia, irritability, or hypervigilance. If these symptoms have persisted less than 1 month, the person may qualify for the diagnosis of acute stress disorder. If the symptoms have persisted for more than 1 month, PTSD would be the more appropriate diagnosis. Estimates vary, but probably 25% of the population have suffered from one of these conditions at some time. Certain forms of severe, prolonged sexual and physical abuse, particularly within families, lead to a variant of PTSD characterized by certain personality deformations, severe depression, somatizing behavior, and a tendency toward panic and other anxiety symptoms. These patients are surprisingly common in the primary care setting—the incidence is probably 2–3%, based on a sample of 300 patients in three family practices (deGruy et al., 1994).

Generalized anxiety disorder is characterized by excessive, uncontrollable, free-floating worry and anxiety. Miriam Welch, described in Case 17-5, exemplifies this condition. In order to meet DSM-IV criteria, this anxiety must have been present for at least 6 months, and must be accompanied by three of the following: muscle tension, fatigue or irritability, difficulty concentrating, insomnia, restlessness. About 5% of adults have met criteria for this disorder at some time, and about twice as many women as men are affected. Unfortunately, the symptoms of anxiety tend to be chronic, and often persist, with variable intensity, over the course of a lifetime. Symptoms of generalized anxiety, whether or not they reach the diagnostic threshold, accompany most medical illnesses, and so anxiety symptoms are extremely common in the medical setting. About 7% of adults in the PRIME-MD Study met criteria for current generalized anxiety disorder, with a site range of 2–13%.

CASE 17-6

Dr. Fletcher looked with dismay over his morning clinic schedule. There, third from the top, was Daria Ruhle. This would be a long morning. Ms. Ruhle faithfully appeared on the schedule at least twice a month; she usually came in with a list of physical complaints at least two pages long, and two or three of these were sure to be severe. She had the thickest chart in the practice, having had innumerable diagnostic workups over the years. All of these workups had been negative, but of course this did little to remove the symptoms themselves, or her concern that there was a physical explanation for these symptoms. In the past year she had been evaluated for recurrent headaches, abdominal pain, leg numbness, blurry vision, nausea, passing out, wrist pain, knee pain, chest pain, weakness, and difficulty urinating.

Somatoform Disorders

The somatoform disorders are characterized by the presence of physical symptoms that cannot be explained by a general medical condition. These symptoms are not intentional and not under voluntary control, and are thereby distinct from Factitious Disorders and Malingering. The symptoms must cause significant functional impairment or result in medical treatment. Only the most severe of the somatoform disorders will be discussed here, namely, somatization disorder.

Somatization disorder is characterized by multiple unexplained physical complaints, as exemplified by Ms. Ruhle in Case 17-6. There is some controversy about the proper diagnostic disposition of patients with multiple somatic complaints, and a number of alternative classifications exist; the DSM-IV requires at least four different pain symptoms, two gastrointestinal symptoms, one sexual symptom, and one pseudoneurological symptom. Somatization disorder in rare in the population: The pooled incidence in the ECA study was 0.13%. Such a rare condition would not ordinarily merit consideration in this overview, but patients affected with this condition are far more common in the general medical setting, and their medical care is extremely expensive. The incidence is about 5–15% in primary care practices, where these patients appear frequently for care. By one estimate, physicians expend nine times as much money on their healthcare than the population average (Smith *et al.*, 1986a). This is generally thought to be related in part to unnecessary diagnostic evaluation by physicians. Somatization disorder has a much higher prevalence among women than men, generally by a ratio of about ten to one (Smith *et al.*, 1985). There are interesting familial patterns associated with this disorder, including somatization and depression in female family members and antisocial characteristics and substance abuse in male family members (Cloninger *et al.*, 1986; Guze, 1993; Guze *et al.*, 1986). There is a strong association between a history of sexual or physical abuse and subsequent somatizing behavior (deGruy *et al.*, 1994).

CASE 17-7

Eric Nelson was a loner. He had grown up as the only child of a drill press operator and a textile mill worker in the Deep South. He had done well through high school, but his classmates hardly knew the sound of his voice. He seemed nice enough, but he certainly kept to himself. In fact, he had never had a friend. During his first semester away from home at college, he began receiving messages through the fillings in his teeth. At first he thought these messages were from his father, but as they became more clear and understandable, he realized that they were from angels warning him about various dangers. He would receive information about which routes to walk on his way to class, and even what to avoid eating and drinking. Soon he began having conversations, aloud, with his guardian angels, and began wearing a ski mask over his face at all times to protect himself from poisonous gases on the campus.

Schizophrenia

Schizophrenia is perhaps the most devastating of the mental illnesses. While there are a number of subtypes of schizophrenia, all are characterized by two or more of the following symptoms:

- Delusions, usually bizarre and often persecutory
- Hallucinations, usually auditory
- Disorganized, loose, tangential speech
- Disorganized, inappropriate behavior

- Negative symptoms such as loss of normal emotional expressiveness, poverty of speech, inability to begin and maintain goal-directed activities

Although schizophrenia is relatively rare, occurring in 1.3% of the population, it tends to appear during late adolescence or early adulthood, completely removes people from their normal spheres of activity, and most of the time causes at least some lifelong impairment. Most people with schizophrenia do not marry, are unemployed or employed at low-level jobs, and have limited social contacts, although there are exceptions to this pattern. Men and women are equally affected. Schizophrenia has a strong familial predilection, although environmental factors also contribute to the appearance of this illness.

Most of the conditions described in this chapter have been characterized as frequent in general medical practice. Schizophrenia is an exception to this rule. While patients with schizophrenia definitely have pronounced physical symptomatology, the mental symptoms are usually so severe and so clearly mental that most of these patients get their care in mental health settings. In fact, the NAMCS data suggest that about one-third of the content of ambulatory psychiatry consists of management of patients with schizophrenia.

SUBTHRESHOLD CONDITIONS

As a general rule, a condition is called a mental illness if two criteria are met: A specified set of symptoms must be present, and these symptoms must collectively cause some sort of impairment. In recent years the assessment of functional health has enjoyed considerable development, so that the measurement of impairment has become much more specific and refined. This development has created an interesting situation in the field of mental health. It turns out that functional impairment frequently occurs before the requisite symptom count threshold has been exceeded. Thus arises the concept of *subthreshold conditions*—symptoms too few or too mild to meet diagnostic criteria, but sufficient to cause significant impairment. This creates quite a sharp dilemma: On the one hand we do not wish to "pathologize" or "medicalize" every twitch and tic, every stress and complaint that occurs in life; on the other hand we do not wish to overlook the plight of people who are suffering significant impairment in their functional health. So there is some instability in the field with respect to the concept of diagnostic threshold, and we can expect that diagnostic criteria will most likely undergo adjustments as clinicians and researchers come to grips with this dilemma.

This issue is most salient with respect to depression, somatization, and perhaps panic and other anxiety disorders.

With respect to depression, severe and persistent symptoms have occurred in up to one-third of the population; minor depression (consisting of at least two of the criterion symptoms for at least 2 weeks) is more common than major depression, and almost as disabling. This is true of the population in general (Robins & Regier, 1991) and of medical patients in particular (Broadhead et al., 1990; Spitzer et al., 1994; Wells et al., 1989).

With respect to somatization, almost 12% of the population meet criteria for lifetime somatization syndrome, consisting of four or more symptoms for men, and six or more for women (Escobar et al., 1989). This is 100 times the incidence of somatization disorder. These patients having somatization syndrome were more likely to be unemployed and to be on welfare than their unaffected counterparts; those who were employed received significantly less pay than employed nonsomatizing people. This pattern repeats in the clinical realm. Subthreshold or abridged somatization is far more common than somatization disorder, and the patients so affected exhibit significantly higher utilization of medical resources and lower levels of functional health than matched nonsomatizing patients.

Sandra Fulcher is a 34-year-old woman with a long history of physical complaints that her physician has been unable to explain: On separate occasions in the past 5 years she has been evaluated for shortness of breath, chest pain, back pain, joint pain, headaches, fatigue, dizziness, blurry vision, nausea, abdominal bloating, burning with urination, pain with intercourse, and painful menstruation. Last visit her physician completed a thorough mental evaluation, and discovered that she met criteria for major depression, panic disorder, and PTSD. The implicated stressor in her diagnosis of PTSD was prolonged, severe sexual abuse by her father when she was a child.

THE PROBLEM OF COMORBIDITY

THE EXTENT AND NATURE OF COMORBIDITY

Case 17-8 illustrates that people with one mental disorder frequently have at least another. The ECA Study made the surprising discovery that all subjects meeting criteria for somatization disorder met criteria for at least one other DSM diagnosis (Robins & Regier, 1991). Those most commonly implicated were phobias, major depression, and panic disorder. This pattern is also found in the medical setting, wherein patients with both somatization disorder and intermediate somatization exhibit an extraordinarily high likelihood of having other mental diagnoses (Brown *et al.*, 1990). Moreover, the mere presence of unexplained physical symptoms increases the likelihood that a primary care patient meets criteria for a mental diagnosis, and this likelihood rises with the number of unexplained symptoms (Kroenke *et al.*, 1994).

We have identified a subset of female patients who meet diagnostic criteria for somatization disorder, who came out of dangerous, abusive families, and who themselves have been abused; these women have an average of over four additional DSM-III-R diagnoses (usually depression, panic, PTSD, other anxiety diagnoses, and substance abuse) and are suffering profound functional impairment (deGruy *et al.*, 1994). This comorbidity is so extensive as to call into question the appropriateness of the diagnosis of somatization disorder. When comorbidity is extensive, one must question whether a more fundamental, comprehensive diagnostic formulation might be more fitting. In this case, some variation of extreme PTSD might more accurately (and more sympathetically) portray this condition.

Somatization is not the only condition implicated in this web of comorbidity. For example, the WHO Study cited earlier demonstrated that all specific psychiatric disorders had comorbidity rates above 50% except alcohol dependence, which had a comorbidity rate of 43% (Ormel *et al.*, 1994). Seventy-one percent of patients with panic disorder had another ICD-10 psychiatric diagnosis, and 62% of patients with a major depressive episode had a comorbid diagnosis.

CASE 17-9

Thomas Layton is a 58-year-old man who suffered a myocardial infarction 3 months ago. His hospital course was uncomplicated, although he was pessimistic about his prospects of returning to a normal life, and he was discharged home to a cardiac rehabilitation program consisting of dietary instruction and a graded exercise regimen. His physician advised him that he should be able to return to normal work activities as a draftsman in about a month. On returning home, however, he expressed increasing pessimism about his future, refused participation in the cardiac rehabilitation program, and showed no interest in returning to work. He became increasingly irritable and agitated and refused visitors. He repeatedly told his wife that "his life was over." Indeed, 4 months after discharge, he died in his sleep.

THE HEALTH CONSEQUENCES
OF MENTAL ILLNESS

MORTALITY

The association between mental illness and mortality has been convincingly and repeatedly demonstrated. The ECA Study documented that people over 55 years of age were four times more likely to die in the ensuing 15 months if they were suffering from major depression than if they were not (Robins & Regier, 1991). In a well-done study of 500 psychiatric outpatients with a wide range of diagnoses followed for an average of 7 years, this cohort had nearly twice the mortality rate of the age-, sex-, and race-adjusted reference population (Martin *et al.*, 1985).

As Mr. Layton's story in Case 17-9 suggests, patients who sustain a myocardial infarction are at increased risk; one study documented a fourfold increased likelihood of death in the following 6 months for those who are depressed at the time of discharge compared with those who are not (Smith *et al.*, 1993). Of course, some of the mortality associated with mental illness is direct: Approximately 15% of patients with severe depression will commit suicide (Fawcett, 1988), and patients with severe panic disorder may be even more likely to kill themselves (Weissman *et al.*, 1989). It is interesting to note that patients with somatization disorder do not appear to be at increased risk of death because of this disorder (Coryell & Norten, 1981).

MORBIDITY

Patients with mental disorders suffer poor health. There are at least two aspects to this relationship. First, mental disorders themselves are associated with significant functional impairment. For example, the MOS study demonstrated that patients suffering from depression are equally or more impaired than comparable patients suffering from medical problems such as hypertension, arthritis, or chronic lung disease (Wells *et al.*, 1989). Even more startling is the finding reported from the PRIME-MD 1000 Study that, among primary care patients, the proportion of functional impairment attributable to mental disorders far outweighs the proportion attributable to physical disorders (Spitzer *et al.*, 1995). In other words, mental disorders themselves seem to cause profound impairment.

The second aspect of this association between mental illness and poor health is related to the comorbidity between mental and medical disorders, such that about two-thirds of patients with a mental diagnosis will have a significant medical problem, with its attendant morbidity (Bridges & Goldberg, 1985; Kroenke *et al.*, 1994). Conversely, patients with medical disorders have a two- to threefold increased likelihood of having a mental diagnosis (Weyerer, 1990). A special case of this mental–medical comorbidity is the peculiar relationship between certain medical disorders, such as stroke or cancer, and mental diagnoses (Wells *et al.*, 1988). It appears that when one has a stroke, for example, one is particularly vulnerable to depression, and when both appear together, the patient is likely to be severely impaired.

USE OF HEALTHCARE RESOURCES

There is a great deal of evidence that patients with mental disorders use more healthcare resources than their unaffected counterparts. Much of this evidence is indirect and in need of confirmation, but several interesting patterns have emerged.

Katon and colleagues conducted a study of distressed high utilizers (top 10% healthcare expenditures) in a primary care setting. Over half were found to qualify for a mental diagnosis (Katon *et al.*, 1990).

Primary care patients with DSM diagnoses show about a twofold increase in healthcare utilization compared with patients without mental diagnoses (Shapiro *et al.*, 1984).

Patients diagnosed with a depressive episode show a rise in visit frequency during the 6 months prior to a diagnosis of depression being made, with a tapering off of visit frequency after the diagnosis has been made and treatment instituted (Widmer & Cadoret, 1978).

Perhaps the most conspicuous utilizers are patients with the diagnosis of somatization disorder. deGruy and colleagues demonstrated that patients selected from a family practice waiting room with this disorder had charts twice as thick, and visit frequencies to the primary care physician nearly twice as great, as matched controls (deGruy *et al.*, 1987). Smith and colleagues studied a group of primary care patients recruited for their conspicuous somatizing behavior, and documented a *ninefold* increased rate of overall expenditure for healthcare, relative to the general population (Smith *et al.*, 1986a).

CASE 17-10

Nadine Carney recognized what was happening to her. She had been down this road before. She and her husband had retired last July, and since moving to her new home on the Gulf Coast, she had not enjoyed the sense of freedom and leisure she had anticipated. In fact, she felt terrible, even though she felt "great": She was growing agitated, irritable, and talkative. She was beginning to stay awake at night, and felt the pressure of thoughts crowding into her head, demanding action. She was beginning to feel as though she was having the most profound, important ideas a human had ever had, and this spelled trouble—her mania was returning. She had been admitted to a private psychiatric hospital 14 years ago, after her symptoms had gotten completely out of control, but had returned to her normal mental state after beginning lithium. She took this medication for 10 years, initially under the direction of her admitting psychiatrist, but eventually her family physician assumed responsibility for monitoring her mental status and her lithium levels; when he retired 3 years ago she simply stopped filling her prescriptions. Now she was getting in trouble again. She knew she needed to begin treatment quickly, before she was "over the edge" again, but didn't know whether to seek psychiatric admission, see a private psychiatrist, visit her family physician, or simply start taking lithium.

RESPONSES TO THE PROBLEM

SOCIETY'S RESPONSE TO MENTAL ILLNESS

One might organize a brief outline of how we as a nation have responded to the problem of mental illness among our citizenry by using as a point of departure the President's Commission on Mental Health, spearheaded by Rosalynn Carter in 1978 (President's Commission on Mental Health, 1978). Prior to this time, several events had occurred that laid the groundwork for the questions raised and programs begun by that commission. In 1961, the Joint Commission on Mental Illness and Health, drawing on census data from mental institutions and early, rough epidemiological data, recommended the Community Health Centers Program as a means of dealing with the mental health needs of the poor and of avoiding unnecessary hospitalization for the mentally ill. Subsequently, many patients with mental illnesses were deinstitutionalized. Concurrently, diagnostic nomenclature and criteria became much more valid and reliable, and by the time DSM-III was developed, it was possible to diagnose the "same" mental disorders across settings. Nevertheless, at the time of the President's Commission, there were still few answers to a number of critically important questions: We knew something about the range of disorders affecting patients currently or formerly in mental institutions, but what proportion of the total national burden of mental illness did this represent? How many of our citizens suffer from mental disorders? In what populations do these disorders occur? What are the health consequences of these disorders? Do these people seek care for their problems? Where? How adequate is the care that is rendered in various settings, and how effective are the treatments even when adequately rendered? A number of ambitious programs were instituted to address these questions, including programs of research and training in the mental health specialty and primary care medical sectors and the extraordinary ECA program, which mapped the mental health of the United States.

While we can be encouraged by the enormous progress in our knowledge about and treatment of mental illness, this progress is seriously deficient in certain areas. At this time only about 20% of patients with mental diagnoses seek help for their condition (Robins & Regier, 1991, p. 341). Moreover, the structure of our healthcare system and our funding priorities practically guarantee that important problems with the care of the mentally ill will persist. The mental health care of children and the elderly is seriously deficient, and we still have a need for improved care of ambulatory patients with serious mental illnesses. Perhaps two of the most important problems are the generally inadequate health insurance benefit for mental health care and the difficulty incorporating mental health care into the incentives and practice structure of the primary healthcare system.

THE CLINICIAN'S RESPONSE TO MENTAL ILLNESS

It is generally conceded that, while most mental health care transpires in the primary care medical setting, the quality and extent of this care are less than optimal. This problem has received extensive discussion recently, and is the subject of considerable research. At the risk of oversimplifying the present state of affairs, I would venture the following summary:

People who present to primary care physicians with mental symptoms and disorders are different from those who appear for care in a mental health care setting. They often present with physical rather than psychological complaints (Bridges & Goldberg, 1985); when this happens, the clinician is less likely to diagnose a mental disorder (Kirmayer *et al.*, 1993). Remember also that comorbidity is extensive, and patients tend to have confusing constellations of symptoms that do not fit very well into the existing classifications.

While primary care physicians tend to have incomplete knowledge of the diagnostic criteria for mental diagnoses (Badger *et al.*, 1994), simple education has little effect on diagnostic accuracy. In fact, provision of diagnostic information alone appears to have little effect on management of mental disorders in primary care (Magruder-Habib *et al.*, 1989).

While protocol-type interventions for specific mental disorders, such as depression (Schulberg *et al.*, 1995) or somatization (Smith *et al.*, 1986b, 1995), have been shown to result in improved outcomes, these have proven difficult to implement in this setting. Even though patients may be extremely resistant to accepting a referral to a mental health professional (Olfson, 1991), they are also resistant to accepting and staying in treatment by their primary care physician (Schulberg *et al.*, 1995). Moreover, even the primary care physician who likes to deal with psychosocial issues faces a number of disincentives, such as a long list of competing demands for the 10–15 minutes allotted for the patient's visit (including dealing with the presenting complaint and with health maintenance issues), the stigma to the patient of a mental diagnosis, and the unwillingness of third parties to pay for mental health services rendered in this setting. Some managed care plans insist that all patients with mental diagnoses be referred to mental health specialists for care, even though the patients refuse to accept the referral.

Nevertheless, there is progress. For example, the PRIME-MD and the SDDS-PC are two of a new generation of instruments that can quickly and accurately make multiple mental diagnoses in the primary care setting. These are powerful case-finding tools that lend a new impetus to the search for effective management strategies within the primary care setting. In fact, several interesting management strategies are currently under investigation, and some have been shown to be effective and cost-effective in the primary care setting, notwithstanding the difficulty of their implementation. For example, Schulberg and colleagues have demonstrated that primary care patients who are randomized into a protocol involving careful administration either of an antidepressant or of psychotherapy, both administered in the primary care setting, fare substantially better than similar patients exposed to usual care (Schulberg *et al.*, 1995). Katon and colleagues demonstrated that primary care patients who receive a consultation visit with a psychiatrist have significantly better outcomes than those receiving usual care (Katon *et al.*, 1995). Smith and colleagues have demonstrated that primary care patients with somatization disorder and with abridged somatization (6–12 unexplained symptoms) benefit if their primary care physician receives a consultation letter from a psychiatrist; group therapy also helps these patients (Smith *et al.*, 1986b, 1995). At this time there are a score of clinical trials under way testing a variety of interventions against mental disorders in the primary care setting; many of these trials are collaborative efforts taking place within the primary care setting.

CONCLUSION

Recently we have learned about the startling degree to which mental disorders affect our nation's health. These disorders are surprisingly common, both in the general population and in various medical settings. They are also surprisingly debilitating. We are accustomed to regarding chronic medical illnesses as causing functional impairment, but mental illnesses have been shown to be as much or more injurious to a person's ability to function normally. Add to this two important barriers: (1) that people do not wish to be known as mentally ill, and will resist seeking care for these problems, and (2) when they do seek care, it is most often in a medical setting, with their mental distress disguised by physical complaints or confounded with physical illness. The training of medical practitioners and the structure of their practices work against the successful management of mental disorders, and the management of these disorders in segregated mental health specialty settings is fraught with problems—the inherent inseparability of the mental and the physical, the resistance of many patients to accepting care in a mental health specialty setting, and the tendency of care to become fragmented and redundant.

Despite these important obstacles, much progress has been made in addressing these problems. We have evolved a reliable and exceptionally powerful diagnostic system for mental disorders. We now have an accurate profile of these disorders and their constituent symptoms as they occur in the population and in various healthcare and mental health care settings. We have begun to learn about the functional consequences of these disorders, and we have begun to learn a great deal about the care people with mental illness need and receive. We continue to discover more efficacious treatments for the various mental disorders, and are likewise learning how to apply these treatments more effectively. Despite the enormous islands of ignorance remaining in our knowledge of mental illness, and the equally enormous discrepancy between the knowledge we have and the service we actually render, we can take hope that sufficient infrastructure, investigators, and providers are in place to feed the stream of progress in the field. We have good reason to be optimistic about the future of this long-neglected domain, even though we have far to go before we can rest assured that the mental health care needs of our citizens and our patients are adequately addressed.

CASES FOR DISCUSSION

CASE 1

Eddie Nelson was having trouble with his bowels. Since his childhood he had had trouble with constipation, and now he knew why. His food was being poisoned by the FBI, who wanted to keep him quiet about their secret operations in the West. For years he had harbored a suspicion that our government was intruding illegally into his life. Two years ago he had joined the CFF, a well-funded and well-organized group dedicated to eliminating these illegal violations of privacy. Lately, however, he had stopped going to meetings and stopped talking to CFF members. The FBI had begun planting distracting thoughts in his head, buzzing about the weather conspiracy and their agents who worked for the television and newspaper companies. He had taken to humming loudly as a way of keeping the buzzing from driving him crazy. He knew that the woman posing as his physician was also trying to poison him with the medication she was giving him, and he avoided taking it whenever possible.

His parents first became worried about a year ago, when he became much more reclusive and suspicious than usual. For almost 6 months prior to his hospitalization, he had refused to leave his room; his mother had sought help for her son when he began defecating in his room to avoid the bathroom, which he believed to be bugged. Initially he had responded dramatically to medication, but lately his old symptoms were returning.

1. *Does Eddie Nelson have a mental disorder? If so, what are the symptoms that suggest mental illness?*
2. *Did he have a mental illness 5 years ago? If not, at what point would you say his mental illness began?*

3. Eddie does not wish to take medication, which he believes steals his awareness of what the FBI is trying to do to him. His parents wish for him to take medication. Is it ethical to force him to take medication over his objections? If his parents wished him left unmedicated, what would be the proper thing to do?

CASE 2

"Twelve more years before retirement. I don't think I can make it. I don't think I can make it for another month. I used to love my work, but now I just don't care. All I want to do is stay in my recliner and watch the tube. Not that I enjoy that either, but I don't feel like doing anything else. I don't have the energy to do anything. I don't eat, I can't sleep, I can't think clearly. I dunno, I give up. I just can't go on living like this." Two months ago Regina Jacobi had been promoted to floor supervisor, a position she had been hoping for 4 years. While this promotion brought new stresses, these were neither unmanageable nor entirely unwelcome. Then her mother died unexpectedly. Shortly thereafter "the color began to go out" of her life, and the symptoms described above began.

1. Does Ms. Jacobi have a mental disorder? If so, what would you call it? If you can't decide or don't know, what additional information would you like to have?
2. What role does stress and loss play in her symptoms? Would the presence of these factors change the way the physician manages this situation?
3. What are the management options here? Is this something that should be handled in the primary care medical setting? In the mental health setting? In the hospital?

CASE 3

Nicole Dunnagan told a hair-raising story. Her life had been normal—boring, even—until last New Year's Eve, when she went to a party at a friend's house. Shortly after midnight she left for home, but was assaulted in the parking lot as she got into her car. Her assailant abducted her at knifepoint, drove her deep into the woods, and brutally raped and beat her. She suffered facial fractures, laryngeal edema from strangulation, a laceration of her right breast, and severe genital trauma. It took her body 6 months to recover, but even after her physical injuries healed, she continued to have nightmares about her ordeal. She awakened almost nightly in a panic, with her heart racing, unable to catch her breath, her stomach in knots. It was hours before she could calm down enough to go back to sleep. She had become so fearful that she couldn't drive any more and refused to go out with her friends. Sounds would startle her, and the very thought of having sex caused her to become physically ill.

1. What is going on here? Is Ms. Dunnagan having a normal reaction? Does she have a mental illness? If so, what?
2. What can be done to help her? Who should do it?
3. What is her prognosis? Does she have a chance to return to her normal, old self?

CASE 4

Veronica Thomas was more worried than ever. Her chest pain was more severe and more frequent, and she wanted some answers. Her cardiologist argued that her age (25 years), her previous normal catheterization, her low risk factor profile, and her atypical symptoms meant her heart was almost surely normal. He refused any further cardiac workup, and suggested she see a gastroenterologist about a GI workup. She did—last week she had an endoscopy, which was normal. Today she is in your office, saying: "I know this pain is not in my head. This pain is real! Something is wrong, and I want you to find out what it is!" You perform a physical examination, which is entirely within normal limits.

1. *What further tests do you want at this point?*
2. *Assume any further tests are also normal. What do you think accounts for Ms. Thomas's pain? How do you explain this to her?*
3. *In 3 weeks Ms. Thomas returns with steady, severe midabdominal pain. Your initial examination is normal. What tests would you order at this point? If these tests are normal, does this suggest a diagnosis?*

CASE 5

Arthur Campbell has returned for his annual visit, to get his medication refilled. He takes an ACE inhibitor for hypertension, which has completely controlled his blood pressure for the past 4 years. Today his pressure is 156/96. He relates that he never missed a dose until last month, when he forgot his pill twice. He says that he has been forgetful lately. This prompts you to ask a series of questions that yield the following facts: Mr. Campbell's forgetfulness seems to be related to a difficulty concentrating; he has been very restless and fidgety, and has begun worrying about things that didn't previously bother him, like his marriage, his kids, his job, and his waning physical capacities. These worries have been present for about 4 months, but more worrisome to him is his loss of interest in his hobbies. He is a gun collector and a hunter, and has not hunted once this season. His sleep, appetite, sex drive, and job performance are unimpaired. On many days he feels fine, but on most days he does not.

1. *Mr. Campbell did not come in complaining of these psychological symptoms, but only wanted his blood pressure medication refilled. Do you regard his symptoms as a problem? Does he have a mental disorder? How will you discuss this with him?*
2. *After a careful diagnostic assessment, you learn that Mr. Campbell has symptoms of depression and anxiety, but meets diagnostic criteria for neither. Does he have a mental illness? How would you chart his problem, and how would you follow it?*
3. *Is treatment indicated for Mr. Campbell's mental symptoms? If so, what treatment?*

———————— RECOMMENDED READINGS ————————

American Psychiatric Association: *Diagnostic and Statistical Manual of Mental Disorders, 4th Edition.* Washington, DC: American Psychiatric Association, 1994.

> This is the current version of the standard psychiatric diagnostic nomenclature and criteria. This volume is dry and somewhat difficult to navigate, but is packed with useful diagnostic clinical material.

American Psychiatric Association: *Diagnostic and Statistical Manual of Mental Disorders, 4th Edition: Primary Care Version (DSM-IV-PC).* Washington, DC: American Psychiatric Association, 1995.

> This is a psychiatric diagnostic manual written for primary care clinicians. It is much simpler and briefer than the full DSM-IV manual, and is organized into diagnostic algorithms that lead the clinician to a diagnosis from presenting symptoms.

Miranda J, Hohmann AA, Attkisson CC, Larson DB (eds): *Mental Disorders in Primary Care.* San Francisco, Jossey–Bass, 1994.

> As the title implies, this interesting volume summarizes what we know, and what we need to know and do, about mental disorders as they occur in the primary care setting.

Robins LN, Regier DA: *Psychiatric Disorders in America: The Epidemiologic Catchment Area Study.* New York, The Free Press, 1991.

> This is a one-volume summary of many of the findings from one of the most ambitious mental health studies ever undertaken, the ECA Study.

CHAPTER 18

C. Special Problems

Sexually Transmitted Diseases

Peggy B. Smith

CASE 18-1

Sarah, an 18-year-old African-American woman, came to the clinic for a pregnancy test. Her test was positive. She was also tested for gonorrhea, chlamydia, and syphilis, and was reactive for syphilis. This was her third pregnancy. She had one living child, a previous abortion, and planned to terminate this pregnancy. All three pregnancies resulted from unprotected intercourse with her 22-year-old boyfriend of $3\frac{1}{2}$ years. This was her second case of syphilis from this partner. She was in denial regarding her partner's infidelity and her risk of pregnancy. She also doubted the diagnosis of syphilis.

—————— INTRODUCTION ——————

As this case indicates, physicians must deal with a number of sensitive and troubling issues when treating patients with sexually transmitted diseases (STDs). After reading this chapter, the student will be able to differentiate between the consequences of various STDs and their impact on the life of the patient, evaluate life circumstances of an individual patient that place him at risk for reinfection with an STD, and identify social values that may act as barriers to effective treatment.

Changing life-styles, serial monogamy, and early initiation of sexual activity have increased the prevalence of STDs. No age group is spared, although 65% of infections are found among individuals 16 to 24 years of age. Despite being viewed by many as an affliction of minorities and the poor, STDs are prevalent among all social, economic, and racial groups.

Social issues as well as epidemiological trends affect the prevalence of STDs and therefore need to be addressed proactively. It is only when these illnesses are evaluated systematically, holistically, and contextually that the patient can be treated effectively.

399

Table 18.1
Sexually Transmitted Diseases[a]

Organism	Disease
Bacteria	
Neisseria gonorrhoeae	Gonorrhea
Haemophilus vaginalis and other anaer-obic bacteria, chlamydia also	Vulvovaginitis, urethritis
Haemophilus ducreyi	Chancroid
Calymmatobacterium granulomatis	Granuloma
Treponema pallidum	Syphilis
Shigella	Dysentery
Salmonella	Gastroenteritis, enteric fever
Group B *Streptococcus*	Neonatal and infant infections
Chlamydia trachomatis	Lymphogranuloma venereum
Trachoma inclusion conjunctivitis agent	Inclusion cervicitis, vaginitis, and urethritis
Fungi	
Candida albicans	Vulvovaginitis
Epidermophyton inguinale	Tinea cruris
Metazoa	
Phthirus pubis	Pediculosis pubis
Acarus	Scabies
Mycoplasma	
Mycoplasma hominis or *T. mycoplasma*	Cervicitis, vaginitis, urethritis
Protozoa	
Trichomonas vaginalis	Vulvovaginitis
Viruses	
Herpes simplex virus type 2	Vulvovaginitis
Papilloma virus	Condyloma acuminatum
Molluscum contagiosum virus	Genital dermatitis
Cytomegalovirus	Cervicitis, urethritis
Hepatitis B	Hepatitis
Human immunodeficiency virus (HIV)	AIDS

[a]Adapted from Smith PB, Mumford DM (eds): *Adolescent Pregnancy: Perspectives for the Health Professional.* Boston, GK Hall & Co, 1980.

As Case 18-1 suggests, a large number of STDs are asymptomatic or have such mild symptoms that they are ignored by the patient. For a subset of individuals, discharges from genital organs, even when malodorous, are seen as normal. Another important point is that some STDs covary; this is often the case with gonorrhea and chlamydia. Because of this covariance, diagnostic procedures have been developed that are sensitive to both infections and should be the screening method of choice.

Another point concerns the way that pregnancy testing and other service options can function as gateways to preventive primary healthcare. Pregnancy testing for women of reproductive age provides a flexible access point to diagnose and treat STDs and other illnesses. A complete physical examination along with appropriate screening for STDs should be routine. Even if the pregnancy test is negative, public health interventions can be initiated. If syphilis is detected, for example, treatment and cure can be initiated so that if another pregnancy is conceived, the fetus will be protected.

Classically, STDs have included syphilis, herpes, chlamydia, and gonorrhea as major entities. HIV/AIDS, by virtue of its form of transmission, has also been added by some to the major category. Since many other diseases are now known to be capable of passage by sexual activity, such as hepatitis B, the list of STDs has grown (see Table 18.1). Most of these infections involve the genital area, but rectal, pharyngeal, and other areas of infection are increasingly common.

With increasing sexual activity, especially by the young, venereal disease incidence continues to rise; for example, the incidence of gonorrhea has increased rapidly over the past 10 years (Hatcher *et al.*, 1990). The increase in gonorrhea in the teenage group has been much faster than in the general population. Moreover, changing legislation on serological screening for marriage licenses in many states, the covariance of sexual intercourse with IV drug use, and the emergence of large homeless populations have changed the typical patient profile of many STDs. For example, it is not unusual for some patients to contract more than one infection, remain with symptoms over an extended period of time, and if treatment is obtained, either refuse to complete the prescription regimen or become reinfected quickly after cure.

In this chapter we will review the major and minor types of STDs: their incidence, their etiology, their symptoms, and the best means of treatment. We then consider how the physician's attitudes, experience, and training can adversely affect the quality of care for patients with STDs. Next we examine the impact of STDs on patients' lives, focusing particularly on the changes brought about in the relationships of patients, their partners, and their physicians. In the fifth section we ask why STDs are so prevalent and consider such factors as survival sex, family dysfunction, sexual abuse, incest, ignorance, taboos, social stigmas, multiple sexual partners, becoming sexually active at a young age, and the asymptomatic nature of many STDs. In the sixth section we focus on a problem long overlooked by physicians, public health officials, and law enforcement officers: the impact of possible infection on victims of sexual assault. Finally, we consider the physician's role in the community and the need for leadership in educating the public about the risks of acquiring STDs and the most realistic means of prevention.

CASE 18-2

A 29-year-old white woman presented in clinic where she had been a patient since 1992, for her annual exam. She reported being sexually active since age 15, being pregnant twice, and having had only one sex partner. No previous STDs had been diagnosed. The patient reported no vaginal discharge but had experienced itching and an odor for 2 weeks. Her cultures for gonorrhea and chlamydia returned with a positive diagnosis. Her partner reported no symptoms.

—————————— MAJOR TYPES OF STDs ——————————

GONORRHEA

Gonorrhea is one of the most common STDs. When one includes reported and nonreported cases there are probably over 3,000,000 persons in the United States infected with gonorrhea (Hatcher *et al.*, 1990). In the United States reinfection and intercourse with multiple partners continue to fuel the disease. Sixty percent of those afflicted with gonorrhea are said to be males, but some authorities place the estimate closer to 50%. Thirty-five percent of women reported to have gonorrhea are adolescent girls 15 to 19 years old, and acute gonococcal infection is on the rise among children and adolescents under the age of 15. Sexual assault and incest contribute significantly to this trend.

Asymptomatic infection of the cervix is the most common form of gonorrhea in women. The symptoms are mild and include vaginal discharge, dysuria, pelvic pain, and uterine bleeding. Uncomplicated gonorrhea is usually limited to the cervix, but disseminated gonorrhea infections may occur. Complicated gonorrhea may involve acute gonococcal salpingitis with fever, chills, abdominal pain during premenstrual intervals, and eventually pelvic inflammatory disease (PID).

Infertility, pain, and ectopic pregnancies often result from this infection. Untreated gonorrhea can scar a woman's tubes and block the transport of a fertilized egg into the uterus. In addition, the CDC reports that in 1988, complications from ectopic pregnancy were the leading cause of pregnancy-related death during the first trimester. Joint and orthopedic problems can be attributed to gonorrhea. The most common form of disseminated gonococcal infection is the arthritis–dermatitis syndrome.

In men, gonorrhea may cause a discharge, urinary symptoms, and pain in the perineal, suprapubic, or inguinal areas. Fever may also be present, along with pain and swelling of the scrotum. Anorectal gonorrhea can result from anal intercourse. This infection is usually asymptomatic but may cause rectal burning, discharge, or bleeding. Another prevalent form of this infection is oropharyngeal gonorrhea. Estimates suggest that 20% of individuals with genital gonorrhea also have an infection in the pharyngeal area.

Women are much more vulnerable to this disease than men. Several authors state that the risk of a woman acquiring gonorrhea from an infected man is 80 to 90%, whereas the man has an estimated 22% risk of being infected by a woman with gonorrhea (Smith & Mumford, 1980). There is also much discussion concerning the difference in symptomatology. Some believe asymptomatic gonorrhea to be present in 80 to 90% of women, but a more likely figure is 50 to 60%. As seen in Case 18-2, men are more likely to be asymptomatic.

Relative resistance of gonorrhea to penicillin varies, and gonorrhea can be resistant to other antibiotics, such as tetracycline. Thus, penicillin or ampicillin treatment failure patients should be monitored after initial treatment and treated with a more powerful antibiotic. Unfortunately, penicillinase-producing *Neisseria gonorrhoeae* (PPNG) has emerged in this country from Asia, so that penicillin can no longer automatically be used as first-line treatment in some areas.

SYPHILIS

In 1988, the total number of reported cases for all ages of primary and secondary syphilis was 40,000 (Hatcher *et al.*, 1990). It should be emphasized that reported cases of syphilis may be considerably fewer than actual or even diagnosed cases. The use of crack cocaine and the exchanging of sex for drugs have increased its prevalence in the heterosexual population. In addition to being transferred sexually, syphilis can be transferred vertically from mother to fetus after the third or fourth month of pregnancy. This form of the disease, called congenital syphilis, occurs in one in every 10,000 pregnancies.

The syphilis spirochetes, found only in humans, are slender corkscrew organisms with 6 to 14 regular spirals. Syphilis is diagnosed through serological testing, the most common test being the Venereal Disease Research Laboratory (VDRL) test. A variety of conditions such as mononucleosis, collagen diseases, malaria, drug addiction, and in some cases pregnancy can cause false positives. Syphilis is usually described as having three stages: primary, secondary, and tertiary syphilis. In addition, a latent phase occurs between the secondary, and tertiary stages. In its early stages syphilis may be unrecognized. It usually takes 3 to 4 weeks of incubation before a chancre or painless sore erupts. The lesion is an ulcer with a clear base and a raised, firm ridge and is found in the genitalia, pharynx, or perianal areas. The VDRL test usually becomes positive 1 or 2 weeks after the chancre is noticed. The spirochete can be found in most lesions, thus making it possible to distinguish the infection from other conditions that have sores, such as genital herpes, lymphogranuloma venereum, or chancroid.

If primary syphilis is not treated, secondary syphilis may follow after a period of a few weeks to 6 months. *Treponema pallidum* may produce systemic signs and symptoms such as fever, myalgia, headaches, loss of appetite, a generalized skin rash, mucous membrane lesions including patches and ulcers, weeping papules in moist skin areas, and generalized nontender lymphadenopathy. Because of the long incubation period and the variety of manifestations, the patients with secondary syphilis may not remember the primary lesion.

Latent or hidden syphilis is the "sleeping" phase that occurs after the subsidence of secondary symptoms but before the appearance of tertiary ones. If symptoms recur in the first 3 to 5 years after primary infection (so-called "relapsing" syphilis), the stage is defined as early latency; if after 5 years, the latent phase. During the latent phase, positive serology persists.

Tertiary syphilis can be benign when it responds to rapid therapy or it can be more damaging, especially where there is central nervous system involvement. Symptoms of neurosyphilis, which is found in 20% of tertiary syphilis cases, is progressive and can be lethal, include dementia, neurologic deficits, and pain. The cardiovascular system may also be involved, with dissection of the ascending aortic arch, universally fatal, being characteristic.

Undetected, syphilis can also cause serious damage to the fetus, midtrimester abortion, or death. As a preventive measure it is recommended that all women be screened in the first and third trimester for this infection. Because of the action of the placenta, the fetus is usually protected from transplacental passage of the infection during the first 4 months of pregnancy.

The fetus infected with congenital syphilis may have a variety of symptoms. Syphilitic pemphigus is usually found on the bottoms of the feet and the palms of the hands. These lesions usually contain the spirochete. Mucous membrane involvement with classic sniffles and enlargement of the spleen and lymph nodes accompanied by anemia are also common. Because the onset of symptoms vary the neonate may not develop signs of congenital syphilis before 2 years of age. Continued evaluation of the newborn during the first year of life is recommended.

HERPES SIMPLEX VIRUSES

The herpes simplex viruses (HSV) consist of a group of at least 25 viruses, five of which are known to infect humans. These infections include HSV types 1 and 2, cytomegalovirus, varicella–zoster, and Epstein–Barr viruses. The last two types usually are not associated with venereal infections.

HSV type 1 causes fever blisters and cold sores, whereas HSV type 2 causes genital lesions and neonatal herpes. Definitive diagnosis of HSV is made through tissue culture, although clinical diagnosis can be made by noting the characteristics of the lesions. Classified into two stages, primary HSV and recurrent or secondary HSV, genital herpes infections are characterized by latency periods and asymptomatic viral shedding stages. In addition, when a person is infected, recurrent lesions often reappear in the same place. Physical and emotional triggers, the presence of an immunosuppressant disease, or increased stress can reactivate the infection.

There is no cure for HSV and its treatment is uncertain, often unsatisfactory, and usually directed toward symptomatic relief. The antiviral drug acyclovir has offered some comfort in reducing initial symptoms and suppressing reoccurring outbreaks. The time-honored remedies of sitz baths and astringent solutions give some comfort. Local analgesic ointments, such as 2% lidocaine, may limit intense pain, but should be used sparingly and for short periods (i.e., less than 2 weeks) to prevent sensitization. Topical acyclovir may be necessary during the ulceration stages but is not as successful as the oral form and is useful only for the first clinical episode. Local antibiotic application to prevent secondary infections is often ineffective. Since *Candida albicans* is a common secondary invader, some authorities recommend nystatin vaginal suppositories.

HSV, if active, can also attack the central nervous system of the neonate during delivery. Neonatal herpes is severe and often fatal. Transmission occurs as the child passes through the birth canal. If a patient with an active case of genital herpes is pregnant, a cesarean section should be performed within 4 hours of the rupture of the membranes to reduce the risk of transmission. The risk of transmission from an infected mother is highest among women with a primary herpes infection but low among women with recurrent herpes. Infants delivered through an infected birth canal should be cultured and followed carefully.

CHLAMYDIA

The chlamydiae are a group of large, intracellular parasites closely related to gram-negative bacteria. Two species exist, *Chlamydia psittaci*, responsible for the disease in birds which may be transferred to humans, and *Chlamydia trachomatis*, which has been implicated in a variety of infections, including pelvic inflammatory disease, nongonococcal urethritis, and epididymitis.

An estimated 4 million new cases of chlamydiae occur annually. Approximately 70% of infected women have few or no symptoms, and asymptomatic infection in women can persist for up to 15 months (Hatcher *et al.*, 1990). Infection can progress in women to involve the upper reproductive tract and may result in serious complications. To identify patients who may have chlamydial infections, the CDC has recommended routine testing based on age, risk behavior, and clinical findings, especially in clinics and group practices that provide reproductive health care to adolescents.

HIV/AIDS

HIV causes a defect in the body's immune system by invading and then multiplying within certain white blood cells. Once released from the infected cells, the virus attacks more cells and multiplies with time. Other infections that activate the immune system, including other STDs, may act as cofactors that speed further multiplication of the virus.

The longer a person is infected with HIV, the more likely the immune system will be impaired, thus leaving the infected person vulnerable to many opportunistic diseases, including cancers and pneumonias. HIV infections persist for the life of the infected individual, as there is no cure.

In the initial stages of the outbreak, gay men were considered at greater risk for the infection. Vigorous educational and behavioral interventions have had some success in leveling the increasing prevalence of this infection among gay men. The heterosexual population now is experiencing a growing infection rate. A combination of factors are often cited, including IV drug use among men and sporadic use of condoms by men. A factor that may contribute to marginal condom usage is the attitudes and practices of the female partners. Women, while knowledgeable as to the need for condom use, may not apply the information to their behavior. Valdiserre *et al.* (1989) found that among women who acknowledged the importance of such practices, only 14% currently used condoms.

During 1994, U.S. health departments reported 80,691 new cases of AIDS to the CDC, which followed the 106,618 new cases reported in 1993 (MMWR, 1995). The number of cases reported in each of these years was significantly greater than that reported in 1992 (47,572), related largely to the expansion of the AIDS surveillance case definition for adolescents and adults implemented on January 1, 1993. The CD4+ T-lymphocyte count is the best laboratory indicator of clinical progression, and comprehensive management strategies for HIV infection are typically stratified by CD4 count. Patients with CD4+ counts > 500 usually do not demonstrate evidence of clinical immunosuppression. Patients with 200–500 CD4+ cells are more likely to develop HIV-related symptoms and to require medical intervention. Patients with CD4+ counts < 200 and those with higher CD4+ counts who develop thrush or unexplained fever are at increased risk for developing complicated HIV disease. The incidence of AIDS-related illnesses increased 3% in 1993 and a similar increase is expected for 1994.

HIV infection has emerged as a major cause of death in young men and women in the United States. In 1989, HIV infection was the sixth leading cause of death among women 25 to 44 years of age. Among men HIV infection is the number one killer in this age group. While men historically have been the gender most affected, the trend is changing. In 1985, 541 cases, about 7% of adult cases, were reported among women, whereas in 1992, 6255 cases, about 14%, were reported among women. Through 1992, more than 27,000 AIDS cases among women in the United States had been reported to the CDC (MMWR, 1995).

Reported AIDS cases associated with heterosexual transmission of HIV have increased steadily among women. Heterosexual contact is considered to be the mode of transmission for persons whose only reported risk is heterosexual contact with a person who is either (1) HIV-infected or at increased risk for HIV infection or (2) born in a country where heterosexual transmission predominates (CDC, 1994b). The number of women reported annually with heterosexually acquired AIDS has increased from less than 100 in 1984 to almost 2500 in 1992. In 1992, almost 40% of all AIDS cases reported in women were attributed to heterosexual contact.

Most women with AIDS are young. About one-quarter of the women reported with AIDS in 1992 were between 20 and 29 years of age at the time of diagnosis. The median period from HIV infection to AIDS is about 10 years. Thus, most of these women were infected as teenagers. Almost half of the women reported with AIDS in 1992 were in their 30s at the time of diagnosis. About 85% of the women with AIDS were of reproductive age, or between 15 and 44 years, at the time of diagnosis (MMWR, 1995).

In 1992, 54% of women reported with AIDS in the United States were black, 23% white, and 21% Hispanic. These percentages have not changed markedly since 1988. In 1992 the incidence of AIDS per 100,000 women was 27 for blacks compared with 13 for Hispanics and 2 for whites. Accordingly, black and Hispanic women had rates approximately 13 and 6 times, respectively, the rate for white women.

About half of these women had a history of sex with an injecting drug user, while the other half had sex with men with other or unspecified risks. Injection-drug use was associated with 45% of the reported AIDS cases in women. In addition, 4% of the women with AIDS reported receipt of blood or blood components, and 12% had other or undetermined risks. Since 1987, the percentage of women with AIDS associated with transfusions has decreased from 12% to 4%, while the percentage of women with AIDS attributed to heterosexual contact has increased from 30% to 39%.

CASE 18-3

Suzie, a 15-year-old Hispanic patient who experienced an induced abortion, had been sexually active since age 13. She had a lifetime total of two sexual partners and currently had the same partner for 18 months. Suzie never tested positive for gonorrhea or chlamydia but had reported a discharge at her previous visit. However, results of serology and cultures were negative. She presented herself to the Family Planning Clinic 1 month prior to her 6-month visit complaining of a discharge with an odor and itching for 2 to 3 days. She reported no "bumps or blisters" on her labia or introitus and she stated that she used condoms occasionally. Her physical exam revealed lesions at the introitus consistent with genital warts. She was treated with trichloroacetic acid one time and was instructed to return to the clinic for additional treatment if needed.

MINOR TYPES OF STDs

CYTOMEGALOVIRUS (CMV)

CMV, a member of the herpes family, is transmitted sexually as well as other ways. More than 80% of adults over 35 years of age in this country have antibodies against CMV. Six to eight percent of sexually active young women are estimated to have CMV in their cervix. CMV has been implicated in some cases of endometritis, cervicitis, PID, and, in men, nonspecific urethritis.

Symptomatic contacts of definitively diagnosed CMV patients may be presumed to have CMV infection as well. Otherwise, definitive diagnosis is difficult to establish because CMV is associated with nonspecific clinical syndromes, and the diagnostic tests are complex and expensive. Definitive diagnosis of CMV infection requires a rise in antibody titer, a positive immunofluorescence test, or identification of the virus in tissues or secretions known to be previously negative in a symptomatic patient. Many healthy individuals shed CMV in their saliva, cervical secretions, urine, semen, breast milk, feces, or blood. Thus, isolating those with known CMV has little value for public health.

CMV is also responsible for the severe, and often fatal, disease of the fetus and newborn called cytomegalic inclusion disease. This disease afflicts approximately 10,000 infants in the United States each year. Infants may also develop conjunctivitis or pneumonia from a mother infected with chlamydia.

Treatment is supportive, nonspecific, and symptomatic. No accepted routine therapy exists for either maternal or neonatal infection. The acquired illness is usually self-limiting among immunocompetent individuals.

In this country, 12,000 to 15,000 babies each year acquire Group B streptococcus infections that are transmitted both sexually and nonsexually. The infection in babies often takes severe, life-threatening forms: septicemia, pneumonia, and meningitis. Approximately half of these babies die. Of those who survive, as many as 50% may develop neurological problems (Hatcher *et al.*, 1990).

CONDYLOMA ACUMINATUM

Condyloma acuminatum (venereal or genital warts) are known to be caused by the human papilloma virus (HPV). Transmission is primarily sexual. Genital warts account for more than one million physician visits annually in the United States (Hatcher *et al.*, 1990). The exact incubation period is unknown, but the lesions are slow growing and may take up to 2 to 3 months to develop after exposure.

The lesions are usually found in the vaginal or cervical area. Condyloma is commonly associated with other infections such as moniliasis and trichomoniasis. The individual lesions are fleshy, pointed, wartlike, soft, and moist, and seem to become less infectious with time. In moist areas the growth may readily spread to adjacent regions. As Case 18-3 suggests, small lesions may not itch, but large ones do. Spontaneous remission of lesions is possible but so too are recurrences. Pregnancy often encourages exuberant growth. Rectal intercourse may result in perianal or rectal warts.

Treatment results for condyloma acuminatum vary and depend somewhat on the size of the lesions, the patient's immune competence, pregnancy status, and perhaps whether other vaginal infections coexist. Podophyllin, in a 10 to 25% solution (often in a tincture of benzoin base), or trichloroacetic acid, as in Case 18-3, may be used on small lesions, but not during pregnancy because of potential toxicity to the fetus. Larger lesions are often treated with laser or electrosurgery.

MOLLUSCUM CONTAGIOSUM

The virus causing molluscum contagiosum is a member of the DNA pox family. It is particularly prevalent in underdeveloped countries and afflicts over 20% of the population in some South Pacific regions. Children are its prime target, but adults can be affected as well. Viral spread is presumably both direct and through the common use of such items as bedding and towels. However, the sexual mode of transmission seems to be increasing in adults and adolescents.

Lesions are 1 to 5 mm, smooth, rounded, firm, shiny flesh-colored to pearly white papules with characteristically umbilicated centers. They are most commonly seen on the trunk and anogenital region and are generally asymptomatic.

Infection is usually diagnosed on the basis of the typical clinical presentation. Microscopic examination of lesions or lesion material reveals the pathognomonic molluscum inclusion bodies. Lesions may resolve spontaneously without scarring. However, they may be removed by curettage after anesthesia. Caustic chemical therapy (podophyllin, trichloroacetic acid, silver nitrate) and cryotherapy (liquid nitrogen) have also been used successfully.

BACTERIAL VAGINOSIS

Bacterial vaginosis, a significant vaginal infection in women, is caused by a mixture of anaerobic organisms. Many women are asymptomatic. Others have mild vulvovaginal irritation with scanty to moderate, gray, slightly malodorous discharge. Anaerobic bacteria often coexist with other virulent organisms in the vagina and hence are often overlooked as a causative agent.

Diagnosis is usually made by smear and culture. Vaginal cells seen under the microscope on a wet mount may have small dark particles adherent to them, called "clue cells." Treatment with metronidazole is greater than 80% effective. Treatment of the male sexual partner is still controversial, although it is useful in women with recurrent infections.

PEDICULOSIS PUBIS (CRAB LICE)

Crab lice (*Phthirus pubis*) are bloodsucking parasites which are more apt to be transmitted sexually than from shared contact with clothes or linen. Adult lice lay eggs (nits) at the base of the pubic skin hair shafts. These eggs hatch in 7 to 9 days and the new lice attach themselves to the skin of the host. Their bites may cause an erythematous papule within a matter of hours. Secondary infection is common.

The usual clinical presenting picture is that of pubic itching or the patient's simply observing lice moving on the skin surface. The lice can be positively identified when seen on a slide under a microscope or with a magnifying glass to view the lice or eggs on the pubic hair.

Treatment is with 1% gamma benzene hexachloride (Kwell) cream, lotion, or shampoo for 12 to 24 hours. Treatment should be repeated in 4 to 7 days to catch any eggs missed on the first application. Sexual partners should also be treated.

CANDIDA ALBICANS

C. albicans is a common saprophyte living in the mouth, vagina, respiratory tract, and intestines. Its presence may be detected from these sites in cultures in 25 to 50% of women. However, mere presence does not necessarily indicate infection.

Predisposing factors to *C. albicans* infections include the use of broad-spectrum antibiotics, oral contraceptives, pregnancy, diabetes mellitus, steroids or other immunosuppressive agents or events, narcotic abuse, perhaps increased carbohydrates in the diet, heat, and moisture. Pantyhose have been identified as contributing agents because they retain heat and are not moisture absorbent.

The organism is an oval, budding, gram-positive yeast. Although *C. albicans* is, in one sense, not communicable since most individuals harbor the organism, it is now being considered a minor STD. Symptoms of candida vulvovaginitis include a discharge, vulval itching, pain, or burning often beginning before menstruation. Painful urination and intercourse are other possible complaints. The vulva is usually red, edematous, and excoriated. The vaginal discharge characteristically is white, thick, and resembles curds of cottage cheese, usually moderate in quantity, but adherent to the vaginal wall.

Diagnosis is based on smears and cultures. Wet mounts may give a rough quantitative estimate of the number of organisms. Treatment of *C. albicans* is often problematic and requires careful attention to predisposing factors. Nystatin is the drug of choice in suppository form. Treatment of male sexual partners is controversial, but useful in women with recurrences, as is condom use.

TRICHOMONIASIS

This flagellated protozoal infection is a common cause of vaginitis in women and is transmitted through sexual intercourse. Sharing of towels, bedding, bathing, and douche equipment may also cause transmission. Infection rates may be as high as 40% in some populations where hygiene is poor.

Diagnosis is made from wet mounts with the treatment of choice being oral metronidazole. This drug should not be used if there is a suspicion of pregnancy or the patient is breast-feeding. To avoid "ping-ponging" the infection, the male partner should be treated simultaneously.

CHANCROID

Chancroid is endemic in many areas of the United States and also occurs in discrete outbreaks. Chancroid, a bacterial STD characterized by genital ulceration, has reemerged in the United States during the last decade. Chancroid has been well established as a cofactor for HIV transmission. As many as 10% of patients with chancroid also may be coinfected with *T. pallidum* or HSV.

Definitive diagnosis of chancroid requires identification of *Haemophilus ducreyi* on special culture media that are not commercially available; even using these media, sensitivity is 80% at best. A probable diagnosis may be made if the person has one or more painful genital ulcers and no evidence of *T. pallidum* infection. Patients should be tested for HIV infection at the time of diagnosis. Patients also should be tested 3 months later for both syphilis and HIV, if initial results are negative.

Treatment involves the use of erythromycin 500 mg taken orally, four times a day for 7 days, or ceftriaxone 250 mg, IM in a single dose. An alternative is trimethoprim/sulfamethoxazole, double-strength tablet (160/800 mg) taken orally, twice a day for 7 days. The susceptibility of *H. ducreyi* to this combination of antimicrobial agents varies throughout the world. The practitioner should evaluate the results of therapy after a maximum of 7 days, and continue therapy until ulcers or lymph nodes have healed. Fluctuant lymph nodes should be aspirated through healthy, adjacent, normal skin. Incision and drainage or excision of nodes will delay healing and are contraindicated. All sexual partner(s) should be simultaneously treated.

HEPATITIS B

Hepatitis B virus (HBV) infection is a common STD. Sexual transmission accounts for one-third to two-thirds of the 200,000 to 300,000 new HBV infections that occurred annually in the United States during the past 10 years. Of persons infected as adults, 6–10% become chronic HBV carriers. These persons are capable of transmitting HBV to others and are at risk for developing fatal complications. HBV leads to an estimated 5000 deaths annually in the United States from cirrhosis of the liver and hepatocellular carcinoma.

Persons known to be at high risk for acquiring HBV should be advised of their risk for HBV infection (as well as HIV infection) and the means to reduce their risk. Persons at specific risk include sexually active homosexual and bisexual men, individuals who have recently acquired another STD, and persons in nonmonogamous relationships. Such individuals should be vaccinated unless they are immune to HBV as a result of past infection or vaccination. There is currently no cure for either acute infections or the carrier state.

CASE 18-4

A white middle-class woman 37 years of age presents herself to her private practice gynecologist for her annual examination and to assess the cause of chronic pelvic pain. During the medical history she reveals that she and her husband have been living apart. CBC, Pap smear, and blood pressure are assessed, but no serology or cultures are taken by the physician. Undiagnosed, the woman has contracted asymptomatic chlamydia and anal gonorrhea.

CASE 18-5

A 25-year-old black woman was seen at her HMO clinic requesting HIV testing. She reported a total of four heterosexual partners in the past 3 years and frequent unprotected vaginal intercourse. She recently began a new sexual relationship and both partners have agreed to HIV screening. Results of her partner's HIV test were negative. However, her HIV test results were positive. She did not plan to tell her family, and her partner was sworn to secrecy. She was referred to an early intervention program.

Two weeks later, the clinic staff received a long-distance collect phone call from her partner. While visiting her grandmother 200 miles away, she became ill, unconscious, and was on a respirator in a small rural community hospital. He reported that the physicians had treated her pneumonia and were surprised that none of the medications were working. The staff told him the pneumonia might be related to her positive HIV status, and that this matter should be discussed with her physicians. The partner stated he had sworn not to tell anyone and therefore could not tell the physicians.

CASE 18-6

A white 50-year-old OB/GYN private practitioner was informed of the presence of trichomoniasis in a black patient. He refused to treat the patient, stating that the disease was "endemic in this population" and "treatment would not be effective."

PHYSICIAN ATTITUDES TOWARD PATIENTS WITH STDs

Physicians often harbor unspoken value judgments and personal expectations concerning how to treat and communicate information about STDs. One perception concerning STDs involves the role of ethnic or social class. In Cases 18-4 and 18-6 the decision to screen and treat were based on stereotypes that a middle class white patient would not need screening and that a black would not benefit from treatment. While certain risk factors may exist, attending physicians should consider every sexually active individual at risk for contracting a an STD. Some physicians hesitate to offer STD screening for married women for fear that the husband may ask why and may, in fact, refuse payment. Nevertheless, STD screening is essential to good primary and reproductive care, especially since a large number of women who have contracted an STD are asymptomatic.

Case 18-5 involves a value judgment about confidentiality and the exceptions about guarding such confidences. While in most cases it is imperative to protect the patient's confidentiality regarding HIV status, physician and patient should discuss at the outset circumstances that might require the waiving of such confidential agreements. In particular, the physician should gain permission to discuss the patient's HIV status with other health professionals involved in her care. Such discussions should be noted in the patient's chart.

411

**PHYSICIAN
ATTITUDES
TOWARD
PATIENTS WITH
STDs**

PHYSICIAN TRAINING

Physician experiences and exposure to STDs can affect knowledge and attitudes which in turn can affect one's ability to diagnose these infections. First, the skills necessary to diagnose new strains of STDs are constantly changing. Improved diagnostic tests and assays developed in the last 10 years require continuing medical education to enhance the ability of practitioners to diagnose and treat such infections. For example, chlamydia, a major disease entity, cannot be diagnosed without reliance on new technology. While such advances may be familiar to young physicians with recent training, these scientific breakthroughs may not reach those physicians with earlier training experiences. In addition, newer and more complicated expressions of STDs may go unnoticed by older practitioners.

Second, many physicians have had limited exposure to human sexuality in their medical training. Many medical schools do not require such courses and their elective status and emphasis on psychosocial issues hinder their attractiveness to budding clinical scientists. Residency requirements in pediatrics, internal medicine, and family medicine now mandate a structured experience including didactic and clinical programs that cover family planning, STDs, and gynecology.

A recent study of residency education suggests additional reforms are needed. Fifty percent of graduates had performed fewer than 20 pelvic examinations, 30% had never prescribed oral contraceptive pills, and 14% lacked a single experience in diagnosing or treating gonorrhea (Braverman & Strasburger, 1994). Only 68% of graduates reported adequate training in sexuality counseling and knowledge, with 64% reporting adequate training in pregnancy and only 46% expressing comfort with abortion counseling.

PHYSICIAN COMFORT LEVEL

Physician discomfort with STDs often relates to personal experience in the area of sexuality. Success in medical and premedical education requires dedication to studies rather than social life and focus on the sciences rather than the humanities. This lack of interpersonal experiences may both retard the development of empathic skills necessary for patient rapport and limit the medical student's understanding of the complexities of sexual decision-making and behavior. For those medical students with little or no sexual experience, treating patients for STDs can create considerable discomfort. In addition, limited sexual exposure can reduce the student's knowledge and raise the student's inhibitions regarding fellatio, anal intercourse, and other alternate forms of sexual expression.

PHYSICIAN SOCIAL ATTITUDES

Healthcare professionals hold widely divergent views regarding the social and moral aspects of treating patients with STDs. One survey found that one-third of physicians believed reproductive services such as screening for STDs should be provided without parental or spousal consent. Another third, however, would require parental and spousal notification and participation (Zackler *et al.*, 1975).

At the heart of this disagreement are cultural and religiously influenced definitions of the purpose of sexuality. Influenced by their backgrounds and beliefs, many medical students fail to appreciate the erotic, as opposed to the reproductive, dimension of sexuality. Unfortunately, medical education has focused almost exclusively on reproductive sexuality, while the erotic function has been either ignored or limited to pathology. Erotic pleasures are an integral part of sexual experience and are independent of the consequences of STDs.

Some healthcare professionals interpret the contraction of an STD as a judgment on the behavior of the infected patient. Such a belief is particularly prevalent when the diagnosis of HIV seropositivity occurs. Other physicians choose to empathize with and advocate for their patients, but feel in conflict with their religious backgrounds and traditions. This conflict is particularly difficult for religiously conservative medical students and residents who must deal with abortion in their training.

CASE 18-7

A 26-year-old Hispanic woman had attended a clinic for general family planning for 4 years. Her sister, a single 17-year-old and also a clinic patient, had a chronically ill 1½-year-old child. The baby was tested and found to be HIV positive. Both sisters were tested and found to be HIV positive. The only risk factor was multiple heterosexual partners.

Following family planning and life-style counseling, a pregnancy test was performed on the older sister. Results were positive. Not interested in a pregnancy termination, she subsequently delivered an HIV-positive baby. Despite counseling, 9 months later she conceived again and delivered another HIV-positive infant.

——— IMPACT OF STDs ON PATIENTS' LIVES ———

Case 18-7 suggests that the consequences of HIV seropositivity often conflict directly with life goals and desires. For such women, especially those who are poorly educated, the decision to avoid childbearing violates cultural norms. The emotional need to be a mother and to acquire the associated social status outweighs the public health or long-term negative consequences of an HIV-positive baby for many women. Educational and counseling efforts must take such issues into account.

Treatment of patients with STDs often requires attention to serious ethical and legal issues. Physicians should discuss the risk of transmission to others and ways of reducing these risks. STD-infected individuals should be counseled to use condoms, preferably in combination with foam. Patients who refuse to protect or notify their partners present an ethical quandary for their physicians. For infections such as HSV and HIV, case laws permit charges and convictions against individuals who knowingly infect others. Regardless of the type of STD, sexual responsibility should be encouraged, but physicians will vary as to the means of doing so.

A patient infected with HSV with primary or recurrent blisters will infect a partner if unprotected intercourse or other forms of sexual activity occur. While abstinence is urged, condom use is mandated if the first alternative is not adopted. Even if an active case is not present, studies suggest that viral shedding of covert lesions occurs among some women.

Thus, the infection can be contracted even if no external lesions are present. Caution dictates continual condom use for such individuals.

Because HIV infections are asymptomatic by definition, at-risk individuals often choose not to be tested to determine their status. Such behavior, though understandable, represents not only psychological avoidance and denial but also, if the patient continues to be sexually active, a shirking of ethical responsibility. Epidemiological projections suggest that as many as 1 million people in the United States are HIV-positive with the largest increases occurring among women and heterosexual populations. The iceberg effect increases the pool of risk to the heterosexual population (Hatcher *et al.*, 1990).

Even more problematic are those heterosexual and homosexual individuals who have tested positive for HIV yet continue to practice unprotected sex. While sexual acting out and irresponsibility are implicit in such behaviors, dislike of condoms is often a contributing factor. Some individuals lie about their status and fear that condom use will reveal their secret. As Case 18-7 indicates, some women choose not to use condoms because they desire to become pregnant. Since transplacental transmission of HIV approximates 30%, the soundness of such decisions is highly questionable.

Most physicians and ethicists agree that HIV infections and other STDs require specific changes in sexual behaviors. Safe sex practices, including the use of condoms, dental dams, and the refraining from rectal intercourse, are recommended. Data indicate that these safe sex practices can reduce the infection risk (Ku *et al.*, 1992).

Because of the chronicity of both HSV and HIV, many people believe that certain interventions may prevent recurrent outbreaks of HSV, which lower an HIV-infected individual's T-cell count. The most commonly recommended interventions include stress reduction, nutritional counseling, and visualization and meditation, as well as acupuncture, massage, and therapeutic touch. Complementary to these methods are support groups, "worried well" groups, and "next step" groups for HIV-positive individuals. In various combinations such behavioral interventions allow individuals to take control of their lives and reduce stress.

Other STDs, while less acute, can still devastate the mental health and personal outlook of the infected individual. In addition to the discomfort, the presence of an STD can negatively affect an individual's sexual self-esteem and self-image. For the conscientious, the possibility of infecting another individual or guilt regarding past behavior can effectively eliminate any interest in sexual activity.

CASE 18-8

A single white woman in her early 20s was hospitalized for the second time with PID. She stated that she was in a monogamous relationship with a man. The continuing etiology of her PID was chlamydia, and her partner had never been treated. The physician informed the partner that the condition would reoccur if he didn't receive treatment, and he agreed to be treated by his partner's physician. Although the male partner received treatment for his infection, subsequent attempts by the couple to conceive were unsuccessful.

PARTNER TREATMENT

When asymptomatic venereal diseases are diagnosed from complications resulting from non- or inadequate treatment, the physician must ascertain whether the patient is still sexually active and whether her partner has been screened and treated concomitantly. In some communities, protocols support the treatment of partners without testing if the woman is symptomatic. Without simultaneous treatment for such conditions, reinfection is almost guaranteed, as illustrated in Case 18-8.

A secondary issue is whether the woman was adequately informed of the need for partner treatment. A good STD treatment protocol is enhanced by a strong educational component. A final consideration is whether access to treatment was convenient for the infected partner. Otherwise, he is unlikely to be cured and he will continue to infect his partner. Typically STD clinics and family planning clinics do not attract asymptomatic partners. In this case special arrangements could be made through the woman's private physician so that services can be accessed in an easy and unobtrusive way.

ASSOCIATION WITH CERVICAL CANCER

Women who have a history of STDs, especially HPV, are at increased risk for cervical cancer, and women attending STD clinics may have additional characteristics that place them at even higher risk. Prevalence studies have found that precursor lesions for cervical cancer occur approximately five times more often among women attending STD clinics than among women attending family planning clinics. The Pap smear is an effective and relatively low-cost screening test for invasive cervical cancer and squamous intraepithelial lesions, the precursors of cervical cancer. An annual Pap is recommended for all sexually active women, especially those with a history of STDs.

CASE 18-9

A 20-year-old white woman is living in an abandoned car with her 26-year-old boyfriend. The patient had been unable to bathe for over a month. She was only able to "wash up" in the sink of a gas station. She presented to the clinic with complaints of a foul vaginal odor. The patient was found to have trichomoniasis and was treated with metronidazole. The patient was instructed to bring her partner in for treatment. After she told him about the infection, she reported that he had beat her. He came the next day for treatment and expressed severe anger about her "infidelity." The staff provided educational information. She denied any partner other than him. He abandoned her because of the infection.

CASE 18-10

Jane, a 13-year-old white girl, was living with her mom, stepfather, and $3\frac{1}{2}$-year-old stepsister when her father came to the home and murdered her mother. Jane witnessed the crime. Her father was captured and convicted. Jane's stepfather began to sexually abuse her stepsister. Jane called Children's Protective Services and the stepfather was prosecuted and imprisoned. Jane, now 14, was "given" to an aunt. Unhappy with the living arrangements, Jane ran away. During this time she became pregnant and put the baby up for adoption. Jane then met Lazaro, her aunt's boyfriend. Jane was rejected by her aunt, and Lazaro, a 27-year-old undocumented worker, went to court and was appointed Jane's legal guardian. They started having sex and he fathered two children. By 16 she had three babies. Periodic STD screening diagnosed recurrent trichomoniasis and gonorrhea.

fighting with Lazaro. She also stated that he was beating the children. She moved
out with a friend but left the three children and said she would come back in a few

Jane then became involved with another illegal alien. She had one abortion
and two more children by age 19. She again tested positive for gonorrhea. The
clinic staff encouraged Jane to have a bilateral tubal ligation, since she was
unsuccessful using contraception. As she could not qualify for subsidized social
services, permanent sterilization services were donated. She became pregnant
again and was scheduled to have a bilateral tubal ligation after delivery. However,
she changed her mind after counseling.

———— WHY DOES THIS PROBLEM EXIST? ————

One of the first steps in providing intervention and treatment for a public health concern, whether it be tuberculosis or an STD, is to evaluate the level of personal control that patients can exercise over their lives. If the basics of survival, food, shelter, and clothing are inadequate, curing a communicable disease will be difficult and the compliance necessary for the completion of a drug regimen will be compromised. In Case 18-9 the lack of running water and facilities for personal hygiene compromised public health compliance. If medical intervention is to be successful, social services must often complement the work of the physician. In Cases 18-9 and 18-10 it is not surprising that STD continued to reoccur.

With regard to STD, homeless individuals and runaway youth are especially vulnerable. In Cases 18-9 and 18-10 the women involved made sexual choices in response to personal needs and to procure the basic commodities of life. This is known as *survival sex*, i.e., sexual intercourse performed in exchange for goods or money.

Another factor that plays a role in the spread of STD is dysfunctional family behavior and the correlate of sexual abuse and incest. A healthy family unit, however it is defined, can provide some prophylaxis for such culturally abnormal behavior. When family units are compromised, some of the taboos associated with interfamilial sexual behavior evaporate. The confidentiality provided by the family unit, unless some other legal transgression is committed, can perpetuate and enhance inappropriate sexual behavior that can involve the contraction of an STD.

In addition to inappropriate sexual behavior, decision-making skills associated with those behaviors are also compromised. In addition to the history of sexual abuse, domestic violence and emotional abuse can also covary with these behaviors. For a variety of reasons, individuals often appear to be paralyzed by their circumstances and cannot mobilize the psychological energy necessary to extract themselves from their surroundings. To be effective in such cases, physicians should be familiar with victim service agencies that can provide emergency care or legal counsel.

Dealing with the chronic nature of STDs requires an appreciation of the various forces that impede treatment. First, many individuals, including those who are highly educated, lack basic understanding of the different types of infections and common means of transmission. Sexual behavior, by its very nature, is shrouded in taboos and values that discourage frank discussion, thus limiting the knowledge and vocabulary necessary to explain the associated aspects of these diseases. Religiosity, personal myths, and ignorance combine to inhibit the development of sound cognitive skills in human sexuality that are the prerequisite for decision-making regarding risky sexual behaviors.

Second, becoming sexually active at an early age and having multiple sexual partners over time enhances the risk of contracting an STD. Surveys conducted over the last 30 years indicate that the age of onset of sexual activity has decreased significantly (Zelnik & Kantner, 1980). In addition, the number of sexual partners has increased during that time among all age cohorts.

A third factor in the increase of certain types of STDs is related to their asymptomatic nature in both the carrier and the individual who becomes infected. Among women, gonorrhea and chlamydia can cause significant damage to the reproductive system without prior signs of the infection. Unfortunately, physicians in private practice may not perform routine screening for these infections, allowing these diseases to go unchecked.

The social stigma attached to being infected with an STD can be a powerful deterrent to seeking treatment. When treatment centers are difficult to access or are lacking in privacy, treatment is likely to be avoided. Inadequate access may justify sending medications home for treatment of the sexual partner.

CASE 18-11

A 20-year-old nulliparous female presented herself to a general health clinic and reported that she had experienced an aggravated sexual assault. The patient reported that the attack was her second sexual experience. A 25-year-old black male was identified as the perpetrator. She said that she had dated him twice before and on this latest occasion he stated that they were going "party hopping." After attending two separate events, he told her that the third party was at a hotel and that it would be the "best ever." After discovering that the hotel room was vacant, she attempted to leave but was forcibly assaulted at gunpoint and was raped orally, vaginally, and anally four times.

He threatened that if she told anyone he would kill her. He also stated that no one would believe her because they had been dating. She did not seek medical treatment for 3 weeks. She subsequently presented herself to the emergency room and was tested for gonorrhea, the result of which was positive. She was then referred to a clinic for a general workup where she was diagnosed with trichomoniasis. After signing a separate consent form she was also tested for HIV. The results came back positive. The patient was visibly upset and because a family member had died of the disease she became very fatalistic about her own demise. Subsequent to counseling, her mother became involved and provided family support so that the woman could attend an HIV-positive support group. The possibility of pressing charges against the man was explored with clinic staff but the family refused because they did not want to undergo the headache of subjecting themselves to the legal process.

——————— SEXUAL ASSAULT ———————

Little attention has been given to the impact of possible infection with an STD or HIV in survivors of sexual assault. This may be related in part to society's conflicting attitudes and beliefs concerning STDs, AIDS, and rape. This problem is compounded in that rape is a crime that is often hidden and underdocumented. The National Women's Study estimated there were 683,000 forcible rapes of adult women in 1991; 22% of rapes were by strangers, and 16% were reported to the police. Significant numbers of adolescents and children are the victims of sexual assaults, often involving multiple encounters. More than half of all rapes (61%) involved victims under the age of 18. In 29% of all forcible rapes, the victims were less than 11, and in 32% between the ages of 11 and 17.

The risk of contracting HIV or other STDs often depends on the health status of the assailant, the type of sexual assault, and the frequency of assaults. The type of sexual exposure (vaginal, anal, or oral), the associated trauma, the presence of other STDs, and the exposure to bodily fluids affect the risk of infection. Gonorrhea, syphilis, or hepatitis B may have per-contact infectivity rates as high as 20%. Compared with these diseases, the estimate of per-contact HIV infectivity rate from male to female via penile–vaginal intercourse is less than two per 1000 contacts.

The presence of lesions or blood from violent assaults may increase the chance of transmission of HIV and other STDs. Genital ulcerative STDs also have been associated with increased infectiousness, as well as susceptibility to HIV. Another factor is the strength of the viral strain. Violence, trauma, and blood exposure or the presence of inflammatory or ulcerative STDs increases the risk.

Physicians counseling rape victims need to educate their patients, help survivors regain a sense of control over their lives, and allow survivors to make decisions regarding STD screening and HIV testing. Information and counseling should be provided in a nondirective manner, offering survivors the opportunity for open-ended discussions of their questions in a nonjudgmental manner.

Some professionals may question whether survivors of sexual assaults should be offered AZT as a prophylactic for HIV infection. Antiretroviral therapy has proven efficacious in inhibiting HIV replication. Many major healthcare facilities offer postexposure zidovudine treatment for workers who sustain injuries with contaminated needles, even though the efficacy of zidovudine in preventing HIV infection after initial exposure remains unproved.

CASE 18-12

A large metropolitan school board in the southern United States, after analyzing the prevalence of STDs and pregnancy in a predominantly Hispanic public high school, passed a resolution for the establishment of a school-based health clinic. The goal was to provide primary health and screening services to the student body and their siblings. Subsequent to board approval local community groups demanded a public meeting. At this forum various parents and community members expressed concern that providing information and services for the treatment of STDs encouraged irresponsible sexual behavior. Furthermore, in spite of the morbidity statistics, the parents insisted that the students were not sexually active and were not at risk for STDs. A great fear was expressed that as part of any prevention strategy condoms would become available on campus. The presence of these items was perceived by a group of parents as sending the wrong message to the community and the students who attended the high school.

Based on the expressed concerns a multidisciplinary team comprised of a pediatrician, psychologist, nurse, health educator, and social worker initiated a series of parent focus groups. At these meetings the various constituencies were given the opportunity to express their concerns. Their input was solicited as to the scope of services to provide and the type of consent procedures required for participation in the medical services.

THE PHYSICIAN'S ROLE
IN THE COMMUNITY

Dealing successfully with STDs will require leadership from the medical community to assuage the public's fears and prejudices. Oftentimes attempts to deal directly with issues associated with sexuality are misconstrued as attempts to provide liberal interpretations of sex education or encouragement to initiate early sexual activity. These fears are exacerbated when one deals with certain cultures. The Hispanic community, for example, has historically maintained a conservative posture on issues relating to human sexuality and STDs. In spite of the increasing prevalence of HIV and STD among this population, Hispanics seem reticent to deal proactively with these delicate subjects. The physician in Case 18-12, in order to provide these proposed services, had to gain the confidence and support of this conservative group.

STD education in the community and in schools, while attempting to reach many individuals, tends to be brief and nonspecific. Community attitudes toward STD and HIV are also problematic. Many communities believe that public education on sexual issues may be a subtle reinforcer of sexual behavior. As a result, misinformation and ignorance abound. Heterosexual populations, for example, find it difficult to concretize their risk because they do not understand transmission issues. In the case of HIV, teens especially may not view AIDS as a "real disease." They have difficulty grasping the notion that a healthy, robust person could transmit a deadly disease. Many adults still identify AIDS as a "gay disease" that does not affect a healthy heterosexual. Risk behaviors such as school drop-out, drug and alcohol use, and sexual misconduct are predictive of nonuse of condoms, STDs, and denial of risk. Persons who engage in these behaviors are difficult to reach and may not appear at healthcare facilities until they are symptomatic.

Scare tactics and calls for abstinence seldom work: Innovative educational programs are needed to motivate the public to practice safer sex. Educational methods appropriate for some populations may be insufficient or even inappropriate for other groups. For example, the gay community is probably more aware that negotiation skills must be learned in making sexual choices, especially as it relates to safe sex. Moreover, certain terms may be interpreted differently. Physicians need to know, for example, that a teen's definition of monogamy may mean being with a person for a week or a month or a year.

Education about STDs must take a positive approach to teaching about all types of sexuality in a manner that is frank and gender appropriate. Use of condoms requires the cooperation of the man, and many men resist using them, leaving their partners vulnerable. Ethnic concepts of sexuality must also be considered when attempting to teach good decision-making skills to high-risk young women. Discussing sex is considered inappropriate in many Latin American communities, making it difficult to educate patients concerning the use of condoms, previous sexual partners, and sexual practices between men and women. This is an example of why cross-cultural training should be an essential part of medical school and residency.

The needs of community populations at risk for HIV infection will increase. Knowledge and preparation for decision-making skills are not sufficient without access to medical, social, and even legal services. Community-minded physicians should also be aware that women face a difficult set of negotiation challenges regarding abstinence or safer sex behaviors. Asking for assistance with condom purchases in stores or pharmacies may not be easy.

Because of the consequences of STDs discussed previously, various efforts have been undertaken to encourage abstinence, postpone sexual involvement, or promote safe sex practices. Such efforts have met with varying levels of success. First, for certain populations, such as adolescents, the risk of acquiring an infection is perceived to be low. It is not surprising that the rates of many STDs are the highest among adolescents (MMWR, 1993a). Second, some population cohorts lack adequate knowledge about diseases and their contagion. Third, there are groups of young adults who express the feelings that they will not live past their 30s, so sexual risk-taking has relatively minor consequences.

Programs developed to enhance life skills associated with sexual decision-making are varied and have different degrees of success. Most programs designed to prevent STDs focus on high-risk individuals who are already sexually active. While some forms of sex education have succeeded at postponing sexual involvement among youth (Ku *et al.*, 1992), training in condom utilization skills is probably a more realistic approach to the problem. Such classes focus on either skills associated with mechanical use or social factors associated with using condoms with a partner. While some change was found in students who participated in these classes (Cohen *et al.*, 1992), large numbers continued with unsafe sexual practices. Some programs have emphasized increasing availability of condoms as perhaps a way of encouraging use (Calsyn *et al.*, 1992). However, even among educated groups such as college students, condoms were not used consistently and those at greatest risk were the least likely to practice safe sex (Oswalt & Matsen, 1993).

CONCLUSIONS

The risks associated with sexual activity are serious and complicated. Past stereotypes are misleading and may inhibit treatment options. Changes in the age of fertility, in the nuclear family, and in the educational and economic opportunities for women have all played a role in increasing exposure of individuals to a variety of STDs.

Epidemiological trends indicate ways STDs are expressed in contemporary populations and suggest strategies physicians should adopt to address them. First, physicians must communicate that all individuals who are sexually active and do not practice safe sex are at risk for HIV/AIDS. Opportunities to stress the risk to patients should be acknowledged and utilized. Testing for such infections, while requiring a separate consent form, should be routine in all primary care settings. In addition to testing, physicians should discuss frankly the availability and use of condoms and the sexual practices of their patients as a routine part of the standard clinical visit. Desensitizing patients and perhaps providing the opportunity to role-play can facilitate safe sex practices.

A second trend is the growing tendency to contract multiple diseases and infections. A patient may have several infections in addition to the one for which treatment is sought. Also, physicians should consider the throat and rectal areas as sites for infection.

A final consideration involves the role that changing life-styles and economics are playing in the transmission of various diseases. Homelessness, drug and alcohol use, and gay life-styles all influence how an individual expresses his sexuality. Traditional models defining sexual behavior are no longer appropriate or broad enough to adequately assess, treat, and prevent STDs.

──────────── **CASES FOR DISCUSSION** ────────────

CASE 1

In October, 1993, a 20-year-old black man came to the clinic concerned about a small sore on his penis and lip. He also reported "flulike" symptoms and a possible weight loss. He was tested for GC, chlamydia, herpes, chancroid, and syphilis. Staff also provided pretest counseling for HIV and he agreed to testing because of unprotected heterosexual contact with 18 partners in the preceding 5 years. He denied or was unaware of his partners' possible risks. He also denied any history of IV drug use or a blood transfusion. Lab results were negative for GC, chlamydia, herpes, chancroid, and syphilis. Results of the HIV test were positive. The young man returned in 2 weeks for posttest counseling and had lost 16 pounds. Posttest counseling was provided and the man agreed to meet an HIV case manager at the county AIDS clinic the next morning. He did not show up and future contacts were unsuccessful. In February, 1994, a female patient came to the family planning clinic with a newspaper obituary of his death from AIDS complications.

1. *Should pre- and posttest counseling be offered to the friends of the HIV-positive adolescent?*
2. *Are there any cultural issues that should be addressed with this population?*
3. *If HIV testing is performed, what consent procedures are required?*

CASE 2

In 1984, Linda, a 13-year-old black female, was brought in by her mom for a rape evaluation regarding an encounter that had occurred 3–4 days earlier. Although she was referred elsewhere, she continued to come for primary care to the clinic. At the next visit, Linda came to the clinic with a gash in her foot requiring stitches. A member of the clinic staff walked to the adjoining housing project where Linda lived to obtain parental consent for treatment. The staff member found the mother in bed with a man. The mom said she would attend to the problem but did not.

At age 16, Linda married an African man and desperately desired to become pregnant. She frequently came in for pregnancy testing. When she was 18, her husband was killed by a car while standing at a bus stop. His survivors received an insurance settlement that was held in trust for her by the executor of the estate, a professor at a nearby university. After the death of her husband, Linda went out of control, associated with drug users, and became a user herself. The next time Linda came in, she had what appeared to be shingles. After a medical history, an HIV-ELISA test was performed and results were positive. The Western blot results were also positive. The staff tried to explain the consequences of being seropositive. However, Linda continued to express her desire to become pregnant. She even reported chewing food and feeding it to an infant in the family.

Linda later brought family members to the clinic and asked the staff to explain HIV. She had a bad cough and purple spots all over her body. She failed to keep her next clinic appointment. The clinic staff tried to locate her because a Pap smear showed severe dysplasia. Linda refused to come in and did not answer any of her correspondence.

1. *Should other tests be performed if the HIV test result is positive?*
2. *What other service options should be offered to this client?*
3. *Are there issues associated with informed consent?*
4. *Are there any reporting requirements that must be addressed?*

CASE 3

A 30-year-old homeless black woman was sexually active with two adult homeless men. She behaved in a manner that suggested schizophrenia and drank on a daily basis. She has been diagnosed with trichomoniasis repeatedly. The indication is that the three of them continue to reinfect each other.

1. *How does the practitioner manage an STD-infected patient who has multiple partners?*
2. *What role does alcohol abuse play in this behavior?*
3. *What sort of social service interventions would be appropriate?*

CASE 4

A 25-five-year-old white woman with mental health problems had been diagnosed with chlamydia four times. She was sent home with doxycycline and instructions. She returned for test of cure, which was still positive. The patient reported that she could only take doxycycline with ice cream, which reduces absorption of the drug. Arrangements to get liquid erythromycin to her were made because of her refusal to comply with the medical instructions.

1. *What are physicians' responsibilities to spouses or partners when STD results continue to be positive? How does a practitioner address frequent reinfections with her patients?*
2. *Are there any other ways to encourage difficult patients to cooperate with treatment regimens?*

CASE 5

In November, 1987, a divorced 37-year-old white businessman developed a sexual relationship with a single woman in Europe. The relationship continued until 1990 when the man subsequently met and married a woman in the United States. In 1991 when his wife was 20 weeks pregnant he received a call from his former lover who revealed that she had tested positive for HIV and suggested that he be tested. His HIV test was positive although he was still asymptomatic. Results of tests for other STDs were negative. His wife tested negative for HIV.

1. *Should the wife be retested for HIV?*
2. *What are some perinatal considerations for the couple?*
3. *What are the issues associated with the sexual relationship of the couple?*

——————— RECOMMENDED READINGS ———————

Hatcher RA, Stewart F, Trussell J, Kowal D, Guest F, Stewart GK, Cates W (eds): *Contraceptive Technology 1990–1992—15th Revised Edition.* New York, Irvington Publishers, Inc, 1992.

> This text provides a comprehensive integration of reproductive health, contraception, and prevention of sexually transmitted disease. Practitioners should consider this a thorough reference on how human reproduction in the life cycle is impacted by a variety of infections, practices, and changing mores.

Morbidity and Mortality Weekly Report: *1993 Sexually Transmitted Diseases Treatment Guidelines.* 42, RR-14, 1993.

This short text describes all current treatment regimens for sexually transmitted diseases. In addition, it provides up-to-date epidemiological trends and changes in contagion and disease expression among various populations.

Carrera M. (ed): *Sex: The Facts The Acts & Your Feelings.* New York, Crown Publishers, Inc, 1993.

This is a comprehensive work generated from experience with college students. It covers a wide array of sexual issues in a direct but tasteful way.

The Boston Women's Health Book Collective (eds): *The New Our Bodies, Ourselves.* New York, Simon & Schuster, Inc, 1981.

This work approaches sexuality from a woman's perspective. The material provides an evaluation of sexuality that empowers women to take control of their sexual decisions.

CHAPTER 19

C. Special Problems

Vulnerable and Indigent Populations

Joshua Freeman, Masie Isabell, Julie Lipkin, Isaiah Perry,
and Anamari Golf

CASE 19-1

Mr. and Mrs. B. are an elderly couple in their 70s. Mrs. B. has rheumatoid arthritis, with deformities of her knees and hands, and she seems to be getting worse. Her arthritis is so advanced that it is too late to prevent joint destruction. She is taking as much medicine as she can tolerate. We decide to do a home visit to assess what is going on and what can be done to help them.

Their home is an old wood frame house that badly needs painting. The heating appears adequate, but the indoor lighting is poor, and probably a safety hazard. The couple welcome us with great appreciation. It is the first time a physician has ever visited their home. They are clearly committed to each other.

After assessing Mrs. B. in the living room, Mr. B. gives us a tour. In their bedroom we see a device made from a funnel resting next to her bed. Mr. B. explains that he invented this device, as his wife is too slow and stiff to go to the bathroom at night and that she has difficulty lifting her hips onto the regular bedpan. This device works well for her. We offer to arrange for a bedside commode, but he politely declines as he feels that his own device is simpler and more likely to prevent urinary incontinence.

Another problem Mrs. B. has is difficulty in ambulation; she is walking less and less, tiring easily, and feeling more insecure about falling. We recommend a wheelchair, but Mr. B. explains that his hall and doorways are too narrow. He has figured out a way around the problem. He shows us an old clerk's office chair on wheels which he uses to wheel his wife from the living room to the kitchen. It is small enough, and although it is a bit awkward to direct the wheels, he manages. We also observe several other creative adaptations and modifications.

We leave in awe. This couple has made extraordinary efforts to survive together and stay in their home. Many other patients in Mrs. B.'s situation would have been institutionalized, but together they came up with creative ideas that were financially reasonable, especially when the standard solutions offered by the healthcare system were inadequate. Clearly, this couple placed great importance on being together and surviving within their means.

INTRODUCTION

Through experiences in dealing with the poor and vulnerable, healthcare providers learn about the inner strengths and resources of people: patients, their families, and their communities. Often, the extended family is an important resource for survival, with nieces and nephews taking care of their aunts and uncles, grandmothers raising their grandchildren, cousins sharing households, and so on. People who live in these stressed environments have organized into community groups working to stop violence and gangs, provide clean, safe, low-cost housing, and otherwise improve their neighborhoods. Healthcare teams need to discover and work with the strengths of these "surviving" families and their communities. Identifying the characteristics of the "survivors" may lead to a better understanding of how strengths can be nurtured in all people. Besides, perhaps Mr. B.'s bedpan could be patented and manufactured!*

All people are vulnerable once they are sick, but some groups of people are more vulnerable to adverse health effects. Members of these groups may have greater risk of exposure to health dangers, have coexisting health, social, or economic problems that magnify the impact of these risk factors, or have limited ability to treat problems early and effectively. While some people, such as Mr. and Mrs. B. in Case 19-1, have done a remarkable job of coping with adversity, our ability to help our patients is enhanced by a better understanding of the characteristics of vulnerable populations. After reading this chapter the student should be able to identify specific characteristics of populations that are more vulnerable to poor health based on ethnicity, income, geography, age, disability, and environment. Second, the student will become familiar with specific data indicating the degree to which this increased vulnerability actually leads to worse health outcomes for these populations. Third, she will be able to identify obstacles to providing quality care to members of these populations, as well as the resources and strengths of "survivors" among these populations. Finally, the student should be able to present and defend several specific suggestions for changes in both medical education and social/health policy to decrease the vulnerability or enhance the health of members of these populations.

CASE 19-2

R. C. is a 73-year-old African-American woman who has Medicare and has been lucky enough to find a local physician who will accept Medicare "assignment," a county hospital-run clinic. However, Medicare does not cover the cost of the

---

*A recommended exercise for students: Do a home visit in a poor community. Make a list of the strengths that exist in the home, the family, and the community. What can other families, communities, and the healthcare system learn?

medications for her hypertension, non-insulin-dependent diabetes mellitus, congestive heart failure, and arthritis, which total over $200 per month. Again she is lucky: She is able to get the medications free at the county hospital. This, however, requires two buses and as much as 2 hours each way. She often does not keep her afternoon appointments in the clinic, arrives late because of the bus, and rushes through appointments to get out early. Frequently, particularly in the winter, she skips appointments altogether and comes for "medication refills" in the morning seeing whatever provider is available, because she wants to be home before it gets dark; she has been mugged once already. Her blood pressure and diabetes mellitus are not well controlled and she has required two hospitalizations in the last year for worsening heart failure.

——— WHAT MAKES A PATIENT VULNERABLE? ———

In general terms, a useful "dictionary" definition of vulnerability is "open to attack" or damage. In the context of this chapter and this book, our focus is specifically on populations with increased vulnerability to healthcare problems. However, many of the characteristics discussed in this section, such as poverty, age, and chronic disease, may make people vulnerable to a variety of other problems that in turn may affect their health. The complex nature of social existence does not permit problems to be easily compartmentalized as "health-related" or "non-health-related." Moreover, members of these populations are the most susceptible to changes in social policy and government spending for social programs, since their very survival—food, housing, healthcare—may be dependent on such programs. This susceptibility is especially concerning in the United States, which, although a wealthy country, does not have a national health system or other broad social programs that characterize many other Western nations.

While indigence, and in addition "medical indigence" (the lack of health insurance or coverage), are definite indicators of increased vulnerability to healthcare problems, they are not the only ones. Age is an important determinant; both children and the elderly have greater vulnerability to health problems, less access, and often need assistance accessing healthcare providers, independent of income or insurance status. Geography affects access to healthcare services, both for rural people and for those in the inner city. Preexisting health status, the presence of disabilities or chronic disease, clearly puts people at higher risk, as does exposure to toxic substances, whether voluntary (smoking, alcohol, or other drugs) or involuntary (air and water pollution, pesticides in food, occupational exposures). In addition, such vulnerabilities, or "risk factors," are rarely seen in isolation. They are frequently combined, as in Case 19-2, to further increase the health risk of people so affected.

HEALTH INSURANCE STATUS

In the United States more than 35 million people were without health insurance in any given month during 1990, representing 13.9% of the population (Woolhandler & Himmelstein, 1992). Not surprisingly, the poor were most likely to be uninsured; 22.3% of those with family incomes under $25,000 per year were uninsured as opposed to 7.7% of those with incomes over $50,000. While young adults 18–39 are most likely to be uninsured (20%), 13% of children under 18 are without insurance despite programs such as Medicaid (Woolhandler & Himmelstein, 1992). Because of Medicare, only 0.9% of people over 64 are uninsured but, as we note from Case 19-2, Medicare does not solve all of the financial barriers to receiving healthcare. Only 7% of the uninsured were unemployed, while 40% were employed and one-third were children of working people. Although members of minority groups are disproportionately uninsured (one-third of Hispanics and 20% of African Americans), 10.7% of non-Hispanic whites were also uninsured (Woolhandler & Himmelstein, 1992).*

INCOME

Poverty is not only associated with less access to healthcare, it is also associated with poor nutrition, poor housing, greater exposure to environmental toxins (such as lead and air pollution), and lower levels of educational understanding about positive health behaviors (Rask *et al.*, 1994; Haan *et al.*, 1987). Not only unemployed people are poor; many full-time, full-year (FT/FY) workers earn less than the poverty level, and the percentage is increasing, from 12% in 1974 to 18% in 1990 (Woolhandler & Himmelstein, 1992). Again, minorities and women are overrepresented among FT/FY workers earning less than poverty levels—13% for whites, 22.4% for blacks, 28.2% for Hispanics, 24.3% for women, and 37% for Hispanic women (Woolhandler & Himmelstein, 1992). The situation is even worse for workers employed part-time or for part of the year.

ENVIRONMENTAL THREATS

Virtually all people on earth are subject to environmental health threats from air and water pollution and pesticides and herbicides in the food supply. However, those living near direct sources of air pollution (factories, highways, dump sites of both toxic and nontoxic waste) or workers exposed to high concentrations of toxic substances are particularly vulnerable (LaDou, 1990; Jaakkola & Miettinen, 1995; Chang *et al.*, 1994; Chao & Wang, 1994; Greer *et al.*, 1993). For people who live in areas where violence is a daily occurrence—and indeed for those who restrict their activities because of a perception of violence, real or not—violence too is an environmental hazard.

LIFE-STYLE

Many substances can be ingested that cause increased vulnerability to health problems. While illegal drugs are the target of much legislative action, the health effects of

---

Medicare is a health insurance program funded and administered by the federal government. It covers primarily the elderly, although blind and disabled people and those with certain chronic diseases (e.g., end-stage kidney disease) are eligible. Medicare usually pays all of the costs of inpatient care, but only part of the cost for outpatient services. Many physicians are reluctant to accept only the amount Medicare pays for services (Medicare assignment). Medicare does not cover the costs of most medications or long-term care, even though the largest number of people requiring long-term care are the elderly.

Medicaid is the health program for the poor, jointly funded by federal and state governments, with the federal government paying 50–70% depending on per capita state income. Services available, and to whom they are available, vary *widely* from state to state. Federal law mandates coverage of certain populations (e.g., families receiving "cash grants"—welfare payments—under the Aid to Families with Dependent Children program) and provision of certain services, but even these can vary widely since states can set quite different income levels for those who are eligible for such payments. In addition, there are a variety of other populations (people making just above poverty-level wages) and services that states can elect to cover, increasing the interstate disparity. Medicaid *does* cover care in nursing homes, known as "long-term care," for the indigent, and this consumes the largest part of the Medicaid budget. Even though the largest percentage of Medicaid *recipients* are dependent children, the largest percentage of *expenditures* go to long-term care.

Table 19.1
Comparison of Various Health Indicators by Race/Ethnicity[a]

Health indicator	All races	Black	Hispanic
Coronary heart disease deaths per 100,000 (1987)	135	163	NA[b]
Cancer deaths per 100,000 (1987)	158 WM	288 BM	NA
	110 WF	132 BF	
Tuberculosis per 100,000 (1988)	9.1	28.3	18.3
Diabetes per 1000 (1987)	28	36	54
Maternal mortality per 100,000 live births (1987)	6.6	14.2	NA
Teen pregnancies per 1000 (age 15-19, 1985)	110	186	158
Homicides per 100,000 men 15–34 (1987)	8.5 (all people)	90.5	53.1
Untreated dental caries children 6–8 (1986)	27%	38%	36%
Prenatal care in 1st trimester (1987)	76%	61.1%	61%
Cigarette smoking > 20 years old (1987)	29%	34%	33%
Mammograms > 40 (1987)	36%	28%	20%

[a]Source: U.S. Public Health Service, *Healthy People 2000* (1991).
[b]NA, not available.

alcohol, sedentary life-styles, high-fat diets, and especially tobacco are much greater (Diacatou *et al.*, 1993; Haan *et al.*, 1987).

ETHNICITY

Minority populations are particularly vulnerable. It is difficult to separate the effects of poverty, physical location, toxin exposure, etc., but for virtually all health indicators identified by departments of public health, the negative impact for minority populations, particularly African-American and Hispanic, is greater than for the population as a whole (Table 19.1) (U.S. Public Health Service, 1991). It is possible that overt or institutionalized discrimination limits access and use of healthcare in addition to other factors.

GEOGRAPHY, AGE, ILLNESS, AND DISABILITY

The physical or social isolation of people living in rural areas and inner cities, the special needs of children and the elderly, and the added burdens of chronic illness and disability are important contributors to health vulnerability. As such they are treated in depth in later sections.

MULTIFACTORIAL VULNERABILITY

All of the risk factors discussed in this section, and a number of others, increase the vulnerability of the people whom they affect. The greater problem is that each of these risk factors—poverty, lack of health insurance coverage, geographic isolation, inner-city living, minority status, toxin exposure, age, chronic disease, and disability—do not vary independently but often occur together. In Case 19-2, our patient was elderly, minority, living in the inner city, geographically (in terms of transportation) isolated from healthcare, vulnerable to community violence, suffering from chronic disease, and had inadequate health insurance.

Children living in the inner city may experience the multiple threats of poverty, community violence, and family disruption. They often live in single-parent families where parents lack access to jobs paying reasonable wages (Diacatou *et al.*, 1993; Haan *et al.*, 1987). Men are often unable to find work and therefore cannot support their families. Men are also discouraged from staying with their families by social policies that prohibit welfare payments to "intact" families, exacerbating the problem of family disruption (Laseter, 1991; Wilson, 1991).

The combination of poverty, inadequate health insurance, geographic isolation from health services, high levels of violence, drug and alcohol use, and disrupted families synergistically contribute to poorer health for the people so affected.

People in rural areas are not only geographically isolated from healthcare settings, but are also disproportionately elderly: again a result of low job availability and consequent out-migration of young people. They are also disproportionately poor and affected with chronic disease.

CASE 19-3

J. R. is a 50-year-old farmer with a history of illness and coronary artery disease for which he is taking medication. On a survey of his farm, which covers 20 miles and is far from the nearest neighbors, he accidentally fell down a cliff. The fall broke his leg and left him hanging on a sharp ledge. He managed to reset and splint the fracture and place a tourniquet to stop the bleeding. Unable to go up or down, he spent all day in the heat and sun without food or water.

After the sun had gone down, a neighbor whom he had contacted that morning noticed that J. R. had not returned and notified the county sheriff's department. A search team on foot and later by air located him. He was lifted from the ledge via a helicopter and taken to the nearest hospital approximately 60 miles away.

—————— GEOGRAPHIC VULNERABILITY ——————

RURAL AREAS

Many rural families live far away from their neighbors. There is limited access to both primary and secondary medical care, with a small clinic in town or hospital in the county. Tertiary care is often accessed via helicopter. The local drugstore is frequently a major source of medical information in rural areas. People who live in such settings often become quite expert at treating many injuries and illnesses without seeking medical attention, although outcomes are not always favorable.

In Case 19-3, J. R. knew a great deal about treating injuries and was able to begin his own treatment before help arrived. Also, he had taken a "routine" precaution and had informed his neighbor of his expected return. He was also very fortunate to be able to tell his story.

Accidents of all types with various degrees of urgency occur in rural areas, in part because of the type of labor, such as farming, ranching, and logging, in which many rural people engage. The long distances to the nearest medical center may delay access to care. In addition, the rural population is increasingly comprised of elderly people, many living alone and some distance from their neighbors. This may lead to minimal interpersonal interaction and promote depression and a feeling of being isolated from society. Some families are without transportation and are dependent on family members or others to meet their daily needs. Family members occasionally resent the inconvenience.

Many hospitals in rural areas lack the medical equipment and personnel to handle life-threatening diseases, such as acute cardiac arrest or acute exacerbation of asthma. Many rural areas also do not have central emergency medical system dispatching services and do not train their citizens in cardiopulmonary resuscitation (CPR) (Becker *et al.*, 1991). Nationwide, only 3% of all patients who have out-of-hospital arrest survive (Hodgetts *et al.*, 1995). Data from Chicago demonstrate that survival rates improve for people who arrest and receive CPR, implying that increasing the percentage of the population trained in CPR would improve survival (Becker *et al.*, 1991).

INNER CITIES

The inner-city neighborhoods of many urban areas have few healthcare facilities, with provider-to-population ratios far lower than for other parts of the metropolitan area (Rask *et al.*, 1994). This results in part from the poverty of these communities, which makes private medical practice less financially attractive. The situation is exacerbated by fear that healthcare providers have of violence against their person and property.

The violence that plagues our inner cities has affected healthcare delivery in numerous ways. Acts of violence are a common sight for the people who live in many inner-city neighborhoods. Patients may not keep their clinic appointments because they are afraid to come out of their homes or afraid to be out of the home after the sun sets for fear of violence. The situation in many public settings, requiring long waits, makes patients very reluctant to come for afternoon appointments, which may result in their being out after dark. Several long waits are often necessary: to register, to see the provider, to get laboratory services, and to get prescriptions. Patient education programs offered in the evenings at local health facilities may get scant attendance because of this fear. This makes these patients increasingly vulnerable because they do not get proper care and follow-up of their many problems.

Patients in urban medical settings are often unemployed and have no insurance. Some receive public aid and have Medicaid, but decreasing reimbursement for services has led to few primary care physicians, and even fewer subspecialists, accepting patients with public aid cards. Transportation poses a problem for people on public aid and fixed incomes. They normally use public transportation to go from home to clinic, and trips for referrals to the hospital consume even more time. Since inner-city clinics often do not have extended hours, the need for residents who are employed to take time off work to come in or bring in a child further complicates the situation. Because of the financial disincentives to private practice, the major sources of care in many of these communities are public city- or county-run clinics, private charity clinics, and community health centers. These sites may have other restrictions, however, including limited laboratory tests and restricted formularies of medications.

CASE 19-4

L. T. is a 12-year-old girl who presents for a sixth-grade school physical complaining of recent breast enlargement. On discovering that her last menstrual period (LMP) was 3 to 4 months previously, you order a urine pregnancy test, which is positive. She has not received any prenatal care as she did not realize she was pregnant. L. T.'s mother feels embarrassed and guilty at her daughter's pregnancy and does not bring her back for additional prenatal care for another 3 months. At that time, you discover that the mother had suspected her own live-in boyfriend of being the father and had immediately thrown him out. She also had not spoken to her daughter for this entire period, and only recently learned that the father was an 18-year-old boy whom her daughter had been seeing; this helped the mother overcome her embarrassment and bring L. T. in for care. L. T. had not yet been tested for syphilis, rubella, HIV, or other sexually transmitted diseases (STDs); her syphilis screen (RPR) was positive. Her weight gain was very poor.

FRAGILE AGE GROUPS

ADOLESCENTS

Case 19-4 is not as atypical as it first may appear. As many as one million U.S. teenagers become pregnant each year (Maurer, 1991). In 1985 the pregnancy rate for girls under 17 was 71/1000; for African Americans the rate was 186/1000, and for Hispanics, 158/1000. Ninety-six percent of pregnant women under 19 are unmarried, and 84% of these pregnancies are unintended (Henshaw *et al.*, 1989; Jones *et al.*, 1986). As in Case 19-4, adolescents who are pregnant are at high risk for not starting prenatal care early, and children born to teenagers are at higher risk for a variety of physical, psychological, and social problems (Singh *et al.*, 1985; Alan Guttmacher Institute, 1987).

Adolescents are at risk for other problems as well. Adolescence is a time of major stress in which the transition from childhood to adulthood leads to experimentation with many of the opportunities life has to offer. Unfortunately, this experimentation includes a number of activities that are detrimental to health, including unprotected sex, use of alcohol, tobacco, and other drugs, and involvement with gangs. The *Healthy People 2000* report indicates that, in 1988, 25% of 12- to 17-year-olds and 58% of 18- to 20-year-olds drink alcohol; for marijuana the percentages are 6.4 and 15.5%, and for cocaine, 1.1 and 4.5%. Thirty percent of adolescents became smokers by age 20 in 1987. Three-fourths of all deaths in the 15–24 age group (99.4/100,000 in 1987) are from auto accidents, and 50% of those involve alcohol. The rate of alcohol use in the 15–24 age group is greater than in any other. Blacks were the only group for whom auto accidents were not the leading cause of death in this age group; homicide, overall the eleventh leading cause of death, is. The 1987 homicide rate was 8.5/100,000; for black males 15–34 years old it was 90.5/100,000. Suicide is also a major problem for adolescents. Although elderly males have the highest successful suicide rate, the rates for teenagers are alarming (10.3/100,000, versus an overall rate of 11.7) and are increasing (U.S. Public Health Service, 1991).

Adolescents frequently lack the maturity of judgment, as well as a belief in their own mortality, to make wise health decisions. In addition, they may develop patterns of behavior such as eating junk food, drinking, and smoking that, even if they do not have negative short-term effects, may increase their risk of disease later in life. Adolescents have the highest rate of STDs of any population group. The overall gonorrhea rate, for example, was 300/100,000 in 1989, but was 1123/100,000 in adolescents (Table 19.2). This rate is largely a result of unsafe sex practices, and often beginning sexual activity before consulting a healthcare provider for counseling and contraception (Washington *et al.*, 1986;

Table 19.2
Incidence of Gonorrhea, 1988[a]

Population group	Gonorrhea incidence (per 100,000)
All races	300
Blacks	1990
Adolescents	1123
Women aged 15–44	501

[a]Source: Centers for Disease Control (1990a).

Centers for Disease Control, 1990a). However, it is important to recognize that the health problems faced by adolescents are not solely the result of their actions, but often involve the actions of adults. This is particularly in the area of pregnancy and STDs. In California in 1993, in three-quarters of births in which one parent was school age, the other was an adult (71% of the births to school-age girls and 23% of births fathered by school-age boys) (Males, 1995). Many pregnant adolescent girls have histories of sexual abuse or rape by family members or adult "boyfriends" 5–10 years older (Gershenson *et al.*, 1989). Thus, it is critical that accurate histories be taken to ensure that responsible adults are identified and the appropriate actions taken. This may include child support, or it may include criminal prosecution for rape or incest, while the pregnant adolescent, the victim, receives the support she requires.

CHILDREN

As noted in the introductory section, children are a particularly vulnerable population. From before birth, they are dependent on others for their care, for their nutrition, for their psychosocial nurturing, and for their immunizations. It is very difficult to take good care of children, even for mature parents with educational and financial resources, support systems, and the best of intentions. Moreover, exposure to a variety of insults in childhood, beginning *in utero* (infections, toxins, lack of immunizations, nondiagnosis of congenital or chronic disease, poor nutrition, neglect, abuse) can have lifelong impact. In general, children are frequently members of the group with multifactor vulnerability; 37 million live in poverty and 9 to 12 million have no health insurance.

The infant death rate in the United States is higher than in virtually every other industrialized country. In some areas, such as the inner city, the numbers are comparable to those in parts of the third world. The overall infant death rate in 1987 was 10.4/1000, while for blacks it was 17.9 (Table 19.3). The percentage of babies of low birth weight (< 2500 g) was 6.9% (12.7% for blacks) and of very low birth weight (< 1500 g), 1.2% (2.7% for blacks) (U.S. Public Health Service, 1991). Infant mortality in the United States is higher than that in virtually all other developed countries (see Table 19.4) and even higher than that in some third world countries, such as Singapore (less than 9/1000) (Woolhandler & Himmelstein, 1992).

Child abuse accounted for 1100 deaths in 1986, half from abuse and half from neglect. There were 1.6 million cases of abuse in 1986, with a rate of 25.2/1000 children under age 18. Of these, the rates were 5.7/1000 for physical abuse, 2.5/1000 for sexual abuse, 3.4/1000 for emotional abuse, and 15.9/1000 for neglect (Westat, Inc., 1988). In addition, only 80% of white children and 50% of black children were immunized against measles before the age of 2 (Centers for Disease Control, 1990b).

Table 19.3

Infant Mortality in United States by Race, 1984[a]

Race	Infant mortality rate (per 1000 live births)
All races	10.4
White	2.9
Black	17.9
American Indian	12.5
Asian	8.8
Hispanic[b]	9.3
Mexican	8.9
Puerto Rican	12.9
Cuban	8.1
Central and South American	8.3
Other and unknown Hispanic	9.6

[a]Source: U.S. Public Health Service, *Healthy People 2000* (1991).
[b]For 23 states and District of Columbia where Hispanic origin of mother was coded on birth certificate.

Diseases such as diarrhea, otitis media, dental caries, accidents, and toxic exposures are major sources of morbidity for children. For example, 3 million children had toxic lead levels (above 15 μg/dl) in 1984; 234,000 had very high levels, over 25 μg/dl. Children in inner cities are at greater risk for lead poisoning (Agency for Toxic Substance and Disease Registry, 1988).

THE ELDERLY

As a group, the elderly have greater health risks for physical, mental, socioeconomic, and societal reasons. Our society is youth-oriented, and the attitudes and values that characterize it play an important role in the way physicians and others treat elderly patients. If we fear growing old and becoming vulnerable, this will affect our attitude toward our older patients. Confronting these attitudes is a critical component of the education of future physicians, for most of us will one day look in the mirror and find ourselves in this fragile age group, vulnerable to the very system we cultivated.

Table 19.4

Infant Mortality in Developed Countries, 1988[a]

Country	Infant mortality (per 1000 live births)
United States	10
Italy	9.3
Australia	8.7
France	7.7
Germany	7.6
Canada	7.2
Japan	4.8

[a]Source: Woolhandler and Himmelstein (1992).

The aging body and mind suffer a reduction in organ reserve and, therefore, in the ability to adapt to stressors. Baseline functioning is usually adequate in healthy elderly persons who continue to lead active, productive lives. However, stresses that would be minimal for younger people, such as a hot day, can cause significant dehydration leading to morbidity and mortality. The elderly often have atypical presentations of disease, which can cause delay or misdiagnosis. For example, an elderly person with pneumonia may present with only acute confusion. Because they have multiple chronic problems, take multiple drugs, and often have altered drug metabolism, adverse drug reactions are more common in the elderly.

The "old-old," those over 85 years, are the fastest growing segment of the population and are often called the frail elderly, because they are also the most likely to suffer from chronic disease and disability. While only about 5% of people over 65 are institutionalized, the frail elderly have such significant losses of function that the rate goes up to 20% (Moon *et al.*, 1990). As a group they are vulnerable to disability and loss of independence, and, consequently, their quality of life becomes compromised.

Physicians and others working in healthcare can have a major impact on maximizing the "healthy years," preventing or slowing the rate of many diseases as opposed to merely prolonging life. This requires an emphasis on disease prevention and health promotion for the elderly, areas that often are ignored (Radecki and Cowell, 1990). In fact, notable deficiencies of medical care have been demonstrated for elderly patients. For example, the longest physician-visit times occur in patients between 45 and 54 years of age and the shortest for those 85 and over, despite the fact these patients often have sensory, ambulatory, and communication impairments (Sloane, 1991).

The quality of these office visits may also leave much to be desired. A decline in screening activities such as breast, pelvic, and rectal exams has been demonstrated with increasing age (Sloane, 1991). Data also suggest that health education and health promotion (counseling on exercise, diet, good health habits) are age-related deficiencies in medical care (Radecki and Cowell, 1990). Studies have shown reduced morbidity, delayed onset of dependency, and improved quality of life when health promotion is instituted as part of routine medical care in the elderly (Radecki & Cowell, 1990). Using data from the 1971–1975 Health and Nutrition Examination Survey (HANES), Heller and colleagues identified a single criterion for assessing the care given elderly patients for five common ambulatory conditions. Applying this criterion, they found high rates of deficiency in the management of angina (46%), dyspnea on exertion (78%), hypertension (26%), hearing impairments (61%), and depression (80%) (Heller *et al.*, 1984). Physicians diagnosed and managed mental health problems less often in the elderly as compared with young adults (Gernan *et al.*, 1987). The Department of Health and Human Services (DHHS) reports that in 1984, 25% of the aged had significant problems with their mental health, and 10–30% of the patients were misdiagnosed with dementing illness (Institute of Medicine, 1987).

Physician guidance in supervising the institutionalized and homebound elderly is declining; more responsibility is being shouldered by the social worker or nurse. In time, lack of adequate supervision can diminish the quality of care (Reuben *et al.*, 1990). Physician services in nursing homes is often characterized as "substandard, superficial, or indifferent" (Moon, 1990; Robbins, 1983). As the elderly population grows, their vulnerability will be exacerbated by insufficient resources within our medical system to care for the expected 65 million elderly in 2030, who will comprise 20% of the population as opposed to the present-day 12%. Even with Medicare insurance benefits, Americans over 65 are vulnerable because they are treated inadequately by physicians and the healthcare system.

Many elderly people also are socioeconomically vulnerable, since they are likely to be on fixed incomes, pensions, or Social Security benefits. While they may have other savings, the interest is not likely to keep up with inflation. Beyond the direct cost of healthcare, health depends on having financial access to adequate housing (e.g., heating, cooling, security), transportation (e.g., accessing services, socialization), and nutrition. The elderly are at risk for social isolation, lack of support when ill, and violence, particularly those who live alone. For those living with relatives, elder abuse/neglect is unfortunately common. Caregivers who control the patient's finances may use them for their own needs or, perhaps in part from frustration with the elder person's dependency, physically or emotionally abuse them. As physicians we need to be aware of all of these problems and provide comprehensive care and advocacy for our patients, just as we hope to have physicians provide comprehensive care and advocacy for us when we are old.

CASE 19-5

M. W., a well-groomed, attractive, 36-year-old woman who is wheelchair bound, comes for her visit via the home transportation provided by the hospital. She is $1\frac{1}{2}$ hours late. She is frustrated and near tears, worrying that she will not be seen. She tells you she got up at 5:30 AM to be ready for the pick up at 6:30 AM. "I was on the van for $3\frac{1}{2}$ hours! They went all over the west side of the city picking up patients."

This is her first visit with you and you hear her story: Nine months ago she was accidentally shot in a drive-by shooting. The injury left her a paraplegic. She had had a part-time job as a sales clerk at a local fashion chain store. She is now on disability. She has a 19-year-old son who is unemployed and had wanted to continue studying at the local community college toward a degree in computer science. Since the accident, however, she is dependent on him and their finances don't permit him to continue school. She expresses guilt about her son's future and frustration in adjusting to these circumstances. She is very proud and independent: "I don't want no 'charity.'" Apparently, her son carries her in and out of the house and down the steps, as there is no ramp. He also helps her get in and out of the bed and the bath, which embarrasses her. She has no sleep problems but does have episodes of fright with palpitations, sweats, and shortness of breath. She notes that she isn't getting out much and no longer goes shopping or over to see her girlfriends for coffee: "They don't have a ramp." She misses dating and wonders if "I'll feel like a woman again."

DISABILITY

Case 19-5 illustrates many of the vulnerabilities related to disability. M. W. has lost much of her social independence as well as her physical function. Although she seems to be coping, she is clearly at risk for depression as well as social isolation. She is at risk for complications of paraplegia such as urinary tract infections and pressure ulcers. She has become dependent on others for coping with the activities of daily living, including her son, who she had hoped would be occupied starting his own adult life; in addition, this is a reversal of normal parent–child roles.

The incidence of disability, defined as loss or limitation in a major activity resulting from a chronic condition, was 9.4% in the U.S. population in 1988. Low-income families, those making less than $10,000 a year, had almost double that rate, 18.9%. Members of minority groups also have higher rates, 13.4% for Native Americans and 11.2% for African Americans. The rate increases with age, to 22.6% for those over the age of 65 from 5.9% in the 18–44 age group (U.S. Public Health Service, 1991). Members of the already vulnerable populations of the poor, minority, and elderly are at further risk of being part of the functionally impaired population as well.

Healthcare resources for the disabled generally come from Medicare and Medicaid. Medicare will not pay for services or equipment that are considered for "comfort," which includes obvious necessities such as hearing aids and eyeglasses. Medicaid will pay for these items; however, a patient must be poor enough to receive Medicaid benefits. If a patient has personal assets, she will be required to "spend down" to the poverty level in order to become Medicaid-eligible. This means the loss not only of all savings but often even one's home. Obviously, these resources may not be adequate, especially for the needs of the disabled that are not directly related to their physical health, but may be related to their quality of life and mental health. Fortunately, there are often other resources available, such as agencies that have different funding sources, including grants. Sometimes services are available on a "sliding scale" based on what the patient can pay.

By their very nature, disabilities are socially isolating and disconcerting, which is one of the biggest hurdles for physicians and patients to handle. In Case 19-5, the patient, M. W., needed extensive remodeling to allow wheelchair access to her home. This included widening doorways and halls, putting in ramps where there are steps, and installing special rails for transferring into and out of bed and bath. The physician learned about and called the HRAIL (Home Repairs for Accessible, Independent Living) program. This organization uses grant money to help remodel homes; clients must meet a qualifying income level. Social workers are a major resource for discovering the various agencies that exist for assistance, but anyone involved, family or friend or healthcare provider, can contact the major organizations handling the needs of the disabled for referral to appropriate agencies. On further investigation the physician learned about other possibilities for M. W., including a "Ready Access Loan" which provides low-interest loans for owners to use for remodeling.

Physicians must make every effort to learn about and address the needs of their handicapped or impaired patients. Vulnerable patients usually need the physician to act as their advocate beyond what typically is expected. More than any standard "medical" prescription, the extra steps taken by M. W.'s physician have the potential for improving the quality of her life and that of her family.

PHYSICAL DISABILITY

The patient in Case 19-5 is an example of an acquired physical handicap/impairment caused by trauma. However, physical problems can be congenital, such as spinal bifida, clubfoot, and infections that are acquired during gestation, e.g., rubella causing deafness, genetic causes, such as muscular dystrophy, or chromosomal causes, such as trisomy 21. Physical disabilities of idiopathic nature can also arise during adulthood, e.g., multiple sclerosis.

By far the most prevalent group of physical impairments are those caused by chronic disease, and these are the conditions that most primary care physicians see most often. Diabetes mellitus can result in multiple amputations and blindness. Hypertension can cause cerebrovascular infarcts. Respiratory and cardiac insufficiency can become severe enough to make their victims bedridden. Advocating for these patients and preventing or slowing the progression of these diseases is the challenge for today's physician.

MENTAL DISABILITY

Mental disabilities may result from congenital mental retardation—genetic, infectious, toxic exposure (e.g., fetal alcohol syndrome), or cerebral palsy. The most prevalent mental disabilities are idiopathic and include schizophrenia, manic depression, and organic dementias such as Alzheimer's disease. Less common etiologies are traumatic causes, skull and brain injuries, infections: meningitis, cerebral abscesses, and encephalitis. Chronic substance abuse is all too common. Both street drugs and alcohol will mentally impair people through both their addictive nature and their direct toxic insults on the cerebrum.

Note that classifying disabilities as physical or mental can be simplistic because these categories are not exclusive; cerebral palsy, for example, is a physical disability that can also have mental effects. Physical and mental problems have a synergistic impact on each other, as the case of M. W. demonstrates.

CASE 19-6

F. T. is a 28-year-old man whom you saw in a neighborhood clinic for tiredness and "not feeling up to my usual self." He also complained of a cold over the last 2 to 3 weeks. His examination and tests indicated acute renal failure. He was advised to be hospitalized immediately for emergency renal dialysis. He refused, but several days later he was taken by ambulance for treatment. While there, the staff observed F. T. holding the hand of his male lover. The patient perceived an immediate change in attitude of the physicians, nurses, and staff to one of hostility and judgmentalism. On learning of the patient's sexual orientation, his physician recommended testing to rule out HIV infection. The patient refused. Overwhelmed by his renal disease and feeling isolated and shunned by the staff, he signed himself out of the hospital. Many of F. T.'s friends had died of AIDS, and he felt certain that he was infected. He felt devastated by the resentment and prejudice of the medical team, from whom he would require treatment for the rest of his life. F. T. became increasingly depressed, stating that he would rather be dead than go through life with this type of treatment. Several days later, he committed suicide.

———— "DIFFERENT" POPULATIONS— ————
VICTIMS OF PREJUDICE

HOMOPHOBIA

The general public as well as many members of the medical profession are still both naive and judgmental concerning HIV disease and the patients who have it. This is compounded by the overt or covert prejudice that often exists against the populations with the greatest prevalence of the disease, homosexual men and injecting drug users. The issues regarding the epidemiology of infection with HIV, including the fact that women infected through heterosexual transmission are the fastest-growing group of people with HIV, are discussed in Chapter 18, "Sexually Transmitted Diseases." The issue here is the negative impact that prejudice and stereotyping have on the quality of healthcare.

In Case 19-6, F. T. may or may not have been infected with HIV; in either case F. T. was not treated humanely by his providers. The physician had not taken an adequate sexual history, and so only found out that F. T. was gay after being informed by the staff. Sexual behaviors may increase the risk for certain diseases; thus, they are an essential part of the data-gathering, problem-solving process. Many healthcare providers find taking a sexual history difficult. Like all new skills, it must be practiced, and if students and residents integrate the sexual history into the routine questions asked of every patient as part of obtaining a database, they will become more comfortable and natural in the process. The negative response of the entire health team to the discovery that F. T. was gay, and at greater risk for HIV disease, could be a reaction to his sexual orientation, fear of the disease, or both. In any case, it was disastrous for the patient. When a patient is very ill, and particularly when he is being asked to consider diagnosis of a terminal disease, the health team must be even more supportive and compassionate. Whatever the *personal feelings* a provider has about a patient's life-style, her *behaviors* must be therapeutic.

F. T.'s response to his disease and fear of HIV infection would be found in any person facing a fatal or potentially fatal disease (Kubler-Ross, 1969). Virtually all such patients develop anxiety, depression, insomnia, somatic concerns, or suicidal thoughts. Appropriate support often requires the assistance of a mental health professional, especially if the adjustment is prolonged, there is a major depression, or the patient is actively suicidal. F. T.'s suicide might well have been prevented if his healthcare providers had shown respect, compassion, and support.

RACISM, SEXISM, AND CLASSISM

In Case 19-6, F. T. felt very isolated as a result of the negative attitudes toward his homosexuality on the part of the staff involved in his care. Prejudice against gay men and lesbian women is common in our society and can affect the quality of care and even the willingness of patients to divulge their sexual preferences or behaviors (Driscoll & Hoffmann, 1984; Schmidt, 1986; Randall, 1988). Other groups, including women, racial minorities, and the poor, may not be able to hide these differences and thus more readily suffer the effects of prejudicial attitudes. This prejudice against people who are perceived as "different" may be overt or insidious and can infect healthcare providers as much as anyone else.

As noted in the introductory section, racial minorities, particularly African-Americans and Hispanics, already suffer worse health than Euro-Americans. Negative attitudes toward people of color on the part of healthcare providers exacerbate this problem and are not acceptable. The fact that racial minorities are underrepresented in the healthcare professions, and particularly among physicians (Society of Teachers of Family Medicine, 1993; Lloyd, 1989; Shea, 1985), means that there is a greater potential for such providers to see minority patients as "other." It requires vigilance to guard against this prejudice and challenge it whenever it occurs.

Sexism is prejudicial attitudes and discriminatory behaviors directed against a majority group, women. The number of women in medicine has been increasing for a long time, and almost as many women as men are in medical school. In many ways, though, medicine remains a male-dominated profession, a characteristic that becomes more evident the "higher" up the medical hierarchy (department chairs, medical directors, deans) one goes. Many of society's attitudes toward women, including their appropriate "roles," attitudes, and behaviors, are shared by some healthcare providers; women in medical professions report greater harassment than do their male peers (Bickel & Ruffin, 1995). Women who do not conform to preconceived notions of what is appropriate in such basic areas as control of their own bodies and lives often receive explicit or implicit criticism from physicians. Women have specific healthcare needs that should be appropriately and sensitively addressed. It is not, however, acceptable for a provider to manifest behaviors that demean women, such as talking to them more condescendingly or making assumptions about their family or professional role differently from the way that provider would treat men. The patient, not the physician, should define the terms by which she will live her life. Physicians should be honest with their patients, listen to their problems and concerns before forming an opinion, and talk to them as they would want to be talked to.

Classism is less frequently discussed than sexism or racism, but it is a real phenomenon. It may be even more insidious, because the absence of vocal protest may make it seem more acceptable. Classism is manifested in part by the exclusion of poor people from many medical practices and settings. However, classism goes beyond that to be, like racism and sexism, manifested in the treatment of patients whom physicians actually do see. It occurs when providers expect less of, have less concern for, or do not fully share information with their patients because of a belief that they are unable to understand key health issues.

Most physicians come from families that are upper or upper-middle class, and they may not be familiar or comfortable with working-class or poor people. Even physicians from lower-class backgrounds are, by their profession, moved into a more privileged sector, and need to be certain that they continue to treat all of their patients with respect and not condescension.

CONCLUSION

In this chapter we have focused on the special needs of populations who are particularly vulnerable to poor health outcomes, populations characterized by their economic status, age, disability, or minority status. We have tried to identify some of the special needs and indicate how often these risk factors are combined to create "multifactorial vulnerability." It is important to understand the epidemiologic data that characterize these populations and the extent to which many risk factors are beyond the control of the individuals involved. In large degree, our ability to improve the health of these populations requires us to work to eliminate the societal causes of poor health and differential health risk.

We also, however, tried to point out the strengths of people in these situations; this is why we began our chapter discussing "survivors." It is important to recognize that "populations" are made up of people, and that people can have enormous character and resilience. Simply surviving in the setting in which some of our "cases" find themselves is a major accomplishment. Identifying the strengths that have facilitated that survival is an effective tool for working with people to improve their health and decrease their risk.

As physicians we are a privileged group, regardless of our background. It is often the most vulnerable who are also the most likely to benefit from a respectful and collaborative physician–patient relationship, in which we combine our knowledge and skills with an ability to listen and an understanding of and respect for the circumstances in which this other person, our patient, exists.

CASES FOR DISCUSSION

CASE 1

A 3-year-old African-American boy is seen in the clinic with complaints of sleeping more than other children, falling when trying to walk, and stomachache. There are three other children under age 6 in the home, who also have vague symptoms but are not as sick as the patient. The child had been discovered chewing on paint chips peeling from the walls of the home. On physical examination, he was a pale, lethargic, limp child. His blood count demonstrated a moderate anemia, and his serum lead level was 65. He was admitted to hospital for chelation therapy and hydration.

1. *The federal government identifies lead poisoning as a major health problem in children, with an estimated 3 million children exceeding the 15 μg/dl threshold in 1984 (U.S. Public Health Service, 1991). Does this seem surprising to you? Why or why not?*
2. *What are sources of lead that put children at risk for lead poisoning? Consider household, environmental, and occupational exposures. Would any of these put adults at risk?*
3. *What would be your next step in finding the source of the lead? How would you prevent reexposure of this child and others?*
4. *If significant costs are involved in cleanup and eradication of the problem, who should pay?*

CASE 2

Immediately following delivery of twins, a 26-year-old woman developed uterine bleeding. She and her husband, both Jehovah's Witnesses, refused blood transfusion, even after all other treatments failed. The patient went into coma. One of the providers was so distraught at the thought of this healthy young woman with two newborns dying needlessly that he unilaterally transfused the patient against her will. The intervention aroused the patient from her coma. When she saw the blood transfusing into her, however, she became distraught and pulled out the IV tubing. She soon relapsed into a coma, and died.

1. *As a provider what would your feelings be if this was your patient?*
2. *Do you think the provider who ordered the blood transfusion was right? Wrong? Was there any justification for his action?*
3. *Sometimes providers are confronted with difficult decisions about whether to intervene with treatments uncertain to provide benefit. In this case, the treatment was virtually certain to provide benefit, but the patient refused. What authority should a medical professional have to make such decisions?*
4. *When you have a patient in a similar situation, how will you feel when she dies? In what way might it change your practice in a future situation?*

CASE 3

M. H., a 27-year-old women who is married and has three children, is coming to you today with the chief complaint of abdominal pain. This is her fourth visit in 6 weeks. Previously she has complained of headaches, malaise, and vaginal discharge. You have found nothing significant on physical exam or laboratory tests, and her symptoms are vague. Today, she states that she continues to have abdominal "aching," which comes and goes and is unrelated to meals. There is no nausea, vomiting, diarrhea, or constipation. Her stool habits are normal. There are no urinary complaints. Her last menstrual period was 4 days ago. Results of physical examination of the abdomen are normal. You proceed with a pelvic exam and you notice a bruise on her left thigh. She shrugs it off saying she had knocked it against a table corner.

1. *What are your hypotheses concerning this patient?*
2. *How would you get a social history of what is happening in the home?*
3. *You ask her about stress and she tells you nervously that she worries she is doing a poor job in the home, never seems to be doing things right like having dinner on time or running out of groceries—"It is so hard with the kids." As she describes her work in the house she becomes tearful and quite self-critical. You finally ask if she is being hit by her husband. Reluctantly, she admits that she is, "but it is my fault, I can't do anything right." Are you required to report this? To whom? If he struck the children, what would the reporting requirements be?*
4. *Do you want to know if there are guns in the house? If there is alcohol or other substance abuse?*
5. *What is her support system? family? friends? religious community? Does her culture accept or tolerate such behavior?*
6. *What would you do next? What resources are available for the patient? What is she likely to do?*

CASE 4

In broken English, the son of a 79-year-old Cambodian man explains that his father has been complaining of abdominal pain and acting somewhat confused. He and the family have waited 5 hours in the emergency room to be seen. The nurse who does triage found his vital signs acceptable and, not being able to obtain much history, put the patient in the less-urgent category. The patient seems anxious. His blood pressure is 136/80, pulse rate 92, temperature 100.3°F. On exam, there is diffuse abdominal tenderness, but no signs of acute abdomen. The urinalysis reveals pyuria (white blood cells) and the dipstick is nitrite positive. You diagnose a urinary tract infection, but also order an abdominal X ray and ultrasound of the gallbladder. You start an intravenous line and give antibiotics. The patient is placed in the hall on the stretcher to await X rays. During this time another 2 hours has elapsed and the son must take his wife and young children home; they have been in the waiting area all day. Since the patient is stable, you approve, and tell him you'll take care of his father. An hour or so later the patient becomes more anxious and begins calling out in Cambodian dialect; no one understands him. The nurses are worried he will fall off the stretcher and place the patient in soft restraints. Vitals signs show a blood pressure of 118/74, pulse rate 98, temperature 101°F. It is a busy night. Two hours later, at 3 AM, the emergency room has calmed down and you look to see if the patient received the X rays. You find the patient on the stretcher in the hall, unresponsive and in full arrest. You call a code.

1. *What happened to this patient? Why was he at risk?*
2. *What may have been the cause of death? Do you think his death was unnecessary?*
3. *How should have things been different? What services, if any, would it have been reasonable for the hospital to provide to help prevent such outcomes?*

CASE 5

J. L. is a 31-year-old woman whom you see for regular gynecologic and obstetric care with no chronic health problems. You delivered her last child, now 18 months old, and you see her other three, who are 10, 8, and 5, for routine care and occasional acute illnesses. The children are well-behaved and generally healthy; thin but not malnourished. You know Mrs. L.'s husband is employed in a non-union, minimum-wage job without benefits; you have seen him only once, for a minor injury. You are concerned about their nutrition and ask the social worker to interview her. She returns with the information that the family food budget is quite insufficient to provide adequate nutrition for the six members of the family. Arrangements are made for the family to receive emergency food assistance (food basket) from a local pantry.

1. *What are the signs of malnutrition in children? How does protein plus calorie deprivation differ from just calorie deprivation? What vitamin deficiencies might you be most concerned about?*
2. *How would you take an adequate nutrition history? What kinds of questions need to be asked?*
3. *What community resources might be available to help families in need? How would you learn about them?*
4. *What health concerns other than nutrition should be raised when finding out a family does not have even enough money for food? How would you go about investigating them?*
5. *What is your reaction to discovering that a full-time worker cannot earn enough to feed his family adequately? Is he lucky to have a job at all? Is this a social problem that needs to be addressed? How might it be addressed?*

CASE 6

S. N., a 54-year-old woman whom you see for management of hypertension, diabetes, and arthritis, comes in accompanied by her three grandchildren, 8, 5, and 4 years old, whom you have never seen. She tells you they are there for physicals required by the state who has placed them in her care because their mother, S. N.'s daughter, was murdered in her home by her boyfriend one week before. S. N. lives in a one-bedroom apartment on a small disability income.

1. *What immediate concerns might you have about the children?*
2. *What kind of services, other than physical examination, might they need? How would you obtain them?*
3. *What problems would you anticipate that she might have in caring for the children? How will her health problems affect, and be affected by, this new situation?*
4. *What will be the financial support for the family? How will S. N.'s disability income be affected?*

CASE 7

A 14-year-old girl is referred to your clinic by a private physician because she has no money. She comes in with her mother, to whom she has just returned after running away to get an abortion. (She refuses to say where.) Results of the physical exam are consistent with an uncomplicated abortion. Her father has been sent to jail for cocaine distribution. Her older sister is a cocaine addict. She has been dating the drug dealer, who is the father of her aborted fetus. The girl denies drug use, but runs away again and is found selling drugs for her boyfriend in a downtown hotel. She finally acknowledges that she does use cocaine, is sent into drug rehabilitation for 6 weeks, and is then sent out of town to school. She is eventually expelled from school for having boys and alcohol in her room. During the next year she becomes pregnant twice more, aborting both times, and is almost stabbed to death by another woman in a fight over the drug-dealer boyfriend. In addition, you find out "through the grapevine" that the girl's mother is selling heroin. When asked about school the girl says to you, "Why do I have to go to school? My boyfriend makes more in one day than you make in a month."

1. *For what medical problems is this girl at risk? What other health risks does she have from her social environment?*

2. *Given her social situation, what is the likelihood that this girl will be able to remain drug and alcohol free? Is there any intervention you can make to increase the likelihood?*
3. *If she does decide to carry a pregnancy to term, is she at increased risk? What would be the prognosis for a child that she delivered?*
4. *What are the potential sources of strength in her life? Despite selling heroin, her mother seems quite concerned about her. Do you think it possible or likely that the mother can be relied on as a support?*
5. *How do you answer her question about your income relative to her drug-dealer boy-friend's?*

RECOMMENDED READINGS

Aday LA: *At Risk in America: The Health and Health Care Needs of Vulnerable Populations in the United States.* San Francisco, Jossey–Bass, 1993.

> As the title indicates, this is a perfect source for further data and analysis of the plight of vulnerable populations. In a very well-referenced work, Dr. Aday develops a comprehensive analysis and taxonomy of the issue. Chapters sequentially address who are vulnerable, how many, why, who pays, etc., and develop proposals for community-oriented health policies.

Abraham LK: *Mama Might Be Better Off Dead.* Chicago, University of Chicago Press, 1993.

> A personal, moving, sobering, and sometimes chilling account of one family's interaction with the healthcare system.

Dula A, Goering S (eds): *"It Just Ain't Fair" : The Ethics of Health Care for African Americans.* Westport, CT: Praeger, 1994.

> A compilation of essays with expert commentary on health and health access, with emphasis on problems faced by African Americans, but with broader implications. Includes chapters on ethics, physicians' responsibilities, HIV, and even the health problems faced by rural whites in Appalachia.

Gesler WM, Ricketts TC (eds): *Health in Rural North America.* New Brunswick, NJ, Rutgers University Press, 1992.

> A thorough and scholarly examination of the general and specific health and health access problems of rural populations, with emphasis on "high-risk" populations, such as children, elderly, and the disabled.

McGinnis JM, Lee PR: *Healthy People 2000* at mid-decade. *JAMA* 273(14):1123–1129, 1995.

> An update on progress toward the *HP2000* goals, from leaders in the Public Health Service.

U.S. Public Health Service: *Healthy People 2000: National Health Promotion and Disease Prevention Objectives.* Washington, DC: U.S. Department of Health and Human Services, 1991. Publication PHS 91-50212.

> The national objectives for the state of the nation's health. This includes baseline data for virtually all major diseases, health impairments, and availability of health services, often subdivided by race, age, gender, or other risk factor. Invaluable source book.

CHAPTER 20

C. Special Problems

Maternal and Child Health

Larry Culpepper, Sara G. Shields, and Mark Loafman

CASE 20-1

Sandy Kopenski is an unscheduled walk-in who appears depressed and upset as Dr. Fields walks into the examining room. Six months ago she had come in with her boyfriend Tom to see Dr. Fields for her first prenatal visit. She is 19 and worked in a nearby factory to pay for tuition at the community college she attended part-time. Dr. Fields has cared for Sandy and her family for years. He knew this unplanned pregnancy had caused considerable tension in the Kopenski family, who always have been outspoken about their strong religious beliefs.

Since Sandy was unsure of her last menstrual period, Dr. Fields performed an ultrasound to help him establish the baby's gestational age. The ultrasound showed a 20-week fetus that appeared to have an abnormality in the continuity of its vertebrae. He referred Sandy to the regional medical center where a targeted ultrasound exam confirmed the presence of a meningomyelocele. She returned to Dr. Fields who explained that the infant might be neurologically impaired and unable to walk or attain control of its bowel and bladder. They discussed options, including termination, and how best to involve her family for support.

The pregnancy continued until 37 weeks of gestation when Sandy went into labor. As planned, she was transferred by ambulance from their community hospital to the medical center in anticipation of the need for neonatal intensive care. The baby was delivered by elective cesarean section and was found to have significant neurologic involvement. The NICU staff was supportive but Sandy felt overwhelmed by the technology, numerous physicians, and the many decisions that had to be made regarding surgery and related care of her infant. Dr. Fields discussed the case with the neurosurgeon and neonatologist and then held a family meeting with the Kopenskis to discuss their options and begin discharge planning. The infant subsequently underwent surgery and was eventually discharged to the care of Sandy, her family, and Dr. Fields. They worked closely with the staff at the regional neurodevelopmental unit and the visiting nurse service. A referral to an early intervention program also was arranged.

Although Sandy appreciates her family's support, she has not resolved her feelings of guilt surrounding the unplanned and out-of-wedlock birth. Her boyfriend Tom is afraid of the baby and is becoming detached. Sandy is becoming increasingly isolated and depressed, and voices her fear that Dr. Fields will be unable to help.

INTRODUCTION

Physicians who provide obstetric services consider the care of women and their families during pregnancy and early childhood one of the most essential and rewarding aspects of practice. The family physician is perhaps the best positioned of all physicians to fulfill the goals of care during this time in a family's life, as defined by the federal Expert Panel on the Content of Prenatal Care (Rosen, 1989). These goals of care include goals for the pregnant woman, the fetus and infant, and the family (see Table 20.1). Success requires that the physician identify and respond in an organized manner to the broad variety of problems that might arise during this time in a family's life. These problems might be of an urgent obstetric or medical nature, of a psychiatric nature, or relate to a family's behaviors and social circumstances.

The preconception and prenatal interval are critical to the health of the fetus and future child, and the care provided during this interval might dramatically alter the entire life of the child and family. Effective preventive interventions can alter conditions that otherwise might lead to permanent disability. In addition, the birth of the first child involves fundamental changes in the relationship between husband and wife; subsequent children further redefine this relationship and the parent–child dynamics of the family.

While this can be a time of growth and joy for the family, it is also a time of risk. Extramarital relationships involving the husband are most likely to start during the first pregnancy. Pregnancy is also a time of heightened risk for physical and emotional abuse

Table 20.1
The Goals of Prenatal Care Defined by the Expert Panel on the Content of Prenatal Care

---

Objectives for the pregnant woman
  • Increase her well-being before, during, and after pregnancy and improve her self-image and self-care
  • Reduce maternal mortality and morbidity, fetal loss, and unnecessary pregnancy interventions
  • Reduce risks to health prior to future pregnancies and beyond childbearing years
  • Promote development of parenting skills
Objectives for the infant
  • Increase well-being
  • Reduce preterm birth, intrauterine growth retardation, congenital anomalies, and failure to thrive
  • Promote healthy growth and development, immunization, and health supervision
  • Reduce neurologic, developmental, and other morbidities
  • Reduce child abuse and neglect, injuries, preventable acute and chronic illness, and need for extended hospitalization after birth
Objectives for the family
  • Promote family development and positive parent–infant interaction
  • Reduce unintended pregnancies
  • Identify for treatment behavior disorders leading to child neglect and family violence

---

(Helton *et al.*, 1987; Newberger *et al.*, 1992). Many women and families are not prepared for the birth of a child and need assistance in fundamental ways. The family physician is often the person to whom a family turns to for help with these issues. Often, effective care of medical and obstetric problems is not possible until psychosocial problems are addressed. For example, the woman who does not have transportation or childcare for her other children, possibly because of a dysfunctional relationship with the father of her children, is not likely to seek early or adequate care for preeclampsia, an often asymptomatic condition involving increased blood pressure and decreased uterine perfusion that can lead to prematurity and low birth weight.

As in Case 20-1, for families with infants born prematurely or with a chronic problem, and for women with chronic medical problems, the coordination of care from prior to conception through pregnancy and from delivery through ongoing care after discharge is important. A young woman with a child who has a congenital defect might find herself cared for initially during pregnancy in her local community and its hospital facilities, then in a tertiary care center by maternal–fetal medicine specialists, delivering at the tertiary care center with subsequent involvement of a neonatologist and neonatal intensive care unit team, and then discharged back to her community with intended follow-up with a variety of pediatric specialists and a community-based team of services for children with special needs. The decisions she must make for her infant, the variety of information she will receive, the feelings of self-blame and guilt for her infant's condition, and the alterations expected for her own life all might be overwhelming.

In these circumstances, the steady presence of a physician who knows the woman and her family, who has developed an understanding of her strengths and ability to cope, as well as her weaknesses, and who is trusted to help with the adjustments and decisions to be made can dramatically alter the outcome for all involved. Thus, core principles of primary care—comprehensiveness, coordination, and continuity—are critical to the provision of high quality care to women, their families, and children during the childbearing years.

CASE 20-2

Catherine Jones related to Dr. Fields the mixed emotions she felt last week as she watched her home pregnancy test turn positive. Although she has wanted a baby for several years, her two previous miscarriages had been devastating. In each case, she developed pain and bleeding late in the first trimester. A thorough evaluation had failed to detect any abnormalities or risk factors for miscarriage. Dr. Fields discussed the various screening tests that were available and set up a schedule of frequent visits to monitor Catherine and her pregnancy. They had already discussed the role of nutrition, life-style modifications, and emotional preparation for pregnancy.

As the pregnancy approached the 10th week, Catherine experienced some painless vaginal bleeding. An ultrasound was reassuring and she was asked to restrict her physical activity. Her employer requested that she either perform her usual duties or take a full medical leave. She asked Dr. Fields to intervene on her behalf.

The bleeding resolved and the pregnancy continued without complication until 32 weeks of gestation when Catherine noticed several episodes of premature contractions. Again, frequent visits and patient education were undertaken along with a series of outpatient visits to the hospital for monitoring.

COMPONENTS OF PRENATAL CARE

As Case 20-2 illustrates, prenatal care involves three basic activities: early and continuing risk assessment, health promotion, and medical and psychosocial interventions in response to risks and problems identified. A comprehensive risk assessment done at initial contact and then regularly updated provides the information around which all other prenatal care is organized. While pregnancy should be viewed as a normal (rather than illness) event, only about 40% of women will be found to have no risk requiring professional intervention (Alexander & Keirse, 1989; Selwyn, 1990). For most mothers, the family physician might need to pursue further investigations and intervene accordingly.

Risk assessment includes history taking, physical examination, and diagnostic tests. Table 20.2 lists the risks that have been documented as influencing birth outcomes (Mohide & Grant, 1989; Rosen, 1989). As can be seen, a great variety of medical, obstetric, nutritional, psychological, health behavior, and social risks can adversely affect pregnancy outcomes. Risks, especially those of a psychosocial nature, are simply characteristics that have been associated with adverse birth outcomes. While they are all markers of poor outcomes, they might not be the direct cause. Instead, as illustrated in Fig. 20.1, such factors might play a role in a complex set of processes leading to poor outcome. The content, timing, and number of prenatal visits will vary depending on the woman's risks.

While risks can be separated into medical (organic) and psychosocial groups, the physician must respond to all risks in an integrated manner. Medical risks can lead to psychosocial risks and vice versa. For example, a woman placed at bed rest early in pregnancy because of a medical complication might lose income and thus require additional support from other family members, leading to other stresses. High levels of stress might in turn lead to blood pressure alterations, increased uterine irritability, and premature labor. For this reason, the biopsychosocial model of care is particularly appropriate for families of reproductive age (Culpepper & Jack, 1993; Ramsey, 1988).

For all women, including those at low risk, a series of health promotion activities is required (Rosen, 1989). These activities are listed in Table 20.3 and can be provided one-on-one or in group settings. Their purpose is to help the woman and her family adjust to the changes that occur during pregnancy and to prepare for the coming of the newborn. They include counseling to promote and support healthy behaviors, education regarding pregnancy and parenting, and provision of information about proposed care. While some activities are likely to be most effective if done early in pregnancy, other become more relevant to the family later in pregnancy. Consequently, some medical and midwifery practices offer both early and late prenatal classes, which may be followed by parenting classes after the birth.

In addition to risk assessment and health promotion, prenatal care includes specific interventions to alter the risks for poor pregnancy outcome, including treating existing medical and obstetric problems, and initiating psychosocial interventions.

CASE 20-3

A 33-year-old woman and her husband, married 3 years, have come to Dr. Fields' office seeking advice and to interview him about being their physician. She has recently attained the seniority at her work that she wanted prior to starting a family. The couple feel they have worked through several difficult relationship issues and are emotionally and financially ready to start a family; they have

Table 20.2
Conditions to Be Targeted during Prenatal Risk Assessment[a]

History
  Sociodemographic
    Age*
    Marital status
    Income and educational level*
    Household size, geographic location
    Level of financial resources for pregnancy*
    Nature of support network for pregnant woman and family*
    Adequacy of housing
    Availability of transportation*
    Availability of childcare
    Fluency and literacy in English language*
    Mental or physical disabilities*
  Psychological
    Major life events and stressors
    Family function*
    Extremes of maternal stress and anxiety*
    Abuse or family violence*
    Mental status and illness*
    Readiness for pregnancy*
    Readiness for parenting (attitudes, knowledge, skills)*
    Adjustment problems*
    Suicide risk*
  Menstrual/gynecologic
    Onset, duration, frequency, and character of menses
    Last menstrual period (LMP) and last normal menstrual period (LNMP)*
    Infections such as pelvic inflammatory disease (PID)*
    Gynecologic surgery
  Contraceptive and sexual
    Whether pregnancy planned or wanted*
    Contraceptive methods used*
    Current sexual relationship, partners
  Past obstetric
    Prior pregnancies, length and timing
    Previous intrauterine growth retardation (IUGR) infant or preterm birth
    High parity, short birth interval*
    Previous hemorrhage
    Stillborn or neonatal death
    Sudden infant death syndrome (SIDS) infant
  Medical and surgical
    Chronic diseases, e.g., diabetes mellitus, hypertension, anemias*
    Prescription medications*
    Infections, e.g., HIV, hepatitis, toxoplasmosis*
    Allergies
    Trauma
    Surgical procedures
    Blood transfusions
  Genetic—individual, spouse, and family
    Repeated spontaneous abortions*
    Chromosomal and other congenital abnormalities*
    Hemoglobinopathies, e.g., sickle-cell anemia*
    Radiation and other toxic substance exposure*
    Multiple births
    Family history of chronic diseases

(Continued)

Table 20.2

(Continued)

Nutrition
    Prepregnancy weight (height-to-weight profile)*
    Diet history with evaluation of adequacy*
    Barriers to adequate nutrition intake, e.g., financial, cultural, food fads,
        pica*
    Special dietary patterns, e.g., vegetarian, lactose intolerance, caffeine*
Behavioral
    Smoking, alcohol, illicit drug use*
    Over-the-counter medications, prescription drugs*
    Rest and sleep patterns*
    Extremes of exercise or physical exertion*
    Dental care*
    History of antisocial behavior*
    Care seeking and compliance*
    Pregnancy wantedness*
Environmental hazards, work hazards, or both
    Exposure to toxins, teratogens*
    Work—occupation, type and level of activity
Current pregnancy to date (first visit)
    Normal signs and symptoms
    LMP and LNMP
    Estimated date of conception, weeks gestation at present time
    Abnormal signs and symptoms, concerns
General physical examination
        Blood pressure
        Breast exam
        Pelvic exam
        Fetal size
        Fetal heart tones
Laboratory tests
    Hemoglobin or hematocrit*
    Blood Rh, Rh negative titer, antibody screen
    Rubella titer (if immunity not previously documented)*
    Syphilis test*
    Pap smear*
    Urine protein and glucose*
    Urine screen for urinary tract infection (UTI), kidney disease
    Gonorrheal culture*
    Hepatitis B titer*
    Screening tests offered to all women*:
        HIV titer
        Drug toxicology
    Screening tests in endemic areas or for women with risk factors*:
        Toxoplasmosis, tuberculosis
        Herpes simplex, varicella
        Chlamydia
        Hemoglobinopathies
        Tay–Sachs
Fetal evaluation
    Confirm gestational age (LMP, uterine size)

*a*Asterisks indicate conditions that are appropriate for preconception identification and inter-
    vention.

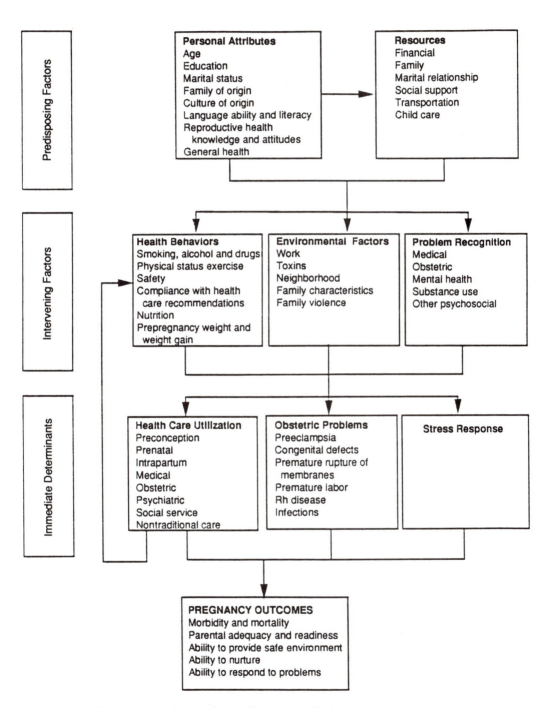

Figure 20.1. Mechanisms by which psychosocial risks affect pregnancy outcomes.

Table 20.3
Health Promotion for Pregnant Women[a]

Counseling to promote and support healthful behaviors
    Nutrition*
    Smoking cessation*
    Avoidance of alcohol*
    Avoidance of illicit drugs*
    Avoidance of teratogens*
    Safer sex*
    Maternal seat belt use
    Work counseling*
    Stress reduction (avoidance of heavy lifting and long standing)*
General knowledge of pregnancy and parenting
    Physiologic and emotional changes of pregnancy
    Sexuality counseling
    Fetal growth and development
    Self-help strategies for common discomforts
    Early pregnancy classes
    Nutrition
    Physiologic changes
    Psychological adaptation
    Exercise for fitness
    Rest and sleep patterns
    Infant car seat and safety
    Preparation for childbirth
    Preparation for parenting
Information on proposed care
    Need for early entry into prenatal care*
    Preparation for screening and diagnostic tests
    Content and timing of prenatal visits needed*
    Need to report danger signs immediately
    Signs and symptoms of preterm and term labor
    Birth plan, expectations, and goals
    Labor onset plans

[a]Asterisks indicate conditions that are appropriate for preconception activity.

bought a house and are saving for private schools. They both want advice and counseling to improve the health of their future child.

PRECONCEPTION CARE

Preconception care is care received by women before they become pregnant to reduce the risk of poor pregnancy outcome. Its components are the same as prenatal care: risk assessment, health promotion, and interventions to reduce risks (Culpepper & Jack, 1991). For an activity to be recommended as a part of preconception care, it must have enhanced value if it is done before conception as compared to waiting until after conception. Conditions for which preconception identification and intervention are appropriate are highlighted in Tables 20.2 and 20.3.

For some risks, intervention is available only if initiated before pregnancy. For others, interventions during pregnancy are available but must be initiated early in the pregnancy. To prevent congenital defects, exposure to teratogens during the first 57 days

Table 20.4
Factors Associated with Beginning and Remaining in Prenatal Care[a]

Characteristics of prenatal care services
1. Individualized psychosocial services available, including feedback and advice
2. Communication patterns
3. Affordable at a reasonable cost or covered by insurance other than Medicaid
4. Geographic accessibility (distance < 1 mile, safe public transportation available)
5. Conservative (traditional birthing arrangements unless previous experience, or social norms associated with innovation)
6. Education and information available
7. Care provided by a multidisciplinary team
8. Care provided by nurse midwives and nurses
9. Availability publicized in news media

The pregnant woman's social network
1. Availability of psychosocial support
2. Social norms support need for care
3. Family supports use of service

Characteristics of the pregnant woman—psychological
1. Satisfied with current health services
2. Feeling of self-competence
3. Positive attitude about care
4. Sense of power
5. Hopeful about the future
6. Absence of depression, denial of pregnancy, fear about the future
7. Low stress level
8. Early developmental and physical stage of pregnancy
9. Expectations about outcome
10. Early acknowledgment of pregnancy
11. Attitude about pregnancy
12. Somatization
13. Accepts innovation only after experience or confirmation by social network

Characteristics of the pregnant woman—social
1. Previous satisfactory experience with high-risk pregnancy or healthcare services
2. Culture
3. Higher social class
4. Length of time since immigration to the United States
5. Higher level of education
6. Being married
7. Informs others about the pregnancy early
8. Availability of social networks
9. Age (>19 years and <35 years)

Characteristics of the pregnant woman—cognitive
1. Higher level of cognitive development

[a]Source: Perez-Woods (1990).

of pregnancy, when most organogenesis occurs, must be eliminated (Moos & Cefalo, 1987). Unfortunately, the very nature of some risks also results in some women not seeking prenatal care until late in pregnancy, if at all. Table 20.4 lists factors associated with women obtaining prenatal care. To reach women who otherwise would not seek prenatal care promptly, physicians can use two strategies: preconception care and working with others to conduct community outreach.

A large portion of neural tube defects are prevented by folate supplementation beginning 1 to 3 months prior to conception (Mulinare *et al.*, 1989), supplementation that did not occur in Case 20-1. Rubella syndrome can be prevented by vaccination of susceptible women prior to pregnancy, but because it involves a live vaccine, vaccination during pregnancy is contraindicated (Centers for Disease Control, 1989). Alcohol consumption during pregnancy is the number one cause of mental retardation; avoidance of unwanted pregnancy among heavy drinkers, or interventions (which may take time) to reduce drinking before pregnancy can eliminate this risk (Herron *et al.*, 1982). For women who smoke, nicotine-containing gum might be a helpful smoking-cessation aid before pregnancy, but is not recommended for use during pregnancy. For women with epilepsy, medications can be altered to remove those with major teratogenic potential. For those who are anorexic or bulimic, interventions that improve nutritional status before conception are important, since underweight women who do not gain adequate weight during pregnancy are at increased risk for fetal death (Naeye, 1979). Genetic counseling before conception allows a couple additional options, e.g., adoption, *in vitro* fertilization, and if needed, can promote early chorionic villous sampling or amniocentesis during pregnancy. Preconception care is appropriate for both men and women, or for couples to consider together.

Perhaps one of the most important preconception risks is the risk of unplanned or unwanted pregnancy. Among married women, 10% of births are unwanted, and an additional 25% are unintended and mistimed: wanted, but not just now. Among unmarried women these percentages are 25 and 40%, respectively (Williams & Pratt, 1989). In some age and socioeconomic subgroups, such as among teenagers, the vast majority of pregnancies are unwanted. Many women, including teenagers, who become pregnant by "leaving it to fate," are not aware of the contraceptive options available to them. The concept of poor investment in pregnancy has been developed to describe the woman with an unwanted pregnancy (DeMuylder *et al.*, 1992; Marsiglio & Mott, 1988; Weller *et al.*, 1987). Such a woman is likely to delay the start of prenatal care, continue the use of alcohol and cigarettes, and engage in behaviors that place her pregnancy at risk. She might delay recognition and care of problems affecting her pregnancy (Joyce & Grossman, 1990). These behaviors are related to adverse outcomes, such as low birth weight at delivery and child abuse after delivery. A child in a family with two unplanned pregnancies is 2.8 times more likely to be abused, and with three unplanned pregnancies the risk increases to 4.6 times, compared to a child in a family with no unplanned births (Zuravin, 1991).

Physicians have numerous opportunities to incorporate preconception care into their practices: during routine periodic health assessments, school, work, and premarital examinations, family planning visits, negative pregnancy test visits, and well-child care for another family member. Unfortunately, many of the women most likely to benefit from preconception care are least likely to have access to it because of the social, financial, health behavior, or psychological risks involved. To reach such women, physicians must work in their communities to make preconception care available in settings where such high-risk women can be reached before becoming pregnant, such as STD clinics, substance abuse treatment centers, women's shelters, halfway houses, and detention centers (Jack & Culpepper, 1990).

CASE 20-4

Shana is 22 years old and Dr. Fields is seeing her for the second time. She was late in her pregnancy and had walked into his office for her first visit the previous week. At that time, the office nurse performed a rapid review of relevant risks, which Dr. Fields subsequently confirmed, and sent blood samples for basic screening lab tests based on her risk status. Shana has had five previous pregnan-

cies, including two that aborted. One of her three children had been born prematurely and subsequently died at home in unclear circumstance at 3 months of age. Her other children were placed in foster care by Child Protective Services. Shana currently smokes two packs a day, drinks regularly, and until midpregnancy supported herself in part through prostitution. She first came to Dr. Fields because she was destitute; her boyfriend had kicked her out of his apartment. She is underweight and had not eaten well in weeks. She complained of burning on urination, and a urinalysis revealed numerous white cells, highly suggestive of a urinary tract infection, which he treated with amoxicillin. An ultrasound and pelvic exam on the first visit indicated a pregnancy of 35 (±3) weeks' gestation, assuming that the fetus was of normal size for gestational age.

Today she returns unhappy with the shelter to which Dr. Fields referred her, in part because of its curfew, and because the shelter's social worker insisted that Shana meet with her regularly. Her laboratory results suggest that she is a hepatitis B carrier. She confides that she has mainlined a variety of substances in the past and uses crack when her boyfriend makes it available. When asked to consent to HIV testing, she declines. Since the weather has improved, she is thinking of leaving the shelter. She also confides that she knows if she can just keep this baby, her life will straighten out.

CARE OF WOMEN AT HIGH RISK

Low birth weight, congenital birth defects, and problems arising during labor and delivery are the major immediate causes of the delivery of newborns who have serious problems with long-term consequences. However, these immediate causes are often preceded by underlying problems that are responsive to prenatal care interventions. These include acute problems, especially infections, and chronic medical conditions, particularly hypertensive disorders and diabetes mellitus, which affect the adequacy of the fetal–placental unit and its ability to maintain a supportive intrauterine environment, and conditions, such as epilepsy, that require chronic medications of a potentially teratogenic nature. In addition, women often have psychosocial risks, including psychological difficulties, social problems, and adverse health behaviors, which can contribute to poor pregnancy outcomes. These latter risks also can lead to problems arising after pregnancy, such as failure to thrive, accidents, and developmental delay.

CONGENITAL DEFECTS

Approximately 3% of newborns are affected by genetic defects. Mendelian (single gene), chromosomal, multifactorial (both high and low heritability conditions), infectious, and environmental etiologies (e.g., radiation, toxin, and drug exposures) contribute to the spectrum of congenital defects (Centers for Disease Control, 1989). The number of chromosomal abnormalities that can be detected in prospective parents is increasing rapidly, as a result of the current emphasis on genome research and advances in DNA probe techniques (Daker & Bobrow, 1989). Ultrasound, MRI, chorionic villous sampling techniques, and early amniocentesis all provide additional diagnostic and therapeutic options once conception has occurred. Early experience with *in utero* therapy for conditions such as fetal urinary tract obstruction, hydrocephalus, or diaphragmatic hernia is promising.

However, the development of genetic screening tests and interventions with potential clinical application result in a variety of considerations for families and their physicians. For many conditions, the undertaking of preconception or prenatal testing for congenital defects currently is limited to those couples known to be at high risk, such as screening for Tay–Sachs disease among Ashkenazi Jews and hemoglobinopathies among those of Greek and Italian descent. For a number of conditions, screening could be of some benefit if routinely performed; this results in a number of controversial issues.

Cystic fibrosis, one of the most common congenital defects, illustrates the complexity of the issues involved in deciding who should be screened. Preconception screening for cystic fibrosis provides a couple with increased options, including not bearing children, artificial insemination, *in vitro* fertilization, surrogate pregnancy, and adoption, as well as conception with early pregnancy testing and selective abortion. Diagnosis during pregnancy does not appear to improve outcomes for infants subsequently born with cystic fibrosis. At least through age 4, there is no evidence that presymptomatic diagnosis of cystic fibrosis is of therapeutic benefit to the child (Lemna *et al.*, 1990).

A three-base-pair deletion in a gene on the long arm of chromosome 7 has been found responsible for 75.8% of cystic fibrosis in the U.S. white population, but only 49, 43, and 30% in Spanish, Italian, and Ashkenazi Jewish populations, respectively (Lemna *et al.*, 1990). A reasonable estimation of the annual cost of medical care for cystic fibrosis patients is $7500, resulting in lifetime costs of about $200,000. A cost–benefit analysis, using 1990 cost estimates, suggests that the cost of avoiding one cystic fibrosis birth by screening all couples during pregnancy would be $2.2 million (Wilfond & Fost, 1990). This estimate assumes that out of 11,100 couples screened, 10 would be identified who are at risk (both parents heterozygotes); that of these, 8 would choose prenatal diagnosis resulting in 2 fetuses identified as having cystic fibrosis, and 1 of these couples would choose to abort.

The potential stigmatization and altered public perceptions of cystic fibrosis possibly resulting from dissemination of cystic fibrosis screening have been identified as areas needing further understanding to enlighten development of public policy. If cystic fibrosis is potentially preventable through screening with subsequent avoidance of pregnancy or abortion, then the public perception might shift toward subtly blaming the parents of children with cystic fibrosis, and decreased support and acceptance of them, including through publicly funded programs. As a consequence of all of these considerations, currently most physicians limit screening for cystic fibrosis and many other conditions to those couples known to be at increased risk because either they or a close relative suffer from it.

In addition to interventions related to genetic screening, physicians can prevent congenital defects through counseling regarding teratogenic exposures at work or around the home, abstinence from alcohol intake during pregnancy, maintenance of adequate folate intake (to prevent neurotubular defects), and tailoring of chronic medications.

LOW BIRTH WEIGHT

Low-birth-weight infants either are born prematurely (before 37 weeks' gestation), have suffered from intrauterine growth retardation (IUGR) and consequently are born small for gestational age (SGA), or both. For all specific birth weight cohorts, the United States has the best rate of infant survival worldwide (Babson, 1989; Evans & Alberman, 1989). However, relative to other developed countries, the United States has had a higher rate of low-birth-weight infants and has seen virtually no decrease in this rate (about 7%) over the past four decades. As a result, its ranking has dropped from having the sixth lowest total infant death rate in 1950–1955, to being twenty-second in recent years (Cole et al., 1989).

Immediate causes of preterm delivery include lethal congenital defects (10–20%); multiple pregnancy, e.g., twins (10%); elective delivery related to an obstetric problem [25–30%, including hypertension/preeclampsia (10–15%), hemorrhage (4–6%), diabetes mellitus (2–3%), IUGR (3–9%), Rh disease (1–2%), and other medical problems (5–10%)]; spontaneous rupture of membranes (SROM) (15–25%); and spontaneous preterm labor (25–35%), including about half complicated by obstetric problems similar to those leading to elective early delivery (Culpepper, 1991; Keirse, 1989). Each of these immediate causes has been linked to risk factors present earlier in pregnancy or before pregnancy. Individual risk factors usually predict multiple immediate causes of low birth weight. A large portion of these are of a psychosocial nature (Institute of Medicine, 1985; Savitz et al., 1991).

Preterm labor occurs with membranes intact, or labor onset and ROM occur together. In addition, once twin pregnancies, fetal deaths, and induced preterm deliveries are excluded, about half of the remaining cases of prematurity start with ROM prior to labor, with labor developing spontaneously or being induced. Preterm labor risk factors include psychosocial ones related to low income, inadequate prenatal care, stress, low social support, and behaviors such as smoking and substance use; acute and chronic medical conditions, including infections; and obstetric problems such as multiple gestation, abruption, and preeclampsia (Keirse, 1989; Klein & Goldenberg, 1990). Of note, studies in other countries have shown that poverty need not be associated with an increased risk of prematurity, as occurs in the United States (Piekkala et al., 1986).

IUGR leads to a 5- to 8-fold increase in fetal death, a 2- to 5-fold increase in neonatal mortality, and a 5- to 10-fold increase in neurologic deficits in surviving offspring. Causes of IUGR are diverse and include factors that affect the integrity of the placental transfer of nutrition, such as maternal hypertension, smoking, drug use, diabetes mellitus, Rh disease, lupus, and other conditions (Kramer, 1987, 1990). Maternal behaviors such as smoking account for over 50% of IUGR. While a theoretical incidence of IUGR of under 1% might be attainable, in high-risk populations incidences of over 10% and even 20% have been found (Goldenberg et al., 1990).

Little national consensus has emerged regarding the diverse approaches to screening, confirmation, monitoring, therapy, and timing of delivery for IUGR. Diagnostic strategies include screening techniques using umbilical height and third trimester ultrasound screening of patients with risk factors and subsequent confirmatory ultrasound investigation. Nonstress test monitoring and fetal growth ultrasound monitoring both have been used to follow fetal well-being. Measurement of fetal and umbilical blood flow by ultrasound Doppler studies holds promise for identifying fetal status, including the need for urgent delivery. The value of bed rest, low-dose aspirin, and home versus hospital care as interventions are all unclear (Crowther & Chalmers, 1989).

Considering all of the causes of low birth weight together, the Institute of Medicine (Institute of Medicine, 1985) concluded that the lack of prenatal care that starts early and is continuous is the most important risk factor. It identified six major reasons for women obtaining inadequate prenatal care: financial constraints (no or inadequate health insurance); inadequate availability of healthcare service providers, especially ones willing to serve socially disadvantaged or high-risk women; insufficient prenatal services and facilities routinely used by high-risk populations, such as community health centers; the experiences, attitudes, and beliefs of pregnant women; poor or absent childcare and transportation services; and inadequate systems to recruit hard-to-reach women into care (Institute of Medicine, 1988).

CASE 20-5

Dr. Fields's next case is Marie Howbarth, a 39-year-old Jehovah's Witness who is returning at 24 weeks' gestation. Dr. Fields has been seeing Mrs. Howbarth weekly to monitor her medical status and fetal development. Mrs. Howbarth has had three previous pregnancies, including a relatively normal first pregnancy, a second pregnancy complicated by deep vein thrombosis, preeclampsia, and gestational diabetes mellitus, and a third pregnancy involving a repetition of the same complications and resulting in a stillbirth at 24 weeks' gestation. Her second child was born premature and requires developmental services for cerebral palsy and borderline mental retardation.

Dr. Fields had counseled the Howbarths regarding the importance of avoiding further pregnancies because of the likely recurrence of the same problems. This pregnancy was unwanted, and considerable tension continues between the Howbarths as a result. Mr. Howbarth is deeply religious and determined that the pregnancy continue with minimal medical intervention; also, he blames his wife for not noticing that her IUD had been spontaneously expelled. Mrs. Howbarth is not as religious, but acquiesces to her husband's wishes. Dr. Fields suspects she would have opted for an abortion if her husband were not involved.

Dr. Fields has monitored fetal growth with monthly sonograms beginning at 12 weeks. In addition, he has maintained Mrs. Howbarth on home injections of heparin, with weekly partial thromboplastin time monitoring, and had planned to begin insulin with home monitoring of blood glucose levels at this visit. Mrs. Howbarth's blood pressure has risen by 15 mm Hg diastolic since 2 weeks ago, and she will need this assessed. Her weight has dropped 2 pounds since last week as well.

However, today Dr. Fields notes that on her heparin diary, this past week Mrs. Howbarth has missed 40% of her doses. When asked about this, Mrs. Howbarth begins crying uncontrollably and notes that she has been unable to sleep or eat, feels terribly guilty about bringing another baby with problems into the world, and has lost all interest in living. When asked about suicidal thoughts, she reveals that she has had almost uncontrollable urges to run her car into the interstate bypass on her way home from picking up her child from the developmental center each afternoon.

RESOURCES REQUIRED TO SERVE HIGH-RISK POPULATIONS

Physicians caring for high-risk women can be most effective in improving pregnancy outcomes, and improving the health of their offspring during childhood, if they have a number of resources available to them. These include the use of a practice record system and information system that promote the comprehensive recognition of women at increased risk and their tracking (Rosen, 1989). The capacity to conduct home visiting, either in person, through the visiting nurse service, or through other community programs, is helpful for further assessing risks identified in the office, and for intervening to reduce a number of risks (Klerman, 1990). Collaboration with community programs that offer special services is crucial to working effectively with certain pregnant women. These include smoking cessation and substance abuse programs, programs for victims of family violence, services for mentally retarded women and those with chronic mental illness, and programs for pregnant teenagers.

For a number of women, especially single parents and women living in poverty, programs to provide social support are important. Social support is postulated as having both direct effects and ones related to its mediation of the effects of stress (Culpepper & Jack, 1993). Stress might result in altered pregnancy outcomes either at birth or later in infancy through several mechanisms (Koeske & Koeske, 1990; Sarason & Sarason, 1985). Stress can divert a woman's or couple's attention from pregnancy and decrease the priority of pregnancy-related issues. This diversion can result in decreased recognition of risks, symptoms, or problems, and decrease the adequacy of response either through delaying or decreasing compliance with care. Stress can have an impact through increasing unhealthy coping behaviors, including smoking, substance use, inadequate rest, and excessive work. It might alter interpersonal relations and decrease the resources available to women. The problems causing stress might concomitantly result in diversion of financial assets. Psychological mediation of effects through increased anxiety, decreased self-esteem, and related alterations has been proposed. The effects of stress have been postulated to be catecholamine, immune system, or hormonally mediated (Ramsey, 1988).

Social support might work to mediate the effects of stress or have unrelated direct effects. This effect can occur through increasing tangible resources such as safe shelter, food, and financial assets, improving the recognition of risks and problems, and improving responses through self-care, care seeking, and compliance with medical recommendations. Social support also might alter psychological mechanisms, or be mediated by biochemical changes. The effects of stress and social support on adverse pregnancy outcomes might occur through their contributing to prenatal problems such as pre-eclampsia, abruption, or preterm labor, or they might have influence on the adequacy of parenting and related infant outcomes.

While the physician with a small number of women requiring such community services might provide or arrange for them personally, the physician working with high-risk populations can be most effective if attached to a team that also includes nursing, social service, and nutritional expertise, as well as the ability to conduct outreach. Such a team might make interventions at the community level, as well as work with individual families. This is important, since communities and neighborhoods themselves may contribute to infant mortality through aspects of social impoverishment (Garbarino, 1990; Turnock & McGill, 1983). For example, infant death rates in the poorest third of Chicago neighborhoods are 5 to 10 times the rate of the most affluent third (Kostelny & Garbarino, 1987). Even when the effect of socioeconomic status has been adjusted for, some neighborhoods stand out as contributing to infant mortality (Garbarino & Sherman, 1980).

The ability of the practice to provide care coordination and case management support is critical to working successfully with high-risk women and their families. Different high-risk families require different types of support (Culpepper, 1995). Some require assistance in the recognition of problems and help in basic decision-making about their care; examples include mentally retarded parents, overwhelmed single parents, and some recent immigrants. A woman who has been subject to spousal abuse may require a provider who identifies not only her risk, but also that to her children. In some cases, the provider needs to make basic decisions for an immobilized woman. Other women might be able to identify problems, but have poor understanding of the consequences likely to be involved, and are unable to set priorities or appropriately follow through with action. A third high-risk group is able to identify the problems and understand the consequences, but is not aware of the resources available or how to use them effectively. Some families simply require information about available resources and encouragement in using them. Finally, some families can manage virtually all of their needs with only occasional support and assistance during particularly difficult times. These families occasionally need the encouragement and advocacy of the helping professionals involved with them.

While in some families the level of function is static and unlikely to change, with others there is potential for growth as the woman or couple involved learns requisite life skills and begins to deal with problems independently. Ideally, the primary care system involved will be responsive to the circumstances of these different types of families and not only ensure appropriate care but concomitantly foster improvement of the functioning of the family unit.

With regard to high-need families, the scope of the primary care system's responsibilities and the adequacy of the medical model are interrelated issues. Not only will the level of involvement in outreach, prioritizing, and decision-making by a case manager vary depending on the family, but also their clinical needs will be diverse over time, and might include traditional primary medical care, dental care, developmental disability services, mental health services such as for substance abuse and behavioral disorders, and preventive services. In addition, the primary care system might need to respond to family dysfunction as a problem in its own right to be able to effectively care for other problems.

In contrast to the diversity of professional services a high-need family might require, primary care clinicians generally follow a medical or biopsychosocial approach. This usually is problem oriented, involving an elucidation of the history and objective findings, collection of additional information through testing, obtaining consultation, or information from others including by home visit, and then development of a therapeutic plan that integrates medical, psychological, and social responses. Within a continuity setting, this then leads to ongoing monitoring of the plan with changes in therapy as needed. The physician generally relates to families in a collaborative–contractual relationship, wherein the physician provides recommendations within a framework in which the woman or family is free to follow or ignore the recommendations, including return for follow-up. The clinician generally views her role as being supportive to the patient, possibly including advocacy in obtaining care from other community agencies. Should a patient not return for follow-up appointments, the clinician might feel little responsibility for aggressive outreach, and indeed might dismiss families who repeatedly miss appointments.

Such a range of physician–patient relationships frequently is too limited for high-need families. Instead, at times adopting the professional relationship modes used by other disciplines is required to work effectively with some families. For example, both mental health and substance abuse treatment providers often must use confrontational tactics with which most primary care clinicians are uncomfortable. Developmental specialists often relate to parents using a developmental model rather than a problem-oriented medical model and engage parents as teachers of their children. A variety of professionals, including those dealing with abusive or neglectful families, use a monitoring and limit-setting style that includes a variety of adverse consequences for noncompliant families. While it is not necessary for the primary care clinician to be highly skilled in all of these modes of relating to patients, nevertheless, they do need to be comfortable with using them on occasion and reinforcing their use by other members of the health team.

CASE 20-6

Katie is a 15-year-old whose parents and younger sisters are also Dr. Fields's patients. Dr. Fields saw Katie's mother recently for worsening migraine headaches and suggested stress reduction classes as well as medication for migraine prophylaxis. Katie has not been seen for a couple of years.

Today Katie has come alone for her appointment, the last one on a busy Thursday afternoon. Dr. Fields greets her and then listens as Katie begins slowly to discuss her main concern: her period is several weeks overdue. With gentle questioning, she acknowledges having intercourse without using contraception. She has many symptoms of pregnancy, and a brief exam of her abdomen reveals an enlarged uterus (halfway to her umbilicus) and audible fetal heart tones. She begins to cry and wonders aloud how she will tell her parents. Dr. Fields offers support and suggests a joint meeting with her parents, stressing the need for the prompt initiation of prenatal care.

——————— ADOLESCENT PREGNANCY ———————

Adolescents are one group of women at increased risk for poor perinatal outcomes whose care demonstrates the principles applicable to many groups of high-risk women. Their increased risk is related to multiple biopsychosocial factors. By understanding and identifying these risk factors prenatally or even preconceptionally, as described earlier, physicians can play an important role in improving adolescent health outcomes in their communities. The rest of this section will focus on issues pertinent to teen pregnancy, but it is also applicable to women with other risk factors.

Adolescent pregnancy is a common public health problem in the United States (Fraser *et al.*, 1995; Goldenberg & Klerman, 1995). In 1989, women under 20 years of age accounted for nearly 13% of births and 25% of abortions in the United States; there are over 1 million teenage pregnancies annually, and over half a million births to teen mothers (Ventura, 1994). Compared with Canada, England, or France, the United States has twice the rate of teen pregnancy. Teen pregnancy rates vary with race in the United States, with over 10% of all births to black women being to those under 18, versus just under 4% of all births to white women. Compared with women 20 to 40 years of age, teens have increased rates of premature delivery, low birth weight, and perinatal complications such as substance use and poor nutrition; they also breast-feed less often and are less likely to use contraception after pregnancy. Teen mothers are less likely to complete high school and more likely to live in poverty.

Primary care physicians are well positioned to respond to the individual and public health impact of teen pregnancy. First, physicians can promote teen pregnancy prevention programs through participation in school health programs and advocacy for education and employment for teens. Second, since they may be the first contact with the health system for teen members of families in their practice, these primary care providers can screen for and help modify many of the risks associated with teen pregnancy. They also might be a key source of contraception. The multifactorial risks associated with teen pregnancy lend themselves to care by clinicians such as family physicians, who are trained to address biomedical and psychosocial issues jointly and to use multidisciplinary resources in addressing these risks.

Working with any high-risk group requires outreach into the community to identify at-risk individuals, preferably prior to development of the undesired outcome for which their risk is increased, in this case pregnancy. For pregnant teens, such outreach includes the physician's contact with school- and church-based health programs, whether that be as simple as knowing the school nurse and being available for questions or referrals, to assisting in the development or staffing of a school clinic. During the care of pregnant teens, one of the key issues is promoting their education, so that outreach includes working with at-risk schools to develop teen-parenting programs, including childcare for teen parents, GED programs, and classes in parenting skills.

To address effectively the multiple biopsychosocial risks associated with adolescent pregnancy, some form of case management is often necessary (Heins *et al.*, 1987). An identified case manager, perhaps a social worker affiliated with a teen-parenting program or a public health nurse, can help the physician coordinate the often multiple referrals needed to provide true comprehensive care to the at-risk pregnant teen; for example, the case manager can assist with transportation to prenatal appointments, encourage adequate nutrition and healthy behaviors, and help plan for postpartum needs such as infant supplies (Buescher *et al.*, 1991; Olds *et al.*, 1986). The case manager might become involved in home visitation during prenatal care to help assess risks and plan interventions. Ideally the case manager acting in concordance with the physician can link the disparate prenatal, intrapartum, and postpartum resources in a community to best serve the pregnant teen and her newborn family.

Part of caring for pregnant teens by necessity involves other members of their families, whether these be biologically or geographically defined; thus, experience in multigenerational care is important (Miller, 1995). The family life-cycle changes that occur with any birth have even more impact when parents are confronting adolescent development simultaneously with becoming grandparents—the effects of "children having children" ripple beyond the teen and the new baby as all family members adjust to their new roles. The new grandparents, especially the new grandmother, might indeed be doing double-parenting once the teen mother returns to school and the newborn needs childcare. The family physician can support the entire family in its adjustments around these issues in ways that promote healthy parenting across generations. This support may include, for example, special support for the teen mother to breast-feed in spite of pressure from her mother who used formula and lacks understanding of basic lactation.

CASE 20-7

Joan is a 29-year-old well-known to Dr. Fields primarily through the well-child care of her only child, 5-year-old Drew, who recently has been diagnosed with attention-deficit hyperactivity disorder (ADHD). Although his parents work hard learning appropriate parenting skills for their active son, Joan as the primary caregiver is often overwhelmed by his behavior and frequently has sought help from Dr. Fields. Today her appointment is for a first prenatal visit; Joan had been ambivalent about having another child after the struggle to cope with Drew's behavior, but she and her husband always have wanted a large family.

Dr. Fields and Joan have a half-hour appointment to review her history, discuss the nausea and fatigue that are currently bothering her at 9 weeks' gestation, and do a focused physical exam to confirm her uterine size. Because she recently has had a complete physical for work, Dr. Fields has current health maintenance records including breast exam and Pap smear, so they can spend most of the visit discussing her history and symptoms and developing a plan for her prenatal care. Dr. Fields notes that Joan looks quite fatigued, and with further questioning she reveals that between her pregnancy symptoms, her husband's recent work-related travels, and Drew's behavior, she has been especially overwhelmed and sleeping poorly. She and Dr. Fields decide that she needs to get more help from both her husband and her mother-in-law, who lives nearby and who often takes Drew for afternoon visits. Joan feels her mother-in-law is better than she is at coping with Drew's behavior.

A month later at her next prenatal visit Joan's mother-in-law and Drew also come along. Joan's fatigue has improved slightly although she is still nauseated frequently. Drew explores the exam room in great detail while awaiting Dr. Fields, but quiets when the physician finds the fetal heart beat. Joan's mother-in-law is teary-eyed with hearing the heartbeat. She ends up attending the rest of Joan's prenatal visits with her, helping settle Drew down in the waiting and exam rooms.

By her third prenatal visit, Joan has begun feeling fetal movement and although this is exciting, she also dreads having to care for a newborn when Drew continues to be so demanding. She and Dr. Fields locate a local support group for parents of kids with ADHD, which meets without the kids one evening a month and with the kids one Saturday afternoon a month.

The next time Dr. Fields sees Joan is just 3 weeks later at an appointment with Drew. She has been to the group and wants a referral to the local university ADHD clinic for Drew to be evaluated for a trial of medication; several of the parents in the group have suggested this clinic. Dr. Fields makes the referral while suggesting that Joan and her husband review the local library's collection of information about ADHD for parents to learn more about the disorder and the potential risks and benefits of the medication. Joan reports continued fatigue but less nausea, and has been trying to take daily walks with Drew.

By her third trimester, Joan and her family have decided to try a placebo-controlled trial of medication for Drew, hoping to have some idea of his response by the time his new sibling arrives. Drew's grandmother, who cares for him after school several times a week to give Joan a break, is opposed to medication and has insisted that his parents work hard around specific behavioral techniques. Dr. Fields has seen the whole family to discuss the clinical trial and offered to follow up on their observations of its success. Drew's behavior has improved somewhat with his grandmother's care, and she agrees to continue providing this after the baby's birth. The family together attends a sibling class that the local childbirth education group sponsors.

WORKING WITH THE FAMILY

Normal pregnancy care involves helping women cope with many of the common symptoms of pregnancy, using lay information as needed, working with community resources around childbirth education and parenting skills, and helping women juggle the demands of working during pregnancy, either in the home or at outside employment. While prenatal care must address biomedical risk factors throughout pregnancy, for most healthy women these risks are minimal, and the majority of prenatal visit time can focus on guiding families through the transitions that come with a new baby.

Encouraging the participation of the rest of the family in the pregnancy and delivery processes is an important role for the clinician as well. Frequently, one challenge is getting the fathers to participate in prenatal care; although societal trends have encouraged fathers to be present in the delivery room, this has not extended into the primary care office as much, sometimes for logistical reasons such as work schedules, and sometimes for family reasons such as estranged or unmarried fathers. The clinician can work around this by offering evening or weekend hours for appointments, by calling the father (with the mother's permission) to ask if he has any concerns or questions, or simply by making a question about the father's involvement or concerns part of each prenatal visit. In addition, during the 9 months of the mother's prenatal care, the clinician can encourage the father to come in for a general checkup as well, to allow him time to discuss his own health issues (McDaniel *et al.*, 1990b).

Another important part of family-oriented pregnancy care is addressing the changes that a new younger sibling will bring into a family. Depending on the age difference among siblings, the parents may need help with issues such as when to have an older child wean, toilet train, or move out of a crib, what childcare plans will work for all of the children, how to cope with sibling rivalry, what to expect with infectious diseases in a larger family, how to plan for care of the older sibling(s) during the childbirth and postpartum times, or whether or not to involve the older child in the birth of her new sibling. The family physician can often use local childbirth education resources for sibling preparation classes and literature to help families with some of these decisions. Other ways to make older children part of the prenatal visits include providing toys or books in the waiting or exam rooms, asking for their help with checking the fetal heartbeat, or asking about their opinions of the new baby's looks or name choices.

When a family is coping during pregnancy with stressful life issues, such as behavior problems with an older child, the family physician can assist by helping them locate resources within or outside their family. This especially might be important in considering postpartum support needs. A physician who has cared for the woman and her other children throughout pregnancy and will continue to follow them all, including the newborn, has particularly important insight into such needs. A physician who understands cross-generational issues can help families find support beyond the immediate nuclear family to face complicated behavioral issues. This might include involving not only the grandparents or other extended family but also community resources such as parent-support groups. Sometimes if the mother is a single parent or the father is unable to be an active participant in the prenatal care, the mother's or father's mother can fill an important support role for the pregnant woman and might provide much lay education about her own childbirth experiences. The family physician should include in routine prenatal care questions about such grandparent participation, particularly since the extended family might be involved at delivery or in the postpartum period.

CASE 20-8

While Dr. Fields is finishing up paperwork one afternoon, his nurse interrupts to say that the translator for Mai, one of their Vietnamese patients, is on the phone reporting that this woman's waters have broken. Mai is a 22-year-old primiparous woman who speaks minimal English and lives with her parents and younger siblings. The father of the baby has returned to Vietnam indefinitely. Through the translator, who works as a patient advocate and labor support person for a community-based organization aiding Southeast Asian refugees, Dr. Fields arranges for Mai to be seen and evaluated.

The translator helps Mai arrange transportation to the office, where Dr. Fields examines Mai and notes that she is in active labor at about 3 cm dilated with ruptured membranes. They walk from Dr. Fields's office across the street to the hospital-affiliated birthing center, where Mai has chosen to give birth in its homelike setting. The translator remains with her, helping her get comfortable in the hospital room and rubbing her back during contractions. Mai's mother comes along but speaks even less English and feels uncomfortable being "in the way" until Dr. Fields through the translator reassures her that her presence is welcome. With support from the advocate, Mai's mother, Dr. Fields, and the nurse, Mai's labor progresses normally and within 4 hours she gives birth to a healthy 6-pound girl. The translator works with Mai and the nurse to help the baby breast-feed right away and to plan for teaching during Mai's short postpartum stay at the center and during her home-based postpartum care.

The birth center works with the local visiting nurse organization, which has a special program for new mothers to help them through the transitions of the first 2 weeks with the newborn. Dr. Fields stays in touch with the visiting nurse and with Mai through the translator in these first weeks to provide breast-feeding support in particular, so that by the time Mai brings the baby back to Dr. Fields's office for her second checkup at 1 month, the baby is thriving.

—— COMMUNITY AND CULTURAL ISSUES ——

Physicians providing perinatal care need to understand community resources for pregnant women and children. This is especially true for communities of potentially higher risk such as adolescents, as described earlier, or communities of diversity where cultural issues might impact on perinatal health.

Physicians also need to understand the potential "low-tech" resources available to them in working with women in labor (Brody & Thompson, 1981; Rosenblatt, 1989; Strobino *et al.*, 1988). Several studies have suggested that the simple presence of a supportive companion in labor can shorten labor and lead to fewer cesarean sections for delivery (Keirse, 1989b; Kennell *et al.*, 1991). This might be particularly true for primiparous women or women who do not speak the same language as their birth attendants (Kennell *et al.*, 1991; Klaus *et al.*, 1986; Sosa *et al.*, 1980). Thus, a physician working in a culturally diverse community might improve her population's perinatal health by working with cross-cultural organizations to train labor advocates. Such advocates can both translate and provide labor support. Modeling the family physician's continuing role in providing care for a new family, advocates also can work with postpartum women and families in the crucial first weeks after a birth.

Family physicians can also support institutional options in labor and delivery care such as the birth center described in Case 20-8. Low-risk women might have more natural childbirth experiences and improved perinatal outcomes if they can labor without continuous electronic monitoring and with freedom to choose different positions.

Another important aspect of immediate postpartum care involves successful initiation and continuation of breast-feeding. Currently about 54% of women giving birth in the United States are breast-feeding when the infant is 1 week old (Lawrence, 1994), and by 6 months only 20% are continuing to breast-feed. While many factors contribute to determining these rates, physicians involved in perinatal care need to emphasize the health benefits for both baby and mother of breast-feeding and need to be well versed in counseling families in common concerns and problems with breast-feeding, especially in the first few weeks postpartum.

As many insurance companies and hospitals move toward early discharge of healthy mothers and babies, physicians need to work with local community resources such as visiting nurse organizations to make sure that these families receive appropriate guidance and timely medical follow-up. Sometimes such follow-up must include both early phone contact with the family and/or visiting nurse, and early postpartum visits for baby and mother, sooner than the traditional 2 and 6 weeks, respectively, or even postpartum home visits by the physician or other clinician. This is especially true for first-time mothers who are breast-feeding, which often takes longer than 24 hours to establish successfully. Labor support advocates can act as a postpartum liaison for the physician, also, modeling the continuity role that family physicians have in perinatal care.

CONCLUSION

Provision of care to families during their reproductive years is a challenging, rewarding, and at times terrifying endeavor. Often the interventions with the greatest impact on a family and its offspring are those low-key efforts designed to lower risks and respond to psychosocial as well as medical and obstetric concerns before crises arise. The drama of labor and delivery requires special skills that are often critical to the health of the mother and infant. They are, however, an extremely limited aspect of the care a family needs in bringing forth new life.

The continuing relationship of a family with a physician who provides comprehensive care from before conception and continuing through childhood offers opportunity for early recognition of risks that otherwise might lead to major problems. Particularly for high-risk families, the physician needs to work closely with other professionals and services in the community. For physicians in high-risk communities, the challenge involves developing and working within a healthcare team and providing leadership to or assisting in the development of a network of services for young families. However, the results can be highly rewarding, particularly for the physician who remains in practice in the same community, caring for families as children grow, and in whose lives they were able to make a difference.

CASES FOR DISCUSSION

All of the cases in this chapter are located in the village of Middletown. It has evolved significantly over the past 20 years from a working- and middle-class, white ethnic suburb of Providence to the ethnically diverse and socioeconomically disadvantaged community it is today. Many of the industries that employed Middletown's citizens have relocated. One large manufacturing plant and two smaller service-oriented firms remain. One of Middletown's two hospitals closed about 5 years ago, leaving Middletown Memorial as the sole healthcare institution servicing the community.

Memorial is a 250-bed, not-for-profit and nonsectarian community hospital that provides full-service primary and secondary care and has an academic affiliation with Bradford Medical School in the Tri-Cities. Memorial Hospital struggles to maintain a "market share" among those with commercial insurance in the surrounding neighborhoods, yet the proportion of patients who are underinsured or uninsured continues to rise.

The businesses in town have enrolled most of their employees in Tri-City HMO, a local branch of a nationwide managed care organization. They have offices in Memorial's professional building. There are also several private practitioners remaining in Middletown who continue to see those patients with commercial insurance and who serve as consultants for the HMO. A community health center was developed 5 years ago in the ambulatory care center of the hospital that closed. This health center has federal and state grants that support its mission of caring for the underserved.

CASE 1

The triage nurse met the paramedics at the ER door. A message from the paramedics had warned that they were en route with a 22-year-old in premature labor. The paramedics gave report as they wheeled the stretcher down the corridor toward the OB unit. Tonya, the patient, thinks her due date is next month. Her contractions started 2 hours ago and she has not received prenatal care and does not have a regular physician. Tonya is crying and writhing in pain.

Debbie, an experienced and reassuring labor nurse, helps to get Tonya admitted. Dr. Smith, the resident on duty, examines Tonya and confirms that she is in active premature labor. Tonya is alone. Her mother wanted to come but could not find anyone to watch Tonya's little brother, who is 11 months old. It was 6:00 PM and Dr. Smith explained that she was going off duty and Dr. Alexander was taking over.

Tonya labored through the evening alone except for Debbie. Dr. Alexander introduced himself and apologetically explained that there were many other patients to attend. Tonya's boyfriend, Johnny, stopped by with one of his friends. The visit felt awkward to him and Tonya was relieved to see him go. They had argued frequently the past few months and Johnny's temper outbursts had turned to violence on more than one occasion. She hoped the baby would make him calm down.

Feeling frightened and alone, Tonya had her baby. The 5-pound baby girl was a few weeks premature and appeared healthy but was taken to the nursery for observation. A drug screen, taken because of the premature labor and lack of prenatal care, is positive for cocaine. Dr. Alexander informed Tonya that if cocaine was found in the baby's system, it would be reported as child abuse. Tonya is discharged the following day while her baby awaited social service evaluation for possible placement. On discharge, Tonya is given Dr. Fields's name and office number for postpartum care.

1. *How could prenatal care affect Tonya's case? Should prenatal care be available to everyone? Is routine prenatal care adequate for Tonya?*
2. *List and determine the appropriate further evaluation of potential risk factors, both medical and psychosocial.*
3. *What is the role of Child Protective Services in this and similar cases? Is there evidence for child abuse? What supports are needed?*
4. *How should the healthcare team encourage the involvement of the baby's father?*

CASE 2

Rosa is a 16-year-old who is in labor. Her baby is also coming a few weeks early, but unlike Tonya, Rosa is not alone. Hector, the baby's father, and Rosa's mother are at her bedside as she labors.

Hector attended childbirth classes with Rosa and went to many of her prenatal visits at the community health center. Hector and Rosa's mother take turns rubbing her back and coaching Rosa through pains. Dr. Thomas, who works at the health center, is also there. He reassures Rosa and her family that the labor is progressing normally and encourages Rosa to focus on the precious little life she is miraculously and courageously bringing into this world.

Feeling frightened but safe and supported, Rosa has her baby. With tears of joy, Hector ceremoniously cuts the cord. Dr. Thomas places the slippery, vigorous 5-pound boy on Rosa's chest. Though 4 weeks premature, the little boy appears healthy and stays in the room with his family. Rosa begins breast-feeding as she had been encouraged to do by the staff at the health center.

The following day, Dr. Thomas discharged Rosa and her baby home. She is seen 3 days later at home by a home care nurse. The baby is thriving on the breast milk but Rosa is frustrated with the breast-feeding and wants to start bottle feedings. Rosa's mother is concerned that the baby is not getting enough milk because Rosa is impatient with the feedings.

Rosa had planned to return to school after a few weeks at home, and has chosen a birth control method. However, the school nurse tells Rosa that she will be tutored at home, and may have to repeat the year. Rosa begins to have conflicts with her mother over the care and discipline of her newborn; Rosa wants to set strict limits, so the baby does not grow up to be spoiled. Hector visits after school but is uncomfortable with the baby and openly annoyed at the conflict between Rosa and her mother.

1. Review the comprehensive care system that Rosa and her family have access to, including: how is it more than routine? and how does it extend the physician's role?
2. What are critical issues requiring continuity between the prepregnancy, prenatal, and postpartum intervals in this family's care? How is such continuity care best organized?
3. Describe the family dynamics. How can Hector be involved? What should Dr. Thomas advise, and how should he approach family members to bring about change?
4. How can Dr. Thomas intervene to help Rosa acquire parenting skills? Consider practical experience, familial modeling, and school- and community-based programs.

CASE 3

Recall Tonya, who delivered a premature baby who was cocaine exposed. There had been little or no prenatal care and Tonya was alone with minimal family support. There was a concern about Johnny, the baby's father, who had become increasingly violent with Tonya. The case had been reported to the Department of Child Protective Services because of the drug abuse. They found no other evidence of abuse and discharged the baby home in the custody of Tonya's grandmother. A case worker was assigned. Tonya had not seen Dr. Fields, and again was encouraged to do so.

One month later, the baby is seen in the local emergency room for a cold and diarrhea. The baby weighs 6 pounds and appears relatively healthy. The baby has not been seen for routine childcare as yet. Tonya and Johnny brought the baby to the ER. The examining physician notices some large bruises on the baby's arms and questions the young parents. They are unsure as to the cause of the bruises and had not noticed them. The cold and diarrhea symptoms are not significant.

1. Consider the alternative societal responses to suspected parenting inadequacies. Which would be appropriate for this family?
2. What obligations and options are there for the ER physician?
3. How could a comprehensive care system influence this family?
4. How should Dr. Fields become involved?

CASE 4

A 21-year-old African-American woman with two previous miscarriages makes an appointment with Dr. Fields to discuss trying to get pregnant again. She is a smoker, and on looking through her chart Dr. Fields sees that she is rubella nonimmune (Dr. Fields tested her at her last contraceptive appointment).

1. *What are some modifiable perinatal risk factors? Discuss smoking and immunizations prior to and during pregnancy.*
2. *What are other risk factors, less modifiable but still important to identify? Discuss genetic counseling around sickle cell disease and race/ethnicity as a risk factor in pregnancy outcomes.*
3. *When should you do preconception care?*
4. *How can primary care practice be organized to support preconception and other preventive and health promotion practices? How can it best work with community-level interventions, including smoking cessation, immunization tracking, sickle cell screening and genetic counseling in the community, psychological concerns, and supporting families around perinatal loss?*

CASE 5

Recall from Case 20-6 the story of Katie, a 15-year-old girl whose family are Dr. Fields's patients. Dr. Fields last saw her 2 years ago. She came to the office by herself with a positive pregnancy test. On further questioning, she had been taking oral contraceptives intermittently and has been feeling fetal movement. She hasn't told her parents yet about the pregnancy. Dr. Fields finds out that she is a smoker. The initial prenatal exam indicates that she is about 18 weeks pregnant; the Pap smear comes back abnormal.

1. *What are some of the public health issues around teenage pregnancy?*
2. *What community resources are needed for school-age mothers?*
3. *How can primary care offices interact with other agencies in caring for pregnant teenagers?*
4. *What are the cross-generational issues for the family's physician?*
5. *What are some of the biomedical issues regarding late prenatal care?*
6. *Discuss the biomedical and practice organizational issues involved in the management of abnormal Pap smears.*

———————— RECOMMENDED READINGS ————————

Enkin M, Keirse MJNC, Renfrew M, Neilsen J (eds): *A Guide to Effective Care in Pregnancy and Childbirth,* London, Oxford University Press, 1995.

> This masterful work is the definitive collection of evidence related to the effectiveness of reproductive healthcare. The work of the Cochrane Center, it has led to an international initiative to promote evidence-based medicine, The Cochrane Collaboration.

Brody H, Thompson JR: The maximum strategy in modern obstetrics. *J Fam Pract* 12:977–986, 1981.
Rosenblatt RA: The perinatal paradox: Doing more and accomplishing less. *Health Affairs,* 1989, pp. 158–168.

> The Brody and Rosenblatt articles describe from different perspectives the dilemmas in applying high-tech approaches to reproductive health at both the individual patient and national policy levels. Together

they provide considerable insight into the controversies facing both clinicians and policymakers as they choose strategies to improve birth outcomes.

Buescher PA, Roth MS, Williams D, Goforth CM: An evaluation of the impact of maternity care coordination on Medicaid birth outcomes in North Carolina. *Am J Public Health* 81(12):1625–1635, 1991.

This article provides convincing evidence of the value of community-based integration of medical and psychosocial care approaches. It provides insight into how services can be organized to respond effectively to the needs of high-risk communities.

Institute of Medicine Committee to Study the Prevention of Low Birthweight: *Preventing Low Birthweight.* Washington, DC, National Academy Press, 1985.

Institute of Medicine Committee to Study Outreach for Prenatal Care: *Prenatal Care: Reaching Mothers, Reaching Infants.* Washington, DC, National Academy Press, 1988.

Institute of Medicine Panel on Adolescent Pregnancy and Childbearing: *Risking the Future: Adolescent Sexuality, Pregnancy, and Childbearing.* Washington, DC, National Academy Press, 1987.

Institute of Medicine Committee on Unintended Pregnancy: *The Best Intentions. Unintended Pregnancy and the Well-Being of Children and Families.* Washington, DC, National Academy Press, 1995.

These Institute of Medicine reports, all of which have executive summaries, are the definitive works related to MCH care of socially high-risk populations in the United States.

Jack BW, Culpepper L: Preconception care: Risk reduction and health promotion in preparation for pregnancy. *JAMA* 264:1147–1149, 1990.

This reference identifies the potential of preconception care to improve birth outcomes and discusses opportunities and impediments to implementing preconception care.

References

AAFP: *Facts about Family Practice*. Kansas City, KS, American Academy of Family Physicians, 1991.

Abel TM, Metraux R, Roll S: *Psychotherapy and Culture*, revised/expanded ed. Albuquerque, University of New Mexico Press, 1987.

Agency for Toxic Substance and Disease Registry. *The Nature and Extent of Lead Poisoning in Children in the U.S.: A Report to Congress*. Washington DC, Department of Health and Human Services, 1988.

AHCPR. *Managing Otitis Media with Effusion in Young Children*. Rockville, Md, Department of Health and Human Services, Public Health Service, Agency for Health Care Policy and Research Publication No. 94–0623, 1994.

Alan Guttmacher Institute. *Blessed Events and the Bottom Line: The Financing of Maternity Care in the United States*. New York, Alan Guttmacher Institute, 1987.

Alexander S, Keirse MJNC. Formal risk scoring during pregnancy, in Chalmers I, Enkin M, Keirse MJNC (eds): *Effective Care in Pregnancy and Childbirth*. London, Oxford University Press, 1989, pp 345–365.

Ambuel B, Brownell E, Hamberger LK: Implementing a community model for training medical students and physicians to diagnose, treat and prevent family violence. Workshop presented at the Second STFM Violence Education Conference, Albuquerque, N Mex, November 1994.

American College of Occupational and Environmental Medicine (ACOEM). The new ACOEM code of ethical conduct. *J Occup Med* 36(1):27–30, 1994.

American Medical Association. Principles of medical ethics, 1957, in Reiser SJ, Dyck AJ, Curran WJ (eds): *Ethics in Medicine: Historical Perspectives and Contemporary Concerns*. Cambridge, Mass, MIT Press, 1977, p 39.

American Medical Association. *Guidelines to the Evaluation of Permanent Impairment*, ed 3. Chicago, American Medical Association, 1988.

American Medical Association, Council on Scientific Affairs. Violence against women. *JAMA* 267:3184–3189, 1992.

American Medical Association. Report of the Board of Trustees (SS, A-93), presented by Scalettar R. Chicago, American Medical Association, 1993.

American Psychiatric Association. *Diagnostic and Statistical Manual of Mental Disorders*, ed 4. Washington, DC, American Psychiatric Association, 1994.

American Psychiatric Association. *Diagnostic and Statistical Manual of Mental Disorders*, ed 4, primary care version (DSM-IV-PC). Washington, DC, American Psychiatric Association, 1994.

American Psychological Association. *Specialty Guidelines for the Delivery of Services in Clinical Psychology, Counseling Psychology, Industrial/Organizational Psychology, and School Psychology*. Washington, DC, American Psychological Association Committees on Professional Standards, 1981.

American Psychological Association Commission on Youth and Violence. *Violence and Youth: Psychology's Response*. Washington, DC, American Psychological Association, 1993.

Anderson P, Cremona A, Paton A, Turner C, Wallace P: Alcohol and risk. *Addiction* 88:1493–1508, 1993.

Apgar WC: *The Crisis Isn't Over—The Continued Need for Affordable Housing in Massachusetts*. Cambridge, Mass, Harvard–MIT Joint Center for Urban Studies, 1991.

Aring C: Sympathy and empathy. *JAMA* 167:448–452, 1958.

Asen KE, Tomson T, Canavan B: *Family Solution in Family Practice.* Lancaster, England, Quay Publishing, 1992.

Babor TF, Kranzler HR, Lauerman RJ: Early detection of harmful alcohol consumption: Comparison of clinical, laboratory, and self-report screening procedures. *Addict Behav* 14(2):139–157, 1989.

Babson SG: Mortality rates. *Pediatrics* 84:402–403, 1989.

Badger LW, deGruy FV, Hartman J, Plant MA, Leeper J, Ficken R, Maxwell A, Rand E, Anderson R, Templeton B: Psychosocial interest, medical interviews, and the recognition of depression. *Arch Fam Med* 3:899–907, 1994.

Baird MA, Doherty WJ: Risks and benefits of a family systems approach to medical care. *Fam Med* 22:396–403, 1990.

Baker LC, Cantor JC: Physician satisfaction under managed care. *Health Affairs* 12 suppl:258–270, 1993.

Balart LA, Ferrante WA: Pathophysiology of acute and chronic pancreatitis. *Arch Intern Med* 142:113–177, 1982.

Balint M: *The Doctor, His Patient, and the Illness.* New York, International Universities Press, Inc, 1957.

Barrett JR. Exercise addiction, in Mellion MB (ed): *Sports Medicine Secrets.* Philadelphia, Hanley & Belfus, 1994, pp 141–144.

Barry KL, Fleming MF: The family physician. *Alcohol Health Res World* 18(1):105–109, 1994.

Basch MF: Empathic understanding: A review of the concept and some theoretical considerations. *J Am Psychoanal Assoc.* 31:101–126, 1983.

Bass MJ, Buck C, Turner L: Predictors of outcome in headache patients presenting to family physicians—A one year prospective study. *Headache* 26:285–294, 1986a.

Bass MJ, Buck C, Turner L: The physician's actions and the outcome of illness. *J Fam Pract* 23:43–47, 1986b.

Beauchamp TL, Childress JF: *Principles of Biomedical Ethics.* London, Oxford University Press, 1989.

Becker HS, Geer B, Hughes E, Strauss A: *Boys in White: Student Culture in Medical School.* Chicago, University of Chicago Press, 1961.

Becker LB, Ostrander MP, Barrett J, Kondos GT: Outcome of CPR in a large metropolitan area—Where are the survivors? *Ann Emerg Med* 20(4):355–361, 1991.

Beckman HB, Markakis KM, Suchman AL, Frankel RM: The doctor–patient relationship and malpractice. Lessons from plaintiff depositions. *Arch Intern Med* 154:1365–1370, 1994.

Beecher HK: *Measurement of Subjective Responses.* London, Oxford University Press, 1959.

Beinfield H, Korngold E: Chinese traditional medicine: An introductory overview. *Altern Ther* 1(1):44–52, 1995.

Bellet PS, Maloney MJ: The importance of empathy as an interviewing skill in medicine. *JAMA* 266:1831–1832, 1991.

Beresford TP, Blow F, Hill E, Singer K, Lucey MR: Comparison of CAGE questionnaire and computer-assisted laboratory profiles in screening for covert alcoholism. *Lancet* 336:482–485, 1990.

Bickel J, Ruffin A: Gender-associated difference in matriculating and graduating medical students. *Acad Med* 70(6):552–559, 1995.

Bindman A, *et al*: Preventable hospitalization and health care access. *JAMA* 274:305–311, 1995.

Bird J, Cohen-Cole SA: The three function model of the medical interview: An educational device, in Hale MS (ed): *Methods in Teaching Consultation–Liaison Psychiatry.* Basel, Karger, 1990, pp 65–88.

Blendon RJ, Leitman R, Morrison I, *et al*: Satisfaction with health systems in ten nations. *Health Affairs* 1990 (Summer), pp 185–192.

Blondell RD: Impaired physicians. *Primary Care* 20:209–219, 1993.

Bloom SW: *The Doctor and His Patient: A Sociological Interpretation.* New York, The Free Press, 1965.

Blum A: Medicine vs. Madison Avenue: Fighting smoke with smoke. *JAMA* 243:739–740, 1980.

Blum A: The AMA tackles smoking: "A strong stand." *NY State J Med* 83:1363–1365, 1983.

Blum A: Targeting of minority groups by the tobacco industry, in Jones L (ed): *Minorities and Cancer.* Berlin, Springer-Verlag, 1989, pp 153–162.

Blum A: The Marlboro Grand Prix: Circumvention of the television ad ban on tobacco advertising. *N Engl J Med* 324:913–916, 1991.

Blum A: Role of the health professional in ending the tobacco pandemic: Clinic, classroom, and community. *JNCI* 12:37–43, 1992.

Blum A: Curtailing the tobacco pandemic, in DeVita VT, Hellman S, Rosenberg SA (eds): *Cancer: Principles and Practice of Oncology*, ed 4. Philadelphia, JB Lippincott Co, 1993, pp 480–491.

Blum A, Solberg E. The role of the family physician in ending the tobacco pandemic. *J Fam Pract* 43(6):697–700, 1992.

Blumenthal D: Health care reform—Past and future. *N Engl J Med* 332:465–468, 1995.

Blumgart HL: Caring for the patient. *N Engl J Med* 270:449–456, 1964.

Blumhagen D: The meaning of hypertension, in Chrisman N, Maretzki TW (eds): *Clinically Applied Anthropology*. Dordrecht, Reidel, 1982, pp 297–323.

Bograd M: The duel over dual relationships. *Fam Ther Networker* 16(6):33–37, 1992.

Bosk CL: *Forgive and Remember: Managing Medical Failure*. Chicago, University of Chicago Press, 1979.

Bouchardy C, Clavel F, LaVecchia C, Raymond L, Boyle P: Alcohol, beer, and cancer of the pancreas. *Int J Cancer* 45(5):842–846, 1990.

Bowlby J: Attachment and loss: Retrospect and prospect. *Annu Prog Child Psychiatry Child Dev*, 1983, pp 29–47.

Boyer LB: Approaching cross-cultural psychotherapy. *J Psychoanal Anthropol* 6:237–245, 1983.

Bradt RC: The launching of the single young adult, in Carter EA, McGoldrick M (eds): *The Changing Life Cycle: A Framework for Family Theory*, ed 2. New York, Gardner Press, 1988, pp 237–253.

Brancati FL: The art of pimping. *JAMA* 262:89–90, 1989.

Branch WT, Suchman A: Meaningful experiences in medicine. *Am J Med* 88:56–59, 1990.

Braverman PK, Strasburger VC: The practitioner's role. *Clin Pediatr* 33(2):100–109, 1994.

Brennan TA: AIDS and the limits of confidentiality: The physician's duty to warn contacts of seropositive individuals. *J Gen Intern Med* 4:242–246, 1989.

Bridges KW, Goldberg DP: Somatic presentation of DSM III psychiatric disorders in primary care. *J Psychosom Res* 29:563–569, 1985.

Broadhead WE, Blazer DG, George LK, Tse CK: Depression, disability days, and days lost from work in a prospective epidemiologic survey. *JAMA* 264:2524–2528, 1990.

Brody H: *Placebos and the Philosophy of Medicine*. Chicago, University of Chicago Press, 1980.

Brody H: *The Healer's Power*. New Haven, Conn, Yale University Press, 1992.

Brody H, Thompson JR: The maximum strategy in modern obstetrics. *J Fam Pract* 12:977–986, 1981.

Brook U, Mendelberg A, Heim M: Increasing parental knowledge of asthma decreases hospitalization of the child: A pilot study. *J Asthma* 30(1):45–49, 1993.

Brown E, Prager J, Lee HY, Ramsey RG: CNS complications of cocaine abuse: Prevalence, pathophysiology, and neuroradiology. *Am J Roentgenol*, 159(1):137–147, 1992.

Brown FW, Golding JM, Smith GRJ: Psychiatric comorbidity in primary care somatization disorder. *Psychosom Med* 52:445–451, 1990.

Brown J, Stewart M, McCracken EC: The patient centered clinical method. II. Definition and application. *Fam Pract* 3(2):75–79, 1986.

Brown R: Identification and office management of alcohol and drug disorders, in Fleming MF, Barry KL (eds): *Addictive Disorders*. St. Louis, Mosby Yearbook Medical Publishers, 1992, pp 25–43.

Bryant BE: *Statistics Abstract of the United States, 110th Edition*. Washington, DC, Bureau of the Census, 1990, p 173.

Buchanan B, Lappin J: Re-storying the soul of the family. *The Family Networker*, November/December 1990, pp 46–52.

Bucher R, Stelling JG: *Becoming Professional*. Beverly Hills, Calif, Sage Publications, Inc, 1977.

Buescher PA, Roth MS, Williams D, Goforth CM: An evaluation of the impact of maternity care coordination on Medicaid birth outcomes in North Carolina. *Am J Public Health* 81(12):1625–1635, 1991.

Bunn WH, Giannini AJ: Cardiovascular complications of cocaine abuse. *Am Fam Physician* 47(5):1072, 1993.

Bureau of the Census. *Historical Statistics of the U.S., Colonial Times to 1970, Bicentennial Edition, Part 2*. Washington, DC, Department of Commerce, 1975.

Bureau of the Census. *Statistical Abstract of the United States*. Washington, DC, Department of Commerce, 1992.

Bureau of Health Care Delivery and Assessment (BHCDA) Office of Shortage Designation. *Guidelines for Health Professional Shortage Area Designation as Established by the National Health Service Corps Revitalization Act of 1990*. Washington, DC, Department of Health and Human Services, Public Health Service, 1990.

Burgess AW (ed): *Rape and Sexual Assault. III. A Research Handbook*. New York, Garland Publishing, Inc, 1991.

Burish TG, Snyder SL, Jenkins RA: Preparation of patients for cancer chemotherapy: Effect of coping preparation and relaxation interventions. *J Consult Clin Psychol* 59(4):518–525, 1991.

Burner S, Waldo D: National health expenditure projection, 1994–2005. *Health Care Financ Rev* 16 (summer):221–242, 1995.

Burstein JM, Levy BS: The teaching of occupational health in US medical schools: Little improvement in nine years. *Am J Public Health* 84(5):846–869, 1994.

Calsyn DA, Meinecke C, Saxon AJ, Stanton V: Risk reduction in sexual behavior: a condom giveaway program in a drug abuse treatment clinic. *Am J Public Health* 82(11):1536–1538, 1992.

Callahan CM, Rivara FP: Urban high school youth and handguns: A school-based survey. *JAMA* 267:3038–3042, 1992.

Campbell TL: *Family's Impact on Health: A Critical Review and Annotated Bibliography.* NIMH Series DN, No. 6, DHHS Publication No. (ADM) 86–1461, 1986. Also published in *Fam Syst Med* 4(2+3):135–328, 1986.

Campbell TL, Patterson J: The effectiveness of family interventions in the treatment of physical illness. *J Marital Fam Ther* 21(4):545–583, 1995.

Candib L: Family life cycle theory. *Fam Syst Med* 7(4), 1989.

Carter EA, McGoldrick M (eds): *The Changing Family Life Cycle: A Framework for Family Therapy.* New York, Gardner Press, 1980.

Carter EA, McGoldrick M (eds): *The Changing Family Life Cycle: A Framework for Family Therapy,* ed 2. New York, Gardner Press, 1988.

Cassell EJ: The nature of suffering and the goals of medicine. *N Engl J Med* 306:639–645, 1982.

Cassell EJ: *The Nature of Suffering and the Goals of Medicine.* London, Oxford University Press, 1991.

Centers for Disease Control. Current trends: Contribution of birth defects to infant mortality: United States, 1986. *MMWR* 38:633–635, 1989.

Centers for Disease Control. *Division of STD/HIV Prevention Annual Report.* Atlanta, U.S. Department of Health and Human Services, 1990a.

Centers for Disease Control. *Morbidity and Mortality Weekly Report* 39:317–318, 1990b.

Centers for Disease Control. Cigarette smoking among adults—United States, 1993. *MMWR* 43(50):925–930, 1994a.

Centers for Disease Control and Prevention. Heterosexually acquired AIDS—United States, 1993. *JAMA* 271: 975–976, 1994b.

Centrella M: Physician addiction and impairment—Current thinking: A review. *J Addict Dis* 13:91–105, 1994.

Chang CC, Ruhl RA, Halpern GM, Gershwin ME: Building components contributors of the sick building syndrome. *J Asthma* 31(2):127–137, 1994.

Chao KY, Wang JD: Increased lead absorption caused by working next to a lead recycling factory. *Am J Ind Med* 26(2):229–235, 1994.

Chappell LT: EDTA chelation therapy should be more commonly used in the treatment of vascular disease. *Altern Ther* 1(2):53–57, 1995.

Charns M: Breaking the tradition barrier: Managing integration in health care facilities. *Health Care Manage Rev* 1:55–67, 1976.

Chelmowski M, Hamberger LK: Screening men for domestic violence in your medical practice. *Wis Med J,* December 1994, pp 623–626.

The Chiropractic Profession: Myths & Facts. Palmerton, Pa, PracticeMakers Products, Inc, 1993.

Chiropractic: State of the Art 1994–1995. Arlington, Va, American Chiropractic Association, 1994.

Chrisman NJ: The health seeking process: An approach to the natural history of illness. *Culture Med Psychiatry* 1:351–377, 1977.

Chrisman NJ, Maretzki TW (eds): *Clinically Applied Anthropology.* Dordrecht, Reidel, 1982.

Christensen JF, Levinson W, Dunn PM: The heart of darkness: The impact of perceived mistakes on physicians. *J Gen Intern Med* 7:424–431, 1992.

Christensen JK, Moller IW, Ronsted P, Angelo HR, Johansson B: Dose–effect relationship of disulfiram in human volunteers: 1. Clinical studies. *Pharmacol Toxicol* 68(3):163–165, 1991.

Chuck JM, Nesbitt TS, Kwan J, Kam SM: Is being a doctor still fun? *West J Med* 159:665–669, 1993.

Clark NM, Feldman CH, Evans D, Levison MJ, Wasilewski Y, Mellins RB: The impact of health education on the frequency and cost of health care use by low income children with asthma. *J Allergy Clin Immunol* 78(1):108–114, 1986.

Cloninger CR, Martin RL, Guze SB, Clayton PJ: A prospective follow-up and family study of somatization in men and women. *Am J Psychiatry* 143:873–878, 1986.

Cluff LE: New agenda for medicine. *Am J Med* 82:803–810, 1987.

Cohen AB, Cantor JC, Barker DC, Hughes RG: Young physicians and the future of the medical profession. *Health Affairs (Millwood)* 9:138–148, 1990.

Cohen CA, Dent C, MacKinnon D, Hahn G: Condoms for men, not women: Results of brief promotion and programs. *Sex Transm Dis* 19(5):245–251, 1992.

Cole S, Hartford R, Bergsjo P, *et al*: International collaborative effort (ICE) on birth weight, plurality, and infant mortality. III: A method of grouping underlying causes of death to aid international comparisons. *Acta Obstet Gynecol Scand* 68:113–117, 1989.

Committee on International Relations, Stein HF: *Us and Them: The Psychology of Ethnonationalism*. Group for the Advancement of Psychiatry, Report No. 123. New York, Brunner/Mazel, 1987.

Consumer Reports on Health, April 1995. *Are herbal remedies good medicine?* Consumer Reports on Health, 1995.

Cook CH: The Minnesota model in the management of drug and alcohol dependency: Miracle, method or myth? Part II. Evidence and conclusions. *Br J Addict* 83:735–748, 1988.

Cooper AE: Duty to warn third parties. *JAMA* 248:431–432, 1982.

Coryell W, Norten SG: Briquet's syndrome (somatization disorder) and primary depression: Comparison of background and outcome. *Compr Psychiatry* 22:249–256, 1981.

Costa AJ, Anetzberger GJ: Elder abuse, in Hamberger LK, Burge S, Graham A, Costa A (eds): *Violence Issues for Health Care Educators*. New York, The Haworth Press, in press.

Coulehan JL, Block MR: *The Medical Interview: A Primer for Students of the Art*. Philadelphia, FA Davis Co, 1992.

Council on Ethical and Judicial Affairs, American Medical Association. Conflicts of interest. Physician ownership of medical facilities. *JAMA* 267:2366–2369, 1992.

Council on Graduate Medical Education (COGME). *Improving Access to Health Through Physician Workforce Reform: Dimensions for the Twenty-first Century*. Washington, DC, Health Resource Services Administration, 1992.

Cowen CP, Cowen H: Transitions to parenthood: His, hers and theirs. *J Fam Issues* 6(4):451–481, 1985.

Crawford R: Healthism and the medicalization of everyday life. *Int J Health Serv* 10:365–388, 1980.

Crawford R: A cultural account of health: Self control, release, and the social body, in McKinlay J (ed): *Issues in the Political Economy of Health Care*. London, Tavistock, 1985, pp 60–103.

Crowther C, Chalmers I: Bed rest and hospitalization during pregnancy, in Chalmers I, Enkin M, Keirse MJNC (eds): *Effective Care in Pregnancy and Childbirth*. London, Oxford University Press, 1989, pp 624–632.

Cullen MR, Rosenstock LS: The challenge of teaching occupational and environmental medicine in internal medicine residencies. *Arch Intern Med* 148(11):2401–2404, 1988.

Culpepper L: Reducing infant mortality: The research gaps. Background report for the HRSA Interagency Committee on Infant Mortality, 1991.

Culpepper L: Primary care provider and system challenges in caring for high-risk children and families, in Grason HA, Guyer B (eds): *Assessing and Developing Primary Care for Children*. Arlington, Va, National Center for Education in Maternal and Child Health, 1995, pp 136–150.

Culpepper L, Jack BW: Preconception care, in Cherry SH, Merkatz IR (eds): *Complications of Pregnancy: Medical, Surgical, Gynecologic, Psychosocial and Perinatal*. Baltimore, Williams & Wilkins Co, 1991, pp 2–15.

Culpepper L, Jack B: Psychosocial issues in pregnancy. *Primary Care* 20(3):599–619, 1993.

Cunningham RM, Stiffman AR, Dore P: The association of physical and sexual abuse with HIV risk behaviors in adolescence and young adulthood: Implications for public health. *Child Abuse Neglect* 18(3):233–245, 1991.

Cushman P, Jacobson G, Barboriak JJ, Anderson AP: Biochemical markers for alcoholism: Sensitivity problems. *Alcoholism Clin Exp Res* 8(3):253–257, 1984.

Daker M, Bobrow M: Screening for genetic disease and fetal anomaly during pregnancy, in Chalmers I, Enkin M, Keirse MJNC, (eds): *Effective Care in Pregnancy and Childbirth*. London, Oxford University Press, 1989, pp 366–381.

Daniels N: Duty to treat or right to refuse? *Hastings Cent Rep*, March–April 1991, pp 36–46.

Debrovner D: Micro medicine. *Am Drug* 208(1):36–41, 1993.

deGruy F, Columbia L, Dickinson P: Somatization disorder in a family practice. *J Fam Pract* 25:45–51, 1987.

deGruy FV, Dickinson L, Dickinson P: Patterns of somatization in primary care. Paper presented at the Eighth Annual NIMH International Research conference on Mental Health Problems in the General Health Care Sector, McLean, Va, 1994.

deMause L: *Reagan's America*. New York, Creative Roots, 1984.

DeMuylder X, Wesel S, Dramaix M, *et al*: A woman's attitude toward pregnancy—Can it predispose her to preterm labor? *J Reprod Med* 37(4):339–342, 1992.

Denton WH: Problems encountered in reconciling individual and relational diagnoses, in Kaslow FW (ed): *Handbook of Relational Diagnoses*. New York, John Wiley & Sons, Inc, 1996, p 450.

Department of Health and Human Services, Public Health Service, Centers for Disease Control, Office on

Smoking and Health. *The Health Consequences of Smoking: Cardiovascular Disease.* A Report of the Surgeon General. DHHS Publication No. (PHS) 82–50179, 1982.

Department of Health and Human Services. *Report of the Task Force on Black and Minority Health.* Washington, DC, DHHS, 1985.

Department of Health and Human Services, Public Health Service, Centers for Disease Control, Office on Smoking and Health. *The Health Consequences of Involuntary Smoking.* A Report of the Surgeon General. DHHS Publication No. (CDC) 87–8398, 1986.

Department of Health and Human Services, Public Health Service, Centers for Disease Control, Office on Smoking and Health. *Reducing the Health Consequences of Smoking: 25 Years of Progress.* A Report of the Surgeon General. DHHS Publication No. (CDC) 89–8411, 1989.

Department of Health and Human Services, Public Health Service, Centers for Disease Control, Office on Smoking and Health. *The Health Benefits of Smoking Cessation.* A Report of the Surgeon General. DHHS Publication No. (CDC) 90–8416, 1990a.

Department of Health and Human Services, Public Health Service, National Institutes of Health, National Cancer Institute. *Smoking Tobacco and Cancer Programs: 1985–1989 Status Report.* NIH Publication No. 90–3107, 1990b.

Department of Health and Human Services, Public Health Service, Centers for Disease Control and Prevention. Asthma—United States 1980–1987. *Morbidity Mortality Weekly Report* 39:493–497, 1990c.

Department of Health and Human Services, Public Health Service, Centers for Disease Control and Prevention. *Preventing Lead Poisoning in Young Children: A Statement by the Centers for Disease Control*, October 1991.

Department of Health and Human Services, National Heart Lung and Blood Institute, National Asthma Education Program. *Teach Your Patients about Asthma: A Clinician's Guide.* Publication No. 92–2737, 1992.

Department of Health and Human Services, Public Health Service, Centers for Disease Control and Prevention. Recommendations and Reports. Assessing the public health threat associated with waterborne cryptosporidiosis: Report of a workshop. *Morbidity Mortality Weekly Report* 44(June 16): 2, 1995b.

Department of Health and Human Services, Public Health Service, Centers for Disease Control and Prevention. Asthma—United States 1982–1992. *Morbidity Mortality Weekly Report* 44:952–955, 1995a.

Department of Labor Bureau of Labor Statistics. *Survey of Occupational Injuries and Illnesses, 1993.* Washington, DC, Government Printing Office, 1995.

DesJarlais DC, Friedman SR, Choopanya K, Vanichseni S, Ward TP: International epidemiology of HIV and AIDS among injecting drug users. *AIDS* 6:1053–1068, 1992.

Deubner DC: A working definition of health and a healthy definition of work. *Semin Occup Med* 2(3):195–200, 1987a.

Deubner DC: Ethics. *Semin Occup Med* 2(3):177–182, 1987b.

Devereux G: *Basic Problems of Ethno-psychiatry*, Gulati BM, Devereux G (trans). Chicago, University of Chicago Press, 1980.

De Vos GA: Afterword, in Reynolds DK: *The Quiet Therapies: Japanese Pathways to Personal Growth.* Honolulu, University of Hawaii Press, 1980.

De Vos GA, Romanucci-Ross L (eds): *Ethnic Identity: Cultural Continuities and Change.* Palo Alto, Calif, Mayfield Publishing Co, 1975.

Dewar MA: Defensive medicine: It may not be what you think. *Fam Med* 26:36–38, 1994.

Diacatou A, Mamalakis G, Kafatos A, Vlahonikolis J, Bolonaki I: Alcohol, tobacco, and father's aggressive behavior in relation to socioeconomic variables in Cretan low versus medium income families. *Int J Addict* 28(4):293–304, 1993.

Dickens BM: Legal limits of AIDS confidentiality. *JAMA* 259:3449–3451, 1988.

Dimsdale JE: Delays and slips in medical diagnosis. *Perspect Biol Med* 27:213–220, 1984.

Dirckx JH: Speaking of illness. *Pharos* 45:22–26, 1982.

Division of Worker Education, Workers' Compensation Commission, State of Connecticut. *Directory of Additional Resources for Injured Employees.* New Haven, Conn, 1989.

Doherty WJ, Baird MA: *Family Therapy and Family Medicine: Toward the Primary Care of Families.* New York, Guilford Press, 1983.

Doherty WJ, Baird MA (eds): *Family-Centered Medical Care: A Clinical Casebook.* New York, Guilford Press, 1987.

Doherty WJ, Campbell TL: *Families and Health.* Beverly Hills, Calif, Sage Family Studies Series, 1988.

Doll R, Hill AB: Lung cancer and other causes of death in relation to smoking: Second report on mortality of British doctors. *Br Med J* 2:1071–1081, 1956.

Driscoll CE, Hoffmann GS: Sexual health care, in Rakel RE (ed): *Textbook of Family Practice,* ed 3. Philadelphia, WB Saunders Co, 1984, pp 1246–1270.

Drossman DA, Leserman J, Nachman G, Li Z, Gluck H, Toomey TC, Mitchell M: Sexual and physical abuse in women with functional or organic gastrointestinal disorders. *Ann Intern Med* 113:828–833, 1990.

Drucker PF: *The Practice of Management.* New York, Harper, 1954.

Dubovsky SL, Schrier RW: The mystique of medical training. *JAMA* 250:3057–3058, 1983.

Dym B (ed): *Working Together: The Newsletter of the Collaborative Family Health Care Coalition* 1(1), 1994.

Eberle S: A progressive agenda for family practice residency training. *Fam Syst Med* 6:371–384, 1988.

Eddy MB: *Science and Health with Key to the Scriptures.* Boston, Published by the author, 1886.

Edinger W, Smucker DR: Outpatients' attitudes regarding advance directives. *J Fam Pract* 35:650–653, 1992.

Eighth Special Report to the U.S. Congress on Alcohol and Health. Department of Health and Human Services, Public Health Service, National Institutes of Health, National Institute of Alcohol Abuse and Alcoholism. Publication No ADM-281-91-0003, 1993.

Eisenberg DM, Kessler RC, Foster C, *et al*: Unconventional medicine in the United States: Prevalence, costs and patterns of use. *N Engl J Med* 328:246–252, 1993.

Eisenberg L, Kleinman AM (eds): *The Relevance of Social Science for Medicine.* Dordrecht, Reidel, 1981.

Emanuel EJ, Dubler NN: Preserving the physician–patient relationship in the era of managed care. *JAMA* 273:323–335, 1995.

Emanuel EJ, Emanuel LL: Four models of the physician–patient relationship. *JAMA* 267:2221–2226, 1992.

Employee Benefit Research Institute: *Sources of Health Insurance and Characteristics of the Uninsured.* Special Report: Issue Brief 158, 1995.

Ende J: Feedback in clinical medical education. *JAMA* 250:777–781, 1983.

Engel GL: The need for a new medical model: A challenge for biomedicine. *Science* 196:129–136, 1977.

Engel GL: The clinical application of the biopsychosocial model. *Am J Psychiatry* 137:535–544, 1980.

Enthoven AC, Singer SJ: Market-based reform: What to regulate and by whom. *Health Affairs*, 1995 (Spring), pp 105–119.

Epstein R: Taking care of. *Arch Fam Med* 3:9–10, 1994.

Epstein RM: Communication between primary care physicians and consultants [see comments]. *Arch Fam Med* 4:403–409, 1995.

Epstein RM, Campbell TL, Cohen-Cole SA, McWhinney IR, Smilkstein G: Perspectives on patient–doctor communication. *J Fam Pract* 37:377–388, 1993.

Erickson EH: *Identity, Youth and Crisis,* ed 2. New York, WW Norton & Co, Inc, 1968.

Escobar JI: Cross-cultural aspects of the somatization trait. *Hosp Community Psychiatry* 38:174–180, 1987.

Escobar JI, Rubio-Stipec M, Canino G, Karno M: Somatic symptom index (SSI): A new and abridged somatization construct. Prevalence and epidemiological correlates in two large community samples. *J Nerv Ment Dis* 177:140–146, 1989.

Evans RG, Barer ML, Marmor TR: *Why are Some People Healthy and Others Not? The Determinants of Health of Populations.* New York, Aldine De Gruyter, 1994.

Evans S, Alberman E: International Collaborative Effort (ICE) on birthweight; plurality; and perinatal and infant mortality. II: Comparisons between birthweight distributions of birth in member countries from 1970 to 1984. *Acta Obstet Gynecol Scand* 68:11–17, 1989.

Ewing JA: Detecting alcoholism: The CAGE questionnaire. *JAMA* 252:1905–1907, 1984.

Faden RR, Beauchamp TL: *A History and Theory of Informed Consent.* London, Oxford University Press, 1986.

Fagin CM: Collaboration between nurses and physicians no longer a choice. Academic Medicine 67(5):295–303, 1992.

Fagin CM: Collaboration between nurses and physicians no longer a choice. *Nurs Health Care* 13(7):354–363, 1992.

Farley E: Family charts: Are they worthwhile? *J Fam Pract* 30:697–700, 1990.

Farrell M, Lewis G: Discrimination on the grounds of diagnosis. *Br J Addict* 85(7):883–890, 1990.

Fawcett J: Predictors of early suicide: Identification and appropriate intervention. *J Clin Psychiatry* 49:7–8, 1988.

Ferraroni M, Negri E, LaVecchia C, DaVanzo B, Franceschi S: Socioeconomic indicators, tobacco and alcohol in the etiology of digestive tract neoplasms. *Int J Epidemiol* 18(3):556–562, 1989.

Fingerhut LA, Ingram DD, Feldman JJ: Firearm and nonfirearm homicide among persons 15 through 19 years of age: Differences by level of urbanization, United States, 1979 through 1989. *JAMA* 267:3048–3052, 1992.

Finkelhor D: Current information on the scope and nature of child sexual abuse. *The Future of Children* 4:31–53, 1994.

Fleming MF, Barry KL: The effectiveness of alcoholism screening in an ambulatory care setting. *J Stud Alcohol* 52(1):33–36, 1991.

Fleming MF, Barry KL (eds): *Addictive Disorders*. St. Louis, Mosby Yearbook Medical Publishers, 1992.

Fleming MF, Barry KL: The effectiveness of brief physician advice with at-risk drinkers: Results of a clinical trial. Unpublished, 1995.

Fleming M, Barry K, Davis A, Kahn R, Riva M: Faculty development in addiction medicine: Project SAEFP: A one-year follow-up study. *Fam Med* 26(4):221–225, 1994.

Fletcher RH, Fletcher SW, Wagner EH: *Clinical Epidemiology—The Essentials*. Baltimore, Williams & Wilkins Co, 1982.

Foster G: Disease etiologies in non-Western medical systems. *Am Anthropol* 78:773–782, 1976.

Foster GM, Anderson BG: *Medical Anthropology*. New York, John Wiley & Sons, Inc, 1978.

Foster Higgins: National survey of employer-sponsored health plans. *Med Benefits* 12:1–2, 1995.

Fox RC: Training for uncertainty, in Merton RK, Reader GG, Kendall P (eds): *The Student Physician*. Cambridge, Mass, Harvard University Press, 1957, pp 207–241.

Fox RC: *The Sociology of Medicine: A Participant Observer's View*. Englewood Cliffs, NJ, Prentice–Hall, Inc, 1989.

Frame PS, Carlson SJ: A critical review of periodic health screening using specific screening criteria. Part 1. Selected diseases of respiratory, cardiovascular, and central nervous systems. *J Fam Pract* 2:29–36, 1975a.

Frame PS, Carlson SJ: A critical review of periodic health screening using specific screening criteria. Part 2. Selected endocrine, metabolic, and gastrointestinal diseases. *J Fam Pract* 2:123–129, 1975b.

Frame PS, Carlson SJ: A critical review of periodic health screening using specific screening criteria. Part 3. Selected diseases of the genitourinary system. *J Fam Pract* 2:189–194, 1975c.

Frame PS, Carlson SJ: A critical review of periodic health screening using specific screening criteria. Part 4. Selected miscellaneous diseases. *J Fam Pract* 2:283–289, 1975d.

Franks P, Culpepper L, Dickinson J: Psychosocial bias in the diagnosis of obesity. *J Fam Pract* 14:745–750, 1982.

Franks P, Clancy CM, Nutting PA: Gatekeeping revisited—protecting patients from overtreatment. *N Engl J Med* 327:424–429, 1992.

Fraser AM, Brockert JE, Ward RH: Association of young maternal age with adverse reproductive outcomes. *N Engl J Med* 332:113–117, 1995.

Freidson E: *Profession of Medicine*. New York, Harper & Row Publishers, Inc, 1970, pp 244–277.

French RM: Interpersonal relations, in *Dynamics of Health Care*, ed 3, New York, McGraw-Hill, 1979, pp 141–143.

Freymann JG: The public's health care paradigm is shifting: Medicine must swing with it. *J Gen Intern Med* 44:313–319, 1989.

Friedman E: Troubled past of "invisible" profession. *JAMA* 264:2851–2858, 1990.

Fuchs V: Has cost containment gone too far? in Lee PR, Estes CL (eds): *The Nation's Health*. Boston, Jones & Bartlett, 1990, pp 253–260.

Fuller AK, Bartucci RJ: Sexual abuse and HIV transmission. *J Sex Educ Ther* 47(1):46–52, 1991.

Fuller RC: The turn to alternative medicine. *Second Opinion* 18(1):11–31, 1992.

Fuller RK, Branchey L, Brightwell DR, *et al*: Disulfiram treatment of alcoholism: A Veteran's Administration cooperative study. *JAMA* 256:1449–1455, 1986.

Gabbard GO, Nadelson C: Professional boundaries in the physician–patient relationship. *JAMA* 273:1445–1449, 1995.

Gallagher DE, Thompson LW, Peterson JA: Psychosocial factors affecting adaptation to bereavement in the elderly. *Int J Aging Hum Dev* 14(2):79–95, 1982.

Gallup Poll (1985) as quoted in Public Health Service. *Healthy People 2000: National Health Promotion and Disease Prevention Objectives*. Washington, DC, 1990, pp 258.

Ganley A: Integrating feminist and social learning analyses of aggression: Creating multiple models for intervention with men who batter, in Caesar PL, Hamberger LK (eds): *Treating Men Who Batter: Theory, Practice and Programs*. Berlin, Springer, 1989, pp 196–235.

Gaquin DA: Spouse abuse. Data from the National Crime Survey. *Victimology* 2:632–642, 1977–78.

Garbarino J: The human ecology of early risk, in Meisels SJ, Shonkoff JP (eds): *Handbook of Early Childhood Interventions*. London, Cambridge University Press, 1990, pp 78–96.

Garbarino J, Sherman D: High-risk neighborhoods and high-risk families: The human ecology of child maltreatment. *Child Dev* 51:188–198, 1980.

Garcia-Preto N: Transformation of the family system in adolescence, in Carter EA, McGoldrick M (eds): *The

Changing Family Life Cycle: A Framework for Family Therapy, ed 2. New York, Gardner Press, 1988, pp 256–281.

Garcia-Preto N, Travis N: The adolescent phase of the family life cycle, in Mirkin MP, Koman SL (eds): *Handbook of Adolescents and Family Therapy.* New York, Gardner Press, 1985, pp 21–38.

Garner HG: *Helping Others through Teamwork.* Washington, DC, Child Welfare League of America, 1988.

Garr DR, Marsh FJ: Medical malpractice and the primary care physician: Lowering the risks. *South Med J* 79:1280–1284, 1986.

Gellert GA, Durfee MJ, Berkowitz CD: Developing guidelines for HIV antibody testing among victims of pediatric sexual abuse. *Child Abuse Neglect* 14:9–17, 1990.

Gelles RJ, Straus MA: *Intimate Violence.* New York, Simon & Schuster, Inc, 1988.

Gerber LA: Career and family dilemmas in doctor's lives. *Fam Med* 17:109–112, 1985.

Gernan PS, Shapiro S, Skinner EH, Von Korff M, Klein LE: Detection and management of mental health problems of older patients by primary care providers. *JAMA* 257:489–493, 1987.

Gershenson HP, Musick JS, Ruch-Ross HS, Magee V, Rubino KK, Rosenberg D: The prevalence of coercive experience among teenage mothers. *J Interpers Viol* 4:204–219, 1989.

Ginzberg E: The monetarization of medical care. *N Engl J Med* 310:1162–1165, 1984.

Glantz S, Parmley W. Passive smoking and heart disease. Mechanisms and risk. *JAMA* 273(13):1047–1053, 1995.

Glazer N, Moynihan DP (eds): *Ethnicity: Theory and Experience.* Cambridge, Mass, Harvard University Press, 1975.

Glick SM: From *Arrowsmith* to *The House of God*, or "Why Now?" *Am J Med* 88:449–451, 1990.

Goldberg BW: Preventing firearm violence, in Hamberger LK, Burge S, Graham A, Costa A (eds): *Violence Issues for Health Care Educators.* New York, The Haworth Press, in press.

Goldbloom R, Battista RN, Haggerty J: Periodic health examination, 1989 Update: 1. Introduction. *Can Med Assoc J* 141(3):205–207, 1989.

Goldenberg RL, Klerman LV: Adolescent pregnancy—another look. *N Engl J Med* 332:1161–1162, 1995.

Goldenberg RL, Davis RO, Nelson KG. Intrauterine growth retardation, in Merktz IR, Thompson JE, Mullen PD, Goldenberg R (eds): *New Perspectives on Prenatal Care.* New York, Elsevier Science Publishing Co, Inc, 1990, pp 461–478.

Goldenson RM, Dunham JR, Dunham CS: *Disability and Rehabilitation Handbook.* New York, McGraw–Hill Book Co, 1978.

Goldstein MK: Physicians and team, in Ham R (ed): *Geriatric Medicine Annual 1989.* Oradell, NJ, Medical Economics Co Book Division, 1989, pp 265–275.

Good BJ, Good MD: The meaning of symptoms: A cultural hermeneutic model for clinical practice, in Eisenberg L, Kleinman A (eds): *The Relevance of Social Science for Medicine.* Dordrecht, Reidel, 1981, pp 165–196.

Gordon GH, Hubbell FA, Wyle FA, Charter RA: Stress during internship: A prospective study of mood states. *J Gen Intern Med* 1:228–231, 1986.

Gostin LO, Lazzarini Z, Alexander D, *et al*: HIV testing, counseling, and prophylaxis after sexual assault. *JAMA* 271:1436–1444, 1990.

Gottlieb BR: Abortion—1995. *N Engl J Med* 332:532–533, 1995.

Government of Canada, Ministry of Health and Welfare. *A New Perspective on the Health of Canadians. A Working Document.* Ottawa, Ministry of Health and Welfare, Government of Canada, 1974.

Grant BF, DuFour MC, Harford TC: Epidemiology of alcoholic liver disease. *Semin Liver Dis* 1988; 8(1):12–25, 1988.

Grantz S, Parmley W: Passive smoking and heart disease. Mechanisms and risk. *JAMA* 273:1047–1053, 1995.

Green CP: *The Environment and Population Growth: Decade for Action.* Population Reports, Series M, No. 10. Baltimore, Johns Hopkins University Population Information Program, 1992.

Greenfield S, Kaplan S, Ware JE Jr: Expanding patient involvement in care. Effects on patient outcomes. *Ann Intern Med*, 102:520–528, 1985.

Greenfield S, Kaplan SH, Ware JE Jr, Yano EM, Frank HJ: Patients' participation in medical care: Effects on blood sugar control and quality of life in diabetes. *J Gen Intern Med* 3:448–457, 1988.

Greenwood CL, Tangalos EG, Maruta T: Prevalence of sexual abuse, physical abuse and concurrent traumatic life events in a general medical population. *Mayo Clin Proc* 65:1067–1071, 1990.

Greer JR, Abbey DE, Burchette RJ: Asthma related to occupational and ambient air pollutants in nonsmokers. *J Occup Med* 35(9):909–915, 1993.

Greist J, Klein M, Erdman H, Bires J, *et al*: Comparison of computer- and interviewer-administered versions of the Diagnostic Interview Schedule. *Hosp Community Psychiatry* 38(12):1304–1311, 1987.

Grieco MS: Birth-marked? A critical view on analyzing organizational culture. *Hum Org* 47:84–87, 1988.

Groves JE: Taking care of the hateful patient. *N Engl J Med* 298:883–887, 1978.

Grube JW, Wallack L: Television beer advertising and drinking knowledge, beliefs, and intentions among school children. *Am J Public Health* 84:254–259, 1994.

Guze SB: Genetics of Briquet's syndrome and somatization disorder. *Ann Clin Psychiatry* 5:225–230, 1993.

Guze SB, Cloninger CR, Martin RI, Clayton PJ: A follow-up and family study of Briquet's syndrome. *Br J Psychiatry* 149:17–23, 1986.

Haan M, Kaplan GA, Camacho T: Poverty and health: Prospective evidence from the Alameda County study. *Am J Epidemiol* 125(6):989–997, 1987.

Hahn RA, Gaines AD: *Physicians of Western Society*. Dordrecht, Reidel, 1985.

Hahn SR, Feiner JS, Bellin EH: The doctor–patient–family relationship: A compensatory alliance. *Ann Intern Med*, 109(1)884–889, 1988.

Halpern J: Empathy: Using resonance emotions in the service of curiosity, in Spiro H, *et al* (eds): *Empathy and the Practice of Medicine*. New Haven, Conn, Yale University Press, 1993, pp 160–173.

Hamberger LK: Confronting violence: Role of the individual family physician. *Am Fam Physician* 48:1012–1014, 1993.

Hamberger LK, Hastings JE: Personality correlates of men who abuse their partners: A cross-validation study. *J Fam Viol* 1:323–346, 1986.

Hamberger LK, Saunders DG, Hovey M: The prevalence of domestic violence in community family practice and rate of physician inquiry. *Fam Med* 24:283–287, 1992.

Hamberger LK, Lohr JE, Bonge D: The intended function of domestic violence is different for arrested male and female perpetrators. *Fam Viol Sex Assault Bull* 10:40–44, 1994.

Hammond EL, Horn D: Smoking and death rates—Report on forty-four months of follow-up of 187,783 men. *JAMA* 166:1294–1308, 1958.

Hanley DQ: Doctors: Rural Rx. Backfires. *Potomac News*, May 9, 1993, p A1.

Harkins E: Effects of empty nest transition on self-report of psychological and physical well-being. *J Marriage Fam* 40:549–556, 1978.

Harper G: Breaking taboos and steadying the self in medical school. *Lancet* 342:913–915, 1993.

Harwood A: The hot–cold theory of disease: Implications for treatment of Puerto Rican patients. *JAMA* 216:1153–1158, 1971.

Harwood A: *Ethnicity and Medical Care*. Cambridge, Mass, Harvard University Press, 1981.

Hatcher RA, Stewart F, Trussell J, Kowal D, Guest F, Stewart GK, Cates W (eds): *Contraceptive Technology 1990–1992—15th Revised Edition*. New York, Irvington Publishers Inc, 1990.

Haugaard JJ, Reppucci ND: *The Sexual Abuse of Children*. San Francisco, Jossey–Bass Inc, Publishers, 1988.

Havens, L: *Making Contact*. Cambridge, Mass, Harvard University Press, 1986.

Health Employer Data Information Set (HEDIS). *New England HEDIS Coalition: 1993 Baseline Performance Profile*. Boston, New England HEDIS Coalition, 1994.

Health Insurance Association of America. *Source Book of Health Insurance Data*. Washington, DC, Health Insurance Association of America, 1995.

Heins HC Jr, Nancy NW, Ferguson JE: Social support in improving perinatal outcome: The Resource Mothers Program. *Obstet Gynecol* 70(2):263–266, 1987.

Heller TA, Larson EB, LoGerlo JP: Quality of ambulatory care of the elderly: An analysis of five conditions. *J Am Geriatr Soc* 32:782–789, 1984.

Helman CG: Feed a cold, starve a fever. *Culture Med Psychiatry* 2:107–137, 1978.

Helton AS, McFarlane J, Anderson ET: Battered and pregnant: A prevalence study. *Am J Public Health* 77:1337–1339, 1987.

Henry J: *Culture against Man*. New York, Random House, Inc, 1963.

Henshaw SK, Kennery AM, Somberg D, Van Vort J: *Teenage Pregnancy in the United States: The Scope of the Problem and State Responses*. New York, Alan Guttmacher Institute, 1989.

Herrington TN, Morse LH: *Occupational Injuries*. St. Louis, Mosby Yearbook Medical Publishers, 1995.

Herron MA, Katz M, Creasy RK: Evaluation of a preterm birth prevention program: Preliminary report. *Obstet Gynecol* 59:452–456, 1982.

HHS News. Rockville, Md, U.S. Department of Health and Human Services, January 31, 1994.

Higgins ES: A review of unrecognized mental illness in primary care: Prevalence, natural history, and efforts to change the course. *Arch Fam Med* 3:908–917, 1994.

Hill CE, Mathews H: Traditional health beliefs and practices among Southern rural blacks: A complement to biomedicine, in Black M, Reed JS (eds): *Social Science Perspectives on the South*. New York, Gordon & Breach Science Publishers, 1981, pp 307–322.

Hill RF, Fortenberry JD, Stein HF: Culture in clinical medicine. *South Med J* 83(9):1071–1080, 1990.

Hillard PJ: Physical violence in pregnancy. *Obstet Gynecol* 66:185–190, 1985.

Hillman BJ, Joseph CA, Mabry MR, Sunshine JH, Kennedy SD, Noether M: Frequency and costs of self-referring and radiologist-referring physicians. *N Engl J Med* 323:1604–1608, 1990.

Hocking B: Anthropologic aspects of occupational illness epidemics. *J Occup Med* 29:526–530, 1987.

Hodgetts TJ, Brown T, Driscoll P, Hanson J: Pre-hospital cardiac arrest—Room for improvement. *Resuscitation* 29(1):47–54, 1995.

Hoffman ML: Interaction of affect and cognition in empathy, in Izard CE, Kagan J, Zajonc RB (eds): *Emotions, Cognitions, and Behavior.* London, Cambridge University Press, 1984, pp 103–131.

Holleman WL, Holleman MC: School and work release evaluations. *JAMA* 260:3629–3634, 1988.

Holleman WL, Edwards DC, Matson CC: Obligations of physicians to patients and third-party payers. *J Clin Ethics* 5:113–120, 1994.

House JS, Landis KR, Umberson D. Social relationships and health. *Science* 241:540–545, 1988.

Hulka BS, Kupper LL, Cassel JC: Determinants of physician utilization. *Med Care* 10:300–309, 1972.

Hultkrantz A: *Shamanic Healing and Ritual Drama: Health and Medicine in Native North American Religious Traditions.* New York, Crossroads, for the Lutheran General Health System, 1992.

Institute for Health Policy, Brandeis University. *Substance Abuse: The Nation's Number One Health Problem; Key Indicators for Policy.* Princeton, NJ, Robert Wood Johnson Foundation, October 1993.

Institute of Medicine. Report: Academic geriatrics for the year 2000. *J Am Geriatr Soc* 35(8):773–791, 1987.

Institute of Medicine Committee to Study Outreach for Prenatal Care. *Prenatal Care: Reaching Mothers, Reaching Infants,* Brown SS (ed). Washington, DC, National Academy Press, 1988.

Institute of Medicine Committee to Study the Prevention of Low Birthweight. *Preventing Low Birthweight.* Washington, DC, National Academy Press, 1985.

Island D, Letellier P: *Men Who Beat the Men Who Love Them.* New York, Harrington Park Press, 1991.

Jaakkola JJK, Miettinen P: Type of ventilation system in office buildings and sick building syndrome. *Am J Epidemiol* 141(8):755–765, 1995.

Jack BW, Culpepper L: Preconception care: Risk reduction and health promotion in preparation for pregnancy. *JAMA* 264:1147–1149, 1990.

Johnson TM: Premenstrual syndrome as a Western culture-specific disorder. *Culture Med Psychiatry* 11(3):337–356, 1987.

Johnson TM, Kleinman A: Cultural concerns in consultation psychiatry, in Guggenheim FG, Weiner MF (eds): *Manual of Psychiatric Consultation and Emergency Care.* New York, Jason Aronson, 1984, pp 275–284.

Jones E, Cawley JF: Physician assistants and health system reform. *JAMA* 271:1266–1272, 1994.

Jones BE: The difference a D.O. makes. Oklahoma City, Times Journal Publishing Co, 1978.

Jones EF, Forrest JD, Goldman N, Henshaw S, Lincoln R, Rosoff JI, Westoff CF, Wulf D: *Teenage Pregnancies in Industrialized Countries: A Study Sponsored by the Alan Guttmacher Institute.* New Haven, Conn, Yale University Press, 1986.

Jones WHS: From "The Physician" and "Decorum," *The Works of Hippocrates,* Cambridge, Mass, Harvard University Press, 1923.

Joyce TJ, Grossman M: Pregnancy wantedness and the early initiation of prenatal care. *Demography* 27(1):1–17, 1990.

Kaplan SH, Greenfield S, Ware JE Jr: Assessing the effects of physician–patient interactions on the outcomes of chronic disease [published erratum appears in *Med Care* 27(7):679, 1989]. *Med Care* 27:S110–S127, 1989.

Karpel MA, Strauss ES: Family secrets, in Karpel MA, Strauss ES (eds): *Family Evaluation.* New York, Gardner Press, 1983, pp 245–263.

Kassirer JP: Our stubborn quest for diagnostic certainty. *N Engl J Med* 320:1489–1491, 1989.

Kassirer JP: What role for nurse practitioners in primary care? *N Engl J Med* 330:204–205, 1994.

Katon W, Kleinman A: Doctor–patient negotiation and other social science strategies in patient care, in Eisenberg L, Kleinman A (eds): *The Relevance of Social Science for Medicine.* Dordrecht, Reidel, 1981, pp 253–279.

Katon W, Kleinman A, Rosen G: Depression and somatization. *Am J Med* 72:127–135, 241–247, 1982.

Katon W, Von Korff M, Lin E, Lipscomb P, Russo J, Wagner E, Polk E: Distressed high utilizers of medical care. DSM-III-R diagnoses and treatment needs. *Gen Hosp Psychiatry* 12:355–362, 1990.

Katon W, Von Korff M, Lin E, Walker E, Simon GE, Bush T, Robinson P, Russo J: Collaborative management to achieve treatment guidelines: Impact on depression in primary care. *JAMA* 273:1026–1031, 1995.

Keefe SE: Real and ideal extended familism among Mexican Americans and Anglo Americans: On the meaning of "close" family ties. *Hum Org* 43:65–70, 1984.

Keirse MJNC: Preterm delivery, in Chalmers I, Enkin M, Keirse MJNC (eds): *Effective Care in Pregnancy and Childbirth*. London, Oxford University Press, 1989, pp 1270–1292.

Keirse MJNC, Enkin M, Lumley J: Social and professional support during labor, in Chalmers I, Enkin M, Keirse MJNC (eds): *Effective Care in Pregnancy and Childbirth*. London, Oxford University Press, 1989a, pp 805–814.

Keirse MJNC, Grant A, King JF: Preterm labour, in Chalmers I, Enkin M, Keirse MJNC (eds): *Effective Care in Pregnancy and Childbirth*. London, Oxford University Press, 1989b, pp 694–745.

Kellerman AL, Rivara FP, Rushforth NB, *et al*: Gun ownership as a risk factor for homicide in the home. *N Engl J Med* 329:1084–1088, 1993.

Kennell JH, Klaus MH, McGrath S, Robertson SS, Hinkley C: Continuous emotional support during labor in a US hospital. *JAMA* 265:2197–2201, 1991.

Keso L, Salaspuro M: Inpatient treatment of employed alcoholics: A randomized clinical trial on Hazelden-type and traditional treatment. *Alcoholism Clin Exp Res* 14(4):584–589, 1991.

Kiecolt-Glaser JK, Fisher LD, Ogrockl P, Stout JC, Spelcher CE, Glaser R: Marital quality, marital disruption, and immune function. *Psychosom Med* 49(1):13–32, 1987.

King L: *The Road to Medical Enlightenment 1650–1695*. New York, American Elsevier, 1970, pp 1–14.

Kingdon JW: *Agendas, Alternatives, and Public Policies*. Boston, Little, Brown & Co, 1984.

Kirmayer LJ, Robbins JM, Dworkind M, Yaffe MJ: Somatization and the recognition of depression and anxiety in primary care. *Am J Psychiatry* 150:734–741, 1993.

Klaus MH, Kennel JH, Robertson SS, Sosa R: Effects of social support during parturition on maternal and infant morbidity. *Br Med J* 293:585–587, 1986.

Klein D, Najman J, Kohrman AF, Munro C: Patient characteristics that elicit negative responses from family physicians. *J Fam Pract* 14:881–888, 1982.

Klein L, Goldenberg RL: Prenatal care and its effect on preterm birth and low birth weight, in Merkatz IR, Thompson JE, Mullen PD, Goldenberg R (eds): *New Perspectives on Prenatal Care*. New York, Elsevier Science Publishing Co, Inc, 1990, pp 501–530.

Kleinman AM: Toward a comparative study of medical systems. *Sci Med Man* 1:55–65, 1973.

Kleinman AM: Explanatory models in health care relationships, in *Health of the Family* (National Council for International Health Symposium). Washington, DC, NCIH, 1975, pp 159–172.

Kleinman AM: Clinical relevance of anthropological and cross-cultural research: Concepts and strategies. *American Journal of Psychiatry* 135:427–431, 1978.

Kleinman AM: *Patients and Healers in the Context of Culture: An Exploration of the Borderland between Anthropology, Medicine, and Psychiatry*. Los Angeles, University of California Press, 1980.

Kleinman AM: The teaching of clinically applied medical anthropology on a psychiatric consultation–liaison service, in Chrisman NJ, Maretzki TW (eds): *Clinically Applied Anthropology: Anthropologists in Health Science Settings*. Dordrecht, Reidel, 1982, pp 83–115.

Kleinman A: The cultural meanings and social uses of illness. *J Fam Pract* 16:539–545, 1983.

Kleinman AM: *The Illness Narratives: Suffering, Healing, and the Human Condition*. New York, Basic Books, Inc, 1987.

Kleinman A, Eisenberg L, Good B: Culture, illness, and care: Clinical lessons from anthropologic and cross-cultural research. *Ann Intern Med*, 88:251–258, 1978.

Klerman GL, Vaillant GE, Spitzer RL, Michels R: A debate on DSM-III. *Am J Psychiatry* 141:539–553, 1984.

Klerman LV: Home visiting during pregnancy, in Merkatz IR, Thompson JE, Mullen PD, Goldenberg R (eds): *New Perspectives on Prenatal Care*. New York, Elsevier Science Publishing Co, Inc, 1990, pp 593–602.

Klonoff-Cohen H, Edelstein S, Lefkowitz E, Srinivassan I, Kaegi D, Chang JC, Wiley KJ: The effect of passive smoking and tobacco exposure through breast milk on sudden infant death syndrome. *JAMA* 273:795–798, 1995.

Kluckhohn F, Strodtbeck F: *Variations in Value Orientations*. Evanston, Ill, Row Peterson, 1961.

Kluft RP: The physician as perpetrator of abuse. *Primary Care* 20:459–480, 1993.

Koeske GF, Koeske RD: The buffering effect of social support on parental stress. *Am J Orthopsychiatry* 60:440–451, 1990.

Koss MP: Rape: Scope, impact, interventions and public policy responses. *Am Psychol* 48:1062–1069, 1993.

Koss MP, Woodruff WJ, Koss PG: Relation of criminal victimization to health perceptions among women medical patients. *Journal of Consulting and Clinical Psychology* 58(2):147–152, 1990.

Koss MP, Koss PG, Woodruff WJ: Deleterious effects of criminal victimization on women's health and medical utilization. *Arch Intern Med* 151:342–347, 1991.

Kostelny K, Garbarino J: *The Human Ecology of Infant Mortality: An Analysis of Risk in 76 Urban Communities*. Chicago, Erikson Institute, 1987.

Kramer MS: For discussion: Birthweight and infant mortality: Perceptions and pitfalls. *Pediat Perinat Epidemiol* 4:381–390, 1987.

Kramer MS: Determinants of low birth weight: Methodological assessment and metaanalysis. *Bull WHO* 65:663–737, 1990.

Krippner S: A cross-cultural comparison of four healing models. *Altern Ther* 1(1):21–29, 1995.

Kristenson H, Ohlin H, Hulten-Nosslin M, Trell E, Hood B: Identification and intervention of heavy drinking in middle-aged men: Results and follow-up of 24–60 months of long-term study with randomized controls. *Alcoholism Clin Exp Res* 7(2):203–209, 1983.

Kroenke K, Spitzer RI, Williams JB, Linzer M, Hahan S, deGruy F, Brody D: Physical symptoms in primary care. Predictors of psychiatric disorders and functional impairment. *Arch Fam Med* 3:774–779, 1994.

Ku LC, Sonenstein FL, Pleck JH: The association of AIDS education and sex education with sexual behavior and condom use among teenage men. *Fam Plann Perspect* 24(3):100–106, 1992.

Kubler-Ross E: *On Death and Dying*. New York, Macmillan Publishing Co, Inc, 1970.

LaDou J (ed): *Occupational Medicine*. Norwalk, Conn, Appleton & Lange, 1990.

Lands WEM, Zakhari S: Alcohol and cardiovascular disease. *Alcohol Health Res World* 14(4):304–312, 1990.

Lang GC: Diabetes and health care in a Sioux community. *Hum Org* 44:251–260, 1985.

La Puma J, Stocking CB, La Voie D, Darling CA: When physicians treat members of their own families. Practices in a community hospital. *N Engl J Med* 325:1290–1294, 1991.

Laseter RL: Black men: Work and family life. Paper presented at the Chicago Urban Poverty and Family Life Conference, University of Chicago, September 24, 1991.

Lassetter J: Educating interns: All in a day's work. *RN* 47:85–86, 1984.

Lawrence R: *Breastfeeding: A Guide for the Medical Profession*. St. Louis, Mosby, 1994.

Lazare A: Shame and humiliation in the medical encounter. *Arch Intern Med* 147:1653–1658, 1987.

Lazare A, Eisenthal S, Wasserman L: The customer approach to patienthood. Attending to patient requests in a walk-in clinic. *Arch Gen Psychiatry* 32:553–558, 1975.

Lazarus RS: *Psychological Stress and Coping Process*. New York, McGraw–Hill Book Co, 1966.

Leaf A: Potential health effects of global climatic and environmental changes. *N Engl J Med* 321:1577–1583, 1989.

Leaf PJ: Psychiatric disorders and the use of health services, in Miranda J, Hohmann AA, Attkisson CC, Larson DB (eds): *Mental Disorders in Primary Care*. San Francisco, Jossey–Bass Inc, Publishers, 1994, pp 377–401.

Lemna WK, Feldman GL, Kerem B-S, *et al*: Mutation analysis for heterozygote detection and the prenatal diagnosis of cystic fibrosis. *N Engl J Med* 322:291–296, 1990.

Levenstein JH, McCracken EC, McWhinney IR: The patient centered clinical method I. A model for the doctor patient interaction in family medicine. *Fam Pract* 1:24–30, 1986.

Levit KR, Cowan CA, Lazenby HC, *et al*: National health spending trends, 1960–1993. *Health Affairs*, 1994 (Winter), pp 14–31.

Levy BS: The teaching of occupational health in United States medical schools: Five-year follow-up of an initial survey. *Am J Public Health* 75:79–80, 1985.

Lin EH: Intraethnic characteristics and the patient–physician interaction. *J Fam Pract* 16:91–98, 1983.

Lin EH, Carter WB, Kleinman AM: An exploration of somatization among Asian refugees and immigrants in primary care. *Am J Public Health* 75:1080–1084, 1985.

Lin EH, Katon W, Von Korff M, Bush T, Lipscomb P, Russo J, Wagner E: Frustrating patients: Physician and patient perspectives among distressed high users of medical services. *J Gen Intern Med* 6:241–246, 1991.

Lindblom CE: *Politics and Markets: The World's Political and Economic Systems*. New York, Basic Books, Inc, 1977.

Linklater D, MacDougall S: Boundary issues. What do they mean for family physicians? *Can Fam Physician* 39:2569–2573, 1993.

Litman TJ: The family as a basic unit in health and medical care. *Soc Sci Med* 8:495–519, 1974.

Lloyd S, Streiner D, Shannon S: Burnout, depression, life and job satisfaction among Canadian emergency physicians. *J Emerg Med* 12:559–565, 1994.

Lloyd SM, Miller RL: Black student enrollment in US medical schools. *JAMA* 261(2):272–274, 1989.

Lock M: Introduction: Health and medical care as cultural and social phenomena, in Norbeck E, Lock M (eds): *Health, Illness, and Medical Care in Japan: Cultural and Social Dimensions*. Honolulu, University of Hawaii Press, 1987, pp 1–23.

Lombard HL, Doering CR: Cancer studies in Massachusetts: Habits, characteristics, and environment of individuals with and without cancer. *N Engl J Med* 198:481–487, 1928.

Lundberg GD: The failure of organized health system reform—now what? *Caveat aeger*—Let the patient beware. *JAMA* 273:1539–1541, 1995.

MacKenzie WR, Hoxie MS, Proctor ME, Gradus MS, Blair KA, Peterson DE, Kazmierczak JJ, Addiss DG, Fox KR, Rose JB, Davis JP: A massive outbreak in Milwaukee of Cryptosporidium infection transmitted through the public water supply. *N Eng J Med* 331:161–167, 1994.

Macquire A: Psychic possession among industrial workers. *Lancet* 2:376–378, 1978.

Madden PA, Grube JW: The frequency and nature of alcohol and tobacco advertising in televised sports. *Am J Public Health* 84:297–299, 1994.

Magruder-Habib K, Zung W, Feussner J, Alling W, Saunders W, Stevens H: Management of general medical patients with symptoms of depression. *Gen Hosp Psychiatry* 11:201–206, 1989.

Majno G: *The Healing Hand.* Cambridge, Mass, Harvard University Press, 1975, pp 156–157.

Makepeace JM: Courtship violence among college students. *Fam Rel* 30:97–101, 1981.

Males MA: Adult involvement in teenage childbearing and STD. *Lancet* 2:64–65, 1995.

Margolis S: Chelation therapy is ineffective for the treatment of peripheral vascular disease. *Altern Ther* 1995; 1(2):53–57, 1995.

Marmot M, Brunner E: Alcohol and cardiovascular disease: The status of the U-shaped curve. *Br Med J* 303:565–568, 1991.

Marsiglio W, Mott FL: Does wanting to become pregnant with a first child affect subsequent maternal behaviors and infant birth weight? *J Marriage Fam* 50:1023–1036, 1988.

Martin D: Domestic violence: A sociological perspective, in Sonkin DJ, Martin D, Walker LEA (eds): *The Male Batterer: A Treatment Approach.* Berlin, Springer, 1985, pp 1–32.

Martin RI, Cloninger CR, Guze SB, Clayton PJ: Mortality in a followup of 500 psychiatric outpatients: I. Total mortality. *Arch Gen Psychiatry* 42:47–54, 1985.

Marx K: *Manifesto of the Communist Party.* London, 1888.

Massachusetts Bureau of Labor Statistics. *Labor Statistics for Massachusetts, New England and the US.* Boston, Massachusetts Labor Statistics Line, 1995.

Massachusetts Department of Education. *Massachusetts Education Statistics.* Malden, Massachusetts Department of Education, 1990.

Massachusetts Department of Public Health. *CHNA 14 Report.* Boston, Massachusetts Department of Public Health, 1995a.

Massachusetts Department of Public Health. *HIV/AIDS Surveillance Monthly Update.* Boston, Massachusetts Department of Public Health, 1995b.

Massachusetts Department of Public Health. *WIC Program Coordination and Outreach Manual.* Boston, Massachusetts Department of Public Health, 1995c.

Massachusetts Office of Public Safety. *Massachusetts Crime Rates for 1992.* Boston, Massachusetts Office of Public Safety, 1993.

Massachusetts Rate Setting Commission. *Improving Primary Care: Using Preventable Hospitalization as an Approach.* Boston, Massachusetts Executive Office of Human Services, Rate Setting Commission, 1995.

Mathew RJ, Wilson WH: Substance abuse and cerebral blood flow. *Am J Psychiatry* 148(3):292–305, 1991.

Maule WF: Screening for colorectal cancer by nurse endoscopists. *N Engl J Med* 330:204–205, 1994.

Maurer HM: The growing neglect of American children. *Am J Dis Child* 145:540–541, 1991.

Mausner JS, Kramer S: Epidemiologic concepts, in *Epidemiologic Concepts in Epidemiology—An Introductory Text.* Philadelphia, WB Saunders Co, 1985, pp 22–42.

May WF: Code, covenant, contract, or philanthropy? *Hastings Cent Rep* 5:29–38, 1975.

May WF. *The Physician's Covenant.* Philadelphia, Westminster Press, 1983.

McAdoo JR: The roles of black fathers in the socialization of black children, in McAdoo H (ed): *Black Families,* ed 2. Beverly Hills, Calif, Sage Publications, Inc, pp 257–259, 1981.

McCullough LB, Ashton CM: A methodology for teaching ethics in the clinical setting: A clinical handbook for medical ethics. *Theor Med* 15:39–52, 1994.

McDaniel SH, Landau-Stanton J: Family-of-origin work and family therapy skills training: Both-and. *Fam Process* 30:459–471, 1991.

McDaniel SH, Campbell TL, Seaburn D: Managing personal and professional boundaries: How to make the physician's own issues a resource in patient care. *Fam Syst Med* 7:1–12, 1989.

McDaniel S, Campbell T, Seaburn D: *Family-Oriented Primary Care: A Manual for Medical Providers.* Berlin, Springer-Verlag, 1990a.

McDaniel S, Campbell T, Seaburn D: The birth of a family: A family-oriented approach to pregnancy care, in *Family-Oriented Primary Care: A Manual for Medical Providers.* Berlin, Springer-Verlag, 1990b, pp 105–122.

McDaniel SH, Hepworth J, Doherty W: *Medical Family Therapy*. New York, Basic Books, Inc, 1992.

McGinnis LS: Alternative therapies. *Cancer* 67(6 suppl):1788–1792, 1991.

McGoldrick M: The joining of families through marriage: The couple, in Carter B, McGoldrick M (eds): *The Changing Family Life Cycle: A Framework for Family Therapy*, ed 2. New York, Gardner Press, 1988a, pp 212–231.

McGoldrick M: Woman and the family life cycle, in Carter B, McGoldrick M (eds): *The Changing Family Life Cycle: A Framework for Family Therapy* ed 2. New York, Gardner Press, 1988b, pp 29–64.

McGoldrick M: Ethnicity and family life cycle, in Carter B, McGoldrick M (eds): *The Changing Family Life Cycle: A Framework for Family Therapy*, ed 2. New York, Allyn & Baron, 1989, pp 69–98.

McGoldrick M, Gerson S: *Genograms in Family Assessment*. New York, WW Norton & Co, Inc, 1985.

McGoldrick M, Heiman M, Carter B: The changing family life cycle, in Walsh F (ed): *Normal Family Processes*, ed 2. New York, Guilford Press, 1993, pp 405–443.

McKegney CP: Medical education: A neglectful and abusive family system. *Fam Med* 21:452–457, 1989.

McKegney CP: Surviving survivors: Caring for patients who have been victimized. *Prim Care Clin North Am* 20:481–494, 1993.

McKinstry B: Paternalism and the doctor–patient relationship in general practice. *Br J Gen Pract* 42:340–342, 1992.

McWhinney IR: Illness, suffering, and healing, in McWhinney IR (ed): *A Textbook of Family Medicine*. London, Oxford University Press, 1989a, pp 73–86.

McWhinney IR: 'An acquaintance with particulars. . . '. *Fam Med* 21:296–298, 1989b.

McWhinney IR: *A Textbook of Family Medicine*. London, Oxford University Press, 1989c.

Mechanic D: *Handbook of health, health care, and health professions*. New York, The Free Press, 1983.

Mederos FR: Men who abuse women and "normal" men: Theorizing continuities and discontinuities. Paper presented at the Third National Family Violence Research Conference, Durham, NH, July 1987.

Mengel M: Physician ineffectiveness due to family of origin issues. *Fam Syst Med* 5(2):176–190, 1987.

Mengel MB, Mauksch LB: Disarming the family ghost: A family of origin experience. *Fam Med* 21:45–49, 1989.

Miller GH: The "less hazardous" cigarette: A deadly delusion. *NY State J Med* 85:313–317, 1985.

Miller R: Preventing adolescent pregnancy and associated risks. *Can Fam Physician* 41:1525–1531, 1995.

Miller RA, Luft HS: Managed care performance since 1980: A literature analysis. *JAMA* 271:1512–1519, 1994.

Millon T, Green C, Meagher R (eds): *Handbook of Clinical Health Psychology*. New York, Plenum Press, 1982.

Miranda J, Hohmann AA, Attkisson CC, Larson DB (eds): *Mental Disorders in Primary Care*. San Francisco, Jossey–Bass, Inc, Publishers, 1994.

Mitchell JM, Sunshine JH: Consequences of physician's ownership of health care facilities—Joint ventures in radiation therapy. *N Engl J Med* 327:1497–1501, 1992.

Mohide P, Grant A: Evaluating diagnosis and screening during pregnancy and childbirth, in Chalmers I, Enkin M, Keirse MJNC (eds): *Effective Care in Pregnancy and Childbirth*. London, Oxford University Press, 1989, pp 66–80.

Mold JW, Stein HF: The cascade effect in the clinical care of patients. *New England Journal of Medicine* 314(8):512–514, 1986.

Moon JB, Davis LE, Eaddy JA, Shacklett GE, Stockton MD: A nursing home rotation in a family practice residency. *J Fam Pract* 30:594–598, 1990.

Moos MK, Cefalo RC: Preconceptional health promotion: A focus for obstetric care. *Am J Perinatol* 4:63–67, 1987.

Morbidity and Mortality Weekly Report. *Chancroid—United States, 1981–1990: Evidence for Underreporting of Cases*. 41(22–3), 1992a.

Morbidity and Mortality Weekly Report. *Community Awareness and Use of HIV/AIDS-Prevention Services*. 41(43):825–829, 1992b.

Morbidity and Mortality Weekly Report. *Ectopic Pregnancy—United States, 1988–1989*. 41(32):591–594, 1992c.

Morbidity and Mortality Weekly Report. *HIV Counseling and Testing Services from Public and Private Providers—United States, 1990*. 41(40):743–752, 1992d.

Morbidity and Mortality Weekly Report. *HIV Infection, Syphilis, and Tuberculosis Screening among Migrant Farm Workers—Florida, 1992*. 41(39):723–725, 1992e.

Morbidity and Mortality Weekly Report. *1993 Sexually Transmitted Diseases Treatment Guidelines*. 42 RR-14, 1993a.

Morbidity and Mortality Weekly Report. *Selective Screening to Augment Syphilis Case-Finding—Dallas, 1991*. 42(22):424–427, 1993b.

Morbidity and Mortality Weekly Report. *Chlamydia Prevalence and Screening Practices—San Diego County, California, 1993.* 43(20):366–375, 1994.

Morbidity and Mortality Weekly Report. *Update: Acquired Immunodeficiency Syndrome—United States, 1994.* 44(4):64–67, 1995.

Morreim EH: *Balancing Act: The New Medical Ethics of Medicine's New Economics.* Dordrecht, Kluwer Academic Publishers, 1991.

Morreim EH: Am I my brother's warden? Responding to the unethical or incompetent colleague. *Hastings Cent Rep*, May–June 1993, pp 19–27.

Morrison MA: Addiction in adolescents. *West J Med* 152:543–546, 1990.

Mulinare J, Cordero JF, Erickson D, Berry RJ: Periconceptional use of multivitamins and the occurrence of neural tube defects. *JAMA* 260:3141–3145, 1989.

Murray RH, Rubel AJ: Physicians and healers—Unwitting partners in health care. *N Engl J Med* 326:61–64, 1992.

Musgrave RA, Musgrave PB: *Public Finance in Theory and Practice.* New York, McGraw–Hill Book Co, 1984.

Naeye RL: Weight gain and the outcomes of pregnancy. *Am J Obstet Gynecol* 135:3–9, 1979.

National Association of Community Health Centers (NACHC). *America's Health Centers.* Washington, DC, National Association of Community Health Centers, 1995.

National Center for Homeopathy Directory: Practitioners, Study Groups, Pharmacies, Resources. National Center for Homeopathy, Alexandria, 1995.

National Institute of Alcohol Abuse and Alcoholism. NIAAA Physician Intervention Guide 1995. For development information contact Francis Cotter, MPH, NIAAA, Willco Building, 600 Executive Blvd, Rockville, Md 20892–7003.

National Institutes of Health. *Respiratory Health Effects of Passive Smoking: Lung Cancer and Other Disorders.* The Report of the U.S. Environmental Protection Agency. Department of Health and Human Services, Public Health Service, National Institutes of Health, Environmental Protection Agency. NIH Publication No. 93–3605, August 1993.

Naumberg E, Franks P, Bell B, Gold M, Engerman J: Racial differentials in the identification of hypercholesterolemia. *J Fam Pract* 36:425–430, 1993.

Neighbour R: Paternalism or autonomy? *The Practitioner* 236:860–864, 1992.

Neugarten B, Kraines RJ: Menopausal symptoms in women of various ages. *Psychosom Med* 27:256–273, 1965, pp 266–273.

Newberger EH, Barkan SE, Lieberman ES: Abuse of pregnant women and adverse birth outcome: Current knowledge and implications for practice. *JAMA* 267:2370–2372, 1992.

Newman NK: Family secrets: A challenge for family physicians. *J Fam Pract* 36:494–496, 1993.

Nga NA: Vietnamese relocation. Department of Family Medicine Grand Rounds, University of Oklahoma Health Sciences Center, Oklahoma City, 23 February 1988.

Nichols MJ: *Family Therapy: Concepts and Methods.* New York, Gardner Press, 1984.

Nomura A, Grove JS, Stemmerman GN, Severson RK: A prospective study of stomach cancer and its relation to diet, cigarettes, and alcohol consumption. *Cancer Res* 50(3):627–631, 1990.

Novack DH: Therapeutic aspects of the clinical encounter. *J Gen Intern Med* 2:346–354, 1987.

Ochsner A, DeBakey ME: Primary pulmonary malignancy: Treatment by total pneumonectomy. Analysis of 79 collected cases and presentation of 7 personal cases. *Surg Gynecol Obstet* 68:435–441, 1939.

O'Connor PO, Selwyn PA, Schottenfeld RS: Medical care for injection drug users with human immunodeficiency virus infection. *N Engl J Med* 331:450–459, 1994.

Ohnishi K, Terabayashi H, Unuma T, Takahashi A, Okuda K: Effects of habitual alcohol intake and cigarette smoking on the development of hepatocellular carcinoma. *Alcoholism Clin Exp Res* 11(1):45–48, 1987.

Ohnuki-Tierney E: Illness and culture in contemporary Japan. London, Cambridge University Press, 1984.

Olds DL, Henderson CR, Tatelbaum R: Improving the delivery of prenatal care and outcome of pregnancy: A randomized trial of nurse home visitation. *Pediatrics* 77:16–28, 1986.

Olfson M: Primary care patients who refuse specialized mental health services. *Arch Intern Med* 151:129–132, 1991.

O'Malley PM, Johnston LD, Bachman JG: Adolescent substance use and addictions: Epidemiology, current trends, and public policy, in *Adolescent Medicine: State of the Art Reviews.* Philadelphia, Hanley & Belfus, 1993, vol 4, pp 227–249.

Organization for Economic Cooperation and Development. *OECD Health Systems: Facts and Trends.* Paris, Organization for Economic Cooperation and Development, 1993.

Ormel J, VonKorff M, Ustun B, Pini S, Korten A, Oldehinkel T: Common mental disorders and disability across cultures. Results from the WHO collaborative study on psychological problems in general health care. *JAMA* 272:1741–1748, 1994.

O'Rourke K: Trust and the patient–physician relationship. *Am J Kidney Dis* 21:684–685, 1993.

Osler W: *Aequanimitas*, ed 3. New York, McGraw–Hill Book Co, 1932. "Aequanimitas," pp 27–32; and "The student life," pp 395–423.

Oswalt R, Matsen K: Sex, AIDS, and the use of condoms: a survey of compliance in college students. *Psychol Rep* 72(1):764–766, 1993.

Pagelow MD: *Family Violence*. New York, Praeger Publishers, 1984.

Parchman ML, Culler S: Primary care physicians and avoidable hospitalizations. *J Fam Pract* 39:123–128, 1994.

Parry KK: Concepts from medical anthropology for clinicians. *Phys Ther* 64:929–933, 1984.

Pauly M: The economics of moral hazard: Comment. *Am Econ Rev*, June 1968.

Peabody FW: Landmark article March 19, 1927: The care of the patient. By Francis W. Peabody. *JAMA* 252:813–818, 1984.

Peachey JE, Annis HM, Bornstein ER, Sykora K, Maglana SM, Shamai S: Calcium carbamide in alcoholism treatment. Part 1. A placebo-controlled, double-blind clinical trail of short-term efficacy. *Br J Addict* 84(8):877–887, 1989.

Peale NV: *A Guide to Confident Living*. Englewood Cliffs, NJ, Prentice–Hall, Inc, 1948.

Pearl R: Tobacco smoking and longevity. *Science* 87:216–217, 1938.

Pellegrino ED: Is truth telling to the patient a cultural artifact? *JAMA* 268:1734–1735, 1992.

Pellegrino ED, Thomasma DC: *The Virtues in Medical Practice*. London, Oxford University Press, 1993.

Pequignot G, Tuyns AJ, Berta JL: Ascitic cirrhosis in relation to alcohol consumption. *Int J Epidemiol* 7(2):113–120, 1978.

Perez-Woods RC: Barriers to the use of prenatal care: Critical analysis of the literature 1966–87. *J Perinat Med* 10:420–434, 1990.

Peteet JR, Ross DM, Medeiros C, Walsh-Burke K, Rieker P: Relationships with patients in oncology: Can a clinician be a friend? *Psychiatry* 55:223–229, 1992.

Peterson LM, Brennan T: Medical ethics and medical injuries: Taking our duties seriously. *J Clin Ethics* 1:207–211, 1990.

Peterson MR: *At Personal Risk: Boundary Violations in Professional–Client Relationships*. New York, WW Norton & Co, Inc, 1992.

Phillips SP, Schneider MS: Sexual harassment of female doctors by patients. *N Engl J Med* 329:1936–1939, 1993.

Piekkala P, Kero P, Erkkola R: Perinatal events and neonatal morbidity: An analysis of 5380 cases. *Early Hum Dev* 13:249–268, 1986.

Pieroni RE: Folk medicine of the black elderly. *Quarterly Contact* [National Caucus and Center on Black Aged, Inc.] 4:7, 1981.

Please Let Me Die. Galveston, Department of Psychiatry, University of Texas, 1974. Videotape.

Pollitt K: The politically correct body. *Mother Jones*, May 1982, pp 66–67.

Poole SR, Schmitt BD, Mauro R: Recurrent pain syndrome in children: A streamline approach. *Contemp Pediatr* 12(1), 1995.

Post-White J: The effects of imagery on emotions, immune functions, and cancer outcome. *Mainlines* 14(1):18–20, 1993.

President's Commission on Mental Health. *Report to the President from the President's Commission on Mental Health* (040-000-00390-8, vol 1). Washington, DC, Government Printing Office, 1978.

Primosch R, Young S: Pseudo battering of Vietnamese children (Cao gio). *J Am Dent Assoc* 101:47–48, 1980.

Quill TE: Partnerships in patient care: A contractual approach. *Ann Intern Med* 98:228–234, 1983.

Quill TE: Recognizing and adjusting to barriers in doctor–patient communication. *Ann Intern Med* 111:51–57, 1989.

Quill TE, Cassel CK: Nonabandonment: A central obligation for physicians. *Ann Intern Med* 122:368–374, 1995.

Quill TE, Williamson PR: Healthy approaches to physician stress. *Arch Intern Med* 150:1857–1861, 1990.

Radecki SE, Cowell WG: Health promotion for the elderly patients. *Fam Med* 22(4):299–302, 1990.

Rakel RE, Blum A: Nicotine addiction, in Rakel RE (ed): *Textbook of Family Practice*, ed 5. Philadelphia, WB Saunders Co, 1995, pp 1549–1564.

Ramsey CR: The family system's influence on reproduction, in Ramsey CN (ed): *Family Systems in Medicine*. New York, Guilford Press, 1988, pp 321–334.

Randall JL: Infectious diseases, in Taylor RB (ed): *Family Medicine: Principles and Practice*, ed 3. Berlin, Springer-Verlag, 1988, pp 563–582.

Rantakallio P: Relationship of maternal smoking to morbidity and mortality of the child up to the age of five. *Acta Paediatr Scand* 67:621–629, 1978.

Rasche C: Domestic murder-suicides: Characteristics and comparisons to nonsuicidal mate killing. Paper presented at the meeting of the American Society of Criminology, Chicago, 1988.

Rask KJ, Williams MV, Parker RM, McNagny SE: Obstacles predicting lack of a regular provider and delays in seeking care for patients at an urban public hospital. *JAMA* 271:1931–1933, 1994.

Rath GD, Jarratt LG, Leonardson G: Rates of domestic violence against adult women by men partners. *J Am Board Fam Prac* 2:227–233, 1989.

Redlich CA, Beckett WS, Sparer J, et al: Liver disease associated with occupational exposure to the solvent dimethylformamide. *Ann Intern Med* 108:680–686, 1988.

Regier DA, Robins LN (eds): *Psychiatric Disorders in America: The Epidemiological Catchment Area Study*. New York, The Free Press, 1991.

Reich WT: Speaking of suffering: A moral account of compassion. *Soundings: An Interdisciplinary Journal* 72:83–108, 1989.

Reiser SJ: Selections from the Hippocratic corpus: 'Oath,' 'precepts,' 'the art,' 'epidemics I,' 'the physician,' 'decorum,' and 'law,' in Reiser SJ, Dyck AJ, Curran WJ (eds): *Ethics in Medicine: Historical Perspectives and Contemporary Concerns*. Cambridge, Mass, MIT Press, 1977, pp 5–7.

Relman AS: The new medical industrial complex. *N Engl J Med* 303:963–970, 1980.

Relman AS: The health care industry: Where is it taking us? in Lee PR, Estes CL (eds): *The Nation's Health*. Boston, Jones & Bartlett, 1994, pp 67–75.

Relman AS, Reinhardt UE: Debating for-profit health care and the ethics of physicians. *Health Affairs*, 1986 (Summer), pp 5–31.

Rest KM, Patterson WB: Ethics and moral reasoning in occupational health. *Semin Occup Med* 1(1):49–57, 1986.

Reuben DB, Noble S: House officer responses to impaired physicians. *JAMA* 263:958–960, 1990.

Reuben DB, Fink A, Vivell S, Hirsch SH, Beck JC: Geriatrics in residency programs. *Acad Med* 65(6):382–387, 1990.

Revised classification system for HIV infection and expanded surveillance case definition for AIDS among adolescents and adults. *Morbidity and Mortality Weekly Report* 41(RR-17):1–19, 1992.

Reynolds RA, Rizzo JA, Gonzalez ML: The cost of medical professional liability. *JAMA* 257:2776–2781, 1987.

Rice DP: Health status and national health priorities, in Lee PR, Estes CL (eds): *The Nation's Health*. Boston, Jones & Bartlett, 1994, pp 45–58.

Rice DP, McKenzie EJ: Cost of injury in the United States: A report to Congress. San Francisco, Institute for Health and Aging, University of California and Injury Prevention Center, The Johns Hopkins University, 1989.

Rice TH, Labelle RJ: Do physicians induce demand for medical services? *J Health Policy Politics Law* 14:587–600, 1988.

Richardson AM, Burke RJ: Occupational stress and job satisfaction among physicians: Sex differences. *Soc Sci Med* 33:1179–1187, 1991.

Richardson M: Mental health services: Growth and development of a system. in Williams SJ, Torrens PR (eds): *Introduction to Health Services*, ed 3. New York, John Wiley & Sons, Inc, 1988, pp 255–277.

Rickert WS: "Less hazardous" cigarettes: Fact or fiction? *NY State J Med* 83:1269–1272, 1983.

Ring ME: *Dentistry. An Illumined History*. New York, Harry N Abrams, 1985.

Ritchie K: The little woman meets son of DSM-III. *J Med Philos* 14:695–708, 1989.

Robbins JA: Training the primary care internist to provide care in skilled nursing facilities. *J Med Educ* 58:811–813, 1983.

Roberts JM: Three Navaho households. Papers of the Peabody Museum of American Archaeology and Ethnology, vol 11, No. 3. Cambridge, Mass, Harvard University Press, 1951.

Robins LN, Regier DA: *Psychiatric Disorders in America: The Epidemiologic Catchment Area Study*. New York, The Free Press, 1991.

Rogers CR: The characteristics of a helping relationship, in Rogers CR (ed): *On Becoming a Person: A Therapist's View of Psychotherapy*. Boston, Houghton Mifflin Co, 1961, pp 39–58.

Rolland JS: *Families, Illness and Disability: An Integrative Treatment Model*. New York, Basic Books, Inc, 1994.

Rosen MG, Culpepper L, Goldenberg RL, Gordis L, Henderson OA, Klein L, Klerman LV: *Caring for Our Future: The Content of Prenatal Care. A Report of the Public Health Service Expert Panel on the Content of Prenatal Care.* Washington, DC, Public Health Service, Department of Health and Human Services, 1989.

Rosenberg L, Slone D, Shapiro S, Kaufman DW, Miettinen OS, Stolley PD: Alcoholic beverages and myocardial infarction in young women. *Am J Public Health* 71(1):82–85, 1981.

Rosenberg ML: Violence prevention. Paper presented at the United States Attorneys Conference, Washington, DC, January 20, 1994.

Rosenblatt RA: The perinatal paradox: Doing more and accomplishing less. *Health Affairs,* 1989, pp 158–168.

Rosenstock L, Cullen MR: *Clinical Occupational Medicine.* Philadelphia, WB Saunders Co, 1986.

Rosenstock L, Cullen MR: *Textbook of Clinical Occupational and Environmental Medicine.* Philadelphia, WB Saunders Co, 1994.

Rosenstock L, Logerfo J, Heyer N, Carter W: Development and validation of a self-administered Occupational Health History Questionnaire. *J Occup Med* 26(1):50–54, 1984.

Rothberg JS: The rehabilitation team: Future direction. *Arch Phys Med and Rehab* 62:407–410, 1981.

Rourke JT, Smith LF, Brown JB: Patients, friends, and relationship boundaries. *Can Fam Physician* 39:2557–2564, 1993.

Rubenstein L: The clinical effectiveness of multidimensional geriatric assessment. *J Am Geriatr Soc* 31(12):758–761, 1983.

Rudebeck CE: General practice and the dialogue of clinical practice: On symptoms, symptom presentations, and bodily empathy. *Scand J Primary Health Care Suppl,* 1992, pp 1–87.

Salgo v. Leland Stanford, Jr. University Board of Trustees, 154 C A 2d 560; 317 P 2d 170.

Saltatos LG, Soranno TM: Alcohol-induced liver disease, in Watson RR (ed): *Biochemistry and Physiology of Substance Abuse,* vol 3. Boca Raton, Fla, CRC Press, 1991, pp 73–92.

Saltzman LE, Mercy JA, O'Carroll PW, Rosenberg ML, Rhodes PH: Weapon involvement and injury outcomes in family and intimate assaults. *JAMA* 267:3043–3047, 1992.

Samuelson PA: *Economics,* ed 11. New York, McGraw–Hill Book Co, 1980.

Sarason IG, Sarason BR: *Social Support: Theory, Research and Applications.* Dordrecht, Martinus Nijhoff Publishers, 1985.

Saunders DG: A typology of men who batter women: Three types derived from cluster analysis. *Am J Orthopsychiatry* 62:264–275, 1992.

Saunders J, Aasland O, Amundsen A, Grant M: Alcohol consumption and related problems among primary health care patients: WHO collaborative project on early detection of persons with harmful alcohol-consumption-1. *Addiction* 88:349–362, 1993.

Savitz DA, Blackmore CA, Thorp JM: Epidemiologic characteristics of preterm delivery: Etiologic heterogeneity. *Am J Obstet Gynecol* 164:467–471, 1991.

Scenic America. *Citizens Action Handbook on Tobacco and Alcohol Billboard Advertising.* Washington, DC, Scenic America, 1990.

Scheiber GJ, Poullier J-P, Greenwald LM: US health expenditure performance: An international comparison and data update. *Health Care Financ Rev* 13(4):1–15, 1992.

Scheiber GJ, Poullier J-P, Greenwald LM: Health spending delivery, and outcomes in OECD countries. *Health Affairs,* 1993 (Summer), pp 120–129. Data from OECD Health Systems: Facts and Trends. Paris, Organization for Economic Development and Cooperation.

Scheiber GJ, Poullier J-P, Greenwald LM: Health system performance in OECD countries, 1980–1992. *Health Affairs* 13:100–112, 1994.

Scheper-Hughes N, Lock MM: The mindful body: A prolegomenon to future work in medical anthropology. *Med Anthropol Q* 1:6–41, 1987.

Scheper-Hughes N, Stein HF: Child-abuse and the unconscious, in Scheper-Hughes N (ed): *Child Survival: Anthropological Approaches to the Treatment and Maltreatment of Children,* Dordrecht, Reidel, 1987, pp 339–358.

Schetky DH, Green AH (eds): *Child Sexual Abuse: A Handbook for Health Care and Legal Professionals.* [See chapters by Finkel, Becker, & Kaplan.] New York, Brunner/Mazel, Inc, 1988.

Schloendorff v. Society of New York Hospital, 211 NY, 1914 (NY Sup Ct).

Schmidt CW: Sexual disorders, in Barker LR, Burton JR, Zieve PD (eds): *Principles of Ambulatory Medicine,* ed 2. Baltimore, Williams & Wilkins Co, 1986, pp 213–227.

Schoenborn CA, Marano M: Current estimates from the National Health Interview Survey: United States 1987, in *Vital and Health Statistics Series 10,* No. 166, Department of Health and Human Services, Publication No. (PHS) 88-1594, 1988.

Schroeder SA: The troubled profession: Is medicine's glass half full or half empty? *Ann Intern Med* 116:583–592, 1992.

Schulberg HC, Block MR, Madonia JJ, Rodriguez E, Scott CP, Lave J: Applicability of clinical pharmacotherapy guidelines for major depression in primary care settings. *Arch Fam Med* 4:106–112, 1995.

Schulz RM, Brushwood DB: The pharmacist's role in patient care. *Hastings Cent Rep* January–February 1991, pp 12–17.

Schwartz GE, Weiss SM: Yale conference on behavioral medicine: A proposed definition and statement of goals. *J Behav Med* 1:3–12, 1978.

Schwartz MA, Wiggins OP: Scientific and humanistic medicine: A theory of clinical methods, in White KW (ed): *The Task of Medicine: Dialogue at Wickenburg*. Menlo Park, Calif, Henry J Kaiser Foundation, 1988, pp 137–171.

Schwenk TL, Romano SE: Managing the difficult physician–patient relationship. *Am Fam Physician* 46:1503–1509, 1992.

Schwenk TL, Marquez JT, Lefever RD, Cohen M: Physician and patient determinants of difficult physician–patient relationships. *J Fam Pract* 28:59–63, 1989.

Seaburn D, Lorenz A, Gunn B, Mauksch L, Gawinski B: *Models of Collaborative Health Care*. New York, Basic Books, Inc, in press.

Selwyn BJ: The accuracy of obstetric risk assessment instruments for predicting mortality, low birth weight, and preterm birth, in Merkatz IR, Thompson JE, Mullen PD, Goldenberg R (eds): *New Perspectives on Prenatal Care*. New York, Elsevier Science Publishing Co, Inc, 1990, pp 39–65.

Selye H: *The Stress of Life*, New York: McGraw–Hill Book Co, 1976 revised edition.

Shaky Statistic: The Number of Uninsured People Is Stirring Confusion in the US Health Care Debate. *Wall Street Journal*, June 9, 1993, A6.

Shapiro S, Skinner EA, Kessler LG, VonKorff M, German PS, Tischler GL, Leaf P, Benham L, Cottler L, Regier DA: Utilization of health and mental health services: Three epidemiologic catchment area sites. *Arch Gen Psychiatry* 41:971–978, 1984.

Shea S, Fullilove MT: Entry of black and other minority students into US medical schools: Historical perspective and recent trends. *N Engl J Med* 313(15):933–940, 1985.

Sheehan KH, Sheehan DK, White K, *et al*: A pilot study of medical student "abuse." *JAMA* 263:533–537, 1990.

Shem S: *The House of God*. New York, Dell Publishing Co, Inc, 1978.

Siegler M: Confidentiality in medicine—A decrepit concept. *N Engl J Med* 307:1518–1521, 1982.

Sigerist HE: The physician's profession through the ages, in Marti-Ibanez (ed): *Henry Sigerist on the History of Medicine*. New York, MD Publications, 1960, pp 3–15.

Simpson M, Buckman R, Stewart M, Maguire P, Lipkin M, Novack D: Doctor–patient communication: The Toronto concensus statement. *Br Med J* 303:1385–1387, 1991.

Singh S, Torres D, Forrest JD: The need for prenatal care in the United States: Evidence from the 1980 national natality survey. *Fam Plann Perspect* 17:118–124, 1985.

Sloane PD: Changes in ambulatory care with patient age: Is geriatric care qualitatively different? *Fam Med* 23(1):40–43, 1991.

Slutsker L: Risks associated with cocaine during pregnancy. *Obstet Gynecol* 79(5):778–789, 1992.

Smith A: *An Inquiry into the Nature and Causes of the Wealth of Nations*. London, 1776.

Smith AC, Kleinman S: Managing emotions in medical school: Students' contacts with the living and the dead. *Soc Psychol Q* 52:56–69, 1989.

Smith GR, Monson RA, Livingston RL: Somatization disorder in men. *Gen Hosp Psychiatry* 7:4–8, 1985.

Smith G Jr, Monson RA, Ray DC: Patients with multiple unexplained symptoms. Their characteristics, functional health, and health care utilization. *Arch Intern Med* 149:69–72, 1986a.

Smith G Jr, Monson RA, Ray DC. Psychiatric consultation in somatizations disorder. A randomized controlled study. *N Engl J Med* 314:1407–1413, 1986b.

Smith GR, Rost K, Kashner TM: A trial of the effect of a standardized psychiatric consultation on health outcomes and costs in somatizing patients. *Arch Gen Psychiatry* 52:238–243, 1995.

Smith JW, Denny WF, Witzke DB: Emotional impairment in internal medicine housestaff: Results of a national survey. *JAMA* 255:1155–1158, 1986

Smith LI, Watts DT, Howell T: *Pharmacy, Drugs, and Medical Care*, ed 4. Baltimore, Williams & Wilkins Co, 1987.

Smith MC, Knapp DA: *Pharmacy, Drugs, and Medical Care*, ed 4. Baltimore: Williams & Wilkins Co, 1987.

Smith NF, Lesperance F, Talajic M: Depression following myocardial infarction. Impact on 6-month survival. *JAMA* 270:1819–1861, 1993.

Smith PB, Mumford DM (eds): *Adolescent Pregnancy: Perspectives for the Health Professional*. Boston, GK Hall & Co, 1980.

Smith RC. Unrecognized responses and feelings of residents and fellows during interviews of patients. *J Med Educ* 61:982–984, 1986.

Snabes MC, Weinman ML, Smith PB: Prevalence of HIV seropositivity among inner-city adolescents in 1988 and 1992. *Tex Med* 90(12):48–51.

Snow LF: Folk medical beliefs and implications for care of patients. *Ann Intern Med* 81:82–96, 1974.

Snow LF: Traditional health beliefs and practices among lower class black Americans. *West J Med* 139:820–828, 1983.

Society for Ambulatory Care Professionals (SACP): Community health centers in Ontario: A paper presented by Ms. Wendy Muckle, Executive Director of the Ontario Community Health Center, 1993.

Society of Teachers of Family Medicine: *Identification and Analysis of Model Family Medicine Training Programs Successful in Increasing Minority Participation, Retention and Practitioners in the Specialty of Family Medicine*, HRSA Contract 240-91-0034, 1993.

Sosa R, Kennell JH, Klaus MH, Robertson SS, Urrutia J: The effect of a supportive companion on perinatal problems, length of labor, and mother–infant interaction. *N Engl J Med* 303:597–600, 1980.

Spiegel D, Kraemer H, Bloom J, Gottheil E: Effect of psychosocial treatment on survival of patients with metastatic breast cancer. *Lancet* (ii):888–891, 1989.

Spiegel J: *Transactions: The Interplay between Individual, Family, and Society*. New York, Science House, 1971.

Spiro H: What is empathy and can it be taught? *Ann Intern Med* 116:843–846, 1992.

Spiro ME: Preface to the second edition, *Buddhism and Society: A Great Tradition and Its Burmese Vicissitudes*, second, expanded edition. Berkeley, University of California Press, 1982 (orig. 1970), pp xi–xix.

Spittle, B: Paternalistic interventions with the gravely disabled. *Aust NZ J Psychiatry* 26:107–110, 1992.

Spitzer RL, Williams JB, Kroenke K, Linzer M, deGruy FV, Hahn SR, Brody D, Johnson JG: Utility of a new procedure for diagnosing mental disorders in primary care. The PRIME-MD 1000 Study. *JAMA* 272:1749–1756, 1994.

Spitzer RL, Kroenke K, Linzer M, Hahn SR, Williams JBW, deGruy FV, Brody D, Davies M: Health-related quality of life in primary care patients with mental disorders: Results from the PRIME-MD 1000 Study. *JAMA* 274:1511–1517, 1995.

Stack CB: *All Our Kin: Strategies for Survival in a Black Community*. New York, Harper & Row Publishers, Inc, 1974.

Stampfer MJ, Colditz GA, Willett WC, Speizer FE, Hennekens CH: A prospective study of moderate alcohol consumption and the risk of coronary disease and stroke in women. *N Engl J Med* 319:267–273, 1988.

Starfield B, Wray C, Hess K, Gross R, Birk PS, D'Lugoff BC: The influence of patient–practitioner agreement on outcome of care. *American Journal of Public Health* 71:127–131, 1981.

Stark E, Flitcraft A, Frazier W: Medicine and patriarchal violence: The social construction of a "private" event. *Int J Health Serv* 9:461–493, 1979.

Starr P: *The Social Transformation of American Medicine*. New York, Basic Books, Inc, 1982.

Starr P: *The Logic of Health Care Reform—Transforming American Medicine for the Better*. Knoxville, Tenn, The Whittle Press, 1995.

Stein HF: Ethanol and its discontents: Paradoxes of inebriation and sobriety in American culture. *J Psychoanal Anthropol* 5:355–377, 1982.

Stein HF: Alcoholism as metaphor in American culture: Ritual desecration as social integration. *Ethos* 13:195–235, 1985a.

Stein HF: An argument for more inclusive context in clinical intervention: The case of family medicine, in Stein HF, Apprey M: *Context and Dynamics in Clinical Knowledge*. Charlottesville, University Press of Virginia, 1985b, pp 78–91.

Stein HF: The annual cycle and the cultural nexus of health care behavior among Oklahoma wheat farming families, in Stein HF, Apprey M: *From Metaphor to Meaning: Papers in Psychoanalytic Anthropology*. Charlottesville, University Press of Virginia, 1987a, pp 156–177.

Stein HF: Farmer and cowboy: The duality of the Midwestern male ethos: A study in ethnicity, regionalism, and national identity, in Stein HF, Apprey M: *From Metaphor to Meaning: Papers in Psychoanalytic Anthropology*. Charlottesville, University Press of Virginia, 1987b, pp 178–227.

Stein HF: In what systems do alcohol/chemical addictions make sense? Clinical ideologies and practices as cultural metaphors. Invited presentation for panel "Toward a Critical Clinical Anthropology," for the 86th Annual Meeting of the American Anthropological Association, Chicago, 1987c [later published in *Soc Sci Med* 30(9):987–1000, 1990].

Stein HF: Review of Koenigsberg RA, The psychoanalysis of racism, revolution and nationalism (New York: The Library of Social Science, 1977/1986). *Can Rev Stud Nationalism* 14:345–347, 1987d.

Stein HF: Where is "the case"? A psychoanalytic–ethnographic inquiry into the boundary of pathology in a spinal cord-injured woman. *J Psychoanal Anthropol* 10:361–383, 1987e.

Stein HF: Substance and symbol, in Galanter M (ed): *Recent Developments in Alcoholism, Volume 11: Ten Years of Progress.* New York, Plenum Press, 1993, pp 153–164.

Stein HF, Apprey M: *Context and Dynamics in Clinical Knowledge.* Charlottesville, University Press of Virginia, 1985.

Stein HF, Apprey M: *From Metaphor to Meaning: Papers in Psychoanalytic Anthropology.* Charlottesville, University Press of Virginia, 1987.

Stein HF, Apprey M: *Clinical Stories and Their Translations.* Charlottesville, University of Virginia Press, 1990.

Stein HF, Hill RF: *The Ethnic Imperative: Examining the New White Ethnic Movement.* University Park, The Pennsylvania State University Press, 1977.

Stein HF, Pontious JM: Family and beyond: The larger context of non-compliance. *Fam Sys Med* 3:179–189, 1985.

Stein LI: The doctor—nurse game. *Arch Gen Psychiatry* 16:699–703, 1967.

Stein LI, Watts DT, Howell T: Sounding board: The doctor–nurse game revisited. *N Engl J Med* 322:546–549, 1990.

Stemmerman GN, Nomura AMY, Chyou P, Yoshizawa C: Prospective study of alcohol intake and large bowel cancer. *Dig Dis Sci* 35(11):1414–1420, 1990.

Stevens R: *In Sickness and in Wealth: American Hospitals in the Twentieth Century.* New York, Basic Books, Inc, 1989.

Stewart MA, McWhinney IR, Buck CW: The doctor/patient relationship and its effect upon outcome. *J R Coll Gen Pract* 29:77–82, 1979.

Stewart M, Brown JB, Weston WW, McWhinney IR, McWilliam CL, Freeman TR: *Patient-Centered Medicine: Transforming the Clinical Method.* Beverly Hills, Calif, Sage Publications, Inc, 1995.

Stoeckle JD, Barsky AJ: Attributions: Uses of social science knowledge in the 'doctoring' of primary care, in Eisenberg L, Kleinman A (eds): *The Relevance of Social Science for Medicine.* Dordrecht, Reidel, 1981, pp 223–240.

Straus MA, Gelles RJ: Societal change and change in family violence from 1975 to 1985 as revealed by two national surveys. *J Marriage Fam* 4:161–180, 1986.

Straus MA, Gelles RJ, Steinmetz SK: *Behind Closed Doors: Violence in the American Family.* Garden City, NY, Anchor Press, 1980.

Strelnick AH, Gilpin M: The family life cycle in the urban context, in Birrer R (ed): *Urban Family Medicine.* Berlin, Springer-Verlag, 1987, pp 27–41.

Strobino DM, Baruffi G, Dellinger WS, *et al*: Variations in pregnancy outcomes and use of obstetric procedures in two institutions with divergent philosophies of maternity care. *Med Care* 26:333–347, 1988.

Suchman AL, Matthews DA: What makes the patient–doctor relationship therapeutic? Exploring the connexional dimension of medical care. *Ann Intern Med* 108(1):125–130, 1988.

Szasz TS, Hollender MH: The basic models of the doctor–patient relationship. *Arch Intern Med*, 97:585–592, 1956.

Tapp JT, Warner RW: The multisystems of view of health and disease, in Schneiderman N, Tapp JT (eds): *Behavioral Medicine: The Biopsychosocial Approach.* Hillsdale, NJ, Lawrence Erlbaum Associates, 1985, pp 1–23.

Tarasoff v. Regents of the University of California, 551 P 2d 334 (Cal 1976) [Cal Sup Ct].

Tatara T: Understanding the nature and scope of domestic elder abuse with the use of state aggregate data: Summaries of the key findings of a national survey of state APS and aging agencies. *J Elder Abuse Neglect* 5:35–57, 1993.

Taylor FW: *The Principles of Scientific Management.* New York, Harper & Brothers, 1911.

Time magazine. Cover story: Revenge of the killer microbes—Are we losing the war against infectious diseases? September 24, 1994, pp 62–69.

Tipton RM: Clinical and counseling psychology: A study of rules and functions. *Prof Psychol* 14:837–846, 1983.

Todd KH, Samaroo N, Hoffman JR: Ethnicity as a risk factor for inadequate emergency department analgesia. *JAMA* 269:1537–1539, 1993.

Tollman S: Community oriented primary care: Origins, evolution, applications. *Soc Sci Med* 32:633–642, 1991.

Tolstoy L: *The Death of Ivan Ilyich.* New York, Bantam Books, Inc, 1981.

Toombs K: *The Experience of Illness.* Boston, Kluwer Academic Publishing, 1992.

Trachtenberg A, Fleming M: Diagnosis and treatment of drug abuse in family practice. *Am Fam Physician*, Summer 1994, monograph.

Trotter RT: Folk medicine in the Southwest. *Postgrad Med* 78:167–179, 1985.

Truman v. Thomas, 165 Cal. Rptr. 308, 611 P.2d 902 (1980), in Faden RR, Beauchamp TL: *A History and Theory of Informed Consent.* London, Oxford University Press, 1986.

Turnock BJ, McGill L: Approaches to reducing infant mortality in Illinois. Part II: Targeting approaches. *Ill Med J* 164:29–32, 1983.

Ullman D: A brief history of homeopathy and its legal status in the U.S., in *Homeopathy Medicine for the 21st Century.* Richmond, Calif, North Atlantic Books, 1988, pp 80–81.

U.S. Bureau of the Census. *Statistical Abstract of the US 1990 Census, 113 ed.* Washington, DC, Bureau of the Census, 1993.

U.S. Department of Justice. *Immigration and Naturalization Service Fact Book: Summary of Recent Immigration Data.* Washington, DC, Department of Justice, U.S. Immigration and Naturalization Service Statistics Division, June, 1994.

U.S. Department of Health and Human Services, National Heart Lung and Blood Institute. Teach your patients about asthma: A clinician's guide. *U.S. Department of Health and Human Services, National Heart Lung and Blood Institute, National Asthma Education Program,* Publication No. 92–2737, 1992.

U.S. Department of Health and Human Services, Public Health Service, Centers for Disease Control and Prevention. Recommendations and Reports. Assessing the public health threat associated with waterborne Cryptosporidiosis: Report of a workshop. *Morbidity Mortality Weekly Report.* 44:June 16, 1995, p 2.

U.S. Environmental Protection Agency. The respiratory health effects of passive smoking: Lung cancer and other disorders. Washington, DC, Office of Health and Environmental Assessment, Office of Research and Development, U.S. Environmental Protection Agency. Publication No. EPA/600/6–90/006F, 1993, pp 7–51.

U.S. Federal Bureau of Investigation. *Crime in the US, 1993.* Washington, DC, Federal Bureau of Investigation, 1994.

U.S. *Federal Register. Poverty Income Guidelines* 60(27):7772, 1995.

U.S. Preventive Services Task Force. The periodic health examination age-specific charts. *Am Fam Physician* 41:189–204, 1990.

U.S. Public Health Service. *Healthy People 2000: National Health Promotion and Disease Prevention Objectives.* Washington, DC, Department of Health and Human Services; 1991. Publication No. PHS 91–50212.

Valdiserri RO, Arena VC, Proctor D, Bonati FA: The relationship between women's attitudes about condoms and their use: Implications for condom promotion programs. *Am J Public Health* 79(4):499–501, 1989.

Veatch RM: Models for ethical medicine in a revolutionary age. What physician–patient roles foster the most ethical relationship? *Hastings Cent Rep* 2:5–7, 1972.

Veldhuis M: Defensive behavior of Dutch family physicians. Widening the concept. *Fam Med* 26:27–29, 1994.

Ventura SJ: Recent trends in teenage childbearing in the United States. *Stat Bull* 75(4):10–17, 1994.

Vincent C, Young M, Phillips A: Why do people sue doctors? A study of patients and relatives taking legal action. *Lancet* 343:1609–1613, 1994.

Waitzkin H, Hubbell FA: Truth's search for power in health policy: Critical applications to community-oriented primary care and small area analysis. *Med Care Rev* 49:161–189, 1992.

Waller JA, Casey R: Teaching about substance abuse in medical school. *Br J Addict* 85(11):1451–1455, 1990.

Walsh F: The family in later life, in Carter EA, McGoldrick M (eds): *The Changing Family Life Cycle: A Framework for Family Therapy* ed 2. Boston, Gardner Press, 1988, pp 311–334.

Warshaw C, Poirier S: Hidden stories of women. *Second Opinion,* October 1991, p 61.

Washington AE, Arno PS, Brooks MA: The economic costs of pelvic inflammatory disease. *JAMA* 255:1735–1738, 1986.

Watkins CE, Lopez FG, Campbell VL, Himmell CD: Counseling psychology and clinical psychology: Some preliminary comparative data. *Am Psychol* 41(6):581–582, 1986.

Watson MF, Protinsky HO: Black adolescents identity development: Effects of perceived family structure. *Fam Relat* 37:288–292, 1988.

Weikel WJ, Palmo AJ: The evolution and practice of mental health counseling. *J Ment Health Couns* 11(1):7–25, 1989.

Weinberg RB, Mauksch LB: Examining family of origin influences in life at work. *J Marital Fam Ther,* 17(3):233–242, 1991.

Weisman AD: *On Dying and Denying: A Psychiatric Study of Terminality.* New York, Behavioral Publications, Inc, 1972.

Weiss KB, Gergen PJ, Crain EF: Inner-city asthma: The epidemiology of an emerging US public health concern. *Chest* 101:362–367, 1992.

Weissman WM, Klerman GL, Markowitz JS, Ouellette R: Suicidal ideation and suicide attempts in panic disorder and attacks. *N Engl J Med* 321:1209–1214, 1989.

Weller RH, Eberstein JW, Bailey M: Pregnancy wantedness and maternal behavior during pregnancy. *Demography* 24:407–412, 1987.

Wells KB, Golding JM, Burnam MA: Psychiatric disorder in a sample of the general population with and without chronic medical condition. *Am J Psychiatry* 145:976–981, 1988.

Wells KB, Stewart A, Hays RD, Burnam A, Rogers W, Daniels M, Berry S, Greenfield S, Ware J: The functioning and well-being of depressed patients. *JAMA* 626:914–919, 1989.

Westat, Inc. *Study Findings: Study of National Incidence of Child Abuse and Neglect*. Washington, DC, Department of Health and Human Services, 1988.

Weyerer S: Relationships between physical and psychological disorders, in Sartorius N, Goldberg D, de Girolamo G, Cost e Silva J, Lecrubier Y, Wittchen U (eds): *Psychological Disorders in General Medical Settings*. Toronto, Hogrefe & Huber, 1990, pp 34–46.

Whippen DA, Canellos GP: Burnout syndrome in the practice of oncology: Results of a random survey of 1,000 oncologists. *J Clin Oncol* 9:1916–1920, 1991.

Whitcomb ME: A cross-national comparison of generalist physician workforce data: Evidence for US supply adequacy. *JAMA* 274:692–695, 1995.

White KL: The Task of Medicine: Dialogue at Wickenburg. Menlo Park, Calif, The Henry J. Kaiser Family Foundation, 1988.

White KL, Williams TF, Greenberg BG: The ecology of medical care. *N Engl J Med* 265:885–892, 1961.

Whiteley JM: Counseling psychology: A historical perspective. *Couns Psychol* 12:3–109, 1984.

Widmer RB, Cadoret RJ: Depression in primary care changes in pattern of patient visits and complaints during a developing depression. *J Fam Pract* 7:293–302, 1978.

Wilensky GR, Rossiter LF: The relative importance of physician-induced demand for medical care. *Milbank Mem Fund Q* 61:252–277, 1983.

Wilfond BS, Fost N: The cystic fibrosis gene: Medical and social implications for heterozyote detection. *JAMA* 263:2777–2783, 1990.

Williams GD, Stinson FS, Brooks SD, Clem D, Noble J: Apparent per capita alcohol consumption: National, state, and regional trends, 1977–1989. NIAAA Surveillance Report No. 20, DHHS Publication No. (ADM) 281-89-0001. Washington, DC, Government Printing Office, 1991.

Williams LB, Pratt WF: Wanted and unwanted childbearing in the United States: 1973–88, National Survey of Family Growth. Washington, DC, Department of Health and Human Services, Public Health Service, 1989.

Williams ME, Williams TF: Evaluation of older persons in the ambulatory setting. *J Am Geriatr Soc* 34:37–43, 1986.

Williams WC: *The Doctor Stories*. Compiled by Robert Coles. New York, New Directions, 1984.

Wilson WJ: Poverty, joblessness, and family structure in the inner city: A comparative perspective. Paper presented at the Chicago Urban Poverty and Family Life Conference, University of Chicago, September 24, 1991.

Wolf PA, D'Agostino RB, Sannel WB, *et al*: Cigarette smoking as a risk factor for stroke: The Framingham Study. *JAMA* 259:1025–1029, 1988.

Wolinsky H, Brune T: *The Serpent on the Staff: The Unhealthy Politics of the American Medical Association*. New York, Tarcher/Purman, 1995.

Woloshin S, *et al*: Language barriers in medicine in the United States. *JAMA* 273:724–728, 1995.

Woolhandler S, Himmelstein DU: *National Health Program Chartbook*, Center for National Health, Monroe, Maine: Common Courage Press, 1992.

World Health Organization. Statistical Indices of Family Health 1976, No. 589:17.

World Health Organization. World AIDS Day. *JAMA* 272:1568, 1994

Wright C, Moore RD: Disulfiram treatment of alcoholism: Position paper of the American College of Physicians. *Ann Intern Med* 111(11):943–945, 1989.

Wyatt GE, Newcomb MD, Riederle MH (eds): *Sexual Abuse and Consensual sex*. Beverly Hills, Calif, Sage Publication, 1990.

Yinger JM: *Religion, Society and the Individual*. New York, Macmillan Publishing Co, Inc, 1957.

Zborowski M: *People in Pain*. San Francisco, Jossey–Bass Inc, Publishers, 1969.

Zelnik M, Kantner F: Sexual activity, contraceptive use and pregnancy among metropolitan area teenagers. *Fam Plann Perspect* 12:230–237, 1980.

Zimmerman MA, Maton KI: Lifestyle and substance use among male African American urban adolescents: A cluster analytic approach. *Am J Community Psychol* 20:121–138, 1992.

Zinn W: The empathic physician. *Arch Intern Med.* 153:306–312, 1993.

Zola IK: Studying the decision to see a doctor. *Adv Psychosom Med* 8:216–236, 1972.

Zuravin SJ: Unplanned childbearing and family size: Their relationship to child neglect and abuse. *Fam Plann Perspect* 23(4):155–161, 1991.

REFERENCES

Index